Functional Training
HANDBOOK

Functional Training
HANDBOOK

Craig Liebenson, DC
L.A. Sports and Spine
Los Angeles, California

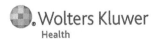
Wolters Kluwer
Health

Philadelphia • Baltimore • New York • London
Buenos Aires • Hong Kong • Sydney • Tokyo

Acquisitions Editor: Brian Brown
Product Development Editor: Dave Murphy
Production Project Manager: Alicia Jackson
Design Manager: Holly McLaughlin
Manufacturing Manager: Beth Welsh
Marketing Manager: Daniel Dressler
Production Services: Integra Software Services Pvt. Ltd.

9 8

Library of Congress Cataloging-in-Publication Data

Functional training handbook [edited by] Craig Liebenson.
   p. ; cm.
   Includes bibliographical references and index.
   ISBN 978-1-58255-920-9
   I. Liebenson, Craig, editor.
   [DNLM: 1. Athletic Performance—standards.   2. Athletic Injuries—prevention & control.   3. Athletic Injuries—rehabilitation.   4. Physical Education and Training.   QT 260]
   RC1235
   617.1'027—dc23

2014009134

Care has been taken to confirm the accuracy of the information present and to describe generally accepted practices. However, the authors, editors, and publisher are not responsible for errors or omissions or for any consequences from application of the information in this book and make no warranty, expressed or implied, with respect to the currency, completeness, or accuracy of the contents of the publication. Application of this information in a particular situation remains the professional responsibility of the practitioner; the clinical treatments described and recommended may not be considered absolute and universal recommendations.

The authors, editors, and publisher have exerted every effort to ensure that drug selection and dosage set forth in this text are in accordance with the current recommendations and practice at the time of publication. However, in view of ongoing research, changes in government regulations, and the constant flow of information relating to drug therapy and drug reactions, the reader is urged to check the package insert for each drug for any change in indications and dosage and for added warnings and precautions. This is particularly important when the recommended agent is a new or infrequently employed drug.

Some drugs and medical devices presented in this publication have Food and Drug Administration (FDA) clearance for limited use in restricted research settings. It is the responsibility of the health care provider to ascertain the FDA status of each drug or device planned for use in their clinical practice.

To purchase additional copies of this book, call our customer service department at (800) 638-3030 or fax orders to (301) 223-2320. International customers should call (301) 223-2300.

Visit Lippincott Williams & Wilkins on the Internet: http://www.lww.com. Lippincott Williams & Wilkins customer service representatives are available from 8:30 am to 6:00 pm, EST.

To Deannie who has been the backbone of this journey.

CONTRIBUTORS

Venu Akuthota, MD
Professor and Vice Chair
Department of Physical Medicine & Rehabilitation
University of Colorado
Denver, Colorado
Director
Spine Center
Spine/Sports
University of Colorado Hospital
Aurora, Colorado

Árni Árnason, PT, PhD
Associate Professor
Department of Physiotherapy & Research
    Centre of Movement Science
School of Health Sciences
University of Iceland
Sports Physiotherapist
Gáski Physiotherapy
Reykjavik, Iceland

Michael Boyle, ATC
Strength and Conditioning Coach
Mike Boyle Strength & Conditioning
Woburn, Massachusetts

Jason Brown, DC
Clinical Director
Brown Integrated Chiropractic
Schodack, New York

Tim Brown, DC
Sports Chiropractic Specialist
Founding Medical Director, Association of
    Volleyball Professionals
Co-Medical Director, Association of
    Surfing Professionals
Founder/Creator of Intelliskin (http://intelliskin.net/)

Stéphane Cazeault, BSc
Director of Strength and Conditioning
Poliquin Group
East Greenwich, Rhode Island

Ken Crenshaw, BS
Head Athletic Trainer
Arizona Diamondbacks
Phoenix, Arizona

Eric Cressey, MA, CSCS
President
Cressey Performance
Hudson, Massachusetts

Jeff Cubos, MSc, DC, FRCCSS(C)
Back On Track Chiropractic & Sport Injury Clinic
Chiropractic Sports Specialist
Spruce Grove, Alberta, Canada

Todd S. Ellenbecker, DPT, MS, SCS, OCS, CSCS
Clinic Director
Physiotherapy Associates
Scottsdale Sports Clinic
National Director of Clinical Research
Physiotherapy Associates
Director of Sports Medicine
Association of Tennis Professionals (ATP) World Tour
Scottsdale, Arizona

Sue Falsone, PT, MS, SCS, ATC, CSCS, COMT
Vice President
Performance Physical Therapy & Team Sports
Athletes' Performance
Phoenix, Arizona
Head Athletic Trainer and Physical Therapist
Los Angeles Dodgers
Los Angeles, California

Michael Fredericson, MD
Professor
Orthopaedic Surgery
Stanford University
Stanford, California
Director
PM&R Sports Medicine Service
Stanford Hospital & Clinics
Redwood City, California

James W. George, DC
Instructor, Chiropractic Science
College of Chiropractic
Logan University
Chesterfield, Missouri

John Gray, RKin, MSc, CSCS
Registered Kinesiologist
Strength and Conditioning Consultant
Movement First, Inc.
Toronto, Ontario, Canada

Cameron Harrison, MD
Department of Physical Medicine & Rehabilitation
University of Colorado School of Medicine
Aurora, Colorado

Ståle Hauge, DC
Chiropractor
Sandefjord Kiropraktikk
Tjodalyng, Norway

Timothy E. Hewett, PhD
Associate Professor
Department of Pediatrics
Cincinnati Children's Hospital
Cincinnati, Ohio

Arthur D. Horne, MEd
Director of Sports Performance
Sports Performance
Northeastern University
Boston, Massachusetts

W. Ben Kibler, MD
Medical Director
Shoulder Center of Kentucky
Lexington Clinic
Lexington, Kentucky

Kyle B. Kiesel, PT, PhD, ATC
Associate Professor
Department of Physical Therapy
University of Evansville
Physical Therapist
ProRehab
Evansville, Indiana

Alena Kobesova, MD, PhD
Lecturer
Department of Rehabilitation and
    Sports Medicine
University Hospital Motol
Second Medical Faculty
Charles University
Medical Doctor
Rehabilitation and Sport Medicine
University Hospital Motol
Prague, Czech Republic

Pavel Kolar, PaedDr, PhD
Professor and Chief
Department of Rehabilitation and Sports Medicine
University Hospital Motol
Second Medical Faculty, Charles University
Head of Clinic
Rehabilitation and Sport Medicine
University Hospital Motol
Prague, Czech Republic

Mark Kovacs, PhD, FACSM, CSCS*D, CTPS
Director
Gatorade Sport Science Institute
Barrington, Illinois
Executive Director
International Tennis Performance Association
Atlanta, Georgia

Robert Lardner, PT
Owner
Lardner Physical Therapy
Chicago, Illinois

Brett J. Lemire, DC, CSCS
Clinic Director
Universal Chiropractic Spine & Sport
Elk Grove, California

Craig Liebenson, DC
L.A. Sports and Spine
Los Angeles, California

Jonathan A. Mackoff, DC
Mackoff Chiropractic & Rehabilitation
Chicago, Illinois

Stuart McGill, PhD
Professor
Department of Kinesiology
Faculty of Applied Health Sciences
University of Waterloo
Waterloo, Ontario, Canada

Gregory D. Myer, PhD, FACSM, CSCS*D
Director, Research and The Human
    Performance Laboratory
Division of Sports Medicine
Cincinnati Children's Hospital Medical Center
Departments of Pediatrics and Orthopaedic Surgery
College of Medicine, University of Cincinnati
Cincinnati, Ohio

Roy Page, MS, DC
L.A. Sports and Spine
Los Angeles, California

Brijesh Patel, MA
Head Strength and Conditioning Coach
Department of Athletics
Qinnipiac University
Hamden, Connecticut

Phillip J. Plisky, PT, DSc, OCS, ATC, CSCS
Assistant Professor and Sports Residency
    Program Director
Doctor of Physical Therapy Program
University of Evansville
Physical Therapist
ProRehab
Evansville, Indiana

**Christopher J. Prosser, BSc, BAppSc
(Chiro), CSSP**
Sports Chiropractor
Global Sport and Spine
Mermaid Beach, Queensland, Australia

Joseph Przytula, ATC, CSCS, CMT
Supervisor of Physical Education,
    Health and Safety
Department of Physical Education
Elizabeth Public Schools
Elizabeth, New Jersey

Neil Rampe, MEd, ATC, CSCS, LMT
Major League Manual and Performance Therapist
Arizona Diamondbacks
Phoenix, Arizona

Michael M. Reinold, PT, DPT, SCS, ATC, CSCS
Champion Physical Therapy and Performance
Boston, Massachusetts

E. Paul Roetert, PhD
Chief Executive Officer
American Alliance for Health, Physical Education,
    Recreation and Dance
Reston, Virginia

Greg Rose, DC
Titleist Performance Institute
Oceanside, California

Koichi Sato, MS, ATC
Director of Sports Performance/Assistant
    Athletic Trainer
Minnesota Timberwolves
Minneapolis, Minnesota

Aaron Sciascia, MS, ATC, PES
Coordinator
Shoulder Center of Kentucky
Lexington Clinic
Lexington, Kentucky

Nathan J. Sermersheim, DC
Spine Center of Ft. Wayne
Fort Wayne, Indiana

Nathan Shaw, ATC, CSCS, RSCC
Major League Strength and Conditioning Coach
Sports Medicine
Arizona Diamondbacks
Phoenix, Arizona

Yohei Shimokochi, PhD, ATC
Associate Professor
Department of Health and Sport Management
Osaka University of Health and Sport Sciences
Osaka, Japan

Charles D. Simpson II, DPT, CSCS
Minor League Physical Therapist
Boston Red Sox
Boston, Massachusetts

Clayton D. Skaggs, DC
Medical Director
Central Institute for Human Performance
St. Louis, Missouri

Adam Sebastian Tenforde, MD
Resident Physician
Division of Physical Medicine and Rehabilitation
Department of Orthopaedics
Stanford University
Stanford, California

Petra Valouchova, DPT, PhD
Lecturer
Department of Rehabilitation and Sports Medicine
University Hospital Motol
Second Medical Faculty
Charles University
Prague, Czech Republic

Ryan Van Matre, DC, MS
Indy Spine and Rehab
Indianapolis, Indiana

Chad Waterbury, MS
Santa Monica, California

Charlie Weingroff, DPT, ATC, CSCS
Physical Therapist, Strength and Conditioning
   Coach, Athletic Trainer
Jackson, New Jersey

Pamela E. Wilson, DC
Wilson Center
Red Bank, New Jersey

FOREWORD

This is an exciting chapter in the history of proactive health through performance. We have arrived at this point in history through a progression that is true of nearly any space. First, there is the identification of need and the science and research to further define and understand the systems involved, then specification into deep subsystems. Next comes sharing through educational mediums in the various disciplines, market awareness, applied career pathways, outcome data, and leaders emerging in each area of expertise. A struggle ensues to determine which career discipline is most powerful, followed by stagnation through isolation, until the next-generation questions why we are doing this in the first place: "Isn't this about helping people achieve their optimal health and performance?" they ask. "And aren't all these systems working in concert within each of us?"

The ***Functional Training Handbook*** (FTH) is positioned as the breakthrough book which bridges the gap between rehab and prehab through performance, acting as the foundation to the next generation of care and understanding. FTH covers a broad spectrum of populations, from the developing child learning basic movement literacy to elite athletes, "weekend warriors," and the aging population. When you look at the All-Star team of contributors, two things will strike you. First, this is a multi-disciplinary group of internationally respected expert practitioners who not only research but, more importantly, apply these methods in the most demanding and measurable environments, from post surgery to professional sports. The second thing you will notice is an impressive performance by the FTH Editor, Dr. Craig Liebenson, who was able to bring this team of experts together and organize their vast knowledge into one integrated and functional approach for the readers' benefit. FTH demonstrates the power of collaboration for the greater good of our respective fields.

Before you dive into FTH, be sure to set aside any preconceived notions, read the chapter authors' backgrounds, and allow yourself to read their chapter with their perspectives in mind. Seek to understand how they

are looking at the problem and helping to solve it. I encourage you to utilize FTH as an applied workbook. Take time after each chapter to summarize three takeaways that directly apply to your situation and clients. This can happen at the end of each chapter or as a summary on the available pages at the beginning or end of FTH. As you do this, you will probably come to the realization, regardless of your educational background or practicing discipline, that the information confirms many of your beliefs. If your key takeaway from FTH is redundant commonalities between the diverse disciplines and practitioners, one would argue we have just taken a giant step forward in upgrading population health and care.

At EXOS, our mission is to upgrade lives. With world-class partners, facilities, technologies, and specialists spanning six continents, we are progressing the intelligence behind human performance wherever necessary. This is our responsibility, and it has given us the honor to learn and work side by side so many of the special people and professionals who made time within their demanding schedules for this book. Their actions should be celebrated. As leaders, they show how we must work together in the best interest of both our clients and the field at all times. Rather than let ego or politics consume energy, we must integrate and apply our knowledge and skills for the needs of each individual client.

The FTH provides us with an insightful literature review on injury prevention, sport-specific and modern athletic development training approaches, off-season systems, and rehabilitation considerations. On behalf of all of us who will benefit from the FTH, I send our deepest gratitude to the editor, Dr. Craig Liebenson, and to all of those who contributed to this work for the passion they put into it. I look forward to witnessing the teamwork and precision each of you will demonstrate in upgrading lives through performance in your current and future work.

Mark Verstegen
President & Founder
EXOS

Functional training and rehabilitation present a popular way to describe approaches to exercise at all levels. "Functional stuff," in a word, is simply more holistic than the current common alternative.

Functional training is often offered as a more complete option in contrast to body part isolation or a highly sport-specific approach.

Really?—let us be honest—that statement is not too hard to get behind; however, building a systematic approach to functional movement health requires more than agreement. Agreement followed by action is easy to track, measure, modify, and improve. Agreement without action actually has the same outcome as non-agreement.

The popularity of "functional (insert your modality here)" might imply that conventional methods of rehabilitation and training fall short in two distinct ways.

One—the conventional rehabilitation solution is incomplete in the resolution or management of dysfunction movement patterns.

Two—the conventional training solution has side effects that might cause or allow dysfunction within fundamental movement patterns.

The functional approach does not discount body part isolation for in-depth evaluation, treatment, and training. Moreover, it also does not address activity and sports specificity or elite performance methods. A functional approach is simply the most efficient and effective entry point. Call it—general physical preparedness or a state of uncomplicated adaptability.

Rehabilitating your knee strength and retaining the dysfunctional limp is an indication that functional movement patterns have not been restored. The strength impairment has been adequately addressed and yet ambulation efficiency is not restored. Likewise, specialization may compromise general functional movement patterns even though a general functional base is the time-tested starting point for greatness. You might find exceptions to this statement, but not a better rule—functional adaptability is the most fertile soil for specialized performance. Staying close to the functional base might also provide great benefit in physical durability, but we will have to be a little smarter to prove it.

Those of us who have dedicated a big part of our practice, teaching, and publishing in defense of function come together on the big ideas even though we may embrace slightly different side paths of the well-traveled road. However, we will reach very close to the common destination. We believe that basic functional movements provide the general base for more advanced physical loads and complex movement tasks. If, however, basic functional movements are dysfunctional at bodyweight, then loads and complex tasks are really not actionable in an efficient and effective manner. The identification of dysfunction justifies more isolated intervention involving anatomical structure, fundamental mobility, motor control, and basic, developmentally significant movement patterns.

To grossly oversimplify, if functional movement patterns are acceptable, then we must impose loads and more complex movements to baseline physical capacity and attempt to improve individual performance in their specific environment. If functional movement patterns are not acceptable, then we must find out why and take action before worrying too much about physical capacity.

Engineering a functional approach requires a blend of science and art. The true functional approach requires a combination of the current best evidence alongside intuitive coaching, wise training, and treating. No engineer will rush the foundation to construct a better building; instead they will obsess on the supporting pillars of the entire thing until they support it.

How can we have a functional approach to movement if we have not clearly identified and defined movement dysfunction? My journey toward a functional approach started a long time ago. At the beginning of that journey, I had to make a decision. I had to trust the functional material and programming presented to me or I had to have a responsible professional way to test the theories and ideas that were proposed under the functional umbrella. I started looking at developmental/ fundamental movement patterns and tried to find the exercise maneuvers and treatments that would restore them efficiently and effectively. I also looked at training methods that produced the unfortunate side effect of gross asymmetry, compromised mobility, or limited motor control. In other words, a loss of the foundation while focussing on a better top floor, if you can appreciate another construction parallel.

Ultimately, we must always validate our journey against the map, compass, and clock—in modern travel, the GPS does it for us. A single gauge points as an indicator of efficiency and effectiveness. The Functional Training Handbook will offer you many ideas about grooving motor patterns, functional restoration, as well as maintaining function in performance situations. Please make sure you have gauges to watch and that you have time to apply what you read. Your observations are extremely valuable when they come from experience in the techniques demonstrated in this text, probably a little less valuable without practical experience. I think we would all agree that opinions formed across time and over real terrain are the ones we prize and respect. Please be of one of those opinions. My wise mentors—starting with my Dad—all articulated that I should hold onto my words, until I had the calluses to back them up. I offer the same advice to you. Dr. Craig Liebenson and his contributors are providing an opportunity that only becomes a lesson with practice and reflection.

This foreword is both a professional and personal thank-you to Craig for his commitment to a better functional model. Welcome to the movement Movement!

Gray Cook, P.T.

The inspiration for the *Functional Training Handbook* came about as a result of the renaissance occurring in rehabilitation and training. We are recognizing the overlapping roles and interdependence of clinicians, trainers, and coaches (see Chapter 3). Corrective exercise and functional training have become popular buzzwords. The book aims to distinguish what is functional about functional training from what is merely popular. With the Internet and social media falsely granting instant expert status on anyone with a loud bullhorn, this book will hopefully give you an ear to what experts with years in the trenches have to say.

Let us start with what functional training is not. It is not sport-specific training which through mimicry trains movement patterns that are replicas of sports maneuvers. Nor is it training on unstable surfaces to "simulate" real-world unpredictability.

What is functional training? It is training with a purpose or goal. By having a clear objective it is inherently client-, athlete-, or patient-centered. Why? Because functional training is designed to help people achieve their goals safely and efficiently.

If we think about or try to define function, the answer becomes "it depends." What is functional depends on an individual's age, sport, injury history, stage of rehabilitation, goals, etc. To many saying "it depends" is a cop-out, but to assume that everyone needs the same tests or exercises is to imagine a world where all people are identical in their physical needs. In fact, we are all unique so what is functional truly depends.

An elderly person may have a high risk for a fall; thus, balance assessment and training would be a functional priority. Women are at risk post-menopausally for osteoporosis; therefore, spinal posture is a key. Young girls and female athletes in sports such as soccer, basketball, or volleyball with sudden starting and stopping and change of direction are at heightened risk for non-contact anterior cruciate ligament injuries so factors which predispose to this (see Chapter 31) should be screened for and addressed. Low back pain is ubiquitous and often follows from improper bending and lifting habits, inadequate lower quarter mobility, or poor motor control of the core; thus, assessing and remediating these key functional deficits are crucial. Individuality is the rule, not the exception.

Clearly, populations have heterogenous rather than homogenous functional requirements. Functional training for a basketball player may require an abundance of frontal plane stability and power work (see Chapters 9 and 26). For a weight lifter it may focus on control of the sagittal plane (see Chapter 16). Meanwhile for a mixed martial arts fighter training will focus on building their rate of force development (see Chapter 28), something which is clearly also of importance in other sports such as baseball, football, sprinting, weight lifting, etc. In contrast, an endurance athlete such as a marathon runner, Iron Man competitor, or triathlete will focus on such traits as running economy (see Chapter 34).

The *Functional Training Handbook* aims to "bridge the gap" between rehabilitation, training, and coaching. Rehab specialists have learned to successfully help patients resume activity and athletes to return to sport. Trainers have learned how to enhance fitness in the general public while their Strength & Conditioning colleagues are able to prepare athletes for the rigorous demands of their sport. If trainers successfully build capacity (strength, endurance, and power) on a foundation of high-quality movement patterns, then skill coaches can focus on biomechanical optimization of the craft of sprinting, kicking, throwing, striking, etc. Most importantly the head coach is now in a position to macro- instead of micro-manage the overall performance aspects of the athlete and team. When the coach can focus on motivating and inspiring each individual on the team to maximize their potential, the most efficient development of the athlete can occur.

Perhaps the most important component of this book is its underlying emphasis on durability. If training is functional, then it will always be as hard as possible, but not harder. Thus, residual adaptation will occur and results will be achieved in the fastest, safest manner possible to develop athleticism throughout the lifespan, during the off-season, and even maintain it in-season (see Chapter 34). This process is always guided by a results-oriented approach (see Chapter 5) called the clinical audit process (CAP). Often described as an assessment-correction-reassessment approach the key is that as the famed Czech Neurologist Dr. Karel Lewit says "the methods should serve the goals."

The CAP involves a rigorous assessment (see Chapters 6 and 22) to find the "weak link." This is the painless dysfunction that is most greatly limiting function in the kinetic chain. Put in other words it is the source of biomechanical overload in the kinetic chain. Once this is identified then a program can be designed that "resets" function so that the painless dysfunction is remediated (see Chapter 7) and performance enhanced in the most efficient manner possible (see Chapter 35). The ***Functional Training Handbook*** strives to free clinicians and trainers from being "prisoners of protocols." Results or outcomes should always trump an output-based approach that blindly follows methods (i.e., "no pain no gain"). In this way, it is my hope that this book will serve as a guide to making rehabilitation, fitness, and athletic development specialists more than just craftsman, but true artists.

"Learn the rules like a pro, so you can break them like an artist"—Pablo Picasso

ACKNOWLEDGEMENTS

It has been a privilege to take this journey from my chiropractic roots to a more broad-based soft tissue injury and athletic development paradigm. As a chiropractor I was introduced to an alternative approach to treating the locomotor system, its particular focus being on role of joint dysfunction in musculoskeletal health. I am indebted in particular to a few of the more revolutionary influences I had in the early 1980s who early on took a more functional than structural approach—Drs. Leonard Faye, Scott Haldeman, and Raymond Sandoz.

At the same time that I was studying this more modern version of chiropractic, I was introduced to the role of soft tissue dysfunction in both pain and movement. I learned of the Nimmo method from the wonderfully observant Chiropractor Richard Hamilton. Then, a key turning point for me was meeting the prolific Osteopath/Naturopath Leon Chaitow who taught me to consider not only muscles, but also fascia as potential "key links." Finally, I was fortunate to learn about perpetuating factors of myofascial trigger points from the legendary Dr. Janet Travell.

With these two pieces in place—joint and soft tissue dysfunction—the next step in the evolution of my understanding came from the great team of Manual Medicine Physicians from Prague. Led by neurologists Pr. Vladimir Janda and Dr. Karel Lewit they successfully framed the musculoskeletal pain problem as one involving the key functional pathology of the motor system—faulty movement patterns. Since 1985, their guidance has steered me toward "keeping an open mind for new ideas that sometimes show that what I thought or believed before was wrong."

As our understanding of rehabilitation of the motor system was growing, other teachers kept emerging: Robin McKenzie, P.T., who welcomed me into the International McKenzie Institute and showed me how painful "markers" could guide our empiric approach to not only more accurately identify a patient's prognosis, but to more efficiently discover the movement "bias" of each patient; Dennis Morgan, D.C., P.T., who was not only trained in P.N.F. but a student of various Scandinavian manual therapy and exercise pioneers. He taught me many of the fundamental principles of what he termed "Stabilization Training" which at that time was taught exclusively in the San Francisco area.

In the 1990s, clinical ideas about stabilization training were finally subjected to scientific scrutiny by my long-time collaborator Pr. Stuart McGill. He emphasized the importance not only of utilizing exercises which challenged muscles while minimizing joint load, but also of spine sparing strategies such as the hip hinge. Within a few years, a new leader emerged within the Prague School of Manual Medicine—Pavel Kolar, P.T., Ph.D. His work based on the Vojta approach to care for children with Cerebral Palsy quickly expanded to include the use of developmental movement patterns to facilitate the emergence of improved, default motor programs for upright posture in both athletes and non-athletes suffering musculoskeletal pain.

Amazingly, while the clinical-rehabilitation world was sharpening its principles and methods for improving the quality of movement patterns, a similar trend began to emerge in the Strength and Conditioning field in the late 1990s. Led by Mark Verstegen, Mike Boyle, and others, it became quickly apparent to clinicians like Gray Cook, P.T., Sue Falsone, A.T.C., P.T., and me that we were in the midst of a Renaissance. Clinicians and trainers were "bridging the gap" between pain and performance. This cross-fertilization exposed me to many of the ideas that are presented within this book.

I have been blessed to have many partners to bounce ideas off of. Drs. Jason Brown, Jeff Cubos, Neil Osborne, Stale Hauge, Phillip Snell; Physical Therapists Robert Lardner, Charlie Weingroff, Clare Frank, Jiri Cumpelik; Athletic Trainers Ken Crenshaw, Koichi Sato; and trainers such as Chad Waterbury and Patrick Ward are just a few individuals that have been instrumental in fostering a culture receptive to the emerging new multidisciplinary paradigm.

This book has had a long gestation period. Chief editor Dave Murphy has stewarded this project with remarkable patience as I have stalled release of the book time and again while I attempted to absorb and test the fast-moving changes in this emerging field. I want to thank my copy editor Martha Cushman who helped immensely smooth out the rough edges of my writing. It is a special honor to have had this opportunity, thanks to my publisher Lippincott Williams & Wilkins, to bring together the remarkably talented and diverse team of experts represented in the *Functional Training Handbook*.

I look forward to seeing the evolution of an integrated approach as you and readers from a broad spectrum of disciplines apply the principles contained in the *Functional Training Handbook* to help their patients, clients, and athletes to be more active and durable, recover faster, become fitter, and enhance their performance.

CONTENTS

The Functional Approach

Training has many different connotations depending on one's perspective. Traditionally, for healthy individuals or athletes it focused on strength, flexibility, or cardiovascular training. Such training would normally be supervised by a personal fitness trainer or strength and conditioning (S&C) coach. This book promotes a different approach in that the aim of training is to promote athletic development (1,2). From the perspective of sustainable athletic development, training is not just limited to strength, flexibility, or cardiovascular domains but also focuses on the fundamental ABC's of agility, balance, and coordination as a foundation for enhanced movement literacy (3).

Ironically, as enhanced movement literacy becomes the goal of athletic development, training not only becomes more functional but also begins to overlap with clinical rehabilitation. It becomes more functional because it is focused on stereotypical movement patterns (i.e., pushing; pulling; squat; lunge) that an athlete uses in all sports instead of isolated motions of specific joints (i.e., bicep curl/elbow flexion; hamstring curl/knee flexion). A bodybuilder may prefer to isolate a muscle to cause hypertrophy, but isolation is not the primary goal for an athlete. An important exercise science principle that highlights the limitations of the isolated muscle or joint approach is the Specific Adaptation to Imposed Demands (SAID) principle. The SAID principle shows that training gains are specific to the movement that is trained (4,5). Therefore, an isolated movement that is trained repetitively does not necessarily transfer any benefit to functional tasks, whereas if fundamental movement skills or movement literacy is trained there is high transfer of benefit to enhanced sport performance as well as injury prevention (6–12).

Clinical rehabilitation of musculoskeletal disorders also traditionally focused on the prescription of repetitive, isolated exercises. For instance, shoulder rehabilitation would involve exercises for the individual rotator cuff muscles with resisted internal and external rotation of the shoulder at different angles of arm elevation (13). This approach has evolved over the past two decades to include greater emphasis on motor control and functional activities (14–16). For instance, rehabilitation of a baseball pitcher with rotator cuff tendinosis or labral insufficiency might draw from a menu involving scapulothoracic stability, closed-chain exercise, core stability, and single leg posterior chain training (17–19). There are parallels in both the rehabilitation and training fields with an evolution toward greater emphasis on motor control with a concurrent lessening of the emphasis on isolation of individual muscles and joints (20,21).

An important process underpinning the emphasis on training functional movement patterns instead of mainly isolating individual muscles and joints is called cortical plasticity. Movements which are repeated are learned by the central nervous system as a new engram. Poor postural habits and adaptations to pain or injury result in compromised movement efficiency. With appropriate training, the body's "software" is updated to address these "viruses." The goal is to "seal" or insulate synaptic pathways for high-quality functional movement patterns. Cortical plasticity occurs via "neural adaptation" at the intracellular level involving structural changes in the glia, binding neurons and myelin surrounding the intersynaptic connections (22–24).

If we only train isolated motions as the SAID principle implies, there will not be an improvement in our functional skills (25). This legacy from bodybuilding by focusing on isolated motions may change our "hardware" by hypertrophying individual muscles, but it will not enhance the quality or efficiency of movement—our "software"—and may even corrupt it by causing or perpetuating muscle imbalances or faulty movement patterns (26–28). Therefore, modern training and rehabilitation both have come to the same conclusion. If we want to achieve sharper resolution motor programs for functional tasks that are relevant for the athlete in the "heat of battle," we should focus on training functional integrated movement patterns rather than merely isolated training of individual muscles and joints (20,21,29–36).

If the goal is to identify and remediate faulty movement patterns, does this mean that we ignore individual joints and muscles? No, frequently there will be a specific dysfunction of a joint (i.e., Acromioclavicular (AC) joint blockage restricting arm adduction), muscle (i.e., tightness of the piriformis restricting hip hinge), or fascia (i.e., anterior chest wall tightness restricting arm elevation overhead) that if corrected will facilitate improved performance. What changes is the way we conceptualize what we are doing. As the famed neurologist from Prague Dr. Karel Lewit said, "our methods should serve our goals." The goal is to improve the functional movement pattern on a subcortical basis. Stretching a tight muscle, manipulating a hypomobile joint, or releasing restricted fascia are possible means to an end, but we want to avoid the trap of "becoming a slave to our methods." For instance, we may train an individual muscle to facilitate it so that it is included in a movement pattern.

Segmental treatment alone, without appreciation of the big picture, will result in the patient or athlete being as lost as their myopic trainer or rehabilitation specialist. When functional assessment of movement patterns is linked to the goals of athletic development, enhancement of performance, or injury prevention then we can select our methods wisely in the service of the athlete's goals.

There are many sacred cows in both the rehabilitation and S&C fields. Such beliefs or practices are considered by some to be exempt from criticism or questioning, despite containing inaccurate dogmas, and this book will attempt to expose some of these myths, while proposing alternative, science-based explanations.

REFERENCES

1. Gambetta V. Athletic Development: The Art & Science of Functional Sports Conditioning. Champaign, IL: Human Kinetics; 2007.
2. Boyle M. Advances in Functional Training. Aptos, CA: On Target Publications; 2010.
3. Balyi I, Hamilton A. Long-Term Athlete Development: Trainability in Childhood and Adolescence. Windows of Opportunity. Optimal Trainability. Victoria: National Coaching Institute British Columbia & Advanced Training and Performance Ltd.; 2004.
4. Sale D, MacDougall D. Specificity in strength training: a review for the coach and athlete. Can J Sport Sci 1981;6:87.
5. Enoka RM. Neuromechanical Basis of Kinesiology. 2nd ed. Champaign, IL: Human Kinetics; 1994.
6. Emery CA, Meeuwisse WH. The effectiveness of a neuromuscular prevention strategy to reduce injuries in youth soccer: a cluster-randomised controlled trial. Br J Sports Med 2010;44:555–562.
7. Myer GM, Faigenbaum AD, Ford KR, et al. When to initiate integrative neuromuscular training to reduce sports-related injuries and enhance health in youth? Am Coll Sports Med 2011;10:157–166.
8. Myer GD, Ford KR, Palumbo JP, et al. Neuromuscular training improves performance and lower-extremity biomechanics in female athletes. J Strength Cond Res 2005;19:51–60.
9. Hewett TE, Myer GD, Ford KR. Reducing knee and anterior cruciate ligament injuries among female athletes: a systematic review of neuromuscular training interventions. J Knee Surg 2005;18:82–88.
10. Hewett TE, Myer GD, Ford KR. Prevention of anterior cruciate ligament injuries. Curr Womens Health Rep 2001;3:218–224.
11. Arnason A, Sigurdsoon SB, Gudmonnson A, et al. Physical fitness, injuries, and team performance in soccer. Med Sci Sports Exerc 2004;2:278–285.
12. Ekstrand J, Gillquist J, Moller M, et al. Incidence of soccer injuries and their relation to training and team success. Am J Sports Med 1983;11:63–67.
13. Jobe FW, Bradley JP, Tibone JE. The diagnosis and non-operative treatment of shoulder injuries in athletes. Clin Sports Med 1989;8:419–438.
14. Kibler WB, McMullen J, Uhl TL. Shoulder rehabilitation strategies, guidelines, and practice. Op Tech Sports Med 2000;8:258–267.
15. Uhl TL, Carver TJ, Mattacola CG, et al. Shoulder musculature activation during upper extremity weight-bearing exercise. J Orthop Sports Phys Ther 2003;33:109–117.
16. Wilk KE, Arrigo C. Current concepts in the rehabilitation of the athletic shoulder. J Orthop Sports Phys Ther 1993;18:365–378.
17. Cools AM, Dewitte V, Lanszweert F, et al. Rehabilitation of scapular muscle balance: which exercises to prescribe? Am J Sports Med 2007;10:1744–1751.
18. Kibler WB, Sciascia AD. Current concepts: scapular dyskinesis. Br J Sports Med 2010;44:300–305.
19. Reinold MM, Escamilla RF, Wilk KE. Current concepts in the scientific and clinical rationale behind exercises for glenohumeral and scapulothoracic musculature. J Orthop Sports Phys Ther 2009;2:105–117.
20. McGill SM. Low Back Disorders: The Scientific Foundation for Prevention and Rehabilitation Champaign, IL: Human Kinetics; 2002.
21. Liebenson C. Functional-Stability Training in Rehabilitation of the Spine: A Practitioner's Manual 2nd ed. Philadelphia, PA: Lippincott Williams & Wilkins; 2007.
22. Fields RD. Myelination: an overlooked mechanism of synaptic plasticity? Neuroscientist 2005;6:528–531.
23. Markham J, Greenough WT. Experience-driven brain plasticity: beyond the synapse. Neuron Glia Biol 2004;4:351–363.
24. Yakovlev PI, Lecours A-R. The myelogenetic cycles of regional maturation of the brain. In: Minkowski A, ed. Regional Development of the Brain in Early Life. Oxford, UK: Blackwell Scientific; 1967:3–70.
25. Rutherford OM. Muscular coordination and strength training, implications for injury rehabilitation. Sports Med 1988;5:196–202.
26. Babyar SR. Excessive scapular motion in individuals recovering from painful and stiff shoulders: causes and treatment strategies. Phys Ther 1996;76:226–238.
27. Ludewig PM, Hoff MS, Osowski EE, et al. Relative balance of serratus anterior and upper trapezius muscle activity during push-up exercises. Am J Sports Med 2004;2:484–493.
28. Smith M, Sparkes V, Busse M, et al. Upper and lower trapezius muscle activity in subjects with subacromial impingement symptoms: is there imbalance and can taping change it? Phys Ther Sport 2008;2:45–50.

29. Cook G. Movement: Functional Movement Systems. Aptos, CA: On Target Publications; 2010.

30. Hewett TE, Stroupe AL, Nance TA, et al. Plyometric training in female athletes. Decreased impact forces and increased hamstring torques. Am J Sports Med 1996;24:765–773.

31. Janda V, Frank C, Liebenson C. Evaluation of muscle imbalance. In: Liebenson C, ed. Rehabilitation of the Spine: A Practitioner's Manual. 2nd ed. Philadelphia, PA: Lippincott Williams & Wilkins; 2007;10:203-225.

32. McGill SM, McDermott A, Fenwick CMJ. Comparison of different strongman events: trunk muscle activation and lumbar spine motion, load, and stiffness. J Strength Cond Res 2009;4:1148–1161.

33. McGill SM, Karpowicz A, Fenwick CMJ, et al. Exercises for the torso performed in a standing posture: spine and hip motion and motor patterns and spine load. J Strength Cond Res 2009;2:455–464.

34. Myer GM, Faigenbaum AD, Ford KR, et al. When to initiate integrative neuromuscular training to reduce sports-related injuries and enhance health in youth? Am Coll Sports Med 2011;10:157–166.

35. Zazulak BT, Hewett TE, Reeves NP, et al. Deficits in neuro muscular control of the trunk predict knee injury risk: a prospective biomechanical-epidemiologic study. Am J Sports Med 2007;35:1123–1130.

36. Zazulak BT, Hewet TE, Reeves NP, et al. The effects of core proprioception on knee injury: a prospective biomechanical-epidemiological study. Am J Sports Med 2007;35:368–372.

The Role of Musculoskeletal Fitness in Injury Prevention in Sport

BIOMECHANICAL LOAD AND INJURIES

When working with athletes, it is important to consider their strengths and weaknesses regarding their sports activity and at the same time to identify athletes who are at risk of sustaining injuries. High-quality training and injury prevention are closely related and both should be sport-specific. The primary aim should be to improve the players' physical fitness, technique, and tactics for their particular sport as well as to reduce their risk of injuries. Injuries usually occur if the biomechanical load becomes higher than the tolerance of the potential structure. This can occur either if the biomechanical load is too high or if the tolerance against a certain biomechanical load is reduced (1).

A too high biomechanical load usually occurs either when a single bout of load is too high for the involved structure to absorb leading to an acute injury or if the load is excessive over a period of time leading to an overuse injury. An example of an excessive biomechanical load is a typical injury mechanism of a lateral ankle sprain in soccer when the involved player is running with the ball. At the moment of injury all of his body weight is on one leg and he receives a laterally directed tackle from an opponent onto the medial side of the ankle or lower leg. No gliding is possible between the shoe and the surface because the cleats fix the shoe to the field and the whole body weight is on the involved leg. This causes a supination or inversion movement of his foot and forces the player to put weight on his supinated or inverted foot. This often results in an injury on the lateral aspect of the ankle, commonly a ligament sprain or even a fracture (2). Another example of an excessive biomechanical load is a well-known injury mechanism of hamstring strains during water skiing. This mechanism usually takes place if the tips of the skies go below the surface of water during a submerged take-off or the skies stick into a wave during towing. This causes a sudden deceleration of the skies. The skier's knees extend and the trunk is pulled forward by the tow rope. This results in a forced hip flexion, followed by an excessive load on the hamstring muscles with a subsequent strain or rupture (3).

Reduced tolerance against a biomechanical load can be caused by many factors. Examples of factors that possibly can lower the tolerance against biomechanical load are if the training status of athletes does not meet the demand of their particular type of sport. That emphasizes that the training methods, as well as the training load, intensity, and progression, are important and need to be sport-specific. The quality of training in junior sports is particularly important when building up different training effects such as strength, flexibility, power, and muscle endurance in a sport-specific manner. Another well-known injury situation is if athletes start high-intensity training or competition too early after a previous injury and the injured structure is not able to tolerate the biomechanical load required. This often results in a recurrent injury.

INJURY MECHANISMS AND RISK FACTORS

Acute injuries are commonly a consequence of specific injury mechanisms together with a sum of different risk factors affecting the athletes. In overuse injuries where the injuries slowly evolve without a clear onset, the injury mechanisms are not always as obvious as in acute injuries. The effect of different risk factors can be variable, depending on many components such as the type of sport, level of play, the athletes' physical and psychological performance, environment, rules of the sport, other risk factors, and injury mechanisms. It is well known that risk factors often interact with each other, which can influence their appearance and strength. Increased age is, for example, a well-documented risk factor for injuries in many types of sport. Older players have usually participated in sport longer than younger players, and often sustained more previous injures. In addition, they most likely have some age-related degenerative changes, and their training volume and intensity may even be reduced compared with younger players, leading to a reduced physical performance and increased risk of fatigue late in training or competition. All of these factors may be related to the amount of risk due to increased age.

Risk factors for injuries can be classified in many ways. Commonly they are classified into intrinsic or person-related risk factors that focus on factors related to the athlete himself, and extrinsic or environmental-related risk factors that relate to factors in the athlete's environment (4,5). Classification into modifiable and nonmodifiable risk factors is also known and is based on the fact that some risk factors are modifiable such as strength imbalance or functional instability, while others are not modifiable such as increased age or race (6). Another method to categorize risk factors is to use a classification based on participation in sport, physical fitness, psychological factors, environmental factors, and unchangeable factors (Table 2.1). Risk factors can be different between athletes and different sports, but they act together and in conjunction with injury mechanisms they predispose athletes to injuries.

Risk Factors Related to Participation in Sport

Sport participation by itself involves some risk of injuries in the sense that factors related to training versus competition, level of participation, coaching, playing position, high-risk periods, player's attention, rules, foul play, and previous injuries can include some risk of injuries.

Training versus Competition

In general, incidence of injuries is higher during competition than during training (7). The reason could be a more intensive and often aggressive play at a higher speed for a longer period of time during competition than during training. This could lead to an increased fatigue response as well as a higher biomechanical load on the athletes, and in many team sports it could lead to more frequent and harder collisions between athletes.

Level of Participation

Many studies have found higher incidence of injuries at a higher than lower level of play (8,9). This may be related to a higher playing intensity, more exposure time during training and match, and a higher training load resulting in a larger biomechanical load on high-level players (9,10). However, studies are also found that show no difference in injury incidence between different levels of play (11), or even higher incidence of injuries at lower levels of play (12,13). This might be due to an inadequate physical performance among players at a lower level of play, less time spent in training, insufficient player technique, or team tactics, leading to a reduced tolerance against biomechanical load among less skilled players. Other factors such as inadequate training condition, as well as psychological factors, may also be of importance (10–12).

Coaching-Related Factors

Playing exposure has been discussed as a possible risk factor for injuries in different kinds of sport. Studies on soccer

TABLE 2.1	Potential Risk Factors for Injuries in Sport[a]

Participation in sport
Training versus competition
Level of participation
Coaching-related factors
- Playing exposure
- Quality of coaching
- Warm-up
Playing position (in team sport)
High-risk periods during the year
Player attention and ball control
Rules and foul play
Previous injuries

Physical fitness
Training specificity
Joint instability
- Mechanical instability
- Functional instability
Muscle strength and strength ratios
Flexibility
Aerobic fitness
Fatigue
Jumping height, power, and speed
Body mass and body mass index

Other risk factors
Psychological factors
Live-event stress
Fighting mentality
Risk-taking behavior
Environmental factors
Field condition
Weather condition
Equipment
Unchangeable factors
Age
Genetic factors
Race
Gender

[a]These factors are related to participation in sport, physical fitness, psychological factors, environment, and unchangeable components.

players have found a lower rate of acute injuries among players who train more or less than the average group in which the highest injury rate incurred (14,15). Studies have also shown a relationship between a high training to match ratio and a lower incidence of injuries (14). It is not surprising that players who train and play soccer for fewer hours sustain fewer injuries, because they are less exposed.

However, players that train more than average could be in a better physical condition, which could increase their resistance against a biomechanical load. Possibly, they also master a better technique and anticipation or awareness of their surroundings, making them more aware of the playing situation and the opponents, and hence better prepared for tackling or collision. These qualities should make them better players, as well as less prone to injury. Players with such qualities are also more likely to be chosen to play by the coach.

Quality of coaching should be an important factor and low-quality coaching has been discussed as a possible risk factor for injuries (14). Research on this topic is scarce, but coaches' education and experience, as well as their cooperation with the medical team if it is available, are probably of importance (16). Sport-specific training should be aimed at making the athlete better prepared for the biomechanical load required in different situations during competition in particular types of sport. Sport-specific training is thought to be an important part of decreasing the injury risk by improving sport-specific conditioning and develop increased fatigue resistance (17). Training intensity as well as training of technique are also important components of preparing the athletes as well as possible for coping with different situations during competition.

Warm-up before training or competition is important in order to prepare the body for an increased biomechanical load, in the sense of both improving the performance of the athletes and reducing the risk of injuries. Warm-up will increase the blood flow and oxygen transport to working muscles, make muscles less viscous and increase their elastic properties, as well as enhance cellular metabolism. It will also decrease the stiffness of the connective tissue, increase range of motion, and even increase speed of nerve impulses (18–20). Several studies, including a recent randomized trial, indicate that structured warm-up can decrease injury risk (21). Several injury prevention programs have been studied that include a structured warm-up as a part of the program (22–24).

Playing Position

In team sports, the playing position can possibly affect the injury rate. Studies are found that indicate such difference, for example, from soccer (25,26). Different playing positions may require different characteristics of the players regarding, for example, running speed, jumping ability, endurance, fatigue resistance, and pivoting. That means that training of players in different playing positions should be aimed at their specific needs.

High-Risk Periods during the Year

When studying risk factors for injuries, some studies have indicated high-risk periods during the year (27). Such high-risk periods could, for example, include training camps during the preseason period, where the amount and intensity of training often is higher than during the preceding period. Other factors such as changes of the playing ground and weather conditions could also play a role. Another period could be the last part of the preseason periods, where the training might be more intensive including a lot of training games or competitions. During the start of the competitive season some teams experience increased injury rate, maybe because of a higher tempo, more games, and, in the northern countries, a change from artificial turf to natural grass in some types of sport. During the end of the competitive season some teams also show an increase in injury rate possible because the players are getting tired (28).

Player's Attention and Ball Control

In ball games where collisions are common, for example, in soccer, Australian Rules football, and other football codes, attention of the exposed player is important. Studies by video analyses of soccer games indicate that many injuries during duels occurred when the attention of the exposed player was focused on the ball either in the air, when the players were attempting to head the ball, or when a player is attempting to control the ball after receiving it. During these situations, the players' attention is often focused on the ball and away from the opponent challenging him for ball possession. Moreover, the exposed players often seemed not to be aware of the opponent at all (29).

Rules and Foul Play

In contact sport, rules can decrease the risk of injuries, and studies have been performed, for example, in volleyball that shows that rule changes as a part of a prevention program can decrease the injury rate (30). In some sport, rule changes have been made to reduce injury risk, for example, in soccer when red card was adopted for tackling from behind. Foul play can also increase the risk of injuries. Studies on soccer players have, for example, indicated that foul play could be responsible for 16% to 28% of all injuries (12,25,27,31). Therefore, fair play has been included in many prevention programs.

Previous Injuries

Previous muscle strains and ligament sprains are one of the best known risk factors for new injuries of the same type and location. Studies on elite, male soccer, and Australian Rules football have found that players with a history of previous groin and hamstring strains are in 2- to 11-fold risk of sustaining new injuries of the same type and location compared with players without a history of such injuries (15,32). Studies have also shown that soccer players with a history of previous ankle or knee sprain have up to fivefold risks of sustaining new ankle or knee ligament sprains of the same location compared with players without such a history (15). The reason for this could be a too early return to high-intensity training or competition (16,33), as well as post-injury structural changes or scar tissue formation in the muscle or tendon (34,35). Such tissue changes may cause decreased strength, elasticity, or neuromuscular coordination, making the muscle or tendon less able to absorb force or biomechanical load, and consequently more prone to re-injury. As for ligament sprains, studies have shown that neuromuscular control, muscle strength, as well as mechanical stability can be reduced after previous injury (33,36–38). All of these factors, independently or combined, can decrease the involved structure's tolerance against biomechanical load and thereby increase the risk of new ligament sprains (39,40).

Risk Factors Related to Physical Fitness

Risk factors related to athletes' physical fitness are important in view of prevention, because they are highly modifiable with sport-specific training.

Training Specificity

To tolerate the biomechanical load required by a specific type of sport the training must be sport-specific. That is, the training must reflect the situations and load during competition. Training methods should improve the players' ability to cope with different situations during competition in their particular type of sport. This is important so that the different tissues can increase their fatigue resistance and tolerance against biomechanical load during the particular type of sport (17).

Joint Instability

Joint instability can be classified as mechanical or functional. Mechanical instability is when ligaments or even the joint capsule is elongated and nonphysiologic movements are possible in the joint. Functional instability is defined as recurrent sprains or the feeling of giving way (36).

Mechanical instability can be a consequence of previous ligament sprains, stretching of ligaments and joint capsule, or generalized joint laxity (14,15,38). Studies on a possible correlation between mechanical instability and risk of new injuries are controversial. Some studies indicate that mechanical instability in ankles and knees could be a potential risk factor for ankle or knee sprains (13,16,33,40), while other studies have not found such correlation (15,41). Therefore, it can be difficult to draw a firm conclusion about the effect of mechanical instability on injury risk. The methods used during testing differ and in most of these studies a multivariate approach has not been used so possible interaction between different risk factors is not detected.

Functional instability can also be a consequence of previous injuries and is thought to be a risk factor for recurrent injuries (15,42). Functional instability of the ankles has been found to be associated with pronator muscle weakness (43) and a longer reaction time of peroneal muscles as compared with functionally stable ankles (37). Some studies indicate that players with an increased stabilometric value (more functional instability) suffer from a higher rate of ankle sprains than those with more stable ankles (39,44). During

a supination load onto the foot, a longer reaction time of the pronator muscles allows the foot to reach an increased supination before these muscles react, which causes an increased biomechanical load that often is higher than these muscles can absorb, resulting in a lateral ankle sprain.

Muscle Strength and Strength Ratios

Many authors have discussed the effect of a decreased strength as a possible risk factor for injuries. Some studies indicate that a decreased hamstring strength or an inadequate hamstring-to-quadriceps strength ratio could be a risk factor for hamstring strains (45). Similarly, studies have found some correlation between a low eversion-to-inversion strength ratio at the ankles and subsequent ankle sprains (41). However, other studies did not confirm any correlation between a decreased strength and injuries (46,47). In recent years, a low eccentric hamstring strength or eccentric hamstring-to-concentric quadriceps strength ratio has been discussed as a possible risk factor for hamstring strains. During high-speed running most hamstring strains are considered to occur right before foot strike when hamstring is working eccentrically or right after foot strike where hamstring is changing from eccentric to concentric muscle work. This is supported by studies that show that the highest electromyographic activity in the hamstring muscles occurs late during the swing phase and right after foot strike (48,49). Slight forward bending during high-speed running, as seen for example when Australian Rules footballers catch the ball, also places an increased mechanical load on the hamstring muscles as well as changes their length during running. This movement has been shown to be associated with increased risk of hamstring strains (17). The effect of muscle fatigue and possibly a reduced reaction time of the fatigued hamstring muscles may also interact with decreased muscle strength and affect the injury rate during high-speed running.

Flexibility

Many believe that muscle tightness is a risk factor for muscle strains, but little evidence supports that belief. Methods of measuring muscle tightness differ between studies, which makes comparison difficult. Most studies to date have found no relationship between short muscles and muscle strains (16,50,51). However, studies are found that indicate some relationship between short hip adductor muscles and adductor strains or overuse injuries in soccer players (15,33), and between short hamstring muscles and muscle strains (52). It is interesting that although decreased flexibility is commonly thought to enhance injury rate in sports, few studies are found that indicate such correlation. The reason can be that most studies published to date only detect strong to moderate association between risk factors and injuries. The studies are too small to detect moderate to small association between risk factors and injuries (53), which suggests the need for large multivariate studies that take into account many possible risk factors. The methods of measuring flexibility are also critical, with respect to comparison.

Aerobic Fitness

It is commonly considered that aerobic fitness contributes to increased player performance and higher intensity of play in many types of sport (54–56). It has also been discussed whether low aerobic fitness could contribute to increased fatigue late in games (55) and possibly increase the risk of injuries because of reduced protective effects of the muscles and altered distribution of forces acting on the muscles, ligaments, cartilages, and bones (57,58). Although many studies have tested the maximal O_2 uptake among soccer players (15,56), no study was found that showed a clear relationship between maximal O_2 uptake and injury risk. However, studies on military recruits have found association between injuries in general and factors like slower run times, lower peak O_2, and fewer pushups (58,59). Although aerobic fitness is assumed to increase player performance, evidence on its importance regarding injury prevention is inconclusive.

Fatigue

Studies are found mainly from soccer, indicating higher incidence of injuries, especially muscle strains, late during each half of matches and training or during the second half of matches (27,47,60). Studies are also found that suggest that moderate or major injuries occur later during matches than minor injuries (47). Muscle fatigue is often used to explain higher risk of injuries late during matches, and this can be supported by studies on animal models, indicating that fatigued muscles are less able to absorb force than non-fatigued muscles (61). Possibly, this reduction in force absorption can affect some mechanical properties in the muscles and reduce their tolerance against biomechanical load, causing fatigued muscles to be more prone to injuries than non-fatigued muscles.

Jumping Height, Power, and Speed

Studies have shown a correlation between jumping height and running speed in athletes (62). More powerful athletes can possibly impose higher force on their muscles, tendons, and joints during, for example, jumping, kicking, sprinting, and changing directions that will increase the biomechanical load on these structures compared with less powerful athletes. Several studies have examined leg power or jumping ability among athletes (15,63), but little or no evidence is found on correlation between leg power and injury rate.

Body Mass and Body Mass Index

Increased body mass increases the load on joints, ligaments, and muscles. That will further increase the biomechanical load during running, jumping, turning, etc. In some types of sport, increased body mass could be a risk factor for some overuse injuries or osteoarthritis because of an increased load on joints in the lower limbs as well as tendons and other working structures.

Other Potential Risk Factors

Some other potential risk factors for injuries have been identified and they can possibly interact with the previously introduced risk factors and make the picture of injury risk more complex.

Psychological Factors

Some studies suggest a correlation between certain psychological factors and injury risk. Factors such as *live-event stress, fighting mentality*, and *risk-taking behavior* have been found to correlate with an increased risk of injuries in soccer, American football, and some other types of sport (64–66).

Environmental Factors

Field and weather conditions can affect the injury rate during training or competition. Different surfaces have different qualities and for outdoor sport weather conditions, for example, rain, snow, evaporation, dry weather, and temperature, can also change the quality of the playing ground. The two main surface-related risk factors have been thought to be the surface hardness (the ability to absorb impact energy) and shoe–surface friction (the footing or grip provided between the surface and the shoe) (67–69). Hard surfaces increase impact forces and can possibly result in an overload of tissues due to a larger single impact or repeated submaximal impact forces (67). Studies also indicate that playing on a harder surface will increase match speed, which again can increase the risk of injuries during sprinting, turning, speed changes, or during harder collisions in contact sports (68,70). For each type of sport, a suitable shoe–surface friction is important. Factors such as characteristics of the playing surface, material and structure of the shoe surface, length and formation of cleats, and weather condition can affect the shoe–surface friction. For sports that require gliding, cutting, or pivoting between shoes and the surface, a too high translational or rotational friction can increase the biomechanical load, leading to an increased risk of ligament sprains in ankles and knees or even a fracture (69). A too low shoe–surface friction can decrease the players' ability to accelerate and decelerate or turn quickly, and increase their risk of slipping when it is not wanted. Under such circumstances injuries such as groin strains can easily occur.

Equipment such as shoes, shin guards, mouth guards, helmets, taping, and braces must meet the requirements of the particular type of sport and playing surface, as well as fit the athletes itself. Inadequate equipments could make the athlete more prone to injuries.

Unchangeable Factors

Some potential risk factors for injuries are not modifiable.

Age

Studies have shown that injury incidence in adolescent or junior athletes increases with age (9,71). In soccer, the oldest high-level junior players often seem to have similar injury incidence as high-level adult players (9,27). Most studies on adult athletes also indicate increased incidence of injuries with increased age (15,47). These findings may be due to several reasons and may not be solely related to age. Older players often have a longer carrier and increased amount of previous injuries, as well as some degenerative changes that could affect their strength, flexibility, joint stability, as well as a weakness at the site of a scar tissue. Older players could also have less fatigue resistance compared with younger players. All these confounding factors could increase the risk of injuries among older players, so although the age itself is not modifiable, some of the factors associated with increased age could be modifiable to the effect of decreasing the risk of injuries in older athletes.

Genetic Factors

Some potential risk factors could be classified as genetic, like anatomical alignment, height, basic structure and strength of connective tissue, cartilages and bones, as well as the basic rate of muscle fiber types. These factors could affect the tolerance against biomechanical load and make athletes more prone or resistant to injuries.

Race is also a genetic factor. Studies have suggested that black soccer players and Australian Rules football players of aboriginal decent sustain significantly more hamstring strains than white players (32,60). The reason can be that these players are generally considered to run faster than the white players and that will generate a higher biomechanical load on their hamstring muscles. The change between concentric and eccentric muscle action will also be faster, which possibly could increase their risk of hamstring strains.

Gender

Most studies indicate a higher rate of knee injuries among female athletes compared with males athletes (47). In soccer, some studies have reported two to eight times higher rate of anterior cruciate ligament (ACL) injuries in female players than in males players (72,73), and these injuries generally occur at a younger age in female players than in males players (74). Possible reasons for this could be: (1) Anatomical factors such as a wider pelvis and increased Q-angle leading to a more valgus at the knees, as well as a smaller intercondylar notch and increased joint laxity (47,75). (2) Hormonal factors have been considered to be potential risk factors for injuries. It has been postulated that estrogen could be an underlying cause of an increased incidence of ACL tears in women compared with men (76). However, studies are not consistent about when the risk is highest during the menstrual cycle (77,78). (3) Training-related and neuromuscular factors have also been considered as a possible reason for increased knee injuries in women. These factors are modifiable such as less muscle strength, altered recruitment patterns between the quadriceps and hamstring muscles that can affect the functional stability of the knee, and different movement patterns and technique during jumping, landing, and cutting (47,79–82). The hip abductor and external rotator strength and recruitment patterns could also be important for controlling adduction and medial rotation at the hip joint, as well as reducing valgus at the knee joint during jumping, landing, or cutting movements. Other risk factors, such as a high shoe–surface friction, increased body mass index, increased fatigue, different injury mechanisms, and genetics, could also interact with these risk factors or situations and affect the injury risk.

Summary of Risk Factors

Injuries occur if the biomechanical load is too high for the involved structure to absorb. An acute injury occurs if a single bout of load is higher than the tolerance of the involved structures and overuse injuries can occur if the total load is excessive over a period of time. The athletes' tolerance against biomechanical load can also be reduced because of many factors often named intrinsic or person-related risk factors. Extrinsic or environmental-related risk factors can also affect the athletes and in combination with their intrinsic risk factors make them more prone to injuries. Risk factors can be classified into factors associated with participation in sport, the athletes' physical fitness, psychological factors, environmental factors, and unchangeable factors. The effect of different risk factors depends on many factors: for example, the type of sport, level of play, the athletes' physical and psychological performance, environment, rules of the sport, other risk factors, and injury mechanisms. The interaction between different risk factors and injury mechanisms can be complex and some of these factors can enhance or diminish the effect of other factors.

PREVENTION OF INJURIES

Importance of Injury Prevention

As previously mentioned, injuries are common in different kinds of sport, but injury incidence, types, and location vary between sports (7,83). Injuries can affect the athletes in many ways.

Severity of Injuries, Athletes' Performance, and Health Consequences

The severity of injuries in sport is usually estimated based on the athletes' duration of absence from matches and training sessions. Injuries can affect the athletes' performance, especially if the injuries are moderate, severe, or recurrent. Most injuries that occur in sport will heal with appropriate rehabilitation, so the athletes can maintain their participation in their sport at the same level as before. However, some injuries may limit the athletes post-injury sport participation so they cannot play at the same level as before or they must quit their sport. Some injuries can also have health consequences, later in life, for example, osteoarthritis following severe knee injuries (84,85). A questionnaire proposed for former English professional soccer players indicated that almost half of the participants retired because of injuries (86).

Psychological effects on the athletes and their families following injuries are also important to be aware of. Some athletes can experience some depression following injuries especially if they miss important competitions that they have extensively prepared for, even for many years. It can also be difficult for some athletes to acknowledge that their teammates or opponents can train and improve their physical performance and skills while the injured athlete must reduce or stop training for some time because of injuries.

Sociological effects should also be considered. Studies have shown that adolescents that participate in sport are less likely to smoke or use alcohol than others at the same age. Sport participation also promotes healthy life in general (87,88). Young athletes that sustain severe injuries in sports that inhibit them from sport participation for an extended period of time like ACL injuries could possibly be at an increased risk for bad influence. Therefore, it is important to find some role for the injured adolescents within the team and maintain their connection with the group.

Team Performance

Injuries of key players in a team can easily affect the team performance, especially if more than one player is injured at the same time. This is particularly noticeable if the group of players is based on a relatively few athletes. A study on soccer players showed a trend toward a better final league standing at the end of the season for teams that showed fewer injury days during the season (89).

Cost of Injuries

Injuries are expensive. Medical treatment and rehabilitation after sport injuries, as well as the loss of competition and working days, sums to an extremely high amount each year that must be paid by the athletes, their families, the teams, or insurance providers (90,91).

When Should Injury Prevention Start?

As noted in the previous section, prevention of injuries is extremely important. In recent years, knowledge about risk factors, their interaction, and confounding has increased in different types of sports. This knowledge provides an important base for preventive measures aiming at reducing the incidence and severity of injuries as well as the risk of injuries.

Injury prevention should start early. Children should learn that preventive measures are a part of training for sport, and injury prevention should be included in the training. If preventive measures start early it will be easier to follow up in adolescent and adult sports. The athletes will also experience the preventive measures as a natural part of the training. An example of injury prevention that should start before puberty is prevention of knee injuries because during or after puberty movement patterns seem to change particularly in female athletes, which appear to increase the risk of severe knee injuries. Such prevention should aim at improving the movement patterns, for example, during jumping, landing, cutting, accelerating and decelerating with neuromuscular training, such as balance and coordination training, as well as strength training, functional exercises, and teaching technical skills both in general and in a sport-specific manner. Information about this concept and the importance of such training should be presented to the athletes and their parents in order to increase their understanding and encourage them to participate in the program.

PREVENTION OF INJURIES IN SPORT

To be able to organize injury prevention, it is important to know the typical risk factors and injury mechanisms for the particular type of sport, as well as the complexity of their interaction and confounding. In recent years, many studies have been conducted in order to increase our knowledge about risk factors and injury mechanisms in different kinds of sports. These studies are an important background for the improvement of prevention strategies, exercises, and programs aimed at reducing the incidence and severity of injuries in sport. However, more large multifactorial studies are needed that take into account many potential risk factors in correlation with different injury situations. That could increase our understanding and build a stronger framework for preventive strategies against various types of injuries in different kinds of sports.

When developing prevention programs one must take into account the biomechanical load during the particular type of sport. One must know the demands of the particular sports placed on the athletes, such as sport-specific movements, running and jumping ability, rules, load during training and competition, as well as typical risk factors and injury mechanisms. Even in the same type of sport, the requirements may be different regarding age, gender, and level of play, playing exposure, playing position, quality of coaching, weather conditions, and playing ground. All these factors should be taken into account and put in the context of the biomechanical load placed on the athletes. The focus of the prevention program should be to increase the athletes' tolerance against the biomechanical load either for injuries in general or for a particular type of injury. The aim of prevention programs should be to decrease the athletes' weaknesses with respect to injuries and thereby decrease the injury risk. This should be confirmed with studies that test the effect of the particular program. Prevention programs should not be too time-consuming, because if they are then it is less likely that they will be completed. The coaches and athletes should also see some performance benefits in the program regarding the particular type of sport (92). An example of such benefits could be increased strength (93–95), increased core stability and technical skills (96,97), and improved neuromuscular control containing balance and coordination (98–100). Injury prevention programs should be a natural part of the training, be performed regularly, and be promoted by the coaches, physical therapists, or athletic trainers.

Prevention programs are usually based on many factors that are considered to affect the risk of injuries, for example, improving balance, coordination, strength, agility and technique, awareness of joint position, movements, or risky playing situations (23,101–103). Because most programs are multidimensional, it is difficult to know which components of these programs are most effective in injury prevention or how they work as they are usually not tested separately (5).

Several studies have been conducted to try out some exercises or programs that could decrease the rate of various injuries in different types of sports. Some of these programs are aimed at decreasing injury incidence in general (21,23), while others focus on preventing injuries of special type or location (94,103). Most of these programs are tried out in specific types of sport: for example, in soccer (22,24,104), Australian Rules football (17), Rugby (105), European handball (21,101), volleyball (30), and alpine skiing (106).

Injury prevention can be classified into two categories: general injury prevention on the one hand, focusing on reducing injuries in general, and specific injury prevention, on the other hand, focusing on special types or locations of injuries.

General Injury Prevention

The aim of general injury prevention should be to reduce injury rate in general for a group of athletes or a team. Such injury prevention should be included in the ordinary training. Components of such training could, for example, include sufficient warm-up, general training of balance and coordination, strength, speed, power, endurance, flexibility, and technique. Adequate training load and intensity considering age, gender, level of play, type of sport, etc., are of high importance. Training and playing on an appropriate playing ground, as well as encouraging the athletes to fair play, is also important. Most studies on general injury prevention programs show reduction in injury rate after performing such programs (21–24), but studies are also found indicating less or nonsignificant effect (107,108), possibly because of low compliance with the prevention programs in these studies.

Specific Injury Prevention

The aim of specific injury prevention should be to reduce the incidence of injuries of a specific type or location. This could be done for either a group or a team and the aim could, for example, be to reduce ACL injuries or knee injuries in general. Individually based screening could also be used in order to identify players at risk for specific or different types or location of injuries. Preventive measures could subsequently be applied for those who are found to be at risk. Studies have been conducted to test the effect of some prevention programs focusing on specific types of injuries; for example, ankle sprains (30,109,110), knee injuries (103), ACL injuries (101,111), hamstring strains (17,94), and groin strains (104). Results from these studies show that preventive measures regarding specific types of injuries are effective and should be recommended, especially in sports with high incidence of such injuries. In a specific prevention, the focus is usually on some of the following factors according to the types and location of injuries.

Improving Sport-Specific Skills and Quality of Coaching

An important part of injury prevention is to improve the athletes' sport-specific skills. Such training is an important part of many prevention programs that have been shown to be effective in preventing, for example, ACL injuries (101,111) and hamstring strains (17). This approach should both improve the sport-specific skills and have a preventive effect, something that every coach and athlete would appreciate. In this context, the quality of coaching is of high importance both for the athletes' basic and specific training, as well as their performance and injury prevention. The training load and intensity must also be suitable for the athletes with regard to their age, gender, training status, etc. The coaches must be aware of high-risk periods during the training that could cause an excessive fatigue response and predispose to acute or overuse injuries. Teaching young athletes appropriate sport-specific skills is an important part of injury prevention and should be emphasized in all types of sport. Examples of such training are teaching and correcting technique during cutting, jumping, and landing in, for example, basketball, team handball, and soccer.

Neuromuscular Training

When soft-tissue injuries occur nerve endings and nerve pathways can be damaged, which can impair the segmental transmission of nerve impulses from proprioceptors located in ligaments or joint capsule. This can affect coordination and joint position sense, as well as alter reflexes, for example, regarding muscle responses that reposition joints back into physiologic range. Such impairments may result in decreased balance and functional instability often represented as the feeling of giving way in joints (112). During the rehabilitation process after injuries, neuromuscular training is important to restore the neuromuscular control for preventing recurrent injuries (42). When preventing injuries, this type of training has been shown to be effective in reducing the rate of recurrent ankle sprains (30,110,113), and as an effective part of preventing programs for ACL injuries of the knee (101,111,114). Neuromuscular training has also been used to increase core stability and functional stability of the shoulder, elbow, and wrist in rehabilitation and as a preventive measure (112). This type of training should include balance exercises at a progressive level of difficulty and should be developed into sport-specific exercises.

Correction of Muscle Imbalance

Strength imbalance between legs or between anterior and posterior muscles of the thigh (H/Q ratio) and a decreased eccentric strength have been considered to be possible risk factors for injuries. Consequently, strength training is a part of many prevention programs. In recent years, an increased emphasis has been on eccentric strength training, which has been shown to have preventive effect, for example, on hamstring strains (94). As mentioned before, little evidence is found in support of decreased flexibility being a risk factor for muscle strains, but short muscles or imbalance in muscle length could possibly predispose to injuries by affecting posture and movement patterns. Such examples could be the combination of short and strong protractor muscles and long and weak retractor muscles of the shoulder girdle. Such combination will increase the protraction of the scapula, affect the movement pattern and stability of the shoulder, and possibly increase the risk of impingement in throwing athletes like team handball players or pitchers in baseball. Therefore, it is important to assess the athletes' posture to detect such conditions. When conducting training programs, it is important to include exercises to correct such posture when present, or use balanced amount of strength and flexibility exercise to avoid such conditions.

External support

External support can be performed with, for example, taping or braces. Ankle support has been shown to reduce the incidence of recurrent ankle sprains, but has not shown a preventive effect on ankles without a previous history of sprains (115). Tape or braces has been recommended during sports activity following ankle sprains to reduce the risk of recurrent sprains until normal ankle function is reached (116). Different methods of taping provide different support and one can adjust the taping with respect to the exact location and support required. Braces are often used instead of taping. They are easier in use for the athletes and do not have to be fixed onto the skin like taping. However, some athletes feel that braces will restrict their ankle movements too much or the ankle will be less stable than with taping.

Helmets and even faceguards have been recommended to decrease the risk of head injuries in many types of sports and in some sport they have become mandatory during competition, for example, in American football, ice hockey, alpine skiing, and snowboarding, as well as in various types of motor sports. Studies have shown that helmets can be effective in preventing head and facial injuries in some types of sport, but less effect is found on concussion risk (117,118).

Other external support such as shin guards has also been shown to be effective in prevention of lower leg injuries in soccer (33), but more recent studies have reported that protective effect of shin guards differs according to types and material (119,120).

Rules and Fair Play

Rules in sport should protect the athletes from foul play, and thereby prevent some serious injuries. Subsequently, rules have been changed to avoid foul play, for example, in soccer as when it was decided that tackles from behind automatically resulted in a red card. Studies have also pointed out that strict rules against late gliding tackles in soccer could prevent some ankle and leg injuries (2). Another example from a study on volleyball players has shown that many ankle injuries occurred when a player landed on an opponent's foot under the net, when landing after blocking or attacking (121). In another study, these authors found that the technique of training and rule changes where players were not allowed to step across the line below the net after attacking or blocking could decrease the rate of ankle injuries (30). Conclusively, rules are important for the protection of the athletes against injuries and rule changes could sometimes have preventive effects. Besides, it is always important to encourage athletes to honor fair play.

Summary of Injury Prevention

Injuries are common in many types of sport. Although most sport injuries heal with appropriate rehabilitation, some injuries can limit the athletes' sport participation or force the athlete to quit in his sport. Injuries can also affect the athletes' physical fitness and have some psychological or social effects as well as affect the team performance. In addition, injuries are expensive for the athletes, their families, the sports clubs, or insurance providers. Consequently, injury prevention is extremely important. Injury prevention should be included in training for sports and start at a young age so that the children learn that injury prevention is a natural part of training for sports. Injury prevention can be classified into general and specific prevention, where general injury prevention focuses on reducing injuries in general, but specific injury prevention focuses on specific types of injuries. Injury prevention and training of sport-specific skills are highly related, something that athletes, coaches, physical therapists, or athletic trainers should appreciate.

REFERENCES

1. Verrall G, Árnason Á, Bennell K. Preventing hamstring injuries. In: Bahr R, Engebretsen L, eds. Handbook of Sports Medicine and Science, Sports Injury Prevention. West Sussex, UK: Wiley-Blackwell; 2009:72–90.

2. Andersen TE, Floerenes TW, Arnason A, et al. Video analysis of the mechanisms for ankle injuries in football. Am J Sports Med 2004;32:69S-79S.

3. Sallay PI, Friedman RL, Coogan PG, et al. Hamstring muscle injuries among water skiers. Functional outcome and prevention. Am J Sports Med 1996;24:130–136.

4. Meeuwisse WH. Assessing causation in sport injury: a multifactorial model. Clin J Sport Med 1994;4:166–170.

5. Bahr R, Krosshaug T. Understanding injury mechanisms: a key component of preventing injuries in sport. Br J Sports Med 2005;39:324–329.

6. Meeuwisse W, Bahr R. A systematic approach to sports injury prevention. In: Bahr R, Engebretsen L, eds. Handbook of Sports Medicine and Science, Sports Injury Prevention. West Sussex, UK: Wiley-Blackwell; 2009:7–16.

7. Hootman JM, Dick R, Agel J. Epidemiology of collegiate injuries for 15 sports: summary and recommendations for injury prevention initiatives. J Athl Train 2007;42:311–319.

8. Nielsen AB, Yde J. Epidemiology and traumatology of injuries in soccer. Am J Sports Med 1989;17:803–807.

9. Inklaar H, Bol E, Schmikli SL, et al. Injuries in male soccer players: team risk analysis. Int J Sports Med 1996;17: 229–234.

10. Ekstrand J, Tropp H. The incidence of ankle sprains in soccer. Foot Ankle 1990;11:41–44.

11. Poulsen TD, Freund KG, Madsen F, et al. Injuries in high-skilled and low-skilled soccer: a prospective study. Br J Sports Med 1991;25:151–153.

12. Peterson L, Junge A, Chomiak J, et al. Incidence of football injuries and complaints in different age groups and skill-level groups. Am J Sports Med 2000;28:S51–S57.

13. Chomiak J, Junge A, Peterson L, et al. Severe injuries in football players. Influencing factors. Am J Sports Med 2000;28:S58–S68.

14. Ekstrand J, Gillquist J, Moller M, et al. Incidence of soccer injuries and their relation to training and team success. Am J Sports Med 1983;11:63–67.

15. Arnason A, Sigurdsson SB, Gudmundsson A, et al. Risk factors for injuries in football. Am J Sports Med 2004;32:5S–16S.

16. Arnason A, Gudmundsson A, Dahl HA, et al. Soccer injuries in Iceland. Scand J Med Sci Sports 1996;6:40–45.

17. Verrall GM, Slavotinek JP, Barnes PG. The effect of sports specific training on reducing the incidence of hamstring injuries in professional Australian Rules football players. Br J Sports Med 2005;39:363–368.

18. Green JP, Grenier SG, McGill SM. Low-back stiffness is altered with warm-up and bench rest: implications for athletes. Med Sci Sports Exerc 2002;34:1076–1081.

19. Rosenbaum D, Hennig EM. The influence of stretching and warm-up exercises on Achilles tendon reflex activity. J Sports Sci 1995;13:481–490.

20. Stewart IB, Sleivert GG. The effect of warm-up intensity on range of motion and anaerobic performance. J Orthop Sports Phys Ther 1998;27:154–161.

21. Olsen OE, Myklebust G, Engebretsen L, et al. Exercises to prevent lower limb injuries in youth sports: cluster randomised controlled trial. BMJ 2005;330:449.

22. Ekstrand J, Gillquist J, Liljedahl SO. Prevention of soccer injuries. Supervision by doctor and physiotherapist. Am J Sports Med 1983;11:116–120.

23. Junge A, Rosch D, Peterson L, et al. Prevention of soccer injuries: a prospective intervention study in youth amateur players. Am J Sports Med 2002;30:652–659.

24. Soligard T, Myklebust G, Steffen K, et al. Comprehensive warm-up programme to prevent injuries in young female footballers: cluster randomised controlled trial. BMJ 2008;337:a2469.

25. Hawkins RD, Fuller CW. Risk assessment in professional football: an examination of accidents and incidents in the 1994 World Cup finals. Br J Sports Med 1996;30:165–170.

26. Boden BP, Kirkendall DT, Garrett WE Jr. Concussion incidence in elite college soccer players. Am J Sports Med 1998;26:238–241.

27. Hawkins RD, Fuller CW. A prospective epidemiological study of injuries in four English professional football clubs. Br J Sports Med 1999;33:196–203.

28. Bahr R. Principles of injury prevention. In: Brukner P, Khan K, eds. Clinical Sports Medicine. 3rd ed. North Ryde, NSW: McGraw-Hill; 2006:78–101.

29. Arnason A, Tenga A, Engebretsen L, et al. A prospective video-based analysis of injury situations in elite male football: football incident analysis. Am J Sports Med 2004;32: 1459–1465.

30. Bahr R, Lian O, Bahr IA. A twofold reduction in the incidence of acute ankle sprains in volleyball after the introduction of an injury prevention program: a prospective cohort study. Scand J Med Sci Sports 1997;7:172–177.

31. Junge A, Chomiak J, Dvorak J. Incidence of football injuries in youth players. Comparison of players from two European regions. Am J Sports Med 2000;28:S47–S50.

32. Verrall GM, Slavotinek JP, Barnes PG, et al. Clinical risk factors for hamstring muscle strain injury: a prospective study with correlation of injury by magnetic resonance imaging. Br J Sports Med 2001;35:435–439.

33. Ekstrand J, Gillquist J. The avoidability of soccer injuries. Int J Sports Med 1983;4:124–128.

34. Noonan TJ, Garrett WE Jr. Injuries at the myotendinous junction. Clin Sports Med 1992;11:783–806.

35. Jarvinen TA, Kaariainen M, Jarvinen M, et al. Muscle strain injuries. Curr Opin Rheumatol 2000;12:155–161.

36. Tropp H, Odenrick P, Gillquist J. Stabilometry recordings in functional and mechanical instability of the ankle joint. Int J Sports Med 1985;6:180–182.

37. Konradsen L, Ravn JB. Prolonged peroneal reaction time in ankle instability. Int J Sports Med 1991;12:290–292.

38. Brynhildsen J, Ekstrand J, Jeppsson A, et al. Previous injuries and persisting symptoms in female soccer players. Int J Sports Med 1990;11:489–492.

39. Tropp H, Ekstrand J, Gillquist J. Stabilometry in functional instability of the ankle and its value in predicting injury. Med Sci Sports Exerc 1984;16:64–66.

40. Beynnon BD, Renstrom PA, Alosa DM, et al. Ankle ligament injury risk factors: a prospective study of college athletes. J Orthop Res 2001;19:213–220.

41. Baumhauer JF, Alosa DM, Renstrom AF, et al. A prospective study of ankle injury risk factors. Am J Sports Med 1995;23:564–570.

42. Zech A, Hubscher M, Vogt L, et al. Neuromuscular training for rehabilitation of sports injuries: a systematic review. Med Sci Sports Exerc 2009;41:1831-41.

43. Tropp H. Pronator muscle weakness in functional instability of the ankle joint. Int J Sports Med 1986;7:291–294.

44. McGuine TA, Greene JJ, Best T, et al. Balance as a predictor of ankle injuries in high school basketball players. Clin J Sport Med 2000;10:239–244.

45. Orchard J, Marsden J, Lord S, et al. Preseason hamstring muscle weakness associated with hamstring muscle injury in Australian footballers. Am J Sports Med 1997;25:81–85.

46. Bennell K, Wajswelner H, Lew P, et al. Isokinetic strength testing does not predict hamstring injury in Australian Rules footballers. Br J Sports Med 1998;32:309–314.

47. Ostenberg A, Roos H. Injury risk factors in female European football. A prospective study of 123 players during one season. Scand J Med Sci Sports 2000;10:279–285.

48. Jonhagen S, Ericson MO, Nemeth G, et al. Amplitude and timing of electromyographic activity during sprinting. Scand J Med Sci Sports 1996;6:15–21.

49. Yu B, Queen RM, Abbey AN, et al. Hamstring muscle kinematics and activation during overground sprinting. J Biomech 2008;41:3121–3126.

50. Watson AW. Sports injuries related to flexibility, posture, acceleration, clinical defects, and previous injury, in high-level players of body contact sports. Int J Sports Med 2001;22:222–225.

51. Soderman K, Alfredson H, Pietila T, et al. Risk factors for leg injuries in female soccer players: a prospective investigation during one out-door season. Knee Surg Sports Traumatol Arthrosc 2001;9:313–321.

52. Witvrouw E, Danneels L, Asselman P, et al. Muscle flexibility as a risk factor for developing muscle injuries in male professional soccer players. A prospective study. Am J Sports Med 2003;31:41–46.

53. Bahr R, Holme I. Risk factors for sports injuries—a methodological approach. Br J Sports Med 2003;37:384–392.

54. Bangsbo J, Lindquist F. Comparison of various exercise tests with endurance performance during soccer in professional players. Int J Sports Med 1992;13:125–132.

55. Wisloff U, Helgerud J, Hoff J. Strength and endurance of elite soccer players. Med Sci Sports Exerc 1998;30:462–467.

56. Helgerud J, Engen LC, Wisloff U, et al. Aerobic endurance training improves soccer performance. Med Sci Sports Exerc 2001;33:1925–1931.

57. Murphy DF, Connolly DA, Beynnon BD. Risk factors for lower extremity injury: a review of the literature. Br J Sports Med 2003;37:13–29.

58. Knapik JJ, Sharp MA, Canham-Chervak M, et al. Risk factors for training-related injuries among men and women in basic combat training. Med Sci Sports Exerc 2001;33:946–954.

59. Jones BH, Bovee MW, Harris JM 3rd, Cowan DN. Intrinsic risk factors for exercise-related injuries among male and female army trainees. Am J Sports Med 1993;21:705–710.

60. Woods C, Hawkins RD, Maltby S, et al. The Football Association Medical Research Programme: an audit of injuries in professional football—analysis of hamstring injuries. Br J Sports Med 2004;38:36–41.

61. Mair SD, Seaber AV, Glisson RR, et al. The role of fatigue in susceptibility to acute muscle strain injury. Am J Sports Med 1996;24:137–143.

62. Kale M, Asci A, Bayrak C, et al. Relationships among jumping performances and sprint parameters during maximum speed phase in sprinters. J Strength Cond Res 2009;23:2272–2279.

63. Rosch D, Hodgson R, Peterson TL, et al. Assessment and evaluation of football performance. Am J Sports Med 2000;28:S29–S39.

64. Dvorak J, Junge A, Chomiak J, et al. Risk factor analysis for injuries in football players. Possibilities for a prevention program. Am J Sports Med 2000;28:S69–S74.

65. Junge A. The influence of psychological factors on sports injuries. Review of the literature. Am J Sports Med 2000;28:S10–S15.

66. Andersen MB, Williams JM. Athletic injury, psychosocial factors and perceptual changes during stress. J Sports Sci 1999;17:735–741.

67. Ekstrand J, Nigg BM. Surface-related injuries in soccer. Sports Med 1989;8:56–62.

68. Orchard J. Is there a relationship between ground and climatic conditions and injuries in football? Sports Med 2002;32:419–432.

69. Olsen OE, Myklebust G, Engebretsen L, et al. Relationship between floor type and risk of ACL injury in team handball. Scand J Med Sci Sports 2003;13:299–304.

70. Norton K, Schwerdt S, Lange K. Evidence for the aetiology of injuries in Australian football. Br J Sports Med 2001;35:418–423.

71. Schmidt-Olsen S, Jorgensen U, Kaalund S, et al. Injuries among young soccer players. Am J Sports Med 1991;19:273–275.

72. Huston LJ, Greenfield ML, Wojtys EM. Anterior cruciate ligament injuries in the female athlete. Potential risk factors. Clin Orthop Relat Res 2000;372:50–63.

73. Bjordal JM, Arnly F, Hannestad B, et al. Epidemiology of anterior cruciate ligament injuries in soccer. Am J Sports Med 1997;25:341–345.

74. Roos H, Ornell M, Gardsell P, et al. Soccer after anterior cruciate ligament injury—an incompatible combination? A national survey of incidence and risk factors and a 7-year follow-up of 310 players. Acta Orthop Scand 1995;66:107–112.

75. LaPrade RF, Burnett QM 2nd. Femoral intercondylar notch stenosis and correlation to anterior cruciate ligament injuries. A prospective study. Am J Sports Med 1994;22:198–202; discussion 3.

76. Griffin LY, Albohm MJ, Arendt EA, et al. Understanding and preventing noncontact anterior cruciate ligament injuries: a review of the Hunt Valley II meeting, January 2005. Am J Sports Med 2006;34:1512–1532.

77. Beynnon BD, Johnson RJ, Braun S, et al. The relationship between menstrual cycle phase and anterior cruciate ligament injury: a case-control study of recreational alpine skiers. Am J Sports Med 2006;34:757–764.

78. Slauterbeck JR, Fuzie SF, Smith MP, et al. The menstrual cycle, sex hormones, and anterior cruciate ligament injury. J Athl Train 2002;37:275–278.

79. Hewett TE, Myer GD, Ford KR. Anterior cruciate ligament injuries in female athletes: part 1, mechanisms and risk factors. Am J Sports Med 2006;34:299–311.

80. Hewett TE, Myer GD, Ford KR, et al. Preparticipation physical examination using a box drop vertical jump test in young athletes: the effects of puberty and sex. Clin J Sport Med 2006;16:298–304.

81. Griffin LY, Agel J, Albohm MJ, et al. Noncontact anterior cruciate ligament injuries: risk factors and prevention strategies. J Am Acad Orthop Surg 2000;8:141–150.

82. Soderman K, Pietila T, Alfredson H, et al. Anterior cruciate ligament injuries in young females playing soccer at senior levels. Scand J Med Sci Sports 2002;12:65–68.

83. Junge A, Langevoort G, Pipe A, et al. Injuries in team sport tournaments during the 2004 Olympic Games. Am J Sports Med 2006;34:565–576.

84. Lohmander LS, Ostenberg A, Englund M, et al. High prevalence of knee osteoarthritis, pain, and functional limitations in female soccer players twelve years after anterior cruciate ligament injury. Arthritis Rheum 2004;50:3145–3152.

85. von Porat A, Roos EM, Roos H. High prevalence of osteoarthritis 14 years after an anterior cruciate ligament tear in male soccer players: a study of radiographic and patient relevant outcomes. Ann Rheum Dis 2004;63:269–273.

86. Drawer S, Fuller CW. Propensity for osteoarthritis and lower limb joint pain in retired professional soccer players. Br J Sports Med 2001;35:402–408.

87. Thorlindsson T, Vilhjalmsson R, Valgeirsson G. Sport participation and perceived health status: a study of adolescents. Soc Sci Med 1990;31:551–556.

88. Pastor Y, Balaguer I, Pons D, et al. Testing direct and indirect effects of sports participation on perceived health in Spanish adolescents between 15 and 18 years of age. J Adolesc 2003;26:717–730.

89. Arnason A, Sigurdsson SB, Gudmundsson A, et al. Physical fitness, injuries, and team performance in soccer. Med Sci Sports Exerc 2004;36:278–285.

90. Dvorak J, Junge A. Football injuries and physical symptoms. A review of the literature. Am J Sports Med 2000;28:S3–S9.

91. Drawer S, Fuller CW. Evaluating the level of injury in English professional football using a risk based assessment process. Br J Sports Med 2002;36:446–451.

92. Steffen K, Bakka HM, Myklebust G, et al. Performance aspects of an injury prevention program: a ten-week intervention in adolescent female football players. Scand J Med Sci Sports 2008;18:596–604.

93. Askling C, Karlsson J, Thorstensson A. Hamstring injury occurrence in elite soccer players after preseason strength training with eccentric overload. Scand J Med Sci Sports 2003;13:244–250.

94. Arnason A, Andersen TE, Holme I, et al. Prevention of hamstring strains in elite soccer: an intervention study. Scand J Med Sci Sports 2008;18:40–48.

95. Mjolsnes R, Arnason A, Osthagen T, et al. A 10-week randomized trial comparing eccentric vs. concentric hamstring strength training in well-trained soccer players. Scand J Med Sci Sports 2004;14:311–317.

96. Holm I, Fosdahl MA, Friis A, et al. Effect of neuromuscular training on proprioception, balance, muscle strength, and lower limb function in female team handball players. Clin J Sport Med 2004;14:88–94.

97. Leetun DT, Ireland ML, Willson JD, et al. Core stability measures as risk factors for lower extremity injury in athletes. Med Sci Sports Exerc 2004;36:926–934.

98. Hewett TE, Myer GD, Ford KR. Decrease in neuromuscular control about the knee with maturation in female athletes. J Bone Joint Surg Am 2004;86-A:1601–1608.

99. Myer GD, Ford KR, McLean SG, et al. The effects of plyometric versus dynamic stabilization and balance training on lower extremity biomechanics. Am J Sports Med 2006;34:445–455.

100. Myer GD, Ford KR, Palumbo JP, et al. Neuromuscular training improves performance and lower-extremity biomechanics in female athletes. J Strength Cond Res 2005;19:51–60.

101. Myklebust G, Engebretsen L, Braekken IH, et al. Prevention of anterior cruciate ligament injuries in female team handball players: a prospective intervention study over three seasons. Clin J Sport Med 2003;13:71–78.

102. Wedderkopp N, Kaltoft M, Lundgaard B, et al. Prevention of injuries in young female players in European team handball. A prospective intervention study. Scand J Med Sci Sports 1999;9:41–47.

103. Hewett TE, Lindenfeld TN, Riccobene JV, et al. The effect of neuromuscular training on the incidence of knee injury in female athletes. A prospective study. Am J Sports Med 1999;27:699–706.

104. Holmich P, Larsen K, Krogsgaard K, et al. Exercise program for prevention of groin pain in football players: a cluster-randomized trial. Scand J Med Sci Sports 2010;20:814-21.

105. Brooks JH, Fuller CW, Kemp SP, et al. Incidence, risk, and prevention of hamstring muscle injuries in professional rugby union. Am J Sports Med 2006;34:1297–1306.

106. Ettlinger CF, Johnson RJ, Shealy JE. A method to help reduce the risk of serious knee sprains incurred in alpine skiing. Am J Sports Med 1995;23:531–537.

107. Engebretsen AH, Myklebust G, Holme I, et al. Prevention of injuries among male soccer players: a prospective, randomized intervention study targeting players with previous injuries or reduced function. Am J Sports Med 2008;36:1052–1060.

108. Steffen K, Myklebust G, Olsen OE, et al. Preventing injuries in female youth football—a cluster-randomized controlled trial. Scand J Med Sci Sports 2008;18:605–614.

109. McGuine TA, Keene JS. The effect of a balance training program on the risk of ankle sprains in high school athletes. Am J Sports Med 2006;34:1103–1111.

110. Verhagen E, van der Beek A, Twisk J, et al. The effect of a proprioceptive balance board training program for the prevention of ankle sprains: a prospective controlled trial. Am J Sports Med 2004;32:1385–1393.

111. Mandelbaum BR, Silvers HJ, Watanabe DS, et al. Effectiveness of a neuromuscular and proprioceptive training program in preventing anterior cruciate ligament injuries in female athletes: 2-year follow-up. Am J Sports Med 2005;33:1003–1010.

112. Kinch M, Lambart A. Principles of Rehabilitation. In: Brukner P, Khan K, eds. Clinical Sports Medicine. 3rd ed. North Ryde, NSW: McGraw-Hill; 2006:174–197.

113. Tropp H, Askling C, Gillquist J. Prevention of ankle sprains. Am J Sports Med 1985;13:259–262.

114. Hewett TE, Ford KR, Myer GD. Anterior cruciate ligament injuries in female athletes: part 2, a meta-analysis of neuromuscular interventions aimed at injury prevention. Am J Sports Med 2006;34:490–498.

115. Surve I, Schwellnus MP, Noakes T, et al. A fivefold reduction in the incidence of recurrent ankle sprains in soccer players using the Sport-Stirrup orthosis. Am J Sports Med 1994;22:601–606.

116. Hansen KJ, Bahr R. Rehabilitation of Ankle Injuries. In: Bahr R, Mæhlum S, eds. Clinical Guide to Sports Injuries. Champaign, IL: Human Kinetics; 2004:419–422.

117. Benson BW, Hamilton GM, Meeuwisse WH, et al. Is protective equipment useful in preventing concussion? A systematic review of the literature. Br J Sports Med 2009;43(Suppl 1):i56–i67.

118. McIntosh AS, McCrory P. Preventing head and neck injury. Br J Sports Med 2005;39:314–318.

119. Bir CA, Cassatta SJ, Janda DH. An analysis and comparison of soccer shin guards. Clin J Sport Med 1995;5:95–99.

120. Francisco AC, Nightingale RW, Guilak F, et al. Comparison of soccer shin guards in preventing tibia fracture. Am J Sports Med 2000;28:227–233.

121. Bahr R, Bahr IA. Incidence of acute volleyball injuries: a prospective cohort study of injury mechanisms and risk factors. Scand J Med Sci Sports 1997;7:166–171.

Bridging the Gap from Rehabilitation to Performance

INTRODUCTION

Traditionally, rehabilitation has focused on assessment of isolated joint pathology and resultant localized treatment of the involved tissue. For example, when someone had shoulder pain, his or her shoulder was evaluated. Treatment focused on decreasing the pain of provocative tissues at the shoulder, via local modalities or manual techniques, and exercises were given to make the shoulder stronger. Once the shoulder felt better, the patient was discharged from physical therapy with a home exercise program. In this model, nothing was done wrong; just everything was not done right. This model treats the "source" of pain, versus finding and treating the "cause" of pain. This lack of acknowledgement of the entire kinetic chain in both evaluation and treatment is the inherent difference between rehabilitating an injury and returning an athlete to sport. Returning an athlete to sport requires a much more comprehensive approach to the evaluation of injured tissue, evaluation of kinetic linking and kinematic sequencing, and resultant prescription of techniques to return an athlete to their sport, perhaps bigger, faster, stronger, and more efficient in their movement than they were prior to injury. This is bridging the gap between rehabilitation and performance.

In today's health care model, specialists are often separated in two ways. First, physically, health care providers for a patient are often located in different facilities, across town, or sometimes even in different towns. When there is a physical separation, the philosophical connection must be strong. If health care providers are more concerned with "who is in charge" of the clients' care, and try to micromanage the other providers, egos become inflated, guards are up, and walls become raised. This creates a philosophy of a self-centered model. What we propose is adopting an athlete-centered model.

WHAT IS AN ATHLETE-CENTERED MODEL?

The athlete-centered model places the athlete at the center core of the program, with all professionals working together to ensure the athlete attains his or her goals. The health care providers leave their letters at the door so to speak, working together as one team with the patients' best interest in mind. Everyone (the doctor, the chiropractor, the physical therapist, the athletic trainer, the massage therapists, the personal trainer, and so on) brings a specialty to the table and can offer insight to help the patient achieve his/her goals. Where the client lies along the performance continuum (Figure 3.1) will depend on who is the "quarterback" of the clients' care at a given time. If the patient is postoperative, the doctor may be the quarterback, dictating precautions and contraindications from the surgery. As the rehabilitation process moves on, the athletic trainer or physical therapist may become the quarterback, as the athlete is improving movement efficiency. At some point when the client is ready to move onto different training movements at various loads and speeds, the performance coach may become the quarterback. And finally, as that athlete begins to work on the technical and tactical aspects of his/her sport, the skill coach may play a lead role, assisting that athlete back to the specifics of their sport and position. Everyone brings something to the table that should be valued and respected with the athletes' best interest in mind. There is no one person that can do everything for the athlete, from the operating room, to skill work and technique work on the field, as well as everything in between. There are many players involved in the process, with certain people wearing larger hats at certain times than others. In the athlete-centered model, everyone is involved in the process. Sometimes the roles of different people are large or small, but everyone is involved, as everyone brings something special to the program. Each health care professional, performance coach, and skill coach must come together, bring their area of expertise, and work together to return the athlete to play. Considering all the things that are involved in returning an athlete to sport or a patient to a high quality of life, there are many things involved that go way beyond the body part of injury (Figure 3.2). Simply rehabilitating that injury is no longer acceptable in this rehabilitation model. Ideally, our athletes return to their sport not only rehabilitated, but as stronger, healthier individuals in general.

Athlete goals are threefold: 1) increase career longevity, 2) increase career productivity, and 3) ownership of their

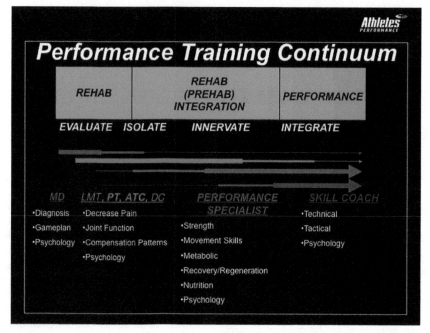

FIGURE 3-1. This continuum depicts how all health care practitioners, performance coaches, and skill coaches can work together in the best interest of the athlete.

injury and treatment via education, to work the strategies set forth, in order to attain his or her personal goals.

HOW DO WE SUCCESSFULLY BRIDGE THE GAP?

Bridging the gap between rehabilitation and performance requires the health care professional (including the MD-medical doctor, LMT-licensed massage therapist, PT-physical therapist, AT-athletic trainer and DC-chiropractor) to understand the performance aspect of training an athlete. Bridging the gap requires the performance specialists, movement

coaches, strength coaches, and skill coaches to understand and respect healing tissue. When these professionals work synergistically in the best interest of the athlete, they will have successfully bridged the gap.

EVALUATION

Functional Anatomy Implications

Core training has gained a tremendous amount of attention in the literature over the last several years (1–3). Clinicians with different backgrounds would agree that some element

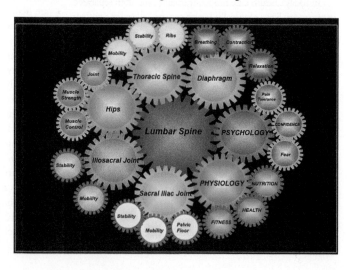

FIGURE 3-2. Many factors can affect training and performance. If one factor is inhibited, it has an effect on the entire unit. There is a constant relationship between each factor working together.

of core strength is important in injury reduction and sport performance, and yet also realize that injury prevention and optimal performance lie much deeper than simple abdominal strength. A combination of mobility, stability, and strength at the shoulders, trunk, and hips is needed to efficiently transfer force from the lower body to the upper body, or vice versa (4–7). These three definable, yet integrated areas are the foundation for all human movement. There is a terrific body of research done on the shoulder, the spine, and pelvis with their associated musculature and function (8–10). There are countless protocols focusing on the rehabilitation or performance enhancement of these areas, but the true synergy lies within their seamless integration (11,12).

Rehabilitation professionals and strength specialists need to move past the simplistic view of the core and look to a more integrated view of pillar strength. Pillar strength is the complete integration of our shoulders, trunk, and hips. Mobility, stability, and strength at each of these individual areas are needed so they can come together to create a conduit for power production and force transfer in the body (13).

When discussing the shoulders, trunk, and hips, there are several things to consider in regard to their relationship with each other. When discussing the "pillar," it is important to realize that there are approximately 63 joints and more than 71 muscles depending on how the individual spinal intrinsics and pelvic floor muscles are counted. All of these are connected via fascial slings that run in the sagittal, coronal, and transverse planes (4). This massive amount of mobile structures creates an intricate system of motor programs, conducting dozens of force couples to work simultaneously together to create a diverse set of seamless movements throughout the kinetic chain.

Movement Assessment

When returning an athlete to sport after injury, one must consider what caused the injury to begin with. Tissue overload due to excessive force or poor positioning and posture is often the reason for both traumatic and nontraumatic injuries. We must identify the cause of pain if we ever hope that the source of pain improves. The body will ultimately follow the path of least resistance during static postures and dynamic movements. People will hang on their ligaments and rest on their joints with minimal effort to support those structures. During movement, athletes become great compensators, focusing on the end goal and not the path it takes to get there. Bridging the gap between rehabilitation and performance is about identifying these faulty postures and compensatory movement patterns that lead to tissue breakdown and teaching the body how to function in what will ultimately be a more efficient manner. Movement efficiency can be viewed as the cornerstone to athletic movement. Athletic movement consists of linear movement, multidirectional movement, jumping, landing,

and transitions from any one of these movements into any other movement.

Most athletes do not need to "be strong." They need sport-specific strength that will support the movement patterns that are required of them day after day, season after season. We should more often than not look at weight room activities as an opportunity to enhance and support the movements required on the field. Traditional strength training and rehabilitation have focused on increasing the strength of an individual. What an athlete needs is power: the ability to do a certain amount of work in a given time or to do more work in the same amount of time. There are several times when an athlete simply may need to train strength for purposes of pure strength. Examples would include someone preparing for the bench test in the National Football League (NFL) combine a power lifter or an Olympic lifter. But true athletic movement is a function of power, and simple strength training will not be enough to improve athletic movement.

Movements can be described and categorized accordingly: *Upper body push* movements can be performed horizontal to the body (bench press) or vertical to the body (military press). *Upper body pull* movements can be performed horizontal to the body (row) or vertical to the body (pull-up). *Lower body push* movements (squats) can be performed single or double leg. *Lower body pull* movements can be hip dominant (Romanian dead lift) or knee dominant (hamstring curl) and can be performed single or double leg. Finally, *rotational* movements can be performed with a stability emphasis (stability chop and lift) or with a propulsive emphasis (rotational row). During program development, all of these movements can be used accordingly to prepare the athlete for movements needed to return to play. Combine these training movements with athletic movement (linear movement, multidirectional movement, jumping, landing, and transitional movements) and you will have a comprehensive program for returning an athlete to their sport. This can be extremely complicated when written out on paper in this manner, but examples are offered throughout this book to break down the movement pattern and sport to which you wish to return your athlete. A proper interplay of mobility, stability, and strength at the proximal segments (shoulders, trunk, and hips) so that the more distal segments (limbs) can move more efficiently is needed. When the hub of the wheel is working properly, the spokes can remain in place. If the hub is broken, the spokes will follow suit.

CONTRACTILE CONTINUUM

When prescribing exercise, many rehabilitation specialists are comfortable prescribing three sets of ten exercises. Three sets of ten is a very comfortable set/rep scheme, where the athlete can work on neuromuscular control, reinforce a movement pattern, and begin to build some strength in an atrophied muscle group or limb. The rehabilitation

FIGURE 3-3. This continuum can be used to describe different types of strength an athlete may use during competition or training.

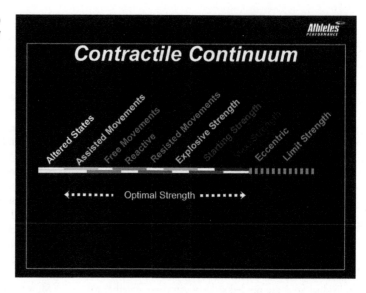

specialist must understand, however, that the athlete does not function in a world of three sets of ten. The athlete functions in a world of varying intensities, varying speeds, and unpredictability. They often must overcome not only force they are creating but forces others are placing on them, pushing them beyond their typical limits of strength, speed, and range of motion. Therefore, therapy must provide varying speeds, intensities, volumes, and external resistances in order to prepare the athlete to return to the playing field. A clinician's interventions must work the contractile continuum (Figure 3.3).

The contractile continuum can be used to describe different types of strength an athlete may use during competition or training. Beginning at the right-hand side of the continuum, we see limit strength. *Limit strength* is strength that is most likely a hormonal, "flight or fight"–type reaction. An example of limit strength would be a grandmother finding the strength to lift a car up off her grandchild who is pinned underneath. These acts of seemingly inexplicable strength cannot be trained and will only be used by the body in emergent or competitive situations. *Eccentric strength* is a lengthening contraction of the muscle and can handle a much greater load than a concentric muscle contraction. *Max strength* is defined by how much mass someone can move compared to their body weight (relative strength) or not compared to their body weight (absolute strength). *Starting strength* is the ability to overcome inertia. *Explosive strength* is the ability to move mass with speed. *Resisted movements* utilize external sources (dumbbells, sleds, other people, etc.) in a planned manner, while reactive strength is not preprogrammed. *Reactive strength* is the ability to react to someone else's movements, while *free movements* are more self-directed motor programs. *Assisted movements* are often described as overspeed training, where someone is being pushed beyond their regular ability to

produce movement. Finally, *altered states* include mediums that affect gravity, such as water. Including various speeds and intensities of movement while working the contractile continuum will allow our athletes the best chance to safely return to play and prepare them for competition. The contractile continuum must be used during program preparation of a rehabilitating athlete.

HOW DO WE MAXIMIZE PERFORMANCE PROGRESSIONS?

This is where the art of rehabilitation, performance, and bridging the gap between the two becomes clearer. Our professions are based on science, but programming and fitting it all together to return an athlete to play is truly the art of therapy and the art of coaching.

Flow and Progressions

Flow is never absolute. Whether talking about a single workout, or a training period, one type of training (e.g., stability) does not stop in order to train another (e.g., power). Many types of movements, contractions, and phases can coexist on any given day or any given training phase. In general, the flow of a workout or training period may be corrective exercise, strength, power, movement skill, and sport skill. Keep in mind, however, that rarely is it divided this nice and neat. No one will have perfect arthrokinematics or muscle firing patterns before they progress to a strength or power phase. No one will have maximum power potential prior to playing his or her sport. At what point does inefficient movement bring cause for concern for an increase in injury potential? This is a difficult question with truly no answer to date. This is what health care and performance professionals have been debating for years, and will continue to debate for years to come. Keeping in mind some simple principles will allow the clinician to progress athletes safely and effectively with minimal risk of setbacks.

Clear and Restore Joint Function

This must be done not only at the source of pain but also at the potential causes of pain. Arthrokinematics of a joint need to be restored and maintained for proper movement patterns to truly occur.

Progressive Tissue Loading

People often think that because someone is an athlete, they can perform higher level exercise earlier on in the rehabilitation process than a nonathlete. Athletes may work through the rehabilitation process more quickly than your average person, but they still need to progress, in order, without skipping a step. When an athlete does not progressively load tissue, tissue becomes irritated, and chronic irritation will cause pain and breakdown. Progressive tissue loading is a concept that needs to be discussed with every rehabilitating athlete. When this concept is not followed, an athlete will feel great one day, and irritated the next. The clinician's tendency will be to chase the ever-changing symptoms, abandoning any formal plan or progressions. Progressively loading tissue will prevent this, gradually allowing tissue to adapt to the stress placed on it. This will allow the athlete to progress through the rehabilitation process at his or her individual pace, no matter how fast or slow that may be.

Rate of Force Development

Progressively allowing an athlete to move at different speeds to learn how to develop force quickly will prepare an athlete to return to the necessary movement patterns for sport (14). Maintaining the same training movement, but altering the speed of which the movement is performed, will bridge that gap between rehabilitation and performance.

Mastery, Then Progression

There is a fine line between challenging an athlete and frustrating an athlete. An athlete must be placed in situations that challenge their tissue and skill level at the time, but allow them eventual mastery so they can feel a sense of accomplishment. A new goal is then created for them to work toward. This happens within individual treatment sessions as well as over time. Allowing them some mastery of skill before progression will satisfy their mental need for competition and goal achievement, fostering a healing environment.

Quality over Quantity

The old adage "you can't teach an old dog new tricks" is very true. It is easier to learn a new skill than to change the way you already do an old skill. This is because when you are learning a new skill, you create new neural pathways and motor programs (14). When you try to relearn an old skill, you must break down old neural pathways before you create new ones, which takes time. During the rehabilitation process, if people perform exercises the wrong way, a poor motor program will be enforced and inefficient movement will be created. When fatigue sets it, and movement efficiency breaks down, it is best to stop the exercise. This again represents the art of coaching. Every exercise will not look perfect. A clinician must decide what they will allow an athlete to work through, versus deciding the exercise is too challenging and picking another one. Quality movements and efficient movement patterns must be emphasized. Compensatory movement patterns cannot prevail. Quality movement patterns are always the priority during rehabilitation and performance.

SO HOW DOES A HEALTH CARE PROFESSIONAL TRULY BRIDGE THE GAP?

The answer is simple; the execution of this answer is not. No matter what capacity we work with athletes in, be it rehabilitation, performance, or skill acquisition and improvement, we all need to understand athletic movement. We need to be able to break down movement patterns, and coach our athletes. The art of coaching comes with time, a dedicated passion to become better, and a desire to find the best verbal, tactile, or neuromuscular cue to illicit the response one is looking for. Simply counting reps, recording a workout, or making someone feel better can no longer be considered good rehabilitation or good strength and conditioning. Athletes are getting bigger, faster, and stronger. When they become injured, a primary objective to them is to play, not only to rehabilitate an injury. When they return to play, they must be prepared to face their competition head on, without reservation. This requires the professional working with the athlete to have an incredible amount of knowledge of the body, anatomy, tissue physiology, arthrokinematics, biomechanics, strength training, conditioning, movement skill, and sport skill. No one person can be an expert in all of these areas. Health care professionals, performance professionals, and sports coaches must come together in order to truly work for the athlete. When everyone works as a team, in an athlete-centered model, the athlete will benefit. Where does rehabilitation end and performance begin? No one can answer that question. That is why a continuum of care is necessary. The athletes should return to their sport faster and more efficient than they were prior to their injury. Bridging the gap from rehabilitation to performance is what each clinician makes of it, by learning from each other and working together. Communicating as One Team for our client, placed at the core of our athlete-centered model, is not an option. Our athletes deserve a team of people working in his or her best interest, to return them to their sport effectively, efficiently, and ethically.

REFERENCES

1. Leetun DT, Ireland ML, Willson JD, et al. Core stability measures as risk factors for lower extremity injury in athletes. *Med Sci Sports Exerc.* 2004;36(6):926–934.
2. Liemon WP, Baumgartner TA, Gagnon LH. Measuring core stability. J Strength Cond Res 2005;19(3):583–586.
3. Sherry M, Best T, Heiderscheit B. Editorial: the core: where are we and where are we going? Clin J Sports Med 2005;15(1):1–2.
4. Myers TW. Anatomy Trains: Myofascial Meridians for Manual and Movement Therapists. New York, NY: Churchill Livingstone; 2008.
5. Sahrmann SA. Diagnosis and Treatment of Movement Impairment Syndromes. St. Louis, MO: Mosby; 2002.
6. Wight J, Richards J, Hall S. Influence of pelvis rotation styles on baseball pitching mechanics. Sports Biomech 2004;3(1)67–83.
7. Young JL, Herring SA, Press JM, et al. The influence of the spine on the shoulder in the throwing athlete. J Back Musculoskeletal Rehabil 1996;7:5–17.
8. Matsuo T, Fleisig GS, Zheng N, et al. Influence of shoulder abduction and lateral trunk tilt on peak elbow varus torque for college baseball pitchers during simulated pitching. J Appl Biomech 2006;22:93–102.
9. Wright J, Richards J, Hall S. Influence of pelvis rotation style on baseball pitching mechanics. Sports Biomech 2004;3(1):67–84.
10. Kibler WB. Biomechanical analysis of the shoulder during tennis activities. Clin Sports Med 1995;14(1):79–85.
11. Hong D, Cheung TK, Roberts EM. A three-dimensional, six-segment chain analysis of forceful overarm throwing. J Electromyogr Kinesiol 2001;11:95–112.
12. McMullen J, Uhl T. A kinetic chain approach for shoulder rehabilitation. J Athletic Train 2000;35(3):329–337.
13. Verstegen M. Core Performance. Emmaus, PA: Rodale; 2004.
14. Bawa P. Neural control of motor output: can training change it? Exerc Sport Sci Rev 2002;30(2):59–63.

Dynamic Neuromuscular Stabilization: Exercises Based on Developmental Kinesiology Models

INTRODUCTION

The etiology of musculoskeletal pain, in particular back pain, is often evaluated from an anatomical and biomechanical standpoint and the influence of external forces (i.e., loading) acting on the spine. However, the evaluation of the forces induced by the patient's own musculature, is often missing. The stabilizing function of muscles plays a critical and decisive postural role and depends on the quality of central nervous system (CNS) control. Kolar's approach to dynamic neuromuscular stabilization (DNS) is a new and unique approach explaining the importance of neurophysiological principles of the movement system. The DNS encompasses principles of developmental kinesiology during the first year of the life; these principles define ideal posture, breathing patterns, and functional joint centration from a "neurodevelopmental" paradigm (1). DNS presents a critical set of functional tests assessing the quality of functional stability of the spinal and joint stabilizers and assisting in finding the "key link" of dysfunction. The treatment approach is based on ontogenetic global postural-locomotor patterns (2,3). The primary goal of treatment is to optimize distribution of internal forces of the muscles acting on each segment of the spine and/or any other joint. In the DNS treatment concept, patient education and participation are imperative to reinforce ideal coordination among all stabilizing muscles.

POSTURAL ONTOGENESIS AND MATURATION OF THE INTEGRATED STABILIZING SYSTEM OF THE SPINE, CHEST, AND PELVIS

Postural ontogenesis entails maturation of body posture and related human locomotion (1–3). Postural muscle function ensures all possible positions in the joints determined by their anatomical shapes and has a strong formative influence on bone and joint morphology. Postural muscle activity is genetically predetermined and occurs automatically during CNS maturation. During newborn stage (Figures 4.1 and 4.2), bones and joints are morphologically immature. For example, the shape of the plantar arch is not well defined (4,5), the chest is shaped like a barrel, the posterior angles of the lower ribs are situated anteriorly relative to the spine, the ribs appear to be more horizontal than in adulthood (6), and the spine is maintained in kyphosis as the spinal lordotic curves have not yet developed (7–9). As the CNS matures, purposeful muscle function increasingly occurs. Muscles controlled by the CNS subsequently act on growth plates influencing the shape of bones and joints. Every joint position depends on stabilizing muscle function and coordination of local and distant muscles to ensure "functional centration" of joints in all possible positions. The quality of this coordination is crucial for joint function and influences not only local but also regional and global anatomical and biomechanical parameters starting in the early postnatal stage.

Ontogenesis demonstrates a very close relationship between neurophysiological and biomechanical principles, which are important aspects in the diagnosis and treatment of locomotor system disorders. This relationship is very apparent in cases where there is a CNS lesion and muscle coordination is affected. The disturbed muscle coordination subsequently alters joint position, morphological development, and ultimately posture (Figure 4.3) (10,11). Postural function and motor patterns are not only the indicators of the stage of maturation, but can point to the fact if the CNS development is physiological or pathological (1–3,12,13). Posture is a term very closely related to early individual development. The quality of verticalization during the first year of life strongly influences the quality of body posture for the rest of a person's life. During early postural ontogenesis, lordotic and kyphotic spinal curves as well as chest and pelvic positions are established. This process corresponds to stabilization of the spine, pelvis, and chest in the sagittal plane at the age of 4.5 months (Figures 4.4 and 4.5). This is followed by the development of phasic locomotor

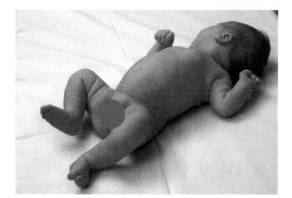

FIGURE 4-1. Typical supine posture of a newborn. Asymmetrical head and body position, showing head predilection (i.e., newborn's preferred head rotation toward one side). Postural immaturity is related to morphological (anatomical) immaturity; underdeveloped chest is short and shaped like a barrel, ventrodorsal chest diameter is larger than the width of the chest, and the posterior angles of the lower ribs are situated anteriorly relative to the spine.

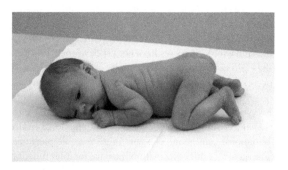

FIGURE 4-2. Typical newborn prone posture, with asymmetrical head predilection position as in supine position. There is no equilibrium as weight-bearing zones have not been defined yet, and the infant cannot hold any segment against gravity. The entire spine is maintained in kyphosis with an anterior pelvic tilt.

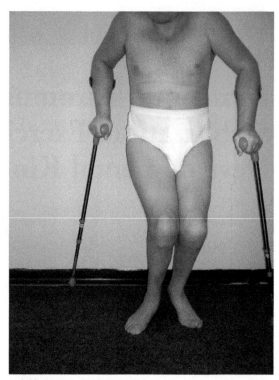

FIGURE 4-3. Postural effects from cerebral palsy (spastic diparesis). Note structural deformities of the hips, knees, and feet as a result of compromised muscle function due to central nervous system lesion.

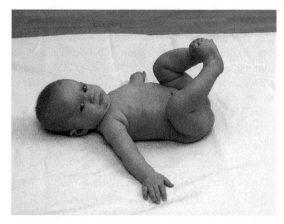

FIGURE 4-4. A 4.5-month physiological infant in supine position. Chest, pelvis, and spinal stabilization in the sagittal plane is fully established and maintained by proportional coactivation between agonists and antagonists (see Figure 4.12 for details). Supine weight-bearing zones include the nuchal line, shoulder blades, sacrum, and upper sections of the gluteal muscles. The infant is able to lift the pelvis above the table as far as the thoracolumbar junction due to established spinal stabilization in the sagittal plane.

function of the extremities, which includes the stepping forward (or reaching, grasping) function and the supporting (or taking off) function (1–3,12). These locomotor function of the extremities develops in two patterns. In the ipsilateral pattern, the leg and arm on the same side serve as a support function (and/or taking off), whereas the other same-sided leg and arm fulfill the phasic, that is, stepping forward and grasping, function (Figure 4.6). Ipsilateral pattern develops from supine position and is later integrated in the process of turning, oblique sitting, and other patterns. On the other hand, in the contralateral pattern, for example, if the right arm functions as a support, then the left leg will also function as a support function at the same time. The left arm has a grasping function and the right leg has a stepping forward function (Figure 4.7). Contralateral pattern develops from prone position and is later integrated in creeping, crawling, or

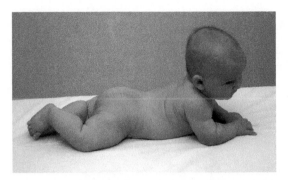

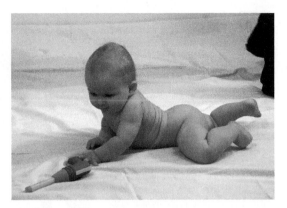

FIGURE 4-5. A 4.5-month physiological infant in prone position. Weight-bearing zones include the medial epicondyles, bilateral anterior superior iliac spine and pubic symphysis. This posture allows the infant to hold the segment (e.g., head or legs) out of the base of support against gravity. When lifting the head, the spine uprights starting at the mid-thoracic segments. Upper thoracic segments functionally belong to the cervical spine.

FIGURE 4-7. Contralateral movement pattern and function of the extremities. The left leg (medial condyle of the knee) provides support while the left arm reaches forward (grasping); the right leg steps forward and the right arm provides support (medial epicondyle of the elbow). Note the reciprocal position of the feet again—the left supporting foot is in plantar flexion and inversion, and the right stepping forward foot is in dorsiflexion and eversion.

gait movement patterns. The ipsilateral and contralateral locomotor patterns of the extremities begin to develop simultaneously after stabilization in the sagittal plane is fully completed, which physiologically corresponds to the age of 4.5 months.

The stepping forward function corresponds to open kinetic chain activities, where the direction of muscle pull is proximal and typically involves movement of the head of the femur or the humerus on a stable acetabulum or glenoid fossa, respectively. The principles are reversed on

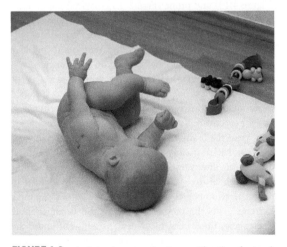

FIGURE 4-6. Ipsilateral movement pattern and function of extremities. Right-sided extremities serve for support and weight bearing while the left arm reaches forward (as in grasping function) and left leg swings forward (as in stepping forward function). Note the "reciprocal" position of the opposite extremities, for example, the right (supporting) foot is in plantar flexion and inversion while the left (stepping forward) foot is in dorsiflexion and eversion. The right arm moves toward pronation, while the left arm moves toward supination.

the supporting side, where the extremity works in a closed kinetic chain. The direction of muscle activity is distal (toward support, i.e., weight-bearing area) and typically involves the movement of the fossa over the stabilized head of the humerus or femur (Figures 4.8 and 4.9).

All afferent systems, including vision (14–16), hearing (17), vestibular (18,19), proprioceptive, and exteroceptive information (20), are integrated in these global patterns of stabilization and stepping forward/supporting extremities' function. In addition, the orofacial system takes part in these complex movement patterns (2,3,12,21). For example, during a throwing action, the athlete automatically places the extremities in a reciprocal position, the eyes and tongue turn toward the same direction as the stepping forward (throwing) arm (eyes preceding the arm movement), enhancing further facilitation and performance of the throwing movement. The athlete shown in Figure 4.10 depicts how all his orofacial muscles are involved in movement, to enhance maximum strength and performance. If the athlete is asked to look in the opposite direction or turn his tongue against the direction of the stepping forward arm movement, it will significantly decrease his sports performance. These principles can be powerfully used in athletic training.

Activation of the stabilizers is automatic and subconscious (the "feed-forward mechanism") and precedes every purposeful movement (Figure 4.11) (22). Any purposeful movement influences global posture and this posture subsequently influences the quality of phasic (dynamic) movement. The integrated stabilizing system of the spine consists of well-balanced activity between deep neck flexors and spinal extensors in the cervical and upper thoracic region. Stability of the lower thoracic and lumbar region depends

FIGURE 4-8.   In an ipsilateral pattern in this case, the left-sided extremities have a stepping forward function. The direction of muscle activity is proximal; the glenoid fossa and acetabulum are relatively fixed and serve as a stable base, while the head of humerus and femur rotates around the stabilized cavity. In other words, the distal segments (extremities) move against a fixed proximal stable base (scapula, pelvis). The opposite is true for the supporting or weight-bearing right arm and leg. The direction of muscle pull is distal; the humerus and femur are now relatively fixed while the glenoid fossa and acetabulum move around them. In other words, the proximal scapula and pelvis move against relatively fixed distal extremities.

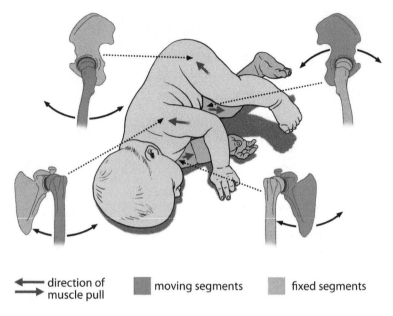

⇐ direction of
⇒ muscle pull

█ moving segments   ▨ fixed segments

on the proportional activity between the diaphragm, pelvic floor, and all sections of the abdominal wall and spinal extensors. The diaphragm, pelvic floor, and abdominal wall regulate intra-abdominal pressure, which provides anterior lumbopelvic postural stability (Figure 4.12) (23–28). In the newborn stage, the diaphragm functions only as a respiratory muscle. Between 4 and 6 weeks of age, the first postural activity occurs; the infant starts to lift his/her head (when prone) and legs (when supine) against gravity and the diaphragm starts to fulfill its dual function as a respiratory and postural muscle. The dual function of the diaphragm is essential for all movements and even more importantly during all types of sports performance (29,30). Under pathological conditions, insufficient postural function of the diaphragm, abnormal recruitment and timing between the diaphragm

and abdominal muscle activity (31), atypical initial chest position (due to imbalanced activity between the upper and lower chest stabilizers, with upper stabilizers dominating), and hyperactivity of the superficial spinal extensors can be observed.

DNS diagnosis is based on comparing the patient's stabilizing pattern to the developmental stabilization pattern of a healthy infant. For example, we compare the patient's supine posture when holding the legs above the table (Figure 4.13) and prone (Figure 4.14) sagittal stabilization during trunk extension test with that of the physiological pattern of a 4.5-month-old baby. The DNS therapeutic system makes use of specific functional exercises to improve spinal and joint stability by focusing on the integrated spinal stabilizing system. However, the primary target is the brain, which must be properly stimulated and conditioned to automatically activate optimal movement patterns necessary for coactivation of the stabilizers. The ultimate strategy is to "train the brain" to maintain central control, joint stability, and ideal quality of the movement restored during therapeutic intervention. This is achieved by activation/stimulation of the stabilizers when placing the patient in primal developmental positions (see the section "Sample Exercises"). As the program advances and becomes more challenging, these ideal movement patterns fall under the patient's voluntary (cortical) control, requiring less assistance from the clinician. Eventually, through repetition of the exercises, the central control establishes an automatic model that becomes a fundamental part of everyday movement. Integration of the ideal pattern of stabilization in sports activities not only decreases the risk of injuries and secondary pain syndromes resulting from overloading but also improves sports performance.

⇐ muscle pull

█ fixed segments

█ moving segments

→ direction of the movement

FIGURE 4-9.   In a contralateral pattern in this case, the left arm and right leg have a supporting function, and the right arm and left leg have a stepping forward function.

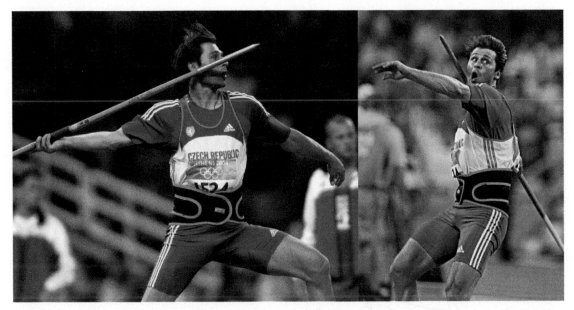

FIGURE 4-10.   Reciprocal function of extremities in a javelin thrower. Note the integration of the orofacial system in the global posture. Eyes and tongue turn toward the same direction as the throwing arm, preceding the throwing action.

MOTOR DYSFUNCTION (ABNORMAL MOTOR PATTERNS) AS AN ETIOLOGICAL FACTOR IN INJURIES AND/OR PAIN SYNDROMES

The anatomy of a muscle is considered to be the decisive factor for muscle strengthening. Specific types of exercise designed for individual muscles are based on the knowledge of the muscle's attachments. Most of fitness machines and benches are based on muscle anatomy. When strengthening muscles, or when analyzing muscle weakness or the muscle's influence on joints, bones, and soft tissues, anatomy and neurobiomechanics of muscles as well as muscle integration into biomechanical chains must be taken into account. CNS control and its associated programs play a critical role in proper integration of these muscle chains (32–34). Under both, static (sitting or lying) and dynamic (locomotion) conditions, individual movement segments must be stabilized by coordinated activity between agonists and antagonists. In other words, a coactivation synergy is necessary and must be trained. Another critical aspect is to train both directions of muscle pull, that is, to train the muscle in both stepping forward (open kinetic chain) and supporting (closed kinetic chain) functions. The most frequent mistake in strength training is that only one direction of muscle activity is trained, for example, the pectoralis is strengthened in open kinetic chain all the time (Figure 4.15), but not in closed chain (Figure 4.16). In brief, it is imperative to train muscles in both, open and closed kinetic chains.

This stabilizing or postural function always precedes any phasic (purposeful) movement (22). Pathology or dysfunction frequently occurs when the muscle is strong enough in its phasic function (or anatomic function) but lacks in its postural (stabilizing) function, thus resulting in postural instability. Poor pattern of stabilization is easily fixed in the CNS, since stabilization is an automatic and subconscious function. Abnormal stabilization is then integrated into any movement and, especially, sports activities (which require strength, speed, and repetition), compromising the quality of movement stereotypes and resulting in overloading, decreased sports performance, and increased risk of injuries. Stereotypical repeated overloading due to poor pattern of stabilization is a frequent primary cause of movement disturbances and pain syndromes. "Practice does not make perfect, it makes permanent," which is true for both, physiological and pathological patterns. Poor methodology of training (or rehabilitation, for that matter) will fix and reinforce poor stereotypes (Figure 4.17).

Postural instability cannot be evaluated merely by manual muscle testing. Functional postural tests must be used. Kolar's approach to DNS explains and demonstrates the importance of the relationship and proper recruitment of all muscular interactions for dynamic stability of the spine and joints and utilizes a series of systematic dynamic tests. The section on sample tests illustrates the most important tests.

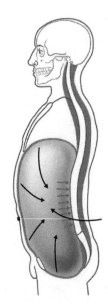

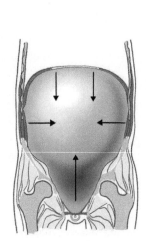

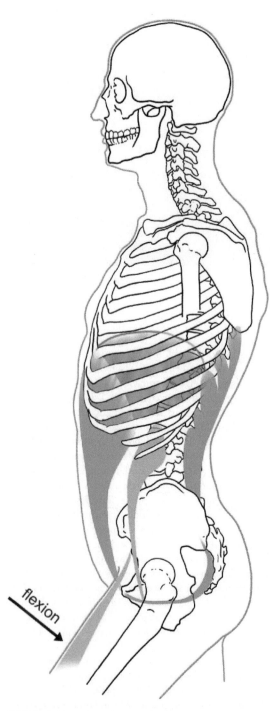

flexion

FIGURE 4-11. "Feed-forward stabilization mechanism." Prior to any phasic or dynamic movement (e.g., hip flexion), the stabilizers must be activated, that is, the integrated function of the trunk-stabilizing muscles (dark areas—diaphragm, pelvic floor, all parts of the abdominal wall, and spinal extensors) precedes the activation of hip flexors (light areas) for dynamic hip flexion.

FIGURE 4-12. In a scheme of stabilization, the cervical and upper thoracic region is stabilized by well-balanced activity between deep neck flexors and spinal extensors. The lower thoracic and lumbar segments are dependent on intra-abdominal pressure regulation providing anterior lumbopelvic postural stability, whereas posterior stabilization is ensured primarily by intrinsic spinal extensors.

BASIC PRINCIPLES FOR EXERCISES

Ideal Initial Posture as a Prerequisite for All Exercises

The quality and efficiency of any movement depends on multiple factors. One of the key factors is the initial body position when performing the exercise. Proper stabilization is critical for all dynamic activities ranging from simple functional tasks to skilled athletic maneuvers (35). In the DNS approach, the initial body position is closely related to the pattern of sagittal stabilization. Ideal posture from a developmental perspective is demonstrated in a physiological baby at 4.5 months of age when sagittal stabilization is completed (see Figures 4.4 and 4.5). Ideal muscle coordination is maximized in this position to provide the best possible biomechanical advantage for movement and muscle performance (strength and power). This initial position can also significantly influence movement execution (sports technique) and hence training and sports performance.

Basic Dynamic Neuromuscular Stabilization Tests for Stabilization

Supine

Place the patient in a supine position with hips and knees flexed 90° above the table. Ask the patient to maintain

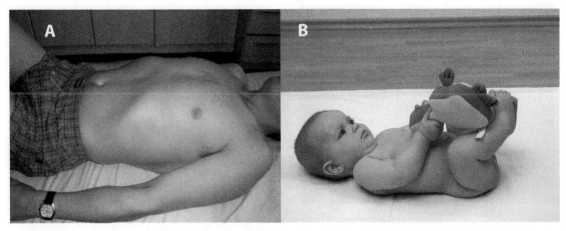

FIGURE 4-13. A comparison of the patient's abnormal supine stabilization pattern (A) with that of a healthy 4.5-month-old infant (B). Compare the following: (1) Head position and activation of neck muscles: The baby's head is supported on a nuchal line with activation of the deep neck flexors. The patient's neck is extended with excessive activation of superficial muscles (sternocleidomastoid, scalenes). (2) Chest position. Note the difference in shape. The infant's chest is in a caudal, neutral position with lower ribs well stabilized. The patient's chest is in more cranial "inspiratory position" with lower ribs flaring out. (3) Back—the infant's entire back adheres to the table (due to sufficient intra-abdominal pressure regulation). The patient's back is extended at the thoracolumbar junction. (4) Abdominal wall—the infant demonstrates proportional activation and contour. The patient demonstrates bulging at the laterodorsal sections of the abdominal wall.

this posture as you gradually remove the support of the legs, while observing the patient's pattern of stabilization (Figure 4.18A). Compare this posture with the physiological 4.5-month old baby posture (Figure 4.18B). Things to look for include the following:

Head: It is in a neutral position, where the nuchal line is the natural weight-bearing zone. If the upper occiput serves as the supporting area, it is often correlated with hyperextension at the cervicocranial junction with hyperactivity of short neck extensors (Figure 4.18C).

Neck: Activity of superficial neck muscles is unnecessary for this posture. Superficial muscles (sternocleidomastoid

[SCM], scalenes, upper trapezius, pectoralis muscles) should be relaxed.

Shoulders: These are relaxed and should not be elevated or protracted. Elevation of the shoulders is often related to hyperactive upper chest stabilizers (SCM, scalenes, upper trapezius, pectoralis muscles) (see Figure 4.18C).

Chest: In neutral position, there should be well-balanced activity between upper (SCM, scalenes, upper trapezius, pectoralis muscles) and lower chest stabilizers (oblique abdominal muscle chains, diaphragm, transverse and rectus abdominis). The most common pathology observed is the chest in

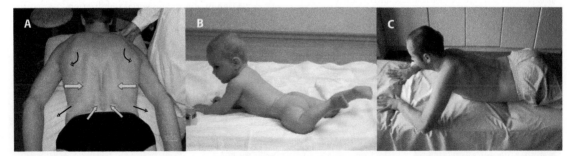

FIGURE 4-14. Comparison of the patient's prone stabilization with that of a healthy prone 4.5-month-old infant (B). (A) Trunk extension test—hyperactivity of scapular external rotators (curved arrows, superficial paraspinal muscles at thoracolumbar junction (thick horizontal arrows) and lumbosacral area). Erector spinae is hyperactive to compensate for insufficient deep spinal stabilizers. Anterior pelvic tilt (thick oblique arrows pointing medially) and bulging of laterodorsal sections of the abdominal wall (thin arrows) are signs of inadequate and/or weak postural function. (C) Retraction of the shoulder blades, hyperextension of cervicothoracic junction, and anterior pelvic tilt. Patient's weight-bearing area is at the level of umbilicus; when compared to the infant's supporting areas, weight bearing is at the level of symphysis. The infant's pelvis is in a neutral position compared to the anterior tilt in the patient.

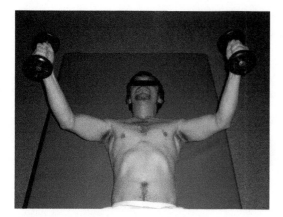

FIGURE 4-15. "Classic" strengthening of pectoral muscles in open kinetic chain. Note the poor pattern of basic stabilization with flaring of the lower ribs and hollowing of the abdominal wall.

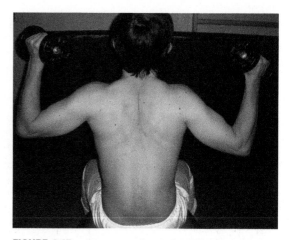

FIGURE 4-17. Poor pattern of sagittal stabilization with scapular retraction and forward drawn position of the head. This exercise on an unstable surface is very challenging and with an added load, the pathological pattern will only be reinforced.

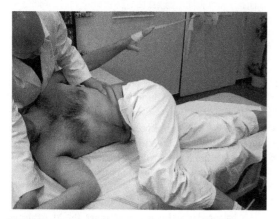

FIGURE 4-16. Strengthening in a reciprocal pattern. Left pectoralis is activated in an open kinetic chain (against resistance) while the right one is trained in a closed kinetic chain; the athlete pronates his right forearm against the therapist's resistance while shifting the weight-bearing zone from deltoid toward the elbow. The body (glenoid fossa) rotates on the fixed humerus. The trunk is lifted against gravity and against the therapist's resistance and rotates toward the right supporting arm. The therapist's left hand helps keep the chest in neutral position and resist the trunk movement at the same time.

a cranial position (inspiratory position) due to dominant and hypertonic upper stabilizers (see Figure 4.18C). Palpate the lower and lateral walls of the chest and try to spring the chest (Figure 4.19). The chest wall should be flexible. If the chest is rigid, soft tissue release may be indicated as a precursor to further training. The posterior angles of the lower ribs should contact the table as they are positioned posterior relative to the spine (see Figure 4.18A,B). However, when these angles are in a less than ideal position, arching of the back (see Figure 4.18C) and flaring of the lower ribs are often observed.

Abdominal wall (test of proportional activation among all sections): Palpate the posterolateral sections (often insufficient), upper part of the rectus abdominis (often hyperactive), and the abdominal wall above the groin (frequently insufficient). Diastasis is a sign of abnormal sagittal stabilization.

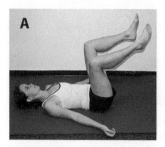
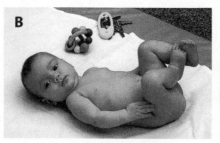
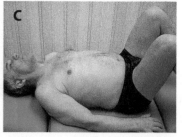

FIGURE 4-18. Supine test with legs above table (90°/90° position = right angle at hips and knees). (A) Physiological pattern in an adult. (B) Ideal model in a 4.5-month healthy infant. (C) Pathological pattern in an adult, with head reclination, neck hyperextension (support on the occiput instead of the nuchal line), sternocleidomastoid hyperactivity, shoulder protraction, "inspiratory" chest position, arching of the lumbar spine due to reduced weight bearing at the thoracolumbar junction, diastasis recti, and anterior pelvic tilt. Stabilization is insufficient.

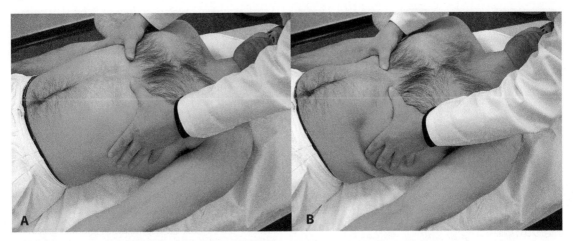

FIGURE 4-19.   (A) "Inspiratory" position of the chest is often fixed and it is difficult to bring the chest to neutral position even passively. (B) Bring the chest to neutral position if possible (pull the chest caudally, do not press it against the table!) and spring the chest. The chest should be flexible and spring back symmetrically. Healthy individuals are able to keep the chest in this position at rest, while still breathing, and during the course of all postural activities.

Thoracolumbar (T/L) junction: This serves as a weight-bearing zone and should be in contact with the table (compare Figure 4.18A–C).

Prone

Place the patient in prone position that corresponds to that of a 4.5-month-old healthy infant (Figure 4.20). Ask the patient to lift the head slightly. Observe the following:

Head: In neutral position, it is elevated a few centimeters above the table.

Neck: When lifting the head, extension should start from the mid-thoracic (T3/4/5) segments. Head reclination (hyperextension of cervicocranial junction) and/or hyperextension of the mid- or lower cervical segments as the CT junction is often fixed or flexed is a sign of abnormal extension stereotype. This poor movement pattern is often related to insufficient coactivation of the deep neck flexors (see Figure 4.20C and Figure 4.23A). Compare the posture to that of a healthy 4.5-month-old

infant (see Figure 4.20B); note the perfect and gradual lengthening of the entire spine including the cervical spine.

Arms: Medial epicondyles serve as weight-bearing zones. The shoulders should be relaxed, and the patient should not raise them.

Shoulder blades: These should be fixed in a "caudal" position due to balance between the upper and lower scapular stabilizers and between scapular adductors and abductors, with the scapula adhering to the rib cage (see Figure 4.20A,B). An elevated scapula suggests the dominance of the upper stabilizers (see Figure 4.20C). Another common abnormality is winging of the lower angle of the scapula. Proper scapular stabilization is dependent on proper support of the medial epicondyles.

Thoracic spine: Observe the lengthening of the spine. Palpate the mid-thoracic spine during head elevation (Figure 4.21). Normally, you should feel segmental movement between T3/4/5/6.

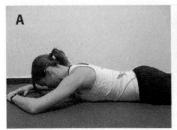
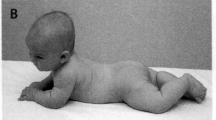
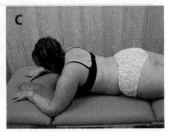

FIGURE 4-20.   Prone test. (A) Physiological pattern in adult. (B) Ideal model in a 4-month-old healthy infant. (C) Pathological pattern in an adult: neck hyperextension, cervicothoracic junction kyphosis, scapular retraction and external rotation, support at the level of the umbilicus instead of the anterior superior iliac spine or symphysis, and pelvic anteversion.

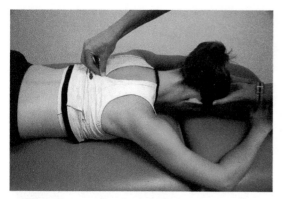

FIGURE 4-21. Palpation of mid-thoracic segments during neck extension test. Neck extension movement pattern should "start" from mid-thoracic spine.

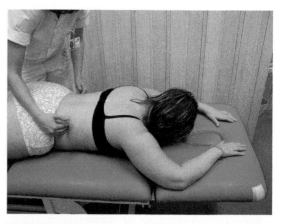

FIGURE 4-22. Neck and trunk extension test, with palpation of laterodorsal sections of the abdominal wall. Symmetrical activation should occur during this movement. Superficial extensors at the thoracolumbar junction will often substitute for insufficient activation of the laterodorsal abdominal muscles (see Figure 4.14A).

Abdominal wall (proportional activity of all its sections): Palpate the laterodorsal portion; there should be slight activation under your fingers (Figure 4.22). Bulging of the lateral walls is a sign of insufficient sagittal stabilization.

Pelvis (stabilized in a neutral position): Both, anterior and posterior tilts are abnormal. Ask the patient to extend the trunk and palpate the sacrum (Figure 4.23A). The sacrum must be stabilized and remain fixed during the movement. If it tilts ventrally, regulation of the intra-abdominal and intrapelvic pressure is often impaired (see Figure 4.23B). The pubic symphysis and the anterior superior iliac spine (ASIS) are naturally weight-bearing zones (see Figure 4.20A,B).

Legs: Observe and/or palpate hamstrings and triceps surae during neck and slight trunk extension. During the initial phase of trunk extension, these muscles should be fairly relaxed.

Standing

Minimal muscle activity is necessary for normal standing posture. Any excessive isometric activity (especially in superficial muscles) is a sign of abnormal posture, which is energy inefficient and may cause overloading of joint segments. Watch (palpate) for muscle tone distribution during primary stance.

The chest must be aligned above the pelvis and the axis of the diaphragm (connecting pars sternalis and costophrenic angle) in the sagittal plane (should be almost horizontal and parallel with the pelvic floor axis) (Figures 4.24A and 4.25B). In this ideal position, the diaphragm may then work against the pelvic floor, especially during any physical strain, in coordination with the abdominal wall, exerting pressure on the

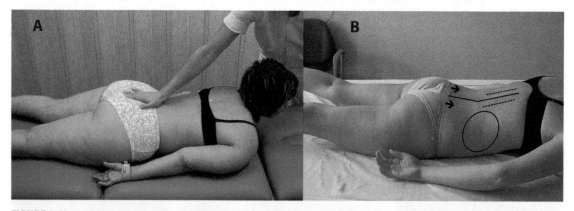

FIGURE 4-23. (A) Trunk extension test, with palpation of the sacrum. The pelvis should maintain neutral position during the test. Postural pelvic instability is indicated if the clinician should feel the patient's sacrum move against his hand in a cranial direction. (B) Abnormal pattern with leg raise: hyperactivity of gluteus maximus, hamstrings, and calf muscles helping to stabilize the trunk during extension and the substitute for insufficient intra-abdominal and intrapelvic pressure regulation. The arrows indicate anterior pelvic tilt, the interrupted lines the hyperactive paraspinal muscles, and the ellipse the hypoactive area.

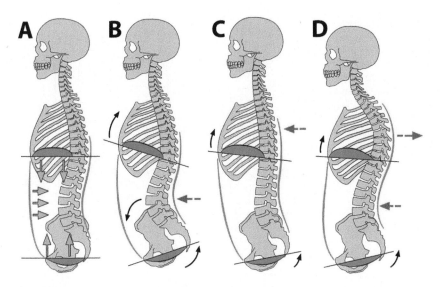

FIGURE 4-24. (A) Physiological position of the diaphragm and pelvic floor. Their axes are horizontal and parallel to one another. (B) "Open scissors syndrome"—oblique axis of the diaphragm and pelvic floor. (C) Forward drawn chest position. (D) Chest aligned behind the pelvis. The light arrows indicate correct muscle activation and direction of increased intra-abdominal pressure from above (diaphragm), below (pelvic floor), and the front and lateral perspective (abdominal wall). The dark arrows indicate movement—abnormal position of the chest and pelvis under pathological conditions. The dashed arrows indicate an abnormal shift of the chest and lumbar spine under pathological conditions.

intra-abdominal contents, thus helping to stabilize lower thoracic and lumbar segments from the front. The following are the most common types of pathologies:

Forward drawn chest position with the chest aligned in front of the pelvis (see Figures 4.24C and 4.25A). This results in constant isometric activity of superficial paraspinal muscles.

Further, chest aligned behind the pelvis (see Figures 4.24D and 4.25C) resulting in a fixed thoracic kyphosis, lack

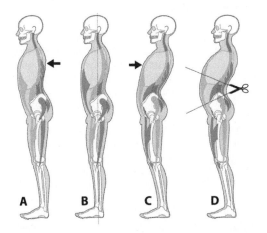

FIGURE 4-25. (A) Forward drawn chest position. (B) Ideal stance position. (C) Chest aligned behind the pelvis. (D) "Open scissors syndrome." The arrows indicate abnormal chest position under pathological conditions.

of segmental movement in mid-thoracic segments, rounded shoulders, short pectoralis major (Figure 4.26D,C).

"Look for open scissors syndrome" (Figure 4.24B and 4.25D), which is the most common postural pathology, with the oblique position of the diaphragm, its anterior attachments more cranial than the posterior attachments (costophrenic part) concurrent with an oblique pelvic axis in sagittal plane as a result of anterior pelvic tilt. This usually is related to lumbar hyperlordosis and hyperactivation of superficial paraspinal muscles. Retraction of the shoulder blades is also a common finding in this syndrome.

Observe muscle tone distribution and contour of the abdominal wall. It should be fairly relaxed when standing. An "hourglass syndrome" can be observed, especially in women. For aesthetic reasons, they perform hollowing of abdominal wall which compromises both, the stabilization and breathing patterns (Figure 4.26B,C).

Respiratory Pattern

Functionally, posture and respiration are interdependent, forming one functional unit (26–30,34,36). Dysfunction in one compromises the other and vice versa. The training of ideal posture must be concurrent with training of the ideal breathing pattern. One of the key prerequisites for physiological spinal stabilization and respiration is the position and dynamics of the chest. Under physiological conditions, the thoracic spine is upright (and elongated), and the chest

FIGURE 4-26. (A) Physiological contour of the abdominal wall. (B and C) "Hour glass syndrome." The dashed lines in A and B indicate the diaphragm. The thin curved arrows indicate abnormal activation of the abdominal wall, the thin upward pointing arrow illustrates cranial movement of the umbilicus under pathological conditions, and the thick arrows illustrate pathological narrowing of the abdominal wall.

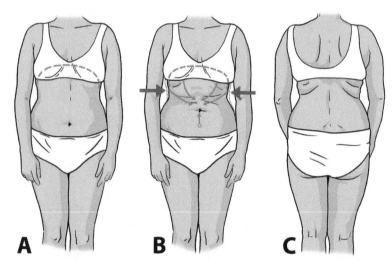

remains in a caudal position during both, inhalation and exhalation (see Figure 4.19B). Accessory respiratory muscles should not be activated for regular, tidal breathing (1,33,34). During inhalation, the lower chest aperture expands proportionally in all directions as the diaphragm drops and flattens out (Figure 4.27A). The clavicles should have a slight upward slope (25°–29°); horizontal position maybe a sign of short (hyperactive) accessory respiratory muscles. Under pathological conditions, the diaphragm is not flattening adequately; it stays in an oblique axis. Excessive cranial/caudal movements can be observed at the sternum (Figure 4.27B).

Between 4-6 weeks of age, when the infant starts to lift the head against gravity when prone or lifts the legs when supine, the diaphragm starts to develop a dual function, simultaneous postural and respiratory function. Physiologically, with every postural activity (both, during breathing and breath holding), the diaphragm descends and flattens out. Its attachments on the lower ribs are stabilized by abdominals, and the centrum tendineum is pulled caudally toward the lower ribs (Figure 4.28B). With dysfunction, however, the diaphragm does not descend adequately during postural activities; the direction of muscle activity reverses and is pulled toward the centrum tendineum (Figure 4.28A), clinically resulting in the "hourglass syndrome" (Figures 4.26B,C and 4.28A).

Testing the Stereotype of Respiration

Supine

The patient is in the hook-lying position or with legs lifted above the table (90° flexion at hips and knees), with the lower legs supported.

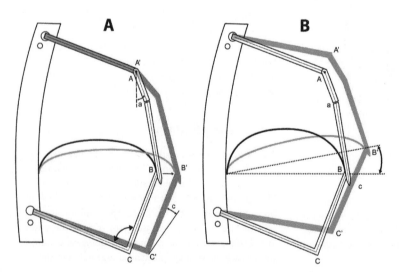

FIGURE 4-27. (A) Healthy breathing pattern. The diaphragmatic axis is almost horizontal. During inhalation, the diaphragm moves caudally while the sternum moves anteriorly. There is proportional expansion of the lower chest (widening of the intercostal spaces). (B) Pathological stereotype of ventilation; the axis of the diaphragm is in an oblique position. The entire chest moves cranially with inhalation and caudally with exhalation with minimal or absent expansion of the lower chest (narrowed intercostal spaces). The lower chest cavity is "locked" with shallow inhalation, subsequently placing increased demands on the accessory muscles of respiration.

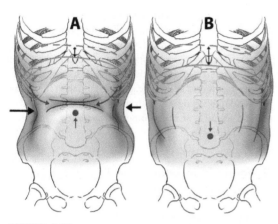

FIGURE 4-28. (A) Pathological postural diaphragmatic activation in the "hour glass syndrome." There is insufficient flattening of the diaphragm and direction of muscle activity toward the centrum tendineum (central tendon), with stiffness of the lower chest and disproportional activation of the abdominal wall toward the umbilicus. The upward pointing dashed arrow indicates a pathological cranial position of the umbilicus. The curved dashed arrows indicate pathological concentric activation of the abdominal wall. The medium arrows indicate abnormal contraction of the diaphragm toward the centrum tendineum. The thick black arrows indicate pathological narrowing of the abdominal wall. (B) Physiological postural diaphragmatic activation: The diaphragm moves caudally, with its attachments fixed and stabilized on the lower ribs by the abdominals; intercostal spaces widen as the lower chest expands, and there is proportional activation of all the sections of the abdominal wall. The medium arrows indicate the correct diaphragm contraction toward the lower ribs (centrum tendineum descending). The dashed arrow indicates the correct neutral position of the umbilicus. In both (A) and (B), the double-ended arrows demonstrate diaphragmatic excursion (greater in B, the physiological case, than in A, the abnormal one).

Observe tidal breathing pattern. Watch and/or palpate accessory respiratory muscles. The muscles should be relaxed. The clavicles should not move cranially and caudally during breathing. Palpate the sternum; it should not shift cranially with every inhalation. The sternum normally remains in a caudal position in the transverse plane during both, inhalation and exhalation.

Palpate the lower intercostal spaces on the lateral aspects of the chest; these spaces should expand or widen with every inhalation.

Palpate the laterodorsal sections of the abdominal wall; these areas should expand with every inhalation. Palpate the abdominal wall above the groin; these areas should expand with every inhalation.

Manually bring the chest (sternum) passively to a caudal position (see Figure 4.19B). While maintaining the sternum in a caudal position, instruct the person to take a breath. The sternum (and your hand) should not be pulled cranially.

Sitting

The same principles apply as for the supine position.

The patient is sitting facing the clinician, with arms and legs relaxed (Figure 4.29). Palpate above the groin and instruct the patient to take a deep breath as if to "breathe into or push against your fingers." During inhalation, the abdominal wall should expand ventrally, caudally, and laterally.

The clinician is behind the seated patient. Palpate posterior aspects of the lower intercostal spaces on both sides and instruct the person to take a deep breath (Figure 4.30). You should feel simultaneous and symmetrical expansion of the lower chest (dorsally and laterally) and widening of the intercostal spaces. There should not be any cranial movement of the chest or trunk.

The clinician stands behind the seated patient. Palpate the laterodorsal aspects of the abdominal wall just below the lower ribs (see Figure 4.30). Instruct the person to breathe in and breathe out. After a full exhalation, instruct the patient to push against your fingers. This is a test for postural function of the diaphragm. The clinician should feel symmetrical and strong expansion of the abdominal wall against his fingers. The expansion is proportional in all directions. If the person is facing the mirror during this test, you should also see ventral expansion of the lower chest and the abdominal wall. Hollowing of the abdominal wall is a sign of abnormal stereotype and paradoxical activation of the diaphragm (see Figures 4.26B and 4.28A).

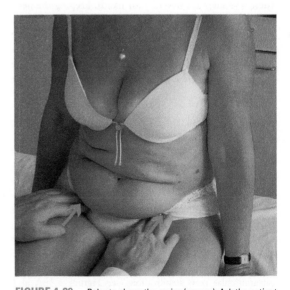

FIGURE 4-29. Palpate above the groins (arrows): Ask the patient to breathe into your fingers and/or to push against your fingers. In both cases, you should feel strong symmetrical activation (lateral, anterior, and caudal) while the umbilicus is stabilized (i.e., not pulled cranially and inward as on the picture where you can see pathological pattern) and the patient should remain relaxed.

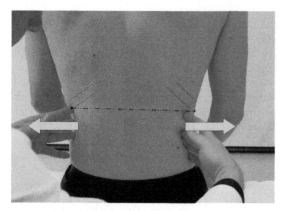

FIGURE 4-30. Diaphragm test. Palpate lower intercostal spaces and below the lower ribs. Ask the patient to breathe into your fingers and/or push into your fingers (arrows; inspiratory diaphragmatic activity) while holding their breath (purely postural activity of diaphragm). In both cases you should feel a strong symmetrical activation. There should not be any concomitant thoracic spine flexion synkinesis or shoulder elevation during the test.

How to Train Optimal Breathing

Begin the training in a supine position with legs bent and feet supported on the table or floor. Place your hands on the side of the patient's lower rib cage and guide the patient how to bring the chest down (see Figure 4.19B). Bring the patient's chest down with your hands (spine should stay in contact with the floor and not flex forward). While inhaling, the patient must expand the lower chest wall sideways toward your hands, keeping the neck and shoulder muscles relaxed as much as possible. When exhaling, allow the chest to relax passively without any contraction of the abdominals. If relaxation of the abdominals during exhalation is difficult, ask the patient to place his/her hands on his abdomen for feedback to monitor for excessive tension.

Progression in Exercise Complexity

All the principles described above should be considered for any exercise prescription in any initial position (lying, sitting, standing, quadruped, oblique sitting, etc.). Regardless of the exercise position, the quality and the pattern of sagittal stabilization require adequate muscle coordination and balance under physiological conditions.

We recommend to begin training in basic, that is, the easiest positions (4.5 month developmental age, prone and supine) in order to reset muscle coordination for deep intramuscular core stabilization (see Figures 4.18A and 4.20A). Any basic position can be advanced by applying resistance and/or by adding limb movement (see Figure 4.16). The amount of applied resistance and the amount of movement have to be matched to the patient's ability to stabilize the core—spine, trunk, pelvis—without any

compensatory movement. The same principle is applied in higher, advanced, or more challenging positions. There are three options to utilize developmental positions during training: 1) training in a particular developmental position itself, 2) training in a transitional phase from one developmental position to another (e.g., from supine to side-lying, from oblique sitting to quadruped), or 3) training only a specific segment of the locomotion phase (e.g., initiation of turning process).

Dynamic Neuromuscular Stabilization Principles for Exercise

The lower the position of the patient to the ground or table, the easier the exercise. For example, it is usually easier to train the proper stereotype of breathing (or any movement, e.g., throwing) in supine than in a quadruped position.

The higher the position is, the more unstable the person becomes; thus, the exercises become more challenging. Hence, progression of the exercise should proceed from lower, more stable to higher or more unstable positions.

For any type of exercise, always choose positions where the person can properly maintain sagittal stabilization and breathing stereotype. If the person exercises with an incorrect stereotype of stabilization and breathing, the pathology will be reinforced as a result of the exercise (see Figure 4.17).

To further challenge the physiological stereotype of stabilization, resistance (e.g., barbell) to the dynamic movements of extremities can be introduced or added. The resistance must be adequate to the person's ability to properly stabilize. If an abnormal stereotype of stabilization or breathing is observed, the resistance should be reduced (see Figure 4.17).

Loading up of the weight-bearing zones can/will assist in stabilization.

Centrate the supporting segments.

To make the exercise more challenging, reduce the number of supporting segments (e.g., in bear position the person is asked to lift one leg or arm, or both contralaterally) (Figure 4.42C,D).

Exercise in various positions (e.g., the tennis player may train the stroke in supine, oblique sitting, or tripod positions).

Have the person focus on the exercise for the purpose of training body awareness.

SAMPLE EXERCISES

Basic Exercises

Supine Position (4.5 Months)

This position corresponds to the position of a 4.5-month-old infant in supine and having the ability to lift its legs

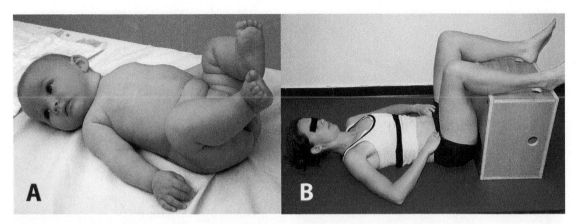

FIGURE 4-31. (A) A 4.5-month-old infant can already hold the legs above the table while stabilizing the core. (B) Basic supine exercise, based on 4.5 months developmental position, with legs supported.

above the table up to 90° in hips and knees (Figure 4.31A). This is a fundamental position for further advanced positions and movements (see Figure 4.31B). All the trunk muscles (abdominals, back muscles, diaphragm and pelvic floor) are well coordinated for integrated spinal stabilization, which is a basic prerequisite for any movement.

Initial Position

In the supine position, the head, chest, spine and pelvis are in a neutral position (see Figure 4.31B); the head is supported on the nuchal line, the neck is neutral, the entire spine maintains contact with the table (floor) without hyperextension. The axis of the chest and the pelvis is parallel and perpendicular to the ground. The shoulders and arms are relaxed. The hips and knees are flexed to 90 degrees. Start with the legs supported under the calves and progress by removing leg support (Figure 4.32).

Exercise Performance

After a few regular breaths, bring the chest into a relaxed position toward the hips. Take a normal breath and direct the breath into the pelvis (pelvic floor). Use your hands to make sure the inhalation goes as far as the groin and increas muscle tension in this area as a result of both, inhalation and voluntary activity. Keep repeating this activity while still breathing in and out. Gradually, lift one leg and then the other leg away from the support. Repeat 3–5 times as long as all body parts are coordinated and maintained in the proper position. You can make the exercise more challenging by moving the legs alternately into extension.

Exercise Errors

These include elevation of the shoulders (shoulder protraction), head and neck hyperextension, chest and rib cage elevation, the belly button being drawn in, using excessive effort, and/or holding the breath.

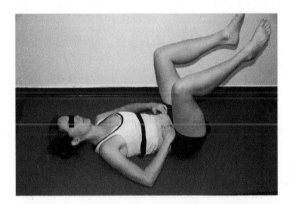

FIGURE 4-32. Basic supine exercise with legs unsupported. Make sure the hips are well centrated during the entire exercise (90° flexion and slight external rotation at the hips). Support or weight bearing is at the level of the upper gluteal muscles. The exercise should be discontinued if the back arches into extension or if the subject is unable to maintain the hip and knee position.

Modification in Supine Position with Thera-Band (Figure 4.33)

Initial Position

The position is identical to the basic supine exercise. Theraband is wrapped around the shins (just under the knees), crossed from the front to the back side, and brought forward around the thighs (just above the knees). The band is held in the palms (wrapped twice), with the free end placed between the thumb and the index finger. Elbows are flexed to 90 degrees. (Figure 4.33A).

Exercise Performance

Maintain the basic supine position with the head, spine, trunk, and pelvis in a neutral position. Breathe into the area above the groin. Supinate your hands while performing external rotation at the shoulders (see Figure 4.33B).

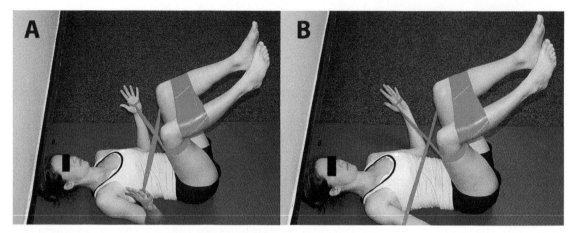

FIGURE 4-33.   Modification of basic exercise in supine using resistive band. (A) Initial position. (B) Exercise performance, with supination and external rotation of the arms against the resistance of the band.

Exercise Errors

These include holding your breath, spine extension, chest elevation, and hip and knee internal rotation.

Prone Position (4.5 Months)

A healthy 4-month-old infant in prone is able to bring its elbows in front of the shoulders, support itself on the medial epicondyles, and lift the head with an upright cervical and upper thoracic spine (Figure 4.34A). This movement is feasible only when the posterior and anterior muscles of the torso work in proportional coactivation (see Figure 4.12) and the shoulder girdle muscles are well coordinated with serratus anterior and the diaphragm to maintain the shoulder blades in a neutral position, "caudal position."

Initial Position

Prone position with elbows in front of shoulders at the level of the ears and the head supported on the forehead (see Figure 4.34B).

Exercise Performance

Position the shoulders caudally and broadly (not retracted). Trunk is supported at the level of the symphysis or ASIS.

Lift the head slightly with cervical and upper thoracic spine upright; the movement should initiate in the mid-thoracic spine between the shoulder blades (see Figure 4.34C).

Exercise Errors

These include hyperextension of the neck (Figure 4.35A), elevation and/or protraction of the shoulders, retraction of the shoulder blades (Figure 4.35B), hyperextension of the T/L junction or lumbar spine and anterior pelvic tilt (see Figure 4.23B).

Modification in Prone Position

Initial Position

The elbows and the forehead are supported on the end of the table, with the lower torso and pelvis lying on a gym ball and the feet resting freely on the floor (Figure 4.36A).

Exercise Performance

Slightly depress the shoulders and press the elbows onto the bench, lift the head slightly from the bench, and press the pelvis slightly into the gym ball (see Figure 4.36B).

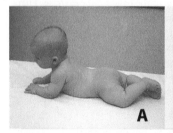
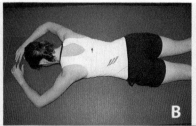
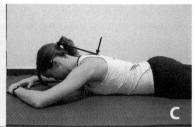

FIGURE 4-34.   (A) Ideal model of 4.5 months prone position. (B) Basic prone exercise, based on 4.5 months developmental position. Initial position. (C) Exercise performance: Lift the head with cervical and upper thoracic spine upright; the movement should be initiated at the mid-thoracic segments (between the shoulder blades [arrow]).

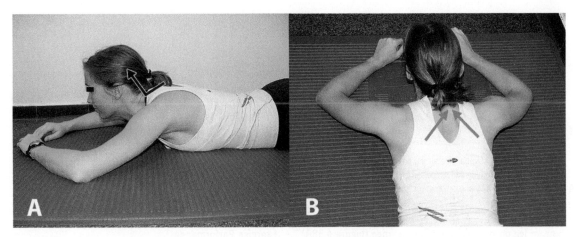

FIGURE 4-35. Poor performance and movement pattern of head extension. (A) Neck hyperextension, with kyphosis of cervicothoracic junction (arrow). (B) Retraction of the shoulder blades (arrows).

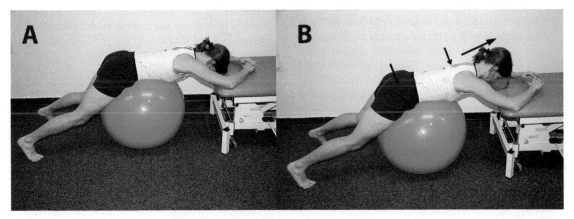

FIGURE 4-36. Modification of basic prone exercise. (A) Initial position with elbows supported on the end of a bench or table, with the lower torso and pelvis supported on the gym ball. (B) During exercise, the head is lifted from the bench with extension starting at the mid-thoracic spine and the pelvis is slightly pressed into the gym ball (arrows).

Exercise Errors

These include shoulder elevation, hyperextension of the lower thoracic and lumbar spine, and flexion of the lumbar spine with posterior pelvic tilt.

Side Sitting Position (7 Months)

This exercise trains the stabilizing function of the supporting shoulder and the functional interplay between the muscles of the shoulder girdles and the lower torso.

Initial Position

This corresponds to the side sitting position of a healthy 7-month-old infant, when the forearm is used for support (Figure 4.37). For exercise, the support is on the forearm (the elbow is located under the shoulder) and on the side of the buttock. The top leg is supported in the front of the

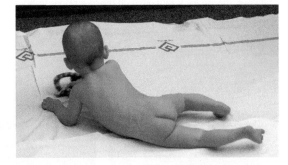

FIGURE 4-37. Healthy 7-month-old infant, showing side sit with support on the forearm. This position is a snapshot of the movement transition from supine or sidelying to quadruped.

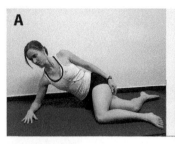
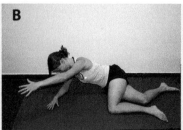
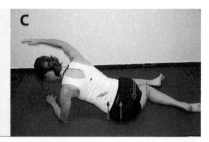

FIGURE 4-38.   (A) Initial side sitting position with the top leg supported on the medial condyle of the knee. (B) Trunk rotation with the top arm elevated, with the top leg still supported on the medial condyle of the knee. (C) Lifting the pelvis in side sitting position; support is shifted from the buttock toward the lateral condyle of the knee (arrows) of the bottom leg.

bottom leg on the medial side of the knee (Figure 4.38A) or on the foot (Figure 4.39A). The entire spine is straight, including the neck and the head.

Exercise Performance

The bottom shoulder is pulled down away from the head. The top arm is raised above the shoulder and the entire trunk rotates forward (Figures 4.38B and 4.39B). Support on the buttock shifts toward the knee (Figures 4.38C and 4.39C). Repetition is performed 3–5 times only as long as all body segments are coordinated and kept in the proper position.

Exercise Errors

The bottom shoulder is elevated and protracted and/or the spine is not uprighted (hyperextended or sagged).

Modification: Side Sitting Position with Hand Support

Initial Position

This corresponds to the oblique sitting position with hand support of an 8-month healthy infant (Figure 4.40A). The supporting hand is placed in line with the pelvis next to the supporting buttock. The bottom leg is semi-flexed at the hip and knee, the top leg is supported on the foot placed in front of the bottom knee. The spine is straight (see Figure 4.40B).

Exercise Performance

Keep the shoulder of the bottom arm depressed and raise the other arm. Lift the pelvis from the supporting position and weight bear on the bottom knee and the foot of the top leg. Movement continues in the forward direction by rotating the torso toward quadruped posture (see Figure 4.40C,D).

Exercise Errors

These include shoulder elevation, spine extension or flexion, weight-bearing elbow hyperextension, and/or the disproportional weight bearing of the supporting hand (overloading of the hypothenar and insufficient weight bearing of the thenar).

Advanced Exercises: Higher Postural (Developmental) Positions

Quadruped Position

The position on all fours is the initial position for crawling when an infant reaches the age of about 9 months (Figure 4.41A). This exercise is important for maintaining straightening of the spine while the extremities are stabilized in a closed kinetic chain. This quadruped position is useful for athletes to train their ability to straighten up the

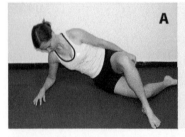
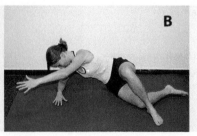
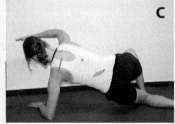

FIGURE 4-39.   (A) Initial side sitting position with the top leg supported on the foot. (B) Trunk rotation with arm reaching forward (the top leg is supported on the foot). (C) Lifting the pelvis in a side sitting position support is shifted from the buttock toward the lateral condyle of the knee of the bottom leg. The arrows on the supporting side indicate that the scapula is fixed in a caudal and abducted position. Note the pattern of scapular stabilization—the lower (supporting) scapula is in caudal position adhering to the rib cage, its medial border parallel with the spine (not elevated or winging).

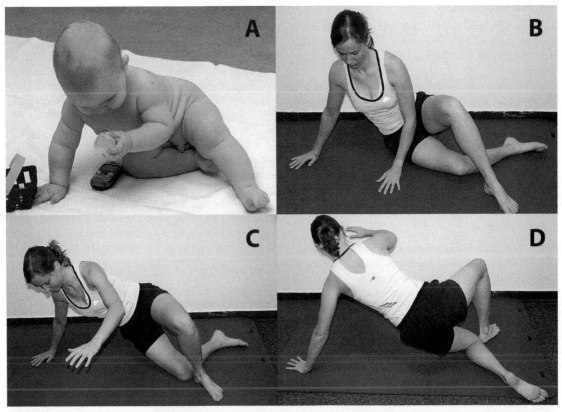

FIGURE 4-40. Side sitting position with hand support. (A) Oblique sitting position in a healthy 8-month-old infant. (B) Initial position for exercise. (C) Exercise performance—lifting the pelvis and loading the bottom knee (front view). (D) Exercise performance—shoulder girdle stabilization. The shoulder blade should not be winging (posterior view).

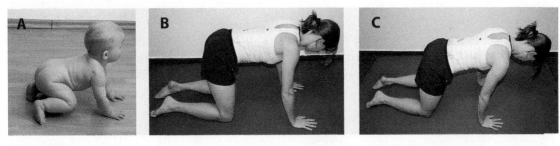

FIGURE 4-41. Quadruped exercise. (A) Quadruped (crawling) position in a healthy 9-month-old infant. (B) Quadruped exercise—initial position. (C) Exercise performance—shifting the trunk forward and backward.

spine with activation of the shoulder, hip, and trunk stabilizers (abdominals, back muscles, diaphragm and pelvic floor).

Initial Position

In order to perform good quality of quadruped position and crawling, the body segments must be properly aligned: the shoulder girdles are positioned over the well-supported hands in a fully loaded neutral/centrated position: weight distribution must be proportional on all metacarpophalangeal joints (equally on the thenar and hypothenar areas). The hip joints are in slight external rotation, positioned above the supported knees, while the shins and feet converge. The entire spine and the trunk are upright (see Figure 4.41B).

Exercise Performance

Push the right hand and left knee (and shin) down to the support and hold for a few seconds. Do the same on the opposite side. Repeat 3–5 times only if the body alignment is correct.

Move the trunk forward and backward 3–5 times. At the same time, keep the shoulders away from ears and focus on elongation of the spine (see Figure 4.41C).

Exercise Errors

These include elevation and protraction of the shoulders, sagging of the torso, extension (lordosis) of the spine, hyperextension of the elbows, and/or disproportional weight bearing through the hands.

"Bear" Position

"Bear" position is a natural transitory position of an infant older than 10–12 months (see Figure 4.42A). The infant uses the "bear" position to transfer from kneeling to squat and to stand up. This exercise is useful to train shoulder stabilizers with a coordinated interplay of the trunk and pelvic muscles.

Initial Position

The support is on hands and feet. The hands are loaded equally on the thenar and hypothenar aspects, shoulders are aligned above the hands, feet are supported on forefeet or on the entire soles (advanced version), and the knees and hips are slightly flexed with the pelvis positioned higher than the head. The spine is elongated without any associated flexion or hyperextension (see Figure 4.42B).

Exercise Performance

Push the right hand and the left foot down to the floor and keep the spine as straight as possible at the same time. Do the same on the opposite side. Repeat a few times.

Push the right hand and the left foot down to the floor and slowly lift the opposite hand and/or foot, while maintaining uprighting of the entire spine and neutral position of the chest at all times (see Figure 4.42C,D).

Exercise Errors

These include disproportional weight bearing of the hands with overloading of the hypothenar aspect and supination of the forearm, elevated and protracted shoulders, sagging

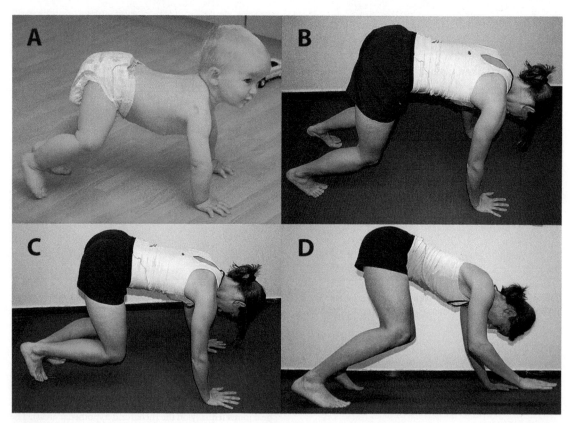

FIGURE 4-42. "Bear" exercise. (A) "Bear" position in a 12-month-old healthy infant (transition from quadruped to standing). (B) "Bear" exercise—initial position. (C) Exercise performance—lifting one leg, while keeping the spine straight and the pelvis level. (D) Exercise performance—lifting one hand while keeping the spine straight and the shoulders level.

trunk, the spine in kyphosis or extension (lordosis), internal rotation at the hips with the knees turned in (valgosity of the knees), disproportional loading of the feet with medial aspect overloaded, and the pelvis dropped on the side of the lifted leg.

Squat

The squat is a transitory or play position for an infant older than 12 months (Figure 4.43A). This exercise is used for training coordination of trunk and hip muscles (ideal training of coactivation between the diaphragm and the pelvic floor). Precise body alignment and focused movement are very important.

Initial Position

It is necessary to stand with the feet apart and positioned at hips' width. The spine, chest, and pelvis are in a neutral position (see Figure 4.43B,C).

Exercise Performance

Perform the movement slowly, with the spine upright and the knees aligned above the big toes (the knee must not shift forward). Gradually, lower the hips to the level of the knees while keeping the arms relaxed at the side or slightly reaching forward. Maintain the posture for a few relaxed respiratory cycles, while directing the inhalation to the lower and lateral part of the chest and down toward the pelvic floor (like "inflating the pelvis") (see Figure 4.43B,C).

Exercise Errors

These include internal rotation at the hips while the knees "cave" into valgosity, anterior pelvic tilt, spinal kyphosis (or lordosis), "inspiratory chest position," and elevated and protracted shoulders.

Dynamic Neuromuscular Stabilization Exercise Modifications for Sports Techniques

Throwing

Prone Exercise on Gym Ball with Bilateral Hand Support

Initial Position

Lie prone over a gym ball and roll forward and reach with the hands to the point when the thighs or the knees are supported on the ball. The head, spine, and the pelvis are kept in a horizontal plane (Figure 4.44A). This position trains basic core and scapular stabilization prerequisite for throwing motion.

Exercise Performance

Move the body forward on stabilized hands as far as you can; keep the spine upright, the shoulder blades adhered to the rib cage, and the chest in neutral position and aligned parallel with the pelvis at all times (see Figure 4.44B). Repeat the rocking forward and backward movement a few times. Make sure your hands are weight bearing proportionally throughout the whole exercise to prevent overloading of the hypothenar part of the hand.

Exercise Errors

These include chest or torso sagging down, elevated shoulders, pelvis that drops into an anterior tilt position, and cervical hyperextension.

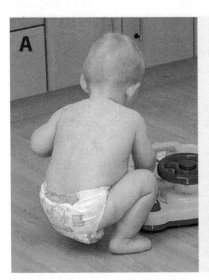
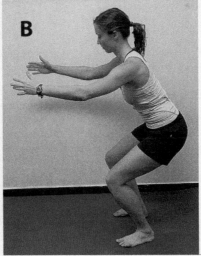
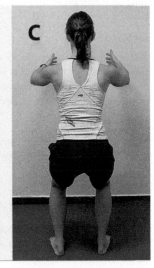

FIGURE 4-43. Squat exercise. (A) Squat position in a 12-month-old healthy infant. (B) Squat exercise—while keeping the back straight, breathing is directed to the lower and lateral parts of the chest (side view). (C) Squat exercise (posterior view)—avoid scapular retraction, forward drawn chest position, and anterior pelvic tilt.

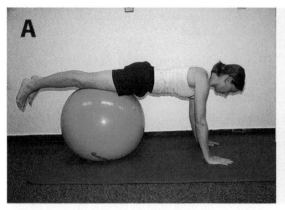 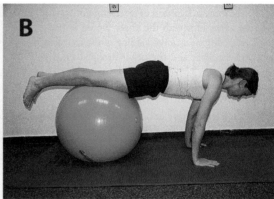

FIGURE 4-44.   Prone exercise on gym ball with bilateral hand support. Initial position, with hands on the floor and legs supported on the gym ball. (A) Shoulders aligned above the hands. (B) Exercise performance—shifting the body forward on fixed hands, keeping the entire body level.

Side Sitting with hand support (See Side Sitting Position, Figure 4.40) can also be used to train optimal muscle coordination in order to achieve stabilization prerequisite for throwing movement

Exercise with Thera-Band in a Standing Position (Forearm and Knee Support Against Wall)

Initial Position

Stand in a corner and support the elbow and the forearm on the wall. The front is slightly bent at the knee and slightly pressed against the wall, whereas the back leg is extended at the knee and loaded on the entire foot—equally on the lateral and medial side (Figure 4.45A).

Exercise Performance

Attach the Thera-band (attached behind) to the free hand and pull it forward at various angles and planes of shoulder elevation (see Figure 4.45B–D).

Exercise Errors

These include shoulder elevation, retraction of shoulder blades, spinal hyperextension or hyperkyphosis, chest elevation or "inspiratory position of the chest," and valgosity of the knee and the hip of the supporting leg.

Kicking

Basic Supine Exercise with Legs Unsupported and Alternately Moved into Extension (See Supine Position Fig. 4-32)

Lunge and One-Leg Stance

Initial Position

This involves standing with a good centration of the feet—equal amount of weight bearing and neutral position of the pelvis, trunk, and entire spine.

Exercise Performance

Lunge forward with the right leg and swing the left arm forward and the right arm backward to a horizontal level

(see Figure 4.46A). Shift the body weight forward to the right leg and extend the knee. In this position, swing the left leg forward to bend the hip and knee to 90°, while bringing the left arm backward and the right arm forward (see Figure 4.46B). Perform a few slow repetitions on each side.

Exercise Errors

These include hyperextension of the spine, "inspiratory" or forward-drawn chest position, "caving in" of the knee and the hip of the lunging leg, the knee of the supporting leg shifting past the big toe (the knee should be aligned above the big toe), and shoulder elevation while swinging the arm.

Jumping, Taking Off

The following already described techniques can be used to train stabilization coordination as a prerequisite for jumping and taking off: Lunge and One-Leg Stance (Figure 4.46)

Squat (See Squat, Figure 4.43)

Lunge on the Step and Taking Off

Initial Position

Lunge forward on the right leg (or the nondominant one for taking off) onto a step at about the height of the left knee. The knee is positioned over the ankle (Figure 4.47A).

Exercise Performance

Load the right foot and unload the left foot from the heel as the left foot is only supported on the toes while maintaining equal weight bearing on both sides of the lunging foot. When weight bearing on the lunging foot, swing both arms up and forward (see on Figure 4.47B). Repeat this movement 5–8 times slowly, focusing on proportional loading of the lunging foot, knee joint centration, and proper positioning of the torso. The Thera-band can be wrapped around the pelvis and attached behind to resist the lunging movement, making the exercise more challenging.

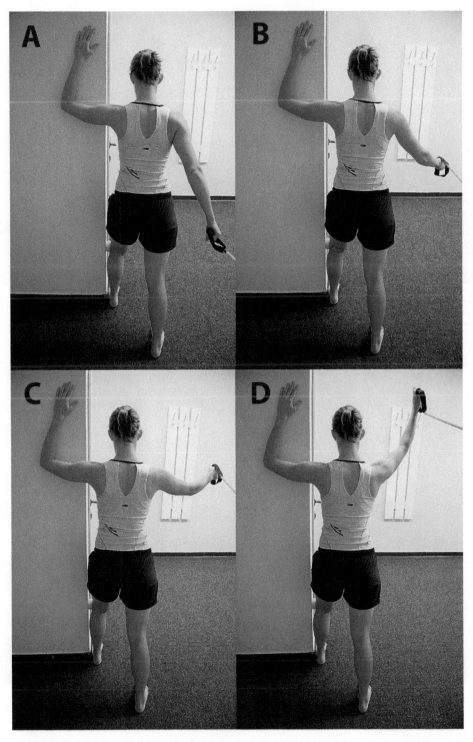

FIGURE 4-45.   Exercise with resistive band when standing with one forearm and knee supported against the wall. (A) Pulling the band in the plane of the body. (B) Pulling the band forward with shoulder abducted. (C–D) Pulling the band forward and upward.

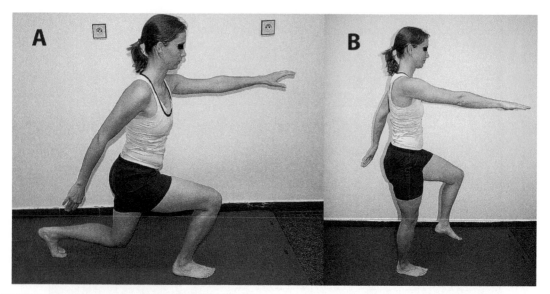

FIGURE 4-46. Lunge—one-leg stance exercise. (A) Forward lunge with reciprocal arm swing. (B) Second phase of the exercise: Switching from a lunge to one-leg stance, while changing the position of the arms.

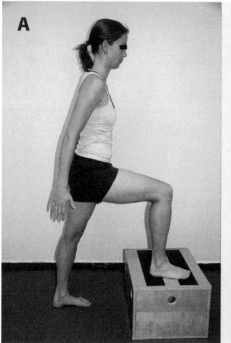 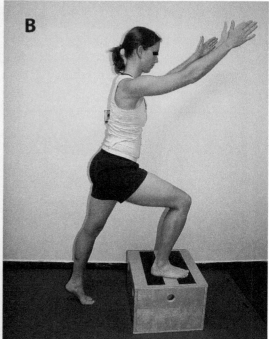

FIGURE 4-47. Lunge exercise on the step. (A) Initial position. (B) Exercise performance—shifting the support from the extended leg toward the lunging leg. Left foot—heel off, weight-bearing lunging (right) foot while swinging both arms forward.

Exercise Errors

These include "caving in" of the knee and the hip of the front leg, the lunging foot not loaded proportionally on both medial and lateral sides, dropping of the nonlunging hip, and an overextended or flexed spine.

Plyometric Exercise

Initial Position

Stand on a step about 30 cm (1 foot) high. Another step 10–15 cm (0.3–0.5 foot) high is placed about 50 cm (1.6 feet) in the front of the first step (Figure 4.48A).

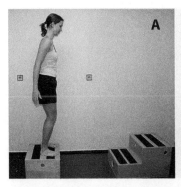
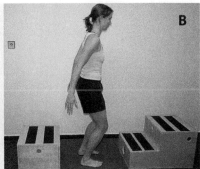
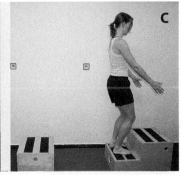

FIGURE 4-48. Plyometric exercise. (A) Initial position. (B) Exercise performance—jumping down from the step with good centration of the spine, hips, knees, and feet. (C) End position of plyometric exercise—after immediate jumping up on the second step.

Exercise Performance

Jump down with both feet between the steps and immediately jump up onto the second step (Figure 4.48B,C).

Exercise Errors

These include chest elevation, anterior pelvic tilt, and a flexed or hyperextended spine.

Shooting (Hockey, Golf)

Bear Exercise (See "Bear" Position, Figure 4.42)

Squat and Twist with Thera-Band

Initial Position

It is necessary to stand with the feet apart, feet and knees pointing out, and the knees slightly bent. The spine is kept upright. A Thera-band is attached to one side and the free part of the band is wrapped with both hands in front of the chest (Figure 4.49A).

Exercise Performance

Rotate the trunk to pull on the Thera-band, while maintaining the pelvis in the original initial position (the pelvis should not rotate!). Keep both feet equally loaded on

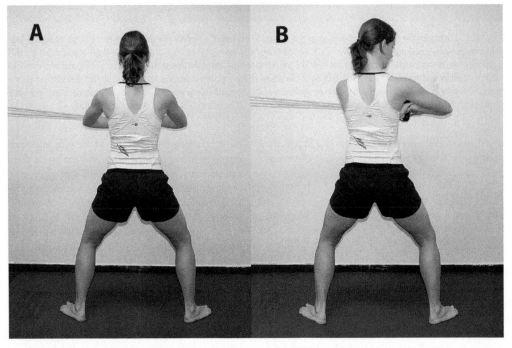

FIGURE 4-49. Squat with trunk rotation against resistance. (A) Initial position. (B) Exercise performance, rotating the trunk while pulling the band.

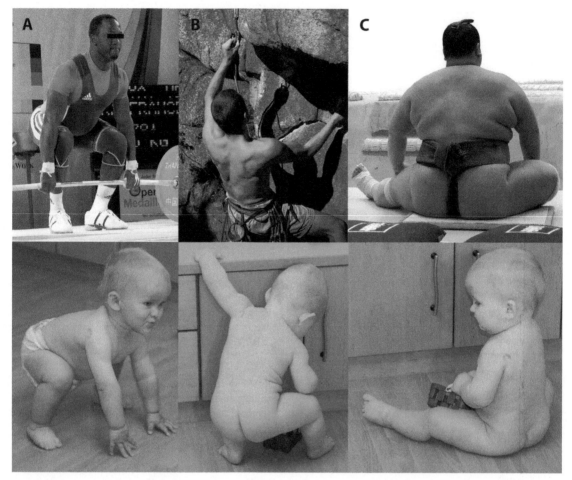

FIGURE 4-50. Comparing the quality of stabilization of and athlete to the one of a healthy infant. (A) Note that the hip, knee, and feet position and stabilization pattern in the weight-lifter and the infant are identical. Note the neutral position of the chest and the shoulder girdles. (B) Note the scapular stabilization pattern (caudal/neutral scapular position) and activation pattern of the lateral and dorsal parts of the abdominal wall are similar in both, the rock climber and the infant. There is no bulging of the lateral abdominal wall unlike the pathological pattern depicted in Figure 4.14A. (C) Note the ideal uprightness of the entire spine in the sitting position of both, the healthy 9-month-old infant and the sumo wrestler. For all of the above six postures, ideal balance between anterior and posterior musculature (including pelvic floor and diaphragm) is necessary.

both lateral and medial sides (see Figure 4.49B). Repeat the exercise slowly or a few times, as long as proper alignment of all body segments is maintained.

Exercise Errors

These include loss of foot contact, rotation of the pelvis, and elevation of the shoulders.

CONCLUSION

During all the exercises described above, DNS principles described in the first two sections of this chapter should be incorporated. In addition to injury prevention, athletes can enhance their sports performance when they understand the developmental principles and functionally centrate the joints during training (Figure 4.50). Those with inadequate body image and compromised functional centration due to pain and protective patterns, anatomical abnormalities, etc., are at higher risk for injuries. Further, their sports performance in terms of maximum speed, strength, and quality will be affected. The ultimate goal of using DNS in both, treatment of athletes and sports training is to stabilize the torso for ideal centration of all the joints for smooth and efficient movement as demonstrated in physiological development.

ACKNOWLEDGMENTS

The authors thank Clare Frank, DPT, and Vanda Andelova, DPT for their assistance in editing the chapter and Lucie Oplova, PT, for her assistance with photographs.

REFERENCES

1. Kolar P. Facilitation of agonist-antagonist co-activation by reflex stimulation methods. In: Liebenson C, ed. Rehabilitation of the Spine—A Practitioner's Manual. 2nd ed. Philadelphia, PA: Lippincott Williams & Wilkins; 2006:531–565.

2. Vojta V. Die zerebralen Bewegungsstörungen im Säuglingsalter: Frühdiagnose und Frühtherapie (Broschiert). Stuttgart: Thieme; 2008.

3. Vojta V, Peters A. Das Vojta—Princip. Berlin: Springer Verlag; 2001.

4. Forriol Campos F, Maiques JP, Dankloff C, et al. Foot morphology development with age. Gegenbaurs Morphol Jahrb 1990;136(6):669–676.

5. Volpon JB. Footprint analysis during growth period. J Pediatr Orthop 1994;14(1):83–85.

6. Openshaw P, Edwards S, Helms P. Changes in rib cage geometry during childhood. Thorax 1984;39(8):624–627.

7. Abitbol MM. Evolution of the lumbosacral angle. Am J Phys Anthropol 1987;72(3):361–372.

8. Lord MJ, Ogden JA, Ganey TM. Postnatal development of the thoracic spine. Spine 1995;20(15):1692–1698.

9. Kasai T, Ikata T, Katoh S, et al. Growth of the cervical spine with special reference to its lordosis and mobility. Spine 1996;21(18):2067–2073.

10. Koman LA, Smith BP, Shilt JS. Cerebral palsy. Lancet 2004;363(9421):1619–1631.

11. DeLuca PA. The musculoskeletal management of children with cerebral palsy. Pediatr Clin North Am 1996;43(5):1135–1150.

12. Orth H. Das Kind in der Vojta-Therapie. München: Elsevier GmbH, Urban & Fischer Verlag; 2005.

13. Zafeiriou DI. Primitive reflexes and postural reactions in the neurodevelopmental examination. Pediatr Neurol 2004;31(1):1–8.

14. Fisk JD, Goodale MA. The organization of eye and limb movements during unrestricted reaching to targets in contralateral and ipsilateral visual space. Exp Brain Res 1985;60(1):159–178.

15. Henriques DY, Medendorp WP, Gielen CC, et al. Geometric computations underlying eye-hand coordination: orientations of the two eyes and the head. Exp Brain Res 2003;152(1):70–78.

16. Gribble PL, Everling S, Ford K, et al. Hand-eye coordination for rapid pointing movements. Arm movement direction and distance are specified prior to saccade onset. Exp Brain Res 2002;145(3):372–382.

17. Kluenter HD, Lang-Roth R, Guntinas-Lichius O. Static and dynamic postural control before and after cochlear implantation in adult patients. Eur Arch Otorhinolaryngol 2009;266(10):1521–1525.

18. Blouin J, Guillaud E, Bresciani JP, et al. Insights into the control of arm movement during body motion as revealed by EMG analyses. Brain Res 2010;1309:40–52.

19. Bresciani JP, Gauthier GM, Vercher JL. On the nature of the vestibular control of arm-reaching movements during whole-body rotations. Exp Brain Res 2005;164(4):431–441.

20. Metcalfe JS, McDowell K, Chang TY, et al. Development of somatosensory-motor integration: an event-related analysis of infant posture in the first year of independent walking. Dev Psychobiol 2005;46(1):19–35.

21. Hixon TJ, Mead J, Goldman MD. Dynamics of the chest wall during speech production: function of the thorax, rib cage, diaphragm, and abdomen. J Speech Hear Res 1976;19(2):297–356.

22. Hodges P. Lumbopelvic stability: a functional model of biomechanics and motor control. In: Richardson C, ed. Therapeutic Exercise for Lumbopelvic Stabilization. Edinburgh: Churchill Livingstone; 2004:13–28.

23. Hodges PW, Eriksson AE, Shirley D, et al. Intra-abdominal pressure increases stiffness of the lumbar spine. J Biomech 2005;38(9):1873–1880.

24. Essendrop M, Andersen TB, Schibye B. Increase in spinal stability obtained at levels of intra-abdominal pressure and back muscle activity realistic to work situations. Appl Ergon 2002;33(5):471–476.

25. Cholewicki J, Juluru K, Radebold A, et al. Lumbar spine stability can be augmented with an abdominal belt and/or increased intra-abdominal pressure. Eur Spine J 1999;8(5):388–395.

26. Hodges PW, Gandevia SC. Changes in intra-abdominal pressure during postural and respiratory activation of the human diaphragm. J Appl Physiol 2000;89(3):967–976.

27. Hodges PW, Sapsford R, Pengel LH. Postural and respiratory functions of the pelvic floor muscles. Neurourol Urodyn 2007;26(3):362–371.

28. Kolar P, Neuwirth J, Sanda J, et al. Analysis of diaphragm movement, during tidal breathing and during its activation while breath holding, using MRI synchronized with spirometry. Physiol Res 2009;58:383–392.

29. Hodges PW, Gandevia SC. Activation of the human diaphragm during a repetitive postural task. J Physiol 2000;522:165–175.

30. Hodges PW, Heijnen I, Gandevia SC. Postural activity of the diaphragm is reduced in humans when respiratory demand increases. J Physiol 2001;537(Pt 3):999–1008.

31. Enoka, ME. Neuromechanics of Human Movement. 3rd ed. Champaign, IL: Human Kinetics; 2002.

32. Lewit K, Kolar P. Chain reactions related to the cervical spine. In: Murphy DR, ed. Cervical Spine Syndromes. New York: McGraw-Hill; 1999:515–530.

33. Lewit K. Manipulative Therapy. Edinburgh: Churchill Livingstone; 2010.

34. Smith CE, Nyland J, Caudill P, et al. Dynamic trunk stabilization: a conceptual back injury prevention program for volleyball athletes. J Orthop Sports Phys Ther 2008;38:703–720.

35. Gandevia SC, Butler JE, Hodges PW, et al. Balancing acts: respiratory sensations, motor control and human posture. Clin Exp Pharmacol Physiol 2002;29(1-2):118–121.

36. Kolar P. The sensorimotor nature of postural functions. Its fundamental role in rehabilitation on the motor system. J Orthop Med 1999;21(2):40–45.

The Clinical Audit Process and Determining the Key Link

INTRODUCTION

The primary goals in patient care or athletic development are to decrease activity intolerances (i.e., walking, sitting, bending), reduce pain, promote fitness, and prevent injury. To enhance function requires an assessment of the patient or athlete's functional capacity and/or movement patterns, in particular, to identify a "key link" or functional pathology. Common faulty movement patterns that should not be missed include dysfunction involving

- Carrying or squatting ability in a lumbar disc patient (1)
- Single leg squat in a patellofemoral pain syndrome patient or to reduce the risk of anterior cruciate ligament injury (2)
- Scapulohumeral rhythm in a rotator cuff syndrome patient (3)
- Cervicocranial flexion in a neck pain or headache patient (4)

But this is just a clinical hypothesis. Each patient is unique, and your patient may be an outlier. To determine this requires an empirical process involving testing, correcting, and retesting. This is termed the clinical audit process (CAP) (Table 5.1) (5–11). When using the CAP it has been shown that "within-session" improvement predicts "between-session" improvement. If posttreatment audit of the patient's mechanical sensitivity (MS) showed improvement, those patients were at least 3.5 times more likely to have between-session improvement (Table 5.2) (12).

The CAP guides care by aiding the musculoskeletal pain specialist in determining what they can do for the patient (modality, manual therapy, or exercise), what the patient can do for themselves (exercise), and the patient's prognosis (12,14–16). Since pain as a rule recurs, it is necessary that a self-care exercise be found which empirically reduces the patient's MS (17). If the patient *only* attributes a successful outcome to manual therapy (or other passive care), then dependency rather than independent function has been achieved (18–21). In order to enhance a patient's motivation to comply with a self-care routine, it is recommended that active care be performed prior to passive care. When the patient sees that their MS is less after active self-care, they will automatically want to do the exercise(s).

According to Cook (13), using a reassessment process is critical to systematic treatment planning (Table 5.3).

THERAPEUTIC TRIAL: THE CLINICAL AUDIT PROCESS

The therapeutic trial begins by performing an active movement assessment to find a painful motion that reproduces the patient's chief complaint (Figure 5.1). The assessment is of active rather than passive motion and includes range of motion, orthopedic (i.e., Kemp's), or functional (i.e., squat) testing. This painful motion is termed the patient's MS. This will be the independent variable in the therapeutic trial. If a patient is not in pain but is seeking preventative care, enhanced fitness (i.e., improved mobility, endurance), or athletic performance gains, then the CAP looks for painless dysfunctional movements instead of MS.

There are two clinical situations in which an MS cannot be found. The first occurs when the patient has **postural** pain. In this case the pain is typically intermittent and aggravated by prolonged static loading (sitting, standing, lying) (20). There is a positional sensitivity, but it takes a prolonged period of static load to elicit any sensitivity. The treatment is a prescription of ergonomic advice/training and microbreaks. In this case, in the course of the typical timeline for a functional evaluation there is no MS.

The second is when pain is due to **central sensitization** (**CS**). In this case the pain is constant and not worse or better with any mechanical loading. There is an MS, but there are no specific movements which increase or decrease the pain. The pain is constant and all movements hurt equally. Patients with CS have a lower pain threshold that leads to allodynia—pain to nonnoxious stimuli such as light pressure (Table 5.4) (22–24). CS patients often are so hypersensitive that they cannot even tolerate lying supine. Pressure alone is sufficient to activate the perception of pain.

CS is a centrally mediated pain that does not require ongoing peripheral injury, inflammation, or irritation since it is a cortical processing dysfunction reflecting neuroplasticity (22,25). These somatosensory changes are likely

TABLE 5.1	Clinical Audit Process

1. **Assess:** identify mechanical sensitivities and painless dysfunctions
2. **Treatment/Training:** convert painless dysfunctions into normal movement patterns
3. **Reassessment:** reevaluate mechanical sensitivities and painless dysfunctions

TABLE 5.2	Mechanical Sensitivity

Definition: Movement or position which reproduces or increases the patient's hallmark symptoms

Synonyms:
- "Marker" test according to Gray Cook in the Functional Movement System (13)
- Functional painful test in the Selective Functional Movement Assessment (13)
- Positive orthopedic test
- Provocative test
- Plus sign

TABLE 5.3	Assessment System Hierarchy According to Cook (13)

- Set a movement path baseline
  - Perform a functional movement screen
- Locate and observe the movement problem
  - Prioritize: find painful "marker" and/or nonpainful dysfunctional movements
- Use corrective measures aimed at the problem
  - Address the most fundamental "painless movement dysfunction first"
- Revisit the baseline
  - Reassess

to be related to dysfunctional motor control (i.e., flexion withdrawal) (23,24). According to Nachemson (26), "various pools of nerve cells in the dorsal columns can be hypersensitized and thus can signal a painful condition even though there is very little peripheral input." The prognosis for patients with CS is guarded. Treatment primarily focuses on motor control training designed to enhance motor control and alter cognitive-behavioral pain expectancies (27,28).

> "If you want your body to feel better, feel your body move better." Diane Jacobs, P.T.

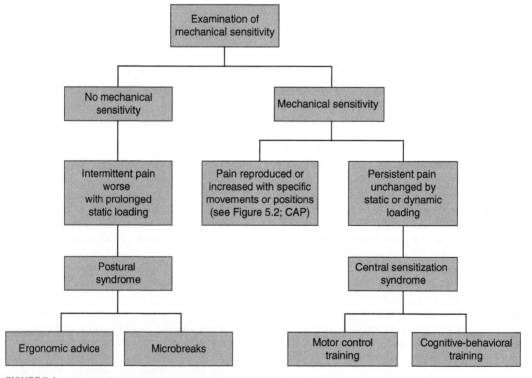

FIGURE 5-1. Algorithm for active movement assessment. CAP, clinical audit process.

TABLE 5.4	Features of Central Sensitization

- Persistent pain that does not demonstrate specific mechanical sensitivities; in other words, all movements and positions are sensitive
- Reactive to light touch—allodynia

If the patient does not have pain due to postural or central processing factors, then it is highly likely that the pain is of a mechanical origin. **Mechanical pain** is confirmed when some movements reproduce the patient's MS and others do not. Once it is established that the patient's pain is behaving mechanically the CAP can begin with a therapeutic trial of exercises aimed at "re-setting" the most significant painless dysfunction. There are three possible responses to this treatment trial (Figure 5.2):

1. MS decreases
2. MS does not change
3. MS worsens

Mechanical Sensitivity Decreases

If the patient's MS decreases after "re-setting" a key painless dysfunction, then you have found a treatment that has created a "within-session" improvement. This predicts a high likelihood of "between-session" improvement in the patient's activity intolerances. If an exercise is found which decreases

the MS during the posttreatment audit, then this should be prescribed as self-care. Patients in this category are confirmed to have **mechanical** pain and a good prognosis.

Fast-Track Care

Finding an exercise that reduces the patient's MS is the beginning, but not always the end. We want to search for the hardest, most functionally relevant exercise that the patient does well. Such a functional approach is constantly shifting over time as we continuously recalibrate where the "edge of capability" is.

The self-care exercise that has been adjudicated is considered to be in the patient's functional training range (FTR)—"the range which is both painless and appropriate for the task at hand" (29). The CAP is a key to expanding the patient's FTR. The exercise in a patient's FTR satisfies these criteria (9):

- Painless (or symptom centralizing)
- Appropriate (good motor control)
- Posttreatment audit that demonstrates a decrease in MS (ideally)

Mechanical Sensitivity Does Not Change

If the patient's MS does not change, then attempt further therapeutic trials to seek an alternative exercise, manual therapy, or modality which reduces the patient's MS. If no

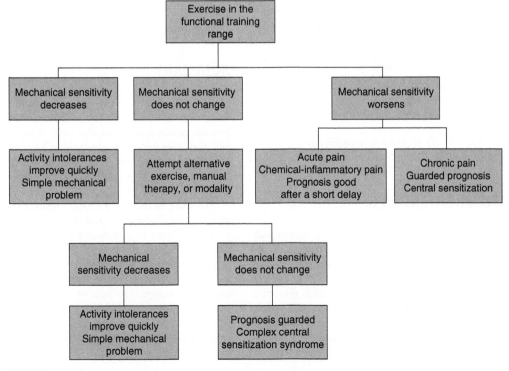

FIGURE 5-2. Algorithm for testing response to a treatment—the clinical audit process.

procedure can be found which changes the patient's MS and the patient has chronic pain, it is likely the patient has **CS** (see above).

Mechanical Sensitivity Worsens

If the patient's MS worsens and the patient has acute pain, it is likely that the pain generator is acting irritably and has a **chemical** component (i.e., inflammatory). In this case the initial treatment is to temporarily "let pain be the guide" and invoke anti-inflammatory strategies (relative rest, ice, fish oil, nonsteroidal anti-inflammatory drugs). The prognosis for this patient is excellent for a speedy recovery after a short delay.

If the MS worsens and the patient is a chronic, recurrent pain patient, it is likely that the pain generator is sensitized from central sources (see above).

Are All Conservative Treatments the Same?

- 181 consecutive patients with sciatica were given active generic exercise or symptom-guided exercise
- Most subjects had suffered sciatica for 1–3 months, with 18% having symptoms for 3–6 months
- 65% of patients had three of more positive nerve root compression signs and thus were surgical candidates
- All had received prior conservative care
- After 8 weeks of treatment, 74% of those that received symptom-guided exercises were back at work in contrast to 60% of those receiving generic exercises
- Those who suffered sciatica for 3–6 months fared just as well as those whose symptoms were of shorter duration

---

Conclusions

1. Failure of conservative care is not an indication for spine surgery.
2. Symptom-guided exercise is more successful than generic exercise.

Albert HB, Mannice C. The efficacy of systematic active conservative treatment for patients with severe sciatica. Spine 2012;37:531–542.

PATIENT CATEGORIES

Fortunately, most patients have pain of a **mechanical** nature, and the prognosis for a speedy recovery is outstanding. In such patients, usually the CAP will find a self-care exercise that is effective on day 1. A subset of mechanical patients have pain of *postural* origin and unless the tissue can be spared from prolonged static overload only minimal improvement will occur. Patients who have strained or injured their tissues will often have a **chemical** or inflammatory component to their pain. Such patients have an

---

TABLE 5.5	Patient Categories

Mechanical
  Static overload—postural
    History alone reveals sensitivity
    Treatment: postural/ergonomic advice
    Prognosis: good
  Dynamic overload
    Examination shows mechanical sensitivity
    Treatment: exercise to address the most relevant painless dysfunction
    Within-session improvement expected
    Prognosis: excellent
Chemical
  Examination shows mechanical sensitivity
  Treatment: relative rest and deinflammation of tissues
  No within-session improvement expected
  Prognosis: excellent, after a short delay
Sensitization (central)
  All movements are painful
  Treatment: motor control and cognitive-behavioral training
  No within-session improvement expected
  Prognosis: guarded

---

excellent prognosis, but recovery will not be immediate and there typically is no self-care exercise in the first few days. A final group of patients who have chronic pain that hurts with all activities have **CS.** Their prognosis is not ideal. Table 5.5 summarizes the features of each clinical category.

SUMMARY

McKenzie (30) sums up the goal of the patient-centered orientation of the CAP: "If you adopt certain positions or perform certain movements that cause your back to 'go out', then if we understand the problem fully we can identify other movements and other positions that, if practiced and adopted, can reverse the process. You put it out—you put it back in."

According to the World Health Organization's revised guidelines on disability, the goal of health care is to enable patients to return to participation and independent functioning in their chosen activities (21,31–35). The specific outcomes used to measure progress toward these goals are the patient's activity intolerances in their home, recreational activities, or occupational activities (e.g., sitting, standing, walking, bending) (36–38). The CAP allows clinicians to adjudicate within-session what treatments are most efficacious, in particular, what self-care the patient can perform to restore function.

Unlike most prescriptive or even evidence-informed approaches, the CAP is truly patient-centered. Whereas a certain prescription of care might be effective for the majority of patients, only the CAP allows care to be customized to an outlier. The patient's own response to a therapeutic trial is used to establish the prescription of self-care. In a nutshell, the treatment recommended is the one that is found through an empirical trial to reduce the patient's MS. In most cases, the clue to finding the patient's "key link" is in finding the most relevant painless dysfunction and then exploring different "resets" until the painless dysfunction is normalized. In this way restoring function is usually found to result in less pain. Thus, the CAP allows the clinician to avoid "chasing the pain" and to focus on the finding and correcting the source of the problem.

REFERENCES

1. Cholewicki J, Silfies SP, Shah RA, et al. Delayed trunk muscle reflex responses increase the risk of low back injuries. Spine 2005;30(23):2614–2620.

2. Hewett TE, Myer GD, Ford KR, et al. Biomechanical measures of neuromuscular control and valgus loading of the knee predict anterior cruciate ligament injury risk in female athletes: a prospective study. Am J Sports Med 2005;33(4):492–501.

3. Kibler WB, McMullen J. Scapular dyskinesis and its relation to shoulder pain. J Am Acad Orthop Surg 2003;11:142–151.

4. Jull G, Kristjansson E, Dalll'Alba P. Impairment in the cervical flexors: a comparison of whiplash and insidious onset neck pain patients. Man Ther 2004;9:89–94.

5. Liebenson CS. Advice for the clinician and patient: functional training part one: new advances. J Bodywork Movement Ther 2002;6(4):248–253.

6. Liebenson CS. Advice for the clinician and patient: spinal stabilization—an update. Part 2—functional assessment. J Bodywork Movement Ther 2004;8(3):199–213.

7. Liebenson CS. Advice for the clinician and patient: spinal stabilization—an update. Part 3—training. J Bodywork Movement Ther 2004;8(4):278–287.

8. Liebenson CS. The importance of the functional examination in patient-centered care for back patients. Kiropraktoren 2005:4–8.

9. Liebenson CS. Rehabilitation of the Spine, Second Edition: A Practitioner's Manual. Baltimore, MD: Lippincott Williams and Wilkins; 2007.

10. Liebenson CS. A modern approach to abdominal training—part III: putting it together. J Bodywork Movement Ther 2008;12:31–36.

11. Liebenson C. The role of reassessment: the clinical audit process. Dyn Chiropractic 2010;28(14).

12. Hahne A, Keating JL, Wilson S. Do within-session changes in pain intensity and range of motion predict between-session changes in patients with low back pain. Aust J Physiother 2004;50:17–23.

13. Cook G, Burton L, Kiesel K, Rose G, Bryant MF. Movement: Functional Movement Systems: Screening, Assessment, Corrective Strategies, Aptos, CA: On Target Publications; 2010.

14. Tuttle N. Do changes within a manual therapy session predict between session changes for patients with cervical spine pain. Aust J Physiother 2005;20:324–330.

15. Tuttle N. Is it reasonable to use an individual patient's progress after treatment as a guide to ongoing clinical reasoning? J Manipulative Physiol Ther 2009;32:396–403.

16. Long A, Donelson R, Fung T. Does it matter which exercise? Spine 2004;29:2593–2602.

17. Croft PR, Macfarlane GJ, Papageorgiou AC, Thomas E, Silman AJ. Outcome of low back pain in general practice: a prospective study. BMJ 1998;316:1356–1359.

18. Harding V, Williams AC de C. Extending physiotherapy skills using a psychological approach: cognitive-behavioural management of chronic pain. Physiotherapy 1995;81:681–687.

19. Harding VR, Simmonds MJ, Watson PJ. Physical therapy for chronic pain. Pain—Clin Updates, Int Assoc Study Pain 1998;6:1–4.

20. McKenzie R, May S. The Lumbar Spine Mechanical Diagnosis & Therapy. Vols 1 and 2. Waikanae, New Zealand: Spinal Publications; 2003.

21. World Health Organization. International Classification of Human Functioning, Disability and Health: ICF. Geneva: WHO; 2001.

22. Cohen ML, Champion GD, Sheaterh-Reid R. Comments on Gracely et al. Painful neuropathy: altered central processing maintained dynamically by peripheral input. (Pain 1992;51:175–194) Pain 1993;54:365–366.

23. Desmeules JA, Cedraschi C, Rapiti E, et al. Neurophysiologic evidence for a central sensitization in patients with fibromyalgia. Arthritis Rheum 2003;48:1420–1429.

24. Juottonen K, Gockel M, Silén T, Hurri H, Hari R, Forss N. Altered central sensorimotor processing in patients with complex regional pain syndrome. Pain 2002;98:315–323.

25. Coderre TJ, Katz J, Vaccarino AL, Melzak R. Contribution of central neuroplasticity to pathological pain: review of clinical and experimental evidence. Pain 1993;52:259–285.

26. Nachemson AL. Newest knowledge of low back pain. Clin Orthop Relat Res 1992;279:8–20.

27. Moore JE, Von Korff M, Cherkin D, et al. A randomized trial of a cognitive-behavioral program for enhancing back pain self-care in a primary care setting. Pain 2000;88:145–153.

28. Vlaeyen JWS, De Jong J, Geilen M, Heuts PHTG, Van Breukelen G. Graded exposure in the treatment of pain-related fear: a replicated single case experimental design in four patients with chronic low back pain. Behav Res Ther 2001;39:151–166.

29. Morgan D. Concepts in functional training and postural stabilization for the low-back-injured. Top Acute Care Trauma Rehabil 1988;2:8–17.

30. McKenzie R. The McKenzie Institute International Pamphlet; 1998.

31. Victorian WorkAuthority—Clinical Framework. http://www.workcover.vic.gov.au/dir090/vwa/home.nsf/pages/chiropractors

32. Abenheim L, Rossignol M, Valat JP, et al. The role of activity in the therapeutic management of back pain: report of the International Paris Task Force on Back Pain. Spine 2000;25:1S–33S.

33. Rundell SD, Davenport TE, Wagner T. Physical therapist management of acute and chronic low back pain using the World Health Organization's International Classification of Functioning, Disability, and Health. Phys Ther 2009;89:82–90.

34. Waddell G, Aylward M. Models of Sickness and Disability. London: Royal Society of Medicine Press; 2010.

35. Waddell G, Burton K. Concepts of rehabilitation for the management of low back pain. Best Pract Res Clin Rheumatol 2005;19:655–670.

36. Liebenson CS. Improving activity tolerance in pain patients: a cognitive-behavioral approach to reactivation. Top Clin Chiropr 2000;7(4):6–14.

37. Liebenson CS, Yeomans S. Outcomes assessment in musculo-skeletal medicine. J Manual Ther 1997;2;67–75.

38. Agency for Health Care Policy and Research (AHCPR). Acute Low-Back Problems in Adults. Clinical Practice Guideline Number 14. Washington, DC: US Government Printing; 1994.

Functional Evaluation of Faulty Movement Patterns

INTRODUCTION

The broad impact of neuromusculoskeletal conditions on society and our limited success in managing them warrants a new approach. We need only look at the low back disability epidemic or the explosive rise in noncontact anterior cruciate ligament (ACL) injuries for evidence of this. The problem is that we are designed to move, yet we move too little (sedentarism), too much (overuse), or with poor quality (faulty movement patterns). Sedentary lifestyle is no longer just a problem of western societies alone but has spread like a virus to the developing nations of the world. "Weekend warriors" along with the fitness trend of more sets, reps, and weight without consideration of quality of movement has led to widespread nonimpact-related musculoskeletal pain (MSP) syndromes from overuse. An inadequate foundation of movement competency or literacy is seen in faulty movement patterns involving fundamental motor programs such as *upright posture, squatting, gait, balance,* and *breathing.* This chapter will describe a new functional paradigm of evaluation.

A functional assessment involves both a history and a functional examination. The history should identify the patient's or athlete's current activities, goals, symptoms, and concerns, as well as his or her past activities and injuries. The examination has two purposes: (1) to identify movements or tissues which are painful and (2) to identify faulty movement patterns where there is painless dysfunction. Recognizing faulty patterns that when repeated can lead to tissue overload and injury is a key component to developing a successful corrective strategy. Beyond assessing movement competency, clinical evaluation should also ascertain any gap between the individual's activity demands and their functional ability (1). This gap may be thought of as a motor control deficit which results in the loss of one's normal stability margin of error. Such a shortfall will not only predispose to injury but lessen performance potential as well.

According to Janda, "Time spent in assessment will save time in treatment" (2). The traditional orthopedic assessment focuses on identifying the site of symptoms and pain generator via provocative testing. Unfortunately,

the orthopedic approach often stops there. In contrast, the functional assessment goes one step further and seeks to identify the source of biomechanical overload. To properly identify the victim and the culprit, it is necessary to distinguish the site of pain from its source (Table 6.1). Treatment is often directed to the site of pain, which is the "victim" of dysfunction, while the source of pain, the true "culprit," goes undetected. Functional assessment takes a deeper look, to avoid the commonly applied, myopic approach.

Functional assessment achieves two main goals: (1) to reassure patients that they do not have significant or ominous pathology and (2) to individualize therapy or training that reduces painful movements and restores function. It has been shown that this type of empirical approach leads to predictable between-session improvement (3–5). This patient or athlete-centered approach is in stark contrast to traditional approaches that follow predetermined protocols, based on a specific diagnosis or isolated findings of weak muscles or restricted mobility.

Treating the biomechanical source of pain instead of the site of symptoms is based on a concept called *regional interdependence* (6–10). This is the theory that dysfunction of one anatomical region is responsible for pain or dysfunction in another, often distant, region. For instance, it has been shown that an ankle sprain leads to a compensatory delay in onset of activation of the gluteus maximus on the injured side. This persists long after the sprain has healed and thus such painless dysfunction must be addressed in rehabilitation (11).

> "After an injury tissues heal, but muscles learn. They readily develop habits of guarding which outlast the injury." Janet Travell (12)

The functional assessment is a "missing link" in the traditional medical-orthopedic assessment of MSP. Janda, Cook, and others have called for the functional assessment of movement patterns to become a "gold standard" for individuals with MSP (13,14). The *overhead squat* and *single leg squat* are two such examples (see Figures 6.18 and 6.20). The overhead squat is invaluable because it screens sagittal plane mobility and stability. In particular mobility of the

TABLE 6.1	Distinguishing the Site vs. the Source of Pain

Site

    Pain generator (tissue)

    Segmental

    Isolated

Source

    Repetitive strain

    Insufficient capacity (i.e., "weak link")

    Faulty movement pattern

    Central sensitization

TABLE 6.2	Red Flags Signs and Symptoms

Age younger than 20 or older than 50 years

Trauma

Recent infection

Past history of carcinoma, long-term steroid use, human immuno-deficiency virus, drug abuse

Failure of 4 weeks of appropriate conservative care

Night pain

Pain at rest

Weight loss unrelated to diet

Malaise

Unremitting flexion restriction

Fever

Motor weakness in lower limbs

Sphincter disturbance

Saddle anesthesia

Source: Waddell G. The Back Pain Revolution. 2nd ed. Edinburgh: Churchill Livingstone; 2004.

ankle, hip, and thoracic spine, as well as stability of the foot, knee, lumbopelvic, shoulder, and neck regions. It also screens a common mechanism of injury for the low back—end-range loading of the lumbar spine in full flexion. The single leg squat is an essential test for most people as it is a window into a person's control of activities dominated by one-legged stance, such as walking and running. It reveals frontal plane issues in the lower quarter kinetic chain, as well as poor core control and posterior chain strength/coordination. Poor control of the single leg squat position has also been shown to be a preventable mechanism of injury for noncontact ACL injuries.

THE LIMITATIONS OF EVALUATING STRUCTURAL PATHOLOGY

Prior to determining an athlete's fitness for participation, a medical evaluation is commonly performed, including general health, past injury history, and recent complaints. Any suspicious findings should be further evaluated to rule out potential "red flags" of serious diseases, such as tumor, infection, fracture, and neurological disease. It has often been assumed that such an evaluation for an individual with pain should routinely include the use of imaging such as X-ray, computed tomography (CT), or magnetic resonance imaging (MRI). However, if a thorough medical history combined with a physical examination is done properly, the likelihood of missing something serious is very small. The "red flags", signs and symptoms from history and examination that would indicate that imaging, laboratory tests, or specialized medical referral is necessary for a low back pain patient are shown in Table 6.2 (15). An additional reason why routine imaging for MSP should be avoided is that the chances of a false-positive test emerging are quite high. The structural findings of these images have poor correlation to pain and function and are commonly found in asymptomatic individuals. Beyond fostering unnecessary treatment and further diagnostic studies, false positives also

lead inexorably to the patient or athlete receiving a more threatening and disabling "label" than is necessary, which has shown to be related to poor treatment outcomes and chronicity (16,17).

Spine

Structural evidence of a lumbar disc herniation in a patient with appropriate symptoms is present over 90% of the time (18–21). Unfortunately, even when utilizing advanced imaging techniques such as myelography, CT, or MRI, the same positive findings are also present in 28% to 50% of asymptomatic individuals (Figure 6.1) (18–23). Similarly, in the neck, the false-positive rate with diagnostic imaging has been reported to be as high as 75% with an asymptomatic population (24,25). Thus, imaging tests have high sensitivity (few false negatives) but low specificity (high false-positive rate) for identifying symptomatic disc problems.

Furthermore, the presence of structural pathology in an asymptomatic individual does not predict a greater likelihood of future problems (26,27). Borenstein et al. conducted MRI examination of 67 asymptomatic people, 31% of whom had abnormality of discs or the spinal canal (26). The MRI findings were not predictive of future low back pain (LBP). Individuals with the longest duration of LBP were not those with the greatest anatomical abnormalities. Carragee et al. studied discograms and reported that a painful disc injection did not predict LBP on follow-up at 4 years (27). While discograms have high sensitivity for identifying tears in asymptomatic patients, it was the psychometric profiles that were found to strongly predict future LBP and work loss.

FIGURE 6-1. False-positive rates for disc hernia-tion with various imaging modalities. Imaging findings of disc abnormalities increase in frequency with age in patients without symptoms. (CT, computed tomography; DJD, degenerative join disease; MRI, magnetic resonance imaging.) From Bigos S, Müller G. Primary care approach to acute and chronic back problems: Definitions and care. In: Loeser JD, ed. Bonica's Management of Pain, 3rd ed. Philadelphia: Lippincott Williams & Wilkins, 2001.

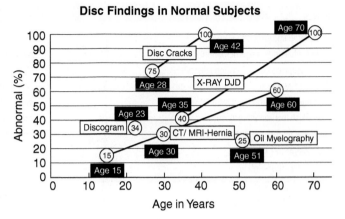

Disc Findings in Normal Subjects

Extremities

Just as in the spine, MRIs have demonstrated high lev-els of structural pathology in the extremities of asymp-tomatic individuals. Fredericson et al. have reported that "asymptomatic elite athletes demonstrate MRI changes of the shoulder (swimmers and volleyball players) and wrist (gymnasts) similar to those associated with abnormalities for which medical treatment and sometimes surgery are advised" (29).

MRIs of the shoulders of 96 asymptomatic individu-als were evaluated to determine the prevalence of findings consistent with a tear of the rotator cuff (30). The over-all prevalence of tears of the rotator cuff in all age groups was 34%. There were 14 full-thickness tears (15%) and 19 partial-thickness tears (20%). These tears were increasingly frequent with advancing age and were compatible with nor-mal, painless, functional activity.

Detailed MRIs of asymptomatic dominant and nondominant shoulders of elite overhead athletes were obtained (31). A 5-year follow-up interview was per-formed to determine whether MRI abnormalities found in the initial stage of the study represented truly clinical false-positive findings or symptomatic shoulders in evolu-tion. Eight of 20 (40%) dominant shoulders had findings consistent with partial- or full-thickness tears of the rota-tor cuff as compared with none (0%) of the nondominant shoulders. Five of 20 (25%) dominant shoulders had MRI evidence of Bennett's lesions compared with none (0%) of the nondominant shoulders. None of the athletes inter-viewed 5 years later had any subjective symptoms or had required any evaluation or treatment for shoulder-related

problems during the study period. Thus, MRI alone should not be used as a basis for operative intervention in this patient population.

The same high false-positive rate with MRIs has been shown in the knee of asymptomatic individuals. Begin-ning in one's thirties, there is degeneration of the meniscus, which increases with age even in asymptomatic people (32). According to De Smet et al., "false-positive MR diagnoses of medial meniscal tears are more common for longitudinal tears than other tear types and are also more common with MR abnormalities at either the superior surface or the menis-cocapsular junction. Spontaneous healing of longitudinal tears accounts for some false-positive MR diagnoses" (33).

Summary

The unfortunate result of using highly sensitive, but not specific tests with high false-positive rates in asymptom-atic individuals or in those with symptoms that do not warrant diagnostic imaging is that patients who may have coincidental findings are labeled as having pathology (15). The musculoskeletal system is not so vulnerable after all and has much greater adaptive potential than it is often given credit for.

A more appropriate use of diagnostic imaging is in patients with a history or examination of red flags for tumor, infection, or fracture or later in care for patients with nerve root or local complaints, which are unresponsive to conser-vative care and may require an invasive procedure such as an epidural steroid injection or other invasive procedure.

STEREOTYPICAL MOVEMENT PATTERNS

Assessment of musculoskeletal function usually consists of evaluation of isolated impairments such as individual mus-cle or joint range of motion (ROM) or strength. But the body works as an integrated system during activities such

TABLE 6.3	Assessment of Musculoskeletal Function

Isolated impairments
Individual joint range of motion
   Biceps curl/elbow flexion strength
   Hamstring curl/knee flexion strength
Integrated functional movement patterns
   Push (horizontal/vertical)
   Pull (horizontal/vertical)
   Squat (2/1 leg)
   Lunge (triplanar)

TABLE 6.5	Top Tier Tests in the Selective Functional Movement Assessment

Cervical range of motion
Upper extremity range of motion
Trunk range of motion
Single leg balance
Overhead squat

as bending, lifting, walking, reaching, grasping, pushing, pulling, etc. (Table 6.3). As such it is the evaluation of movement that is crucial, yet poorly understood. Janda detailed the specific assessment of a core set of fundamental movement patterns (Table 6.4) (13). More recently, Gray Cook has created a functional movement screen (FMS) that can also be used to identify basic movement pattern faults which are upstream of a person's musculoskeletal problem (14). Furthermore, Cook has proposed a selective functional movement assessment (SFMA) to help orient the provider by prioritizing tests through the use of an algorithm (Table 6.5).

> A famous saying: "The brain does not think in terms of individual muscles. It thinks in terms of movement patterns."

Functional ability includes establishing stability within the functional range for the specific, relevant task. If a joint is unstable, then injury risk will be heightened. A stable joint is one where the muscles are able to handle the various forms of strain typically encountered. When a joint is stable, agonist–antagonist coactivation helps to maintain functional joint centration against expected and unexpected perturbations (34–36). Adequate movement competency (intermuscular coordination) as well as sufficient movement capacity must be present for the unique activity

TABLE 6.4	Janda's Movement Patterns

1. Hip abduction
2. Hip extension
3. Trunk flexion
4. Arm abduction
5. Head/neck flexion
6. Push-up

Source: Janda V, Frank C, Liebenson C. Evaluation of muscle imbalance. In: Liebenson C, ed. Rehabilitation of the Spine: A Practitioner's Manual. Philadelphia, PA: Lippincott Williams & Wilkins; 2007.

demands the individual faces. Stability results from having the necessary movement literacy or competency to perform skilled movement with appropriate agility, balance, and coordination, while also having sufficient capacity to handle large loads and endure potentially fatiguing challenges. For instance, landing a jump with medial knee collapse and lifting by stooping instead of squatting are examples of unskilled movements that will predispose to injury and limit performance. While the ability (i.e., competency) to avoid these common mechanisms of injury is necessary, so too must the capacity to do so when fatigue is present.

Poor movement patterns are easily recognized by virtue of the de-centration of relevant joints during movement. They also can be predicted or anticipated by the presence of certain postural signs. A number of the most common signs of faulty movement patterns in the locomotor system will be highlighted here (13).

Cervicocranial (C0-C1)

A forward head posture can be correlated with insufficiency of the deep neck flexors (longus colli/capitis) (Figure 6.2). The typical movement pattern fault involves poor motor control of nodding of the head or C0-C1 flexion, in particular poking of the chin (Figure 6.3). This has been found to be correlated with chronic headaches and neck pain of either traumatic or insidious onset (37–40).

Scapulohumeral

Shrugged or rounded shoulder(s) are a common postural finding due to muscle imbalance between overactivity in shoulder girdle elevators and inhibition of shoulder girdle depressors (Figure 6.4). A rounded shoulder posture typically leads to a chain reaction with shoulder shrugging being the first consequence. The typical movement pattern fault occurs when the shoulder girdle shrugs up during the early part of arm abduction (Figure 6.5) (13,41–43). This is termed the "setting phase" and occurs during the first 45° of arm abduction. It has been shown that excessive or early shrugging is correlated with a muscle imbalance involving overactivity of the upper trapezius and underactivity of the lower trapezius and serratus anterior muscles (44). In turn this is seen commonly in shoulder impingement syndromes (45).

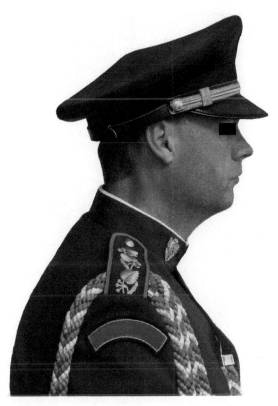

FIGURE 6-2. Forward head posture.

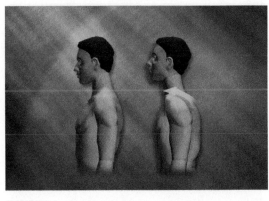

FIGURE 6-4. Rounded shoulders.

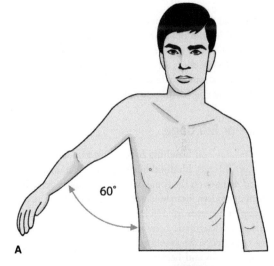

A

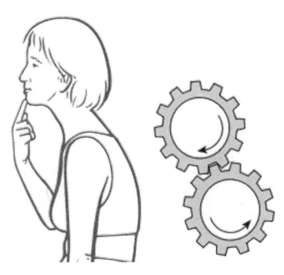

FIGURE 6-3. Poking of the chin. From Pavlu D, Petak-Kruerger S, Janda V. Brugger methods for postural correction. In: Liebenson C, ed. Rehabilitation of the Spine: A Practitioner's Manual. 2nd ed. Philadelphia, PA: Lippincott Williams & Wilkins; 2006.

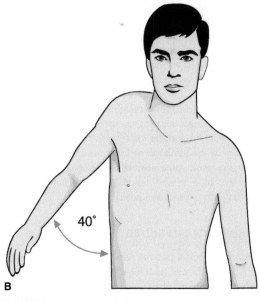

B

FIGURE 6-5. Shoulder shrug with arm abduction: (A) normal; (B) faulty.

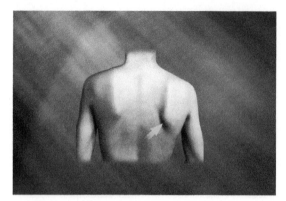

FIGURE 6-6. Winging scapula.

A related problem occurs in the scapulothoracic joint as the medial-inferior border becomes winged due to serratus anterior inhibition (Figure 6.6) (13,42,43). According to Kibler and McMullen, this is termed as scapular dyskinesia and is found commonly in overhead athletes with shoulder problems (see also Chapter 32) (46).

Anterior Rib Cage

Both posture and breathing have a powerful effect on the anterior rib cage. Ideally the anterior rib cage hangs in a relaxed manner on the spine. Unfortunately, due to sedentarism in modern lifestyle (e.g., prolonged sitting), the thoracic spine becomes fixed in kyphosis. This in turn inhibits normal diaphragmatic breathing and leads to compensatory upper chest breathing which results in the rib cage being lifted up and held in an inspiratory position. This easily becomes fixed as a subcortical motor program with significant deleterious effects, as Lewit says, "respiration is the most common faulty movement pattern" (47).

When chest breathing predominates the chest becomes fixed in an inspiratory position. This results in an anterior rib cage posture with a steep slope or upward tilt (Figure 6.7) (48). The combination of fixed upper thoracic kyphosis, faulty breathing, and lifted anterior-inferior rib cage contributes to Janda's lower crossed syndrome or what Kolar calls "open scissors" at the thoracolumbar and lumbopelvic junctions (Figure 6.8). With normal thoracic spine posture and diaphragm function, the lower anterior ribs should be more caudal with the diaphragm in a horizontal position.

Lumbopelvic Junction

The normal posture of the lumbar spine is slight lordosis. A loss of the natural lumbar curve has been correlated with poor mobility of the hips (49). Loss of normal hip extension mobility has been shown to be associated with a history of disabling LBP (7). Other researchers have also

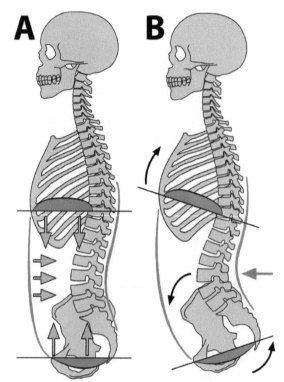

FIGURE 6-7. Horizontal diaphragm. (A) horizontal; (B) tilted upward.

found this association (50,51). The typical movement pattern fault involves insufficient postural control of "neutral" lumbar lordosis during sitting, bending, or lifting (Figure 6.9). This has been found to correlate with LBP or injury (52). Certain times of the day are known to carry a higher risk such as in the morning due to variations in disc hydration (53). Patients can benefit from this knowledge as avoidance of early morning flexion has been shown to be a successful treatment for acute LBP (54).

Instability in the spine can result in a loss of equilibrium such that the center of mass of the trunk is not easily maintained over its base of support—the feet (55,56). Stability and mobility go hand in hand. Often stiff joints or tight muscles alter movement patterns so that instability results. For instance, if there is a loss of posterior hip flexibility/mobility, it will not be possible to avoid end-range lumbar spine flexion during a deep squat. The trunk will lean forward and weight may shift to the balls of the feet. Agonist–antagonist muscles in the spine will show a higher amount of co-contraction as they attempt to maintain a "neutral" spine posture (57–59).

Knee

The knee has a tendency to collapse medially into an excessive valgus position (Figure 6.10). This is correlated with

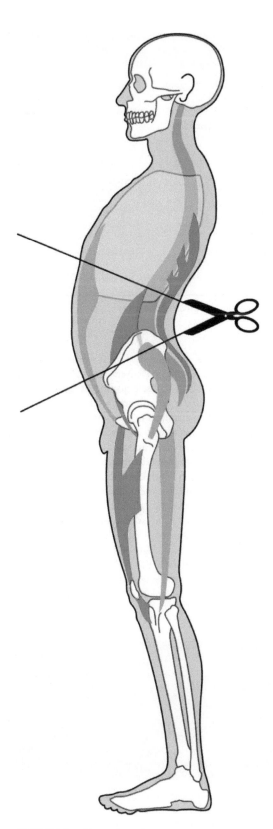

FIGURE 6-8.   "Open scissors."

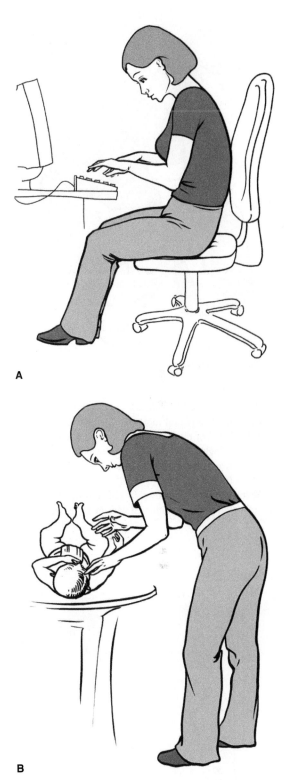

A

B

FIGURE 6-9.   Lumbosacral flexion with sitting (A), bending (B), and lifting (C). From Liebenson C, ed. Rehabilitation of the Spine: A Practitioner's Manual. 2nd ed. Philadelphia, PA: Lippincott Williams & Wilkins; 2006.

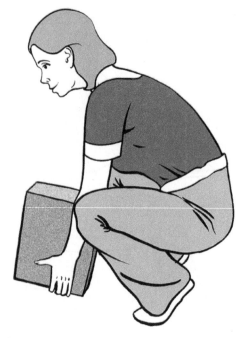

c

FIGURE 6-9.   (Continued)

insufficiency of the hip abductor muscles such as the glu-teus medius. The typical movement pattern fault involves medial collapse of the knee during landing a jump or per-forming a single leg squat. This faulty pattern has been found to correlate with ACL injury as well as patellofemoral problems (60–64).

Women have been shown to utilize different muscu-lar activation patterns compared with men (i.e., decreased

TABLE 6.6	Information from Janda's Hip Abduction Movement Pattern Assessment
What is agonist–antagonist–synergist–stabilizer relationship (muscle imbalance)?	Gluteus medius inhibition, adductor tightness, QL and TFL substitution, core insufficiency
What are the typical faulty movement patterns?	Short adductors > limited hip abduction mobility
	Tight iliotibial band > compensatory hip flexion
	Overactive QL > compensatory hip hike
Which joint tends to stiffness?	Hip abduction
Which muscle(s) tend to tightness?	Adductor, TFL, QL
Which muscle tends to inhibition?	Gluteus medius, core
Where is the repetitive strain?	Hip, knee, sacroiliac joint

QL, quadratus lumborum; TFL, tensor fascia latae.

gluteus maximus and increased rectus femoris muscle activity) during landing maneuvers (65). Decreased hip muscle activity and increased quadriceps activity were concluded to be likely contributors to the increased sus-ceptibility of female athletes to noncontact ACL injuries. Quadriceps dominance involving preferential activation of the quadriceps versus hamstrings (60) or strength imbal-ance between stronger quadriceps and weaker hamstrings (66) has been shown to correlate with ACL injury.

For each movement pattern, there are distinct find-ings that give us invaluable clinical information linking tight muscles, inhibited muscles, and joint dysfunction (Table 6.6). Hip abduction is one of the more illustrative faulty movement patterns (Figure 6.11).

For each pain generator that is due to repetitive strain, there is a movement pattern fault that is the source of bio-mechanical overload in the kinetic chain (Table 6.7).

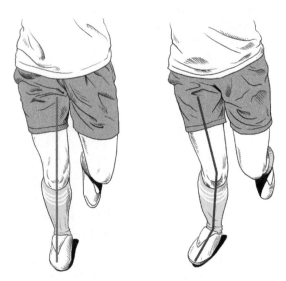

FIGURE 6-10.   Medial collapse of the knee.

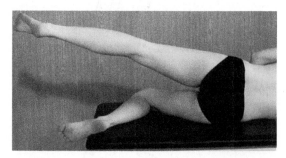

FIGURE 6-11.   Hip abduction. From Liebenson C, ed. Rehabilitation of the Spine: A Practitioner's Manual. 2nd ed. Philadelphia, PA: Lippin-cott Williams & Wilkins; 2006.

TABLE 6.7	Relationship between Key Sources of Biomechanical Overload and Painful Joints	
Painful Joints	**Faulty Posture**	**Faulty Movement Pattern**
Arch/Heel	Forward drawn posture	Forward lean
Knee	Valgus knee	One-leg squat, squat
Hip	Pelvic unleveling	Hip abduction, one-leg squat
Lumbar disc	Slump, inspiratory position of anterior chest wall	Squat, front plank, IAP
Lumbar facet	Lower crossed syndrome	Hip extension, IAP
Cervicocranial	Head forward	Neck flexion, IAP
Glenohumeral	Rounded/shrugged shoulder	Scapulohumeral rhythm, arm lifting test, wall angel
Upper ribs	Slump	Breathing
Temporomandibular joint	Chin protrusion	Mouth opening

IAP, intra-abdominal pressure test.

THE ROLE OF STIFFNESS AND MUSCLE IMBALANCES

When we evaluate the kinetic chain it becomes apparent that certain areas have a greater stability need, whereas others have a greater mobility need. Excessive stiffness is a typical problem for the thoracic spine, hip, and ankle, whereas the cervicocranial, scapulohumeral, lumbar spine, and knee joints have a tendency to become unstable.

A hallmark area where stiffness occurs and can be a source of biomechanical overload elsewhere in the kinetic chain is the thoracic spine. The mid-thoracic spine has a tendency to become fixed in kyphosis (see Figure 6.9a). Sedentary postures and improper training methods with an overemphasis on push training of the chest versus pull training of the back are possible culprits. Often this fixed kyphosis is "upstream" of other functional pathologies such as the C0-C1 and scapulohumeral faulty movement patterns described above, as well as other faults such as during overhead squat or with breathing (40,47,67–71).

Thoracic spine posture has been shown to influence the biomechanics of the shoulder (72). Muscle force is 16.2% less in the 90° abducted arm position in individuals with a slouched versus erect thoracic posture. There is a 23.6° decrease in shoulder abduction range of motion (ROM) in the slouched posture. Scapular kinematics are significantly influenced by thoracic spine posture. For instance, there is less scapular posterior tilt (posterior and caudal movement of the scapulae) when slouched. Impingement patients have been shown to have reduced scapular posterior tilt during shoulder elevation when compared with asymptomatic individuals (73).

One aspect of a slumped posture is rounding of the shoulder forward (see Figure 6.4). This overstretches the anterior capsule and tightens the posterior capsule. Harryman et al. have reported that posterior capsular tightness results in anterosuperior migration of the humeral head, thus leading to subacromial impingement (74).

Bullock et al. have shown that an erect sitting posture increases active shoulder flexion ROM in subjects with impingement syndrome (75). In the slouched posture, mean shoulder flexion ROM was 109.7°, whereas in the erect posture it was 127.3°.

It has been reported that a fixed kyphotic posture or tight posterior shoulder capsule will need to be mobilized in order for the patient to gain proper control of the scapulothoracic articulation (76–78). Boyles et al. have shown that T4-8 manipulation is a successful treatment for shoulder impingement syndrome (79). Similarly, different researchers have independently shown that thoracic spine manipulation is effective for treating neck pain (80,81).

When we take a step back and see that each area of the body has its own unique tendency to either become stiff or unstable, this helps in our clinical planning (82). Janda is credited with pioneering the idea that certain muscles tend to "tightness" and others to inhibition and that this will affect movement patterns in a predictable manner (Table 6.8) (13,83). From these observations emerged the classic Janda syndromes—upper cross, lower cross, and layer (or stratifications) (Figures 6.12–6.14).

This discovery was made possible by the fact that in paralytic conditions such as stroke or spinal cord injury, certain muscles were typically paralyzed and in spastic conditions a different set of muscles were found to be in contracture (83). This is designed to enhance survival and it turns out the same tendencies are present in the healthy population simply to a lesser degree. In fact, modern society by virtue of increasing sedentarism promotes muscle imbalance. Even "fitness" training following the body building philosophy of isolating individual muscles, rather than training movement patterns, actually reinforces faulty movement patterns and compensatory muscle imbalances. Today we see this paradigm referred to as the "joint-by-joint approach" (Table 6.9; Figure 6.15) (84). It is easy to see the similarity between Janda's layer syndrome and Boyle's "joint-by-joint approach."

TABLE 6.8	Predictable Muscle Imbalances According to Janda	
Prone to "Tightness" or Overactivity	**Inhibition Prone**	**Faulty Movement Pattern**
Gastroc-soleus	Sole of foot—quadratus plantae	Forward lean, squat
Thigh adductors	Hip abductors—gluteus medius	Hip abduction, one-leg balance or squat
Hip flexors	Hip extensors—gluteus maximus	Hip extension; one or two leg squat
Thoracolumbar erector spinae	Abdominal wall	Planks (front or side), hip extension
Shoulder girdle elevators (upper trapezius and levator scapulae)	Lower and middle trapezius, latissimus dorsi	Scapulohumeral rhythm, side plank
Pectorals	Serratus anterior	Push-up, overhead squat
Sternocleidomastoid	Deep neck flexors	Head/neck flexion, curl up

ASSESSMENT

All providers are faced with the problem of identifying what area to address first. The locomotor system is made up of mechanical links which function to carry out an infinite variety of tasks. Central nervous system control, somatosensory input, and muscular output frame the potential for this powerful machinery of life. When we train the locomotor system, the threat of injury hangs over our craft. The challenge is to identify painful markers, mechanical sensitivities (MS), painless dysfunctions, or signs of abnormal motor control (AMC) (see Chapter 5). We then train our patients or athletes to increase their functional abilities by erasing their painless dysfunctions. Simplified, one could say "you are only as strong as your weakest link."

Merely stretching and/or strengthening of isolated segments may yield positive results, but is often insufficient to enhance performance and may fail to improve durability. The art of training the locomotor system consists of seeing the mechanical linkage system and its underlying neurologic control and finding patterns of dysfunction responsible for limiting performance and precipitating

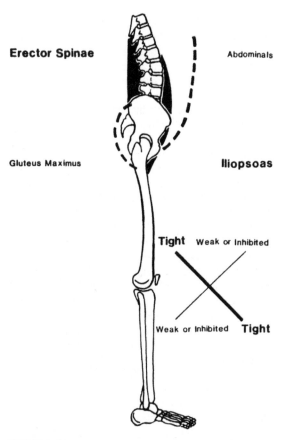

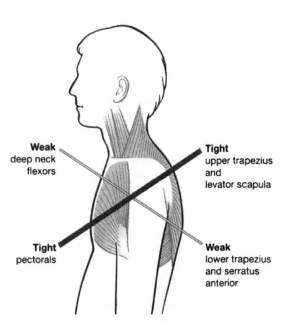

FIGURE 6-12. Upper cross. From Liebenson C, ed. Rehabilitation of the Spine: A Practitioner's Manual. 2nd ed. Philadelphia, PA: Lippincott Williams & Wilkins; 2006.

FIGURE 6-13. Lower cross. From Liebenson C, ed. Rehabilitation of the Spine: A Practitioner's Manual. 2nd ed. Philadelphia, PA: Lippincott Williams & Wilkins; 2006.

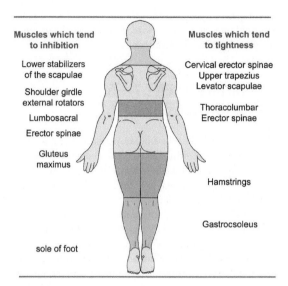

Muscles which tend to inhibition

Lower stabilizers of the scapulae

Shoulder girdle external rotators

Lumbosacral

Erector spinae

Gluteus maximus

sole of foot

Muscles which tend to tightness

Cervical erector spinae
Upper trapezius
Levator scapulae

Thoracolumbar Erector spinae

Hamstrings

Gastrocsoleus

FIGURE 6-14. Layer or Stratification Syndrome (alternating areas of hypo & hypertrophy).

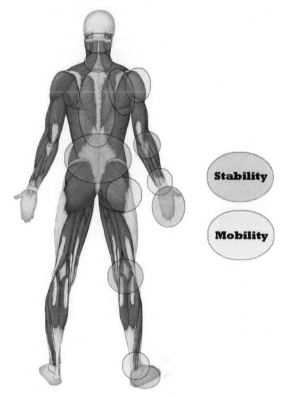

Stability

Mobility

FIGURE 6-15. Joint-by-joint approach.

injury. This is a functional, holistic approach that acknowledges regional interdependence in the locomotor system. We attempt to determine where mechanical load is most pernicious to the body. A history of constrained postures or repetitive activities should be uncovered. Additionally, examination of how the body moves should seek to identify where the linkage system is not handling even simple movements with appropriate motor control, or, when basic levels of competency are assured, when capacity breaks down under load, repetitions, or speed.

From the rehabilitation world, Lewit provides valuable insight about the need for thorough functional assessment, "Many doctors whose methods include treating only function and concomitant reflex changes are thinking only in terms of the method, not in terms of the clinical object to which the method is applied, i.e. to disturbed function, which seems very elusive. Yet to treat mainly at the site of symptoms, or pain, is to fail, if the trouble is disturbed function .... The practitioner may well feel the ground

slipping from under him, which is *why the patterns of chains based on empirical observation help by providing a rational approach to systematic clinical examination directed at disturbed function*" (47).

The body should be viewed as a linkage system whereby one link in the chain can have an effect on even distant links. Kibler et al. describe a functional kinetic chain approach which helps, for example, understand how subtalar hyperpronation can affect not only the foot and ankle but the knee, lumbar spine, or even shoulder stability (Table 6.10) (85). The kinetic chain approach highlights the regional interdependence of different links in the body (10). Herring famously said, "signs and symptoms of injury abate, but these functional deficits persist ... adaptive patterns develop secondary to the remaining functional deficits" (86).

Functional training should focus on the source of biomechanical overload rather than just where weakness or

TABLE 6.9	The "Joint-by-Joint Approach"
Needs Mobility (Stiff)	**Needs Stability (Unstable)**
Ankle	Foot
Hip	Knee
Thoracic	Lumbopelvic
	Cervical
	Shoulder

Source: Boyle M. Advances in Functional Training. Aptos, CA: On Target Publications; 2010.

TABLE 6.10	Kinetic Chain
Chief complaint	
Pain generator (tissue site of pain)	
Source of biomechanical overload	
Functional adaptation	

tightness exists. Too often athletes receive an endless array of exercises to "fix" a problem. For instance, a knee issue will be addressed with various stretching or strengthening exercises but the injury does not respond because the problem was coming from another link in the kinetic chain! If subtalar hyperpronation is the cause of medial collapse of the knee and valgus overload, then no local approach to the knee itself is going to help. Therefore, a functional evaluation should identify the source of biomechanical overload in the kinetic chain *before* a training plan commences so that the "key link" can be unmasked.

> Lewit stated, "I don't touch a patient until I have examined everything. I want to know what is the relevant chain. I begin with a general picture, not a single lesion" (47). In other words, think globally, but act locally.

Performing a screening examination of AMC is the quickest way to identify areas of increased strain or sources of weakness. This will also enable the clinician to see patterns of compensation and thus determine the "key link" through empirical trial.

Once we have identified a faulty movement pattern we can see the holistic picture of dysfunction for our athlete. For instance, if the lower back is sensitive and during the Janda hip extension test hip extension is limited, but excessive motion is occurring in the lumbar spine in hyperextension and rotation, then clear treatment targets emerge (87). Rather than stretching or providing manual therapy to the lower back, training will be focused at the key dysfunctional links in the kinetic chain. The hip stiffness would be addressed with hip joint mobilization and/or psoas lengthening. The spine instability would be addressed with bracing training and "neutral" spine control exercises during twisting or extension challenges such as pushing, pulling, squat, and balance reach training.

Practice-Based Problem

Since impairments (dysfunction) are so common, how can the provider avoid focusing on coincidental functional pathology?
As Lewit stated, "the objective of remedial exercise is a faulty motor pattern or stereotype which has been *diagnosed* and is considered *relevant* to the patient's problem." However, "remedial exercise is always time consuming, and time should not be wasted ... We should not attempt to teach patients ideal locomotor patterns, but only correct the fault that is causing the trouble" (47).

Many dysfunctions (impairments) are secondary and should be audited for improvement, but they should not be targeted with specific interventions. For instance, a tight upper trapezius muscle is typically secondary to faulty workstation ergonomics and a stiff upper thoracic kyphosis.

The trapezius tightness is a functional adaption and not a cause of biomechanical overload. Training should be aimed at the workstation and kyphosis.

THE MAGNIFICENT 7—A FUNCTIONAL SCREEN

This section will describe how to perform a sample functional screen to prioritize dysfunctional findings and identify a "key link" to address with treatment or training. While there are many functional tests that one should know (see Rehabilitation of the Spine DVD and Chapters 34 & 35), it is important to possess a screening examination to identify major dysfunctions and then progress toward more targeted assessments or "break-outs" that will elucidate where treatment is most likely to be efficacious (14). Screening is often performed to detect disease in asymptomatic people, but can also be performed using inexpensive exams to guide further assessment. The Magnificent 7 (Mag 7) is an example of a practical and valuable screen that can be used in both symptomatic and asymptomatic individuals for both of these purposes. The Mag 7 aims to identify key signs of MS or AMC and includes assessment of tests related to fundamental human functions. If we take a helicopter view the *fundamental functions* that are tested are **breathing**, **upright posture**, and **gait**. It also possesses challenge to all three planes of motion (sagittal, frontal, and transverse) and allows creation of a hierarchy of problems and paired solutions based on the involved functions and planes. To draw out future problems, the Mag 7 contains several common injury mechanisms including lumbosacral flexion during bending (Squat test) and valgus collapse of the knee (1 leg squat test).

Evaluating breathing is essential because without it we could not live. According to Lewit, it is "the most important movement pattern" (47). Coordinated breathing relates directly to abdominal function and core stability. The diaphragm and abdominals are in a reciprocal relationship. Along with the pelvic floor and deep spinal intrinsic muscles they help regulate intra-abdominal pressure (IAP) by forming the ceiling, floor and ring around the lumbar spine and abdomen. Faulty breathing usually results in chest breathing and overactivity in accessory muscles of respiration such as upper trapezius and scalenes. Less common, but more dysfunctional would be paradoxical breathing.

Tests: Breathing, IAP

Upright bipedal posture is one of the features that are unique to human beings. Like speech and larger brain size, upright posture, or control of the *sagittal plane*, occurred for the first time in the biological kingdom approximately 200,000 years ago. It is "hard-wired" into our nervous system and by 4.5 years of life is mature. Yet with our modern, sedentary lifestyle this motor program is corrupted into a slumped, slouched posture, which predisposes to headache, neck pain, shoulder impingement syndromes, and LBP.

Tests: Wall Angel, Squat

Since humans are designed to move, our most stereo-typical function is gait. Approximately 85% of normal cadence gait occurs in single leg stance. Thus, Janda has suggested that the fundamental posture of humans should be assessed in single leg stance rather than double leg stance (87). Single leg stance requires motor control in the *frontal* and *transverse planes* with significant proprioceptive demands on the feet and ankles. Its assessment highlights pronatory dysfunction, valgus collapse of the knee issues, and dysfunction involving lateral stability of the pelvis.

Tests: 1 Leg Squat, 1 Leg Balance

As a window into both posterior chain function and *transverse plane* stability, the single leg bridge is a simple screening test. Many injuries such as sports hernia, lumbar disc syndromes, and abdominal strains occur in athletes playing baseball, hockey, tennis, etc., with high torsional stress. Control of the transverse plane is crucial (88), in particular, anti-rotation stiffness, since today's athletes are bigger, stronger, and faster than those just a few decades ago, but they do not necessarily possess the sufficient motor control to handle this additional horsepower (1,82,84).

Test: 1 Leg Bridge

Grading a Test

When grading the tests of this screening examination, a standardized grading scheme such as developed by Cook is important (Table 6.11). In this scheme pain is distin-guished from discomfort in the following way. A feeling of stretch is defined as discomfort, whereas any other sensa-tion is by default termed painful. According to Cook, when in doubt give the lower score (14). Any test which scores as a 0 requires a detailed clinical evaluation and this MS, or marker test, can be used as a benchmark for progress in a clinical setting. Any test with a 1 or a 2/3 painless asym-metry (painless dysfunction) requires functional correction such as stabilization or mobilization. The goal is fastest to a symmetric 14, not 21 (14). According to Lewit, "the goal is not to teach perfect movement patterns, but to correct the key fault that is causing the trouble" (47). We will keep this goal in mind as we review the results of the Mag 7.

TABLE 6.11	Cook's Scoring—Functional Movement Screen*

0—pain

1—unable to perform movement

2—performs movement with compensation (imperfect)

3—movement performed without compensation (perfect)

*For each test, note symmetry or asymmetry.
Source: Cook G, Burton L, Kiesel K, Rose G, Bryant MF. Movement: Functional Movement Systems: Screening, Assessment, Corrective Strategies. Aptos, CA: On Target Publications; 2010.

Importance of Assessing Habitual Movement Patterns

In any examination or assessment, it is essential to get valuable and reliable information. In both the FMS and SFMA, a distinguishing feature is the emphasis on evaluat-ing functional patterns rather than isolated impairments. Cook states, "the hallmark of the SFMA design is the use of simple basic movements to expose natural reactions and responses by the patient" (14). One issue with respect to functional assessment is how much to cue the subject. With detailed instruction, we tend toward evaluating abilities rather than habits.

Janda states, "During movement pattern testing, minimal verbal cues should be used which test an individual's habitual way of performing a movement. If the cues are too 'leading,' then the test will be of the subject's ability to learn how to perform the movement correctly, rather than how they are habitually performing it" (13).

Frost and colleagues recently completed a study of the FMS in a large group of firefighters. To avoid "training the test" and ensure that habitual movement patterns were evaluated, minimal cues were given. "Aside from the stan-dard verbal instructions, no specific cues were given and participants were blinded to the test objectives, scoring cri-teria and their screen results. The firefighters were graded on how they chose to perform rather than how they could perform the tasks given minimal feedback or coaching. No rationale was given as to the general purpose of the screen to ensure that each individual's task performance was as natural as possible" (89).

Understanding the relationship between isolated impairments, functional movement patterns (i.e. compe-tency), strength/endurance/power (i.e., capacity), isolated impairments (i.e., capacity), and performance is a "holy grail" in injury prevention, rehabilitation, and athletic performance. Moreside and McGill found that training-induced improvements in hip ROM—changing what par-ticipants *could do* following 6 weeks of passive and active stretching—had no influence on what the participants *actually habitually did* during a battery of screening tasks. It appears that improving ROM impairments do not auto-matically lead individuals to use the newfound mobility in their normal activities (e.g., walking, bending, squat-ting). The "take home" message is that movement patterns must be retrained after mobilization procedures to ensure a change in how people use their newfound ROM (90). The future of rehabilitation and training is concerned with establishing a link between baseline tests of how a person habitually moves and corrective measures to enhance per-formance. This in turn becomes a springboard for athletic development (see Chapter 34). During movement pattern assessment, the goal is to achieve the most authentic pattern

TABLE 6.12	The Magnificent 7 (Mag 7)

1. Range of motion
2. T4 mobility screen (wall angel)
3. Overhead squat
4. Single leg balance
5. Single leg squat
6. Single leg bridge
7. Breathing/core

possible to best serve as a window to evaluate the central nervous system.

Keeping in mind the importance of minimal cueing, the next section will explain the specific performance of the Mag 7 (Table 6.12 and Appendix). Realize that this is an un-loaded examination and that when repetitions, load, or speed is added poor patterns often improve while good patterns often deteriorate. Before anyone is qualified for load or speed these variables must be tested.

Range of Motion (70)

In the first test screen trunk ROM, or if there is a painful joint, assess the ROM of that joint (i.e., shoulder, hip) (Figure 6.16). See the Appendix, which uses the lumbar spine as an example, for scoring.

T4 Mobility Screen: Wall Angel Position (70)

To start, the person stands with the back against a wall with feet shoulder width apart and slightly forward of wall (Figure 6.17). Make sure the

- Arms are externally rotated/supinated and at shoulder height
- Buttocks are against the wall
- Back of head is against the wall with chin tucked to achieve a horizontal gaze
- Elbows are against the wall
- All five fingers are against the wall

Then attempt to

- Flatten wrist while maintaining all five fingers and the elbows on the wall
- Flatten the spine to the wall (This should be achieved with rib crunch and not a posterior tilt of the pelvis.)

See Appendix for scoring.

Overhead Squat (14)

Squatting occurs at about a year of life in the Sumo position and requires upright posture in the thoracic spine along

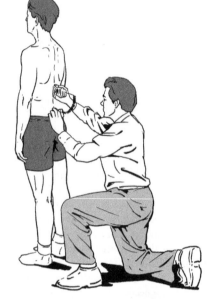

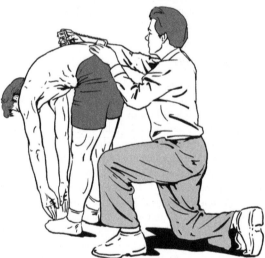

FIGURE 6-16.   Range of motion in lumbar spine.

with mobility in key areas such as the mid-thoracic spine and posterior hip capsule. Performed improperly during lifting tasks, it is a leading factor in the etiopathology of LBP due to disc disorders. The so-called "athletic posture" associated with the ready position in most sports (i.e., tennis, basketball, golf) is basically a squat. It is one of the most popular exercises, yet very commonly individuals will say, "I can't squat." Most trainers and rehabilitation experts know this means the individual most likely does not know how to squat correctly. Finally, passing an unloaded squat test does NOT qualify a person to add load. Adding load is a critical test in it's own right, therefore if the screen seeks to determine an individual's worthiness

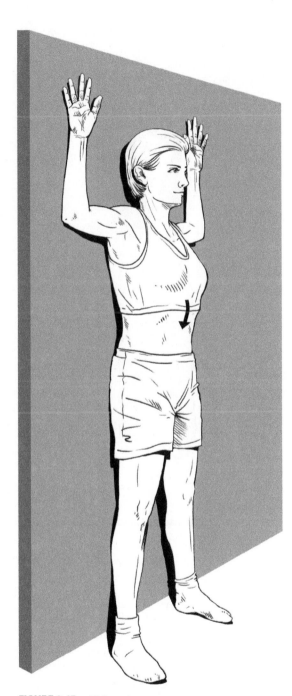

FIGURE 6-17. Wall angel.

to "go under the bar" how the spine behaves under load must also be assessed.

Have the person (Figure 6.18)

- Stand with feet shoulder width apart
- Raise arms overhead
- Squat down slowly until hips are below knees

Or use an alternate method with a dowel:

- Hold a dowel on top of head with elbows at 90°
- Raise dowel overhead

See Appendix for scoring.

For the reasons discussed above squat testing is amongst the most important in any movement screen. However, due to individual variability in hip joint anatomy certain individuals with "Scottish" hips may not be able to achieve the same depth as others (1). So long as an individual can identify the safe depth for their squat - where they can avoid losing the "neutral" lumbar spine posture - and stay in that functional training range then they are qualified to add repetitions, load , and/or speed. For this reason the Mag 7 scoring of the squat as a 1 should not be considered an absolute contra-indication for adding further challenge. The key is to find the range where the individual can maintain "neutral lordosis" and a) progress that range, and b) add repetitions, load, and/or speed within that range.

Every case is unique so that specific qualifications for assuring competency and therefore readiness for capacity training is not black and white. Clinical status, past history activity demands, anatomy (i.e. hip joint and disc), etc all factor into the decision-making.

To determine anatomical integrity for deep squatting there are two tests. One, supine palpation of the hip mobility with hip flexed at and beyond 90° hip flexion (1). Second, is the quadruped rocking manouvre to see at what moment the lumbar spine begins to flex. Hip width can be varied to look for anatomical clues regarding where the feet should be placed during squats (1).

Single Leg Balance Test (91–93)

- Have the patient stand on one leg and look straight ahead (with arms folded). The person can choose preferred one-leg stance position (Figure 6.19).
- Perform eyes open (EO) first, then use this instruction:
  - Stand on 1 leg & look straight ahead, focusing on a spot on the wall in front of you
  - Now, keep balancing, with eyes closed (EC)
  - Visualize the spot in front of you

The patient gets up to five tries on each leg, with a maximum of two EO trials and three EC trials. To save time perform only 1 repetition with EO and 2 with EC.

- Stop test if the patient maintains balance for 30 seconds
- Record time when subject
  - Hops
  - Moves foot
  - Reaches out and touches something with either hand

See Appendix for scoring.

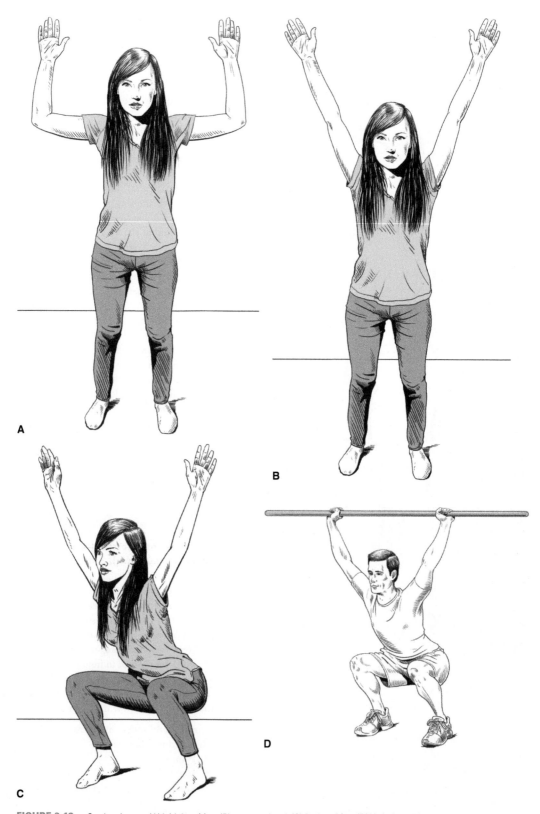

FIGURE 6-18. Overhead squat: (A) initial position; (B) arms overhead, (C) final position, (D) Variation with dowel.

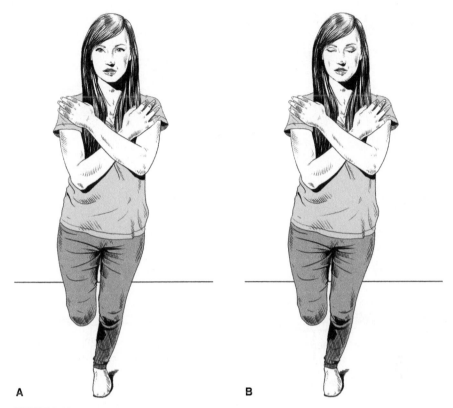

FIGURE 6-19.   Single leg balance: (A) eyes open; (B) eyes closed.

Single Leg Squat Test (60,70)

The single leg squat requires balance, strength, and frontal plane stability. It highlights the common compensatory dysfunction of quadriceps dominance. The single leg squat is a highly challenging test and predictive of knee injury due to valgus collapse of the knee (60,61). This assessment is much more challenging and sensitive than merely balancing on one leg. Passing an unloaded single leg squat test does not qualify a person to add speed or change of direction challenge. Adding speed such as landing a single leg box drop or single leg hopping or adding change of direction such as in "cutting" or decelerating a sprint are necessary in order to qualify a persons readiness for "return to sport". When modified, it is a great posterior chain exercise (e.g., single leg dead lift or box squat). All athletes should learn to train on a single leg even if they are concerned with developing power in their upper extremities such as pitching.

Have the patient (Figure 6.20)

- Squat to approximately 30° knee flexion
- Or perform off step (8″ or 20 cm high) with non-weight-bearing leg straight until heel gently touches floor. This is a typical stair step height.

See Appendix for scoring.

Single Leg Bridge

Have the patient (Figure 6.21)

- Lie supine with knees bent (approximately 90°)
- Push through heels allowing pelvis to lift to neutral
- Begin with alternating knee extension (three repetitions)
- Progress to single leg bridge with thighs parallel (three repetitions)
- Score right or left based on the supporting leg

See Appendix for scoring.

Respiration/Core (47,67,68,70,94–96)

Take the following steps:

- Observe habitual breathing in the upright (sitting or standing), recumbent, and supine triple flexion unsupported postures.
- Initially, avoid cueing the breath (Ideally, inspect while patients are unaware they are having their breathing assessed.)
- Finally, in the triple flexion position
  - Support the head if necessary to ensure a horizontal face line (i.e., avoid cervicocranial hyperextension)
  - Support the legs

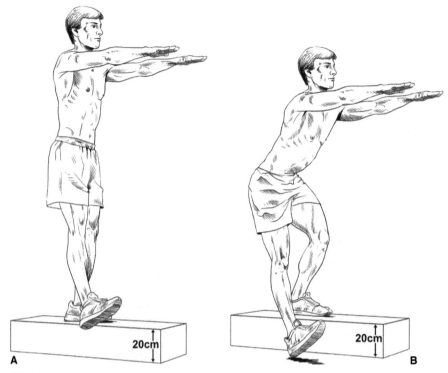

FIGURE 6-20. Single leg squat: (A) initial position; (B) final position.

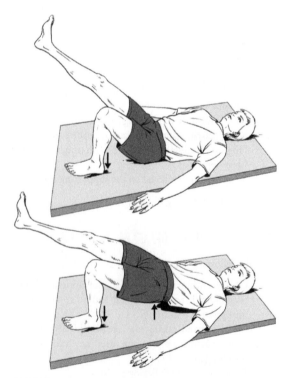

- Cue the subject to actively hold the rib cage in caudal depression
- Withdraw support from the legs after requesting the subject to hold the legs up
- Observe movement in the rib cage during inhalation and exhalation
- See Appendix for scoring. Illustrations of selected conditions: in upright or recumbent positions during inhalation, the rib cage or clavicle moves cephalad (Figures 6.22 and 6.23): 1 point
  - Paradoxical breathing: during inhalation the abdomen goes in (Figures 6.24 and 6.25): 1 point
  - During the cued triple flexion test: cephalad movement of the anterior-inferior rib cage (Figure 6.26): 1 point
  - Movement performed without compensation (note horizontal pattern) (Figure 6.27) and caudal anterior-inferior rib cage position (Figure 6.28): 3 points

After Performing a Functional Screen

It is important to create clinical groupings after performing a functional screen (Table 6.13). In interpreting the results of the functional screen, always prioritize to any test which is painful. This is termed the "marker" or MS. No training of this pattern occurs, but this should be reassessed for improvement after training or therapy. The marker

FIGURE 6-21. Single leg bridge.

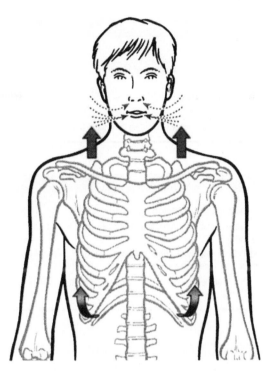

FIGURE 6-22. Faulty breathing pattern due to elevation of the rib cage: upright. From Liebenson C, ed. Rehabilitation of the Spine: A Practitioner's Manual. 2nd ed. Philadelphia, PA: Lippincott Williams & Wilkins; 2006.

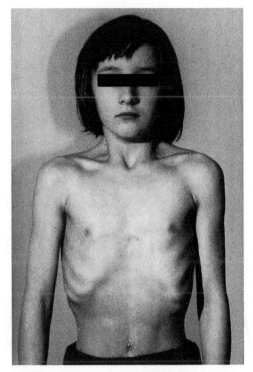

FIGURE 6-24. Paradoxical breathing—upright. From Liebenson C, ed. Rehabilitation of the Spine: A Practitioner's Manual. 2nd ed. Philadelphia, PA: Lippincott Williams & Wilkins; 2006.

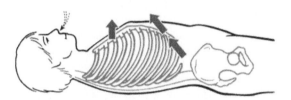

FIGURE 6-23. Faulty breathing pattern due to elevation of the rib cage: recumbent.

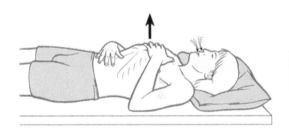

FIGURE 6-25. Paradoxical breathing—recumbent (on inhalation, belly moves in instead of out).

test should be distinguished from any tests which demonstrate painless dysfunction, also known as AMC (test with a score of 1). The painless dysfunction should be "re-set" with exercises in the individual's functional training range. This is the "painless range which is appropriate for the task at hand."

You can prioritize to sagittal (wall angel, overhead squat, breathing/IAP), frontal (one-leg balance or squat), or transverse (one-leg bridge) plane dysfunction for a variety of reasons:

- Sagittal plane: sedentary person due to excessive kyphosis from prolonged sitting
- Frontal plane: runner, soccer, or basketball player due to single leg stress
- Transverse plane: golf or tennis, hockey, baseball player due to repetitive torsion stress

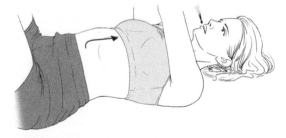

FIGURE 6-26. Triple flexion cephalad rib cage after cueing.

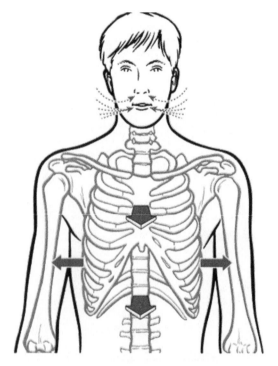

FIGURE 6-27. Normal breathing.

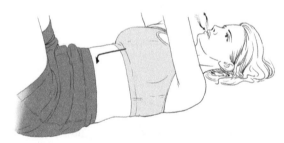

FIGURE 6-28. Caudal anterior-inferior rib cage position.

TABLE 6.13	Clinical Groupings

At least one test a 0: patient

At least one test a 1 or any asymmetries: at-risk individual

≥14 with all symmetric twos and threes: fit individual

After normalizing any fundamental AMC, reassess the MS using the painful test to see whether it is improved (Table 6.14). If it is, then progress from a movement competency foundation to the goal of building movement (or functional) capacity. An excellent rule of thumb is to distinguish between a primary mobility or stability problem (Table 6.15).

TABLE 6.14	Progression of Corrective Training

Identify painful tests

Identify and correct painless dysfunction in fundamental tests of all three planes

Reassess painful tests

If painful tests are improved, then progress from reestablishing movement competency to building movement capacity

TABLE 6.15	Mobility or Stability?

Mobility: active and passive testing positive

    Active prone hip extension and modified Thomas tests are both positive

Stability: only active testing positive (normal or hypermobile range of motion on passive testing)

    Active prone hip extension test positive, whereas modified Thomas test is negative

ADDITIONAL FUNCTIONAL TESTS

For fit individuals, the functional screen may not be sufficiently challenging to unmask their "weak link." They typically require additional testing to properly evaluate more demanding movements, such as with added load or speed, in order to reduce risk with strenuous activities or to establish athletic development goals to enhance their performance. What follows is a description of individual tests that provide an example of the different tests that can be performed when the functional screen is not capturing the necessary information. Functional testing is an evolving art and science, and this list is not intended to describe every test proposed by different experts. Rather, it is the authors' overview of a set which has shown to be valuable in practice along with many recommended in "evidence-based" sources. The reader is encouraged to keep an open mind and explore other tests such as the FMS and SFMA collections, drop box test, gait analysis, Dynamic Neuromuscular Stabilization evaluation, McGill's loaded examination (i.e. rope pull, loaded squat, box jump, and so on (1,13,14,60).

> A screening evaluation of AMC should include variables such as load and speed in order to qualify a person for higher level challenges or "return to sport".
> Ikeda DM, McGill SM. Can altering motions, postures, and loads provide immediate low back pain relief. Spine 2012;37:E1469–1475.

Basic testing should be divided into those that evaluate the domains presented in Table 6.16 (see also Table 6.17).

TABLE 6.16   Functional Testing Domains

Domains	Components	Sample Tests
Fundamental movement patterns	Upright posture, breathing, one-leg stance	One-leg stance balance, breathing, wall angel
Functional movement patterns	Scapulohumeral rhythm, squat, lunge, horizontal and vertical push/pull	Vele, overhead squat, single leg squat, inline lunge, hip abduction, active straight leg raise, seated hip flexion, arm abduction, trunk lowering from a push-up, neck flexion, C0-C1 flexion
Physical capacity	Range of motion, strength, endurance, cardiovascular endurance	Range of motion, side and front plank endurance, trunk flexor endurance, step test, treadmill test, repetition max test of push/pull/lift/etc
Athletic performance	Agility, power, speed	Three-cone drill, 5-10-5, 60-yard dash, vertical leap, broad jump, medicine ball chest pass, repeat sprint test

TABLE 6.17   Examples of Additional Screening Tests for Abnormal Motor Control

Vele's forward lean

Lunge test

Y balance test

Janda's hip abduction

Active straight leg raise

Seated hip flexion

Janda's hip extension

Side plank endurance (capacity test)

Front plank endurance (capacity test)

Trunk flexor endurance (capacity test)

Stability shear test

Intra-abdominal pressure test

Arm lifting test

Push-up

Arm abduction

Head/neck flexion

C0-C1 flexion

Mouth opening

Vele's Forward Lean

Purpose

- To assess the stability of the transverse arch of the foot and sagittal plane stability during a forward lean

Procedure (Figure 6.29)

- Have subject barefoot
- Lean forward from the ankles without bending at the waist

Signs of Failure

- Check for delayed or absent gripping and asymmetry
- Check for failure to lean from the heels or maintain the body in a plank position

Inline Lunge Test (14)

Purpose

- To evaluate lower extremity pain and/or LBP. Assess sagittal, frontal, and transverse plane control

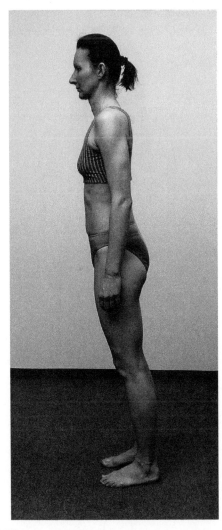

FIGURE 6-29.   Vele's forward lean. From Liebenson C, ed. Rehabilitation of the Spine: A Practitioner's Manual. 2nd ed. Philadelphia, PA: Lippincott Williams & Wilkins; 2006.

Procedure (Figure 6.30)

- Hands at side
- Step forward far enough so that heel of front foot should be 1–2″ in front of rear knee
- Step in line
- Balance for 2–3 seconds
- Then, rise back up to a standing position

Score

Check for excursion and motor control:

- Patellofemoral shear
- Hyperpronation
- Trunk flexion
- Balance

If positive, possible treatments to consider include lunges (with cueing or reactive training), psoas stretches and anterior hip capsule mobilization, or frontal plane and/or transverse plane stabilization.

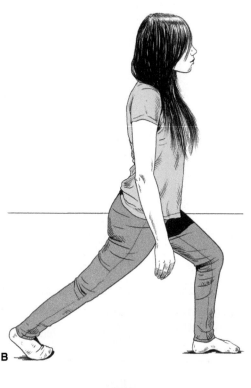

B

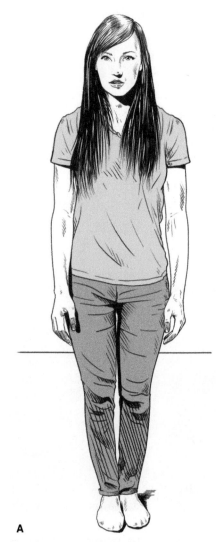

A

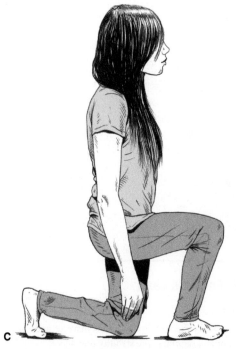

C

FIGURE 6-30. Lunge (A–C).

Y Balance Test (97–101)

Purpose

- To assess single-limb dynamic balance. The lower quarter Y balance test protocol evolved from the star excursion balance test.
- Upper quarter Y balance test: mobility, strength, and control are simultaneously challenged at the limit of balance control.
Procedure and Signs of Failure

Janda's Hip Abduction Movement Pattern (13,47,102)

Purpose

- To assess frontal plane stability

Procedure (see Figure 6.13)

- Side lying with lower leg flexed at hip and knee
- Pelvis perpendicular to the table
- Slowly raise leg straight up to the ceiling
- Perform resisted strength test with leg prepositioned in 20°–30° of pure hip abduction

Signs of Failure

- Pass/fail criteria: failure if the first 20° occurs with the following:
  - Hip flexion—tensor fascia latae substitution
  - Hip external rotation—piriformis substitution
  - Cephalad shift of pelvis (from initiation)—quadratus lumborum substitution
  - Pelvic rotation—substitution pattern indicating gluteus medius weakness
  - Reduced ROM in abduction—adductor tightness
  - Grade muscle strength _/5

Active Straight Leg Raise (70,103–106)

Purpose

- To assess core stability during supine hip flexion.

Procedure (Figure 6.31)

- Supine: have patient perform a straight leg raise 20 cm up from table.
- Patient may place hands under small of back to palpate loss of pressure and trunk rotation with the hands.

Signs of Failure

- Note if there is
  - Sacroiliac joint pain
  - Significant trunk rotation toward raised leg
  - Increased lordosis
  - Improved response with active bracing
- If the test is negative, add resistance and grade _/5

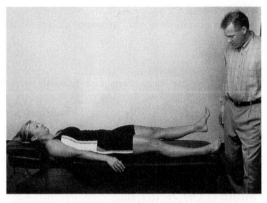

FIGURE 6-31. Active straight leg raise. From Liebenson C, ed. Rehabilitation of the Spine: A Practitioner's Manual. 2nd ed. Philadelphia, PA: Lippincott Williams & Wilkins; 2006.

Seated Hip Flexion Test (96)

Purpose

- To assess frontal and sagittal spine stability during seated hip flexion.

Procedure (Figure 6.32)

- Evaluator stands behind patient
- Subject's feet should not touch the ground
- Hands on thighs, with palms up
- Ask the subject to lift one knee up (about 3–4″ or 10 cm)
- Observe thoracic spine and trunk
- Observation may be repeated from the front
- Evaluator may add slight overpressure resistance to subject's knee as it is lifted up

Signs of Failure

- Shoulder unleveling
- Back bending, side bending, and/or rotation of the torso

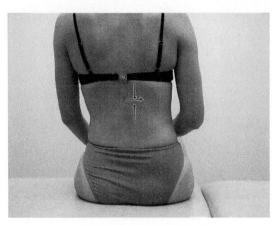

FIGURE 6-32. Seated hip flexion. From Liebenson C, ed. Rehabilitation of the Spine: A Practitioner's Manual. 2nd ed. Philadelphia, PA: Lippincott Williams & Wilkins; 2006.

- Pelvic torque/rotation
- Hyperactivation of the paraspinal muscles/trunk extension
- Hip hike
- Umbilical deviation
- Stabilizing leg recruitment with internal femoral rotation
- Asymmetrical hip flexor strength when offering resistance (can be graded _/5)
- Weak activation of the lateral abdominal muscles

Janda's Hip Extension Movement Pattern (13,47,70,107,108)

Purpose

- To assess coordination during hip extension.

Procedure (Figure 6.33)

- Prone
- Raise leg toward ceiling
- Perform resisted strength test (with leg in ~10° of hip extension)
- Note: patient may place hands under pelvis (ASIS) and palpate loss of pressure and trunk rotation with the hands.

Signs of Failure

- Pass/fail criteria: failure if at initiation
  - anterior pelvic tilt, lumbar hyperextension, or trunk rotation toward raised leg within first 10° of leg raising at the hip joint
  - delayed activation of the gluteus maximus
  - knee flexes—hamstring substitution
- Grade muscle strength _/5

Side Plank Endurance (109,110)

Purpose

- To identify an endurance deficit or asymmetry in the lateral stabilizers of the spine.

Procedure (Figure 6.34)

- Perform test on each side
- Raise pelvis from floor until spine is aligned
- Only feet and forearm/hand are on floor
- Evaluator times ability to maintain position

Signs of Failure

- Record time to failure
  - When pelvis begins to lower, cue to raise up again.
  - The second time pelvis drops from its peak height, the time is recorded as the failure time.
- Normative data (109)
  - Less than 45 seconds is dysfunctional (mean minus the standard deviation)
  - A side-to-side difference in time of greater than 5% is dysfunctional

Front Plank Endurance (110)

Purpose

- To identify an endurance deficit in the anterior stabilizers of the spine while maintaining a front plank.
- This is an alternative to the side plank endurance test if shoulder pain precludes performance of the test.

Procedure (Figure 6.35)

- Perform test on forearms and toes with forearms in a V position
- Raise torso from floor until it is horizontal
- Ability to maintain horizontal position is timed

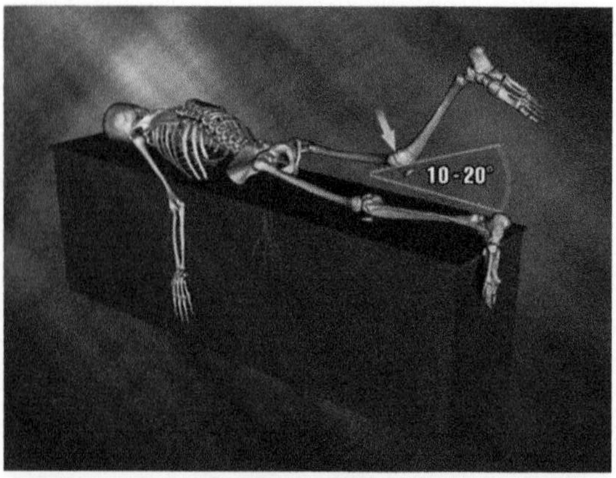

FIGURE 6-33.   Janda's hip extension. From Liebenson C, ed. Rehabilitation of the Spine: A Practitioner's Manual. 2nd ed. Philadelphia, PA: Lippincott Williams & Wilkins; 2006.

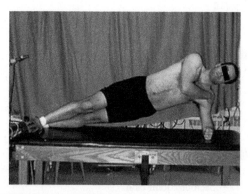

FIGURE 6-34.   Side plank endurance. From Liebenson C, ed. Rehabilitation of the Spine: A Practitioner's Manual. 2nd ed. Philadelphia, PA: Lippincott Williams & Wilkins; 2006.

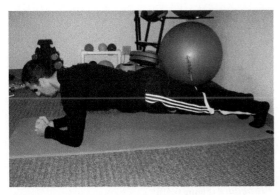

FIGURE 6-35. Front plank endurance.

Signs of Failure

- Record time to failure
  - When torso begins to lower, cue subject to raise up again.
  - The second time the torso drops from its peak height the time is recorded as the failure time.
- Normative data (109): less than 55 seconds is dysfunctional (mean minus the standard deviation)

Trunk Flexor Endurance (109,110)

Purpose

- To identify an endurance deficit in abdominal wall musculature while maintaining the trunk at a 50° angle.

Procedure (Figure 6.36)

- Leaning supported on 50° wedge
- Feet anchored by tester
- Wedge is pushed back 4″ and patient must maintain spinal alignment
- Ability to maintain position is timed

Signs of Failure

- Record time to failure (when trunk leans back into wedge). Patient is given cues if position is lost, multiple cues can be given until failure occurs
- Normally this endurance time is longer than the side bridge endurance time, but weaker than the trunk extensor endurance time
- Less than 50 seconds is dysfunctional (109)

Stability Shear Test (82)

Purpose

- To identify a patient who is likely to improve with stabilization exercise.

Procedure (Figure 6.37)

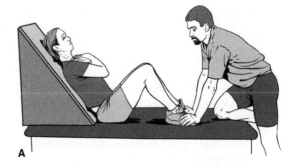

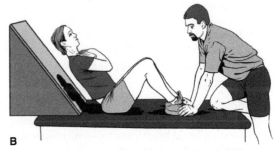

FIGURE 6-36. Trunk flexor endurance. (A) Initial position; (B) test position.

- Subject is prone with hips at edge of table and feet dangling off table
- Clinician performs posterior to anterior compressions
- If painful, then have subject raise legs up and recheck sensitivity

Interpretation

- If posterior to anterior compressions are now less painful with legs extended, stabilization training is indicated since muscle activity decreased pain
- If patient is not better with leg raising it does not mean stabilization is contraindicated, but patient will be more complex and progress slower

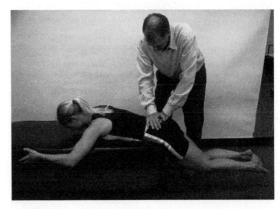

FIGURE 6-37. Stability shear. From Liebenson C, ed. Rehabilitation of the Spine: A Practitioner's Manual. 2nd ed. Philadelphia, PA: Lippincott Williams & Wilkins; 2006.

Intra-abdominal Pressure Test (96)

Purpose

- To assess the ability of the deep stabilization system (DSS) to handle load. The DSS refers to coordinated activity of the diaphragm, pelvic floor, abdominal wall, and spinal intrinsic muscles during loaded tasks.

Procedure (Figure 6.38)

- Subject lays supine (alternative position is seated)
- Hips/knees 90°/90°
- Evaluator supports legs
- Passively bring chest into caudal position
- Support at thoracolumbar junction
- Ask subject to actively hold this position
- Then, gradually remove support from legs

Signs of Failure

- Subject cannot hold caudal position
- Subject cannot keep support at thoracolumbar junction (avoid hyperextension)—will observe thoracolumbar hyperextension
- Minimal or absent activity in lateral-dorsal abdominal wall

Arm Lifting Test (96)

Purpose

- To assess coordination of the DSS during arm elevation overhead.

Procedure (Figure 6.39)

- Supine (or standing)
- The standard is in supine position—to relax the paraspinals.
- Subject lifts both arms slowly

Signs of Failure

- Thorax lifts cranially (unable to maintain expiratory rib position)
- Increased lordosis

Push-Up (13,43,70,111)

Purpose

- To assess scapulothoracic stability in the closed kinetic chain.

Procedure (Figure 6.40)

- In a push-up position from toes or knees
- Slowly lower and then raise the trunk up

Signs of Failure

- Scapulae retracts
- Scapulae wings
- Shoulders shrug

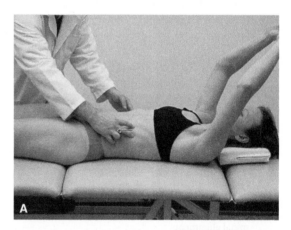

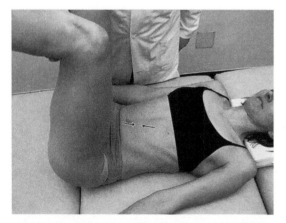

FIGURE 6-38. Intra-abdominal pressure test—normal. From Liebenson C, ed. Rehabilitation of the Spine: A Practitioner's Manual. 2nd ed. Philadelphia, PA: Lippincott Williams & Wilkins; 2006.

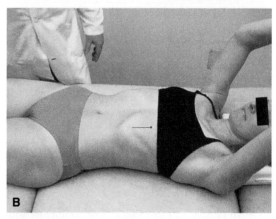

FIGURE 6-39. Arm lifting test: (A) correct; (B) incorrect. From Liebenson C, ed. Rehabilitation of the Spine: A Practitioner's Manual. 2nd ed. Philadelphia, PA: Lippincott Williams & Wilkins; 2006.

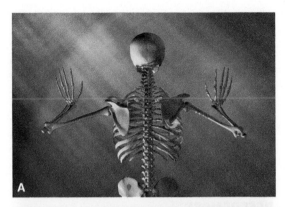

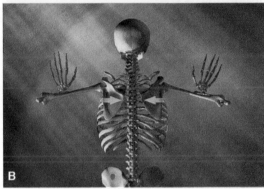

FIGURE 6-40. Push-up: (A) winging; (B) retraction.

Arm Abduction—Scapulohumeral Rhythm (13,41,43,44,47,70)

Purpose

- To identify abnormal movement during an arm abduction maneuver.

Procedure (see Figure 6.5)

- Arm at side, elbow bent 90°, and wrists in neutral position
- Slowly raise arm (abduction)

Signs of Failure

- During the "setting phase," first 60°, the shoulder should not elevate

Janda's Neck Flexion Coordination Test (13,37,40,70)

Purpose

- To identify coordination during head/neck flexion.

Procedure (Figure 6.41)

- Slowly raise head up from table toward chest

Signs of Failure

- Chin protrusion
- Sternocleidomastoid muscle overactivity
- Shaking

Cervicocranial Flexion (37,38)

Purpose

- To identify poor motor control during an isometric cervicocranial flexion endurance test.

Procedure (Figure 6.42)

- Patient demonstrates nodding motion. If patient is unable then clinician models motion on patient until he or she is able
- Inflate cuff to 20 mmHg
- With the chin nod motion, patient increases pressure to 22 mmHg and holds for 10 seconds
- Patient tries to increase pressure to 24, 26, 28, and 30 mmHg holding for 10 seconds with a rest period after each new level

Signs of Failure

- A positive test occurs with
  - overactivation of the superficial neck muscles
  - inability to hold a constant pressure at specific test level
  - an inability to achieve higher pressure levels (26–30 mmHg)

Mouth Opening Test (112)

Purpose

- To assess coordination during jaw opening, in particular the retrusion capability of the masticatory muscles.

FIGURE 6-41. Janda's neck flexion coordination test. From Liebenson C, ed. Rehabilitation of the Spine: A Practitioner's Manual. 2nd ed. Philadelphia, PA: Lippincott Williams & Wilkins; 2006.

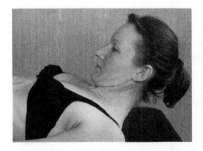

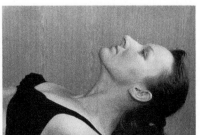

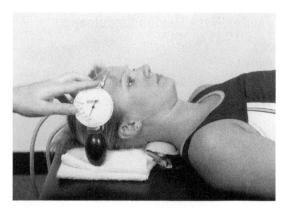

FIGURE 6-42. Cervicocranial flexion. From Liebenson C, ed. Rehabilitation of the Spine: A Practitioner's Manual. 2nd ed. Philadelphia, PA: Lippincott Williams & Wilkins; 2006.

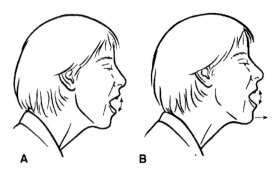

A   **B**

FIGURE 6-43. Mouth opening test (A and B). From Liebenson C, ed. Rehabilitation of the Spine: A Practitioner's Manual. 2nd ed. Philadelphia, PA: Lippincott Williams & Wilkins; 2006.

Procedure (Figure 6.43)

- Patient is instructed to open the mouth fully

Signs of Failure (Pass/Fail Criteria)

- Chin protrusion
- Decreased ROM (less than three knuckles vertical clearance)
- Head extension

CONCLUSIONS

It is crucial to be able to find faulty movement patterns or painless dysfunctions in order to accelerate pain management, rehabilitation, and athletic development. Identifying the underlying problem is the first step in establishing a foundation in movement competency. This in turn is a springboard for building the requisite functional capacity that an athlete requires. There are myriad methods to restore function, but without assessment and reassessment the health care provider or exercise specialist will never know if they are successful. In fact, a "gold standard" outcome or goal must be established to adjudicate that the improved function was relevant and not merely coincidental. In pain management the goal is a reduction in activity intolerances and MS. In rehabilitation, it is improvement in AMC (painless dysfunction). In athletic development, it is improvement in an independent measure of athleticism such as agility, speed, or power. Performing a motor control assessment, improving function, and finally auditing relevant outcomes is a logical way to offer athlete or patient-centered care.

REFERENCES

1. McGill SM. Ultimate Back Fitness and Performance. 4th ed. Waterloo, Canada: Backfitpro Inc.; 2009. ISBN 0-9736018-0-4. www.backfitpro.com
2. Janda V. Evaluation and Treatment of Faulty Movement Patterns. Los Angeles College of Chiropractic Visiting Scholar's Symposia; 1988.
3. Hahne A, Keating JL, Wilson S. Do within-session changes in pain intensity and range of motion predict between-session changes in patients with low back pain. Aust J Physiother 2004;50:17–23.
4. Tuttle N. Do changes within a manual therapy session predict between session changes for patients with cervical spine pain. Aust J Physiother 2005;20:324–330.
5. Tuttle N. Is it reasonable to use an individual patient's progress after treatment as a guide to ongoing clinical reasoning? J Manipulative Physiol Ther 2009;32:396–403.
6. Mascal CL, Landel R, Powers C. Management of patellofemoral pain targeting hip, pelvis, and trunk muscle function: 2 case reports. J Orthop Sports Phys Ther 2003;33:647–660.
7. McGill S, Grenier S, Bluhm M, et al. Previous history of LBP with work loss is related to lingering deficits in biomechanical, physiological, personal, psychosocial and motor control characteristics. Ergonomics 2003;46:731–746.
8. Powers CM. The influence of abnormal hip mechanics on knee injury: a biomechanical perspective. J Orthop Sports Phys Ther 2010;40:42–51.
9. Sciascia AD, Kibler WB. Conducting the "non-shoulder" shoulder examination. J Musculoskel Med 2006;23(8):582–598.
10. Wainner RS, Whitman JM, Cleland JA, Flynn TW. Regional interdependence: a musculoskeletal examination model whose time has come. J Orthop Sports Phys Ther 2007;37(11):658–660.
11. Bullock-Saxton JE, Janda V, Bullock MI. The influence of **ankle** sprain injury on muscle activation during hip extension Int J Sports Med 1994;15:330–334.
12. Travell J. Basic Principles of Myofascial Pain. DC Dental Society; 1985.
13. Janda V, Frank C, Liebenson C. Evaluation of muscle imbalance. In: Liebenson C, ed. Rehabilitation of the Spine: A Practitioner's Manual. Philadelphia, PA: Lippincott Williams & Wilkins; 2007:203–225.

14. Cook G, Burton L, Kiesel K, Rose G, Bryant MF. Movement: Functional Movement Systems: Screening, Assessment, Corrective Strategies. Aptos, CA: On Target Publications; 2010.

15. Waddell G. The Back Pain Revolution. 2nd ed. Edinburgh: Churchill Livingstone; 2004.

16. Bogduk, N. What's in a name? The labeling of back pain. Med J Aust 2000;173:400–401.

17. Kendrick D, Fielding K, Bentler E, et al. Radiography of the lumbar spine in primary care patients with low back pain: randomized controlled trial. BMJ 2001;322:400–405.

18. Boden SD, Davis DO, Dina TS, et al. Abnormal magnetic-resonance scans of the lumbar spine in asymptomatic subjects. J Bone Joint Surg [Am] 1990;72:403.

19. Hitselberger WE, Witten RM. Abnormal myelograms in asymptomatic patients. J Neurosurg 1968;28:204.

20. Bell GR, Rothman RH, Booth RE. A study of computer-assisted tomography. Spine 1984;9:548.

21. Wiesel SE, Tsourmans N, Feffer HL, et al. A study of computer-assisted tomography. I. The incidence of positive CAT scans in an asymptomatic group of patients. Spine 1984;9:549.

22. Brandt-Zawadzki MN, Jensen MC, Obuchowski N, et al. Interobserver and intraobserver variability in interpretation of lumbar disc abnormalities: a comparison of two nomenclatures. Spine 1995;20:1257–1263.

23. Jensel MC, Brant-Zawadzki MN, Obuchowki N, et al. Magnetic resonance imaging of the lumbar spine in people without back pain. N Engl J Med 1994;2:69.

24. Boden SD, McCowin PR, Davis DO, et al. Abnormal magnetic-resonance scans of the cervical spine in asymptomatic subjects. J Bone Joint Surg 1990;72A:1178–1184.

25. Teresi LM, Lufkin RB, Reicher MA, et al. Asymptomatic degenerative disk disease and spondylosis of the cervical spine: MR imaging. Radiology 1987;164:83–88.

26. Borenstein DG, O'Mara JW, Boden SD, et al. The value of magnetic resonance imaging of the lumbar spine to predict low-back pain in asymptomatic subjects. J Bone Joint Surg 2001;83-A:1306–1311.

27. Carragee EJ, Barcohana B, Alamin T, et al. Prospective controlled study of the development of lower back pain in previously asymptomatic subjects undergoing experimental discography. Spine 2004;29:1112–1117.

28. Baras JD, Baker LC, Health A. Magnetic resonance imaging and low back pain care for Medicare patients. Millwood 2009;28(6):w1133–w1140.

29. Fredericson M, Ho C, Waite B, et al. Magnetic resonance imaging abnormalities in the shoulder and wrist joints of asymptomatic elite athletes. PMR 2009;1(2):107–116.

30. Sher JS, Uribe JW, Posada A, et al. Abnormal findings on magnetic resonance images of asymptomatic shoulders. Bone Joint Surg Am 1995;77(1):10–15.

31. Connor PM, Banks DM, Tyson AB, et al. Magnetic resonance imaging of the asymptomatic shoulder of overhead athletes: a 5-year follow-up study. Am J Sports Med 2003;31(5):724–727.

32. Guten GN, Kohn HS, Zoltan DJ. False positive MRI of the knee: a literature review study. WMJ 2002;101(1):35–38.

33. De Smet AA, Nathan DH, Graf BK, et al. Clinical and MRI findings associated with false-positive knee MR diagnoses of medial meniscal tears. AJR Am J Roentgenol 2008;191(1):93–99.

34. Cholewicki J, McGill SM. Mechanical stability of the in vivo lumbar spine: implications for injury and chronic low back pain, Clin Biomech 1996;11(1):1–15.

35. Cholewicki J, Panjabi MM, Khachatryan A. Stabilizing function of the trunk flexor-extensor muscles around a neutral spine posture. Spine 1997;22:2207–2212.

36. Stokes IAF, Gardner-Morse M, Henry SM, Badger GJ. Decrease in trunk muscular response to perturbation with preactivation of lumbar spinal musculature. Spine 2000;25:1957–1964.

37. Jull G, Kristjansson E, Dall'Alba P. Impairment in the cervical flexors: a comparison of whiplash and insidious onset neck pain patients. Man Ther 2004;9:89–94.

38. Hodges P, Jull G. Spinal segmental stabilization training. In: Liebenson C, ed. Rehabilitation of the Spine: A Practitioner's Manual. Philadelphia, PA: Lippincott Williams & Wilkins; 2007:585–611.

39. Trelealvan J, Jull G, Sterling M. Dizziness and unsteadiness following whiplash injury: characteristic features and relationship with cervical joint position error. J Rehabil Med 2003;35:36–43.

40. Liebenson CS. Advice for the clinician and patient: functional reactivation for neck pain patients. J Bodywork Movement Ther 2002;6(1):59–68.

41. Babyar SR. Excessive scapular motion in individuals recovering from painful and stiff shoulders: causes and treatment strategies. Phys Ther 1996;76:226–238.

42. Liebenson C. Self-management of shoulder disorders—part 1. J Bodywork Movement Ther 2005;9:189–197.

43. Liebenson C. Shoulder disorders—part 2. J Bodywork Movement Ther 2005;9:283–292.

44. McQuade KJ, Dawson JD, Smidt GL. Scapulothoracic muscle fatigue associated with alterations in scapulohumeral rhythm kinematics during maximum resistive shoulder elevation. J Orthop Sports Phys Ther 1998;28:74.

45. Smith M, Sparkes V, Busse M, Enright S. Upper and lower trapezius muscle activity in subjects with subacromial impingement symptoms: is there imbalance and can taping change it? Phys Ther Sport 2008;10(2):45–50.

46. Kibler WB, McMullen J. Scapular dyskinesis and its relation to shoulder pain. J Am Acad Orthop Surg 2003;11:142–151.

47. Lewit K. Manipulative Therapy in Rehabilitation of the Motor System. 2nd ed. London: Butterworths; 1991.

48. Kolar P, Sulc J, Kyncl M, et al. Postural function of the diaphragm in persons with and without chronic low back pain. J Orthop Sports Phys Ther 2012;42(4):352–362.

49. Cholewicki J, McGill SM. Mechanical stability of the in vivo lumbar spine: implications for injury and chronic low back pain. Clin Biomech 1996;11(1):1–15.

50. Kujala UM, Taimela S, Salminen JJ, Oksanen A. Baseline arthropometry, flexibility and strength characteristics and future low-back-pain in adolescent athletes and nonathletes. A prospective, one-year, follow-up study. Scand J Med Sci Sports 1994;4:200–205.

51. Van Dillen LR, Sahrmann SA, Norton BJ, et al. The effect of active limb movements on symptoms in patients with low back pain. J Orthop Sports Phys Ther 2001;31:402–413.

52. Cholewicki J, Simons APD, Radebold A. Effects of external trunk loads on lumbar spine stability. J Biomech 2000;33(11):1377–1385.

53. Adams MA, Dolan P, Hutton WC. Diurnal variations in the stresses on the lumbar spine. Spine 1987;12:130.

54. Snook SH, Webster BS, McGorry RW, Fogleman MT, McCann KB. The reduction of chronic nonspecific low back pain through the control of early morning lumbar flexion. Spine 1998;23:2601–2607.

55. Reeves NP, Narendra KS, Cholewicki J. Spine stability: the six blind men and the elephant. Clin Biomech 2007;22(3):266–274.

56. Reeves NP, Cholewicki J. Expanding our view of the spine system. Eur Spine J 2010;19(2):331–332.

57. Cholewicki J, Panjabi MM, Khachatryan A. Stabilizing function of the trunk flexor-extensor muscles around a neutral spine posture. Spine 1997;22:2207–2212.

58. Panjabi MM. The stabilizing system of the spine. Part 1. Function, dysfunction, adaptation, and enhancement. J Spinal Disord 1992;5:383–389.

59. Cholewicki J, Silfies SP, Shah RA, et al. Delayed trunk muscle reflex responses increase the risk of low back injuries. Spine 2005;30(23):2614–2620.

60. Hewett TE, Myer GD, Ford KR, et al. Biomechanical measures of neuromuscular control and valgus loading of the knee predict anterior cruciate ligament injury risk in female athletes: a prospective study. Am J Sports Med 2005;33(4):492–501.

61. Hewett TE, Myer GD, Ford KR. Anterior cruciate ligament injuries in female athletes: part 1, mechanisms and risk factors. Am J Sports Med 2006;34:299–311.

62. McLean SG, Walker K, Ford KR, et al. Evaluation of a two dimensional analysis method as a screening and evaluation tool for anterior cruciate ligament injury. Br J Sports Med 2005;39(6):355–362.

63. Powers CM. The influence of altered lower-extremity kinematics on patellofemoral joint dysfunction: a theoretical perspective. J Orthop Sports Phys Ther 2003;33:639–646.

64. Myer GD, Ford KR, Barber Foss KD, et al. The incidence and potential pathomechanics of patellofemoral pain in female athletes. Clin Biomech 2010;25:700–707.

65. Zazulak BT, Ponce PL, Straub SJ, et al. Gender comparison of hip muscle activity during single-leg landing. J Orthop Sports Phys Ther 2005;35(5):292–299.

66. Baratta R, Solomonow M, Zhou BH, et al. Plyometric training in female athletes. Decreased impact forces and increased hamstring torques. Am J Sports Med 1988;16(2):113–122.

67. Lewit K. Relation of faulty respiration to posture, with clinical implications. JAOA 1980;79:75–79.

68. Liebenson CS. Advice for the clinician and patient: mid-thoracic dysfunction (Part One): overview and assessment. J Bodywork Movement Ther 2001;5:2.

69. Liebenson CS. Advice for the clinician and patient: mid-thoracic dysfunction (Part Three): clinical issues. J Bodywork Movement Ther 2001;5:4.

70. Liebenson C, Skaggs C, Fonda S, Deily S. Integrated approach to the cervical spine. In: Liebenson C, ed. Rehabilitation of the Spine: A Practitioner's Manual. Philadelphia, PA: Lippincott Williams & Wilkins; 2007:852–886.

71. Janda V. Some aspects of extracranial causes of facial pain. J Prosthet Dent 1986;56:484–487.

72. Kebaetse M, McClure P, Pratt NA. Thoracic position effect on shoulder range of motion, strength, and three-dimensional scapular kinematics. Arch Phys Med Rehabil 1998;80:945–950.

73. Lukasiewicz AC, McClure P, Michener L, et al. Comparison of 3-dimensional scapular position and orientation between subjects with and without shoulder impingement. J Orthop Sports Phys Ther 1999;29:574–586.

74. Harryman DT II, Sidles JA, Clark JM, et al. Translation of the humeral head on the glenoid with passive glenohumeral motion. J Bone Joint Surg 1990;72A:1334–1343.

75. Bullock MP, Foster NE, Wright CC. Shoulder impingement: the effect of sitting posture on shoulder pain and range of motion. Man Ther 2005;10:28–37.

76. Godges JJ, Matson-Bell M, Shah D, Thorpe D. The immediate effects of soft tissue mobilization with PNF on shoulder external rotation and overhead reach. J Orthop Sports Phys Ther 2003;33:713–718.

77. Tyler TF, Nicholas SJ, Ory T, Gleim G. Quantification of posterior capsule tightness and motion loss in patients with shoulder impingement. Am J Sports Med 2000;28: 668–673.

78. Young JL, Herring SA, Press JM, et al. The influence of the spine on the shoulder in the throwing athlete. J Back Musculoskel Rehab 1996;7:5–17.

79. Boyles RE, Ritland RM, Miracle BM, et al. The short-term effects of thoracic thrust manipulation on patients with shoulder impingement syndrome. Man Ther 2009;14: 375–380.

80. Cleland JA, Childs JD, Fritz JM, Whitman JM, Eberhart SL. Development of a clinical prediction rule for guiding treatment of a subgroup of patients with neck pain: use of thoracic spine manipulation, exercise, and patient education. Phys Ther 2007;87:9–23.

81. Herman M, Thomas T, Tai-Hing L. The effectiveness of thoracic manipulation on patients with chronic mechanical neck pain—a randomized controlled trial. Man Ther 2011;16:141–147.

82. McGill SM. Low Back Disorders: The Scientific Foundation for Prevention and Rehabilitation. Champaign, IL: Human Kinetics; 2002.

83. Janda V. Muscles, central nervous motor regulation and back problem. In: Korr IM, ed. The Neurobiologic Mechanisms of Manipulative Therapy. New York, NY: Plenum Press; 1978:27–41.

84. Boyle M. Advances in Functional Training. Aptos, CA: On Target Publications; 2010.

85. Kibler WB, Herring SA, Press JM. Functional Rehabilitation of Sports and Musculoskeletal Injuries. Gaithersburg, MD: Aspen; 1998.

86. Herring SA. Rehabilitation of muscle injuries. Med Sci Sports Exerc 1990;22:453–456.

87. Janda V. On the concept of postural muscles and posture in man. Aust J Physiother 1983;29:83–84.

88. Gray G. Lower Extremity Functional Profile. Adrian, MI: Wynn Marketing; 1995.

89. Frost DM, Beach TAC, Callaghan JP, McGill SM. Using a movement screen to evaluate the effectiveness of training. J Strength Cond Res 2011:1620–1630.

90. Moreside JM, McGill S M. Improvements in hip flexibility and/or core stability does not transfer to function. Phys Ther Journal of Strength & Conditioning Research. 2013;27(10):2635–2643.

91. Maribo T, Iverson E, Andresen N, Stengaard-Pedersen K, Schiottz-Christensen B. Intra-observer and interobserver reliability of one leg stand test as a measure of postural balance in low back pain patients. Int Musc Med 2009;31:172–177.

92. Bohannon RW, Larkin PA, Cook AC, Gear J, Singer J. Decrease in timed balance test scores with aging. Phys Ther 1984;64:1067–1070.

93. Byl N, Sinnot PL. Variations in balance and body sway in middle-aged adults: subjects with healthy backs compared with subjects with low-back dysfunction. Spine 1991;16:325–330.

94. Travell J, Simons D. Myofascial Pain and Dysfunction, The Trigger Point Manual: The Upper Extremities. Baltimore, MD: Williams & Wilkins; 1983.

95. Chaitow L, Delany JW. Clinical Application of Neuromuscular Techniques. Volume 1: The Upper Body. London: Harcourt Publishers; 2000.

96. Kolár P. Facilitation of agonist-antagonist co-activation by reflex stimulation methods. In: Liebenson C, ed. Rehabilitation of the Spine: A Practitioner's Manual. 2nd ed. Philadelphia, PA: Lippincott; 2007:532–565.

97. Plisky PJ, Rauh MJ, Kaminski TW, Underwood FB. Star Excursion Balance Test predicts lower extremity injury in high school basketball players. J Orthop Sports Phys Ther 2006;36(12):911–919.

98. Lehr ME, Plisky PJ, Kiesel KB, Butler RJ, Fink M, Underwood FB. Field expedient screening and an injury risk algorithm predicts non-contact[Q71] lower extremity injury in collegiate athletes. Sports Health. (in review).

99. Gribble PA, Hertel J, Plisky PJ. Using the star excursion balance test to assess dynamic postural control deficits and outcomes in lower extremity injury. J Athl Train (in press).

100. Gorman PP, Plisky PJ, Butler RJ, et al. Upper quarter Y balance test: reliability and performance comparison between genders in active adults. J Strength Cond Res 2012;26(11):3043–3048.

101. Plisky PJ, Gorman P, Kiesel K, Butler R, Underwood F, Elkins B. The reliability of an instrumented device for measuring components of the Star Excursion Balance Test. NAJSPT 2009;4(2):92–99.

102. Nelson-Wong E, Flynn T, Callaghan JP. Development of active hip abduction as a screening test of identifying occupational low back pain. J Orthop Sports Phys Ther 2009;39:649–657.

103. Mens JM, Vleeming A, Snijders CJ, et al. Reliability and validity of the active straight leg raise test in posterior pelvic pain since pregnancy. Spine 2001;26:1167–1171.

104. Liebenson C, Karpowicz A, Brown S, et al. The active straight leg raise test and lumbar spine stability. Phys Med Rehabil 2009;1(6):530–535.

105. O'Sullivan PB, Beales DJ, Beetham JA, et al. Altered motor control strategies in subjects with sacroiliac joint pain during the active straight-leg-raise test. Spine 2002;27:E1–E8.

106. Pool-Goudzwaard A, Vleeming A, Stoeckart C, Snijders CJ, Mens MA. Insufficient lumbopelvic stability: a clinical, anatomical and biomechanical approach to "a-specific" low back pain. Man Ther 1998;3:12–20.

107. Hu Y, Wong YL, Lu WW, Kawchuk GN. Creation of an asymmetrical gradient of back muscle activity and spinal stiffness during asymmetrical hip extension. Clin Biomech 2009;24:799–806.

108. Vogt L, Banzer W. Dynamic testing of the motorial stereotype in prone hip extension from the neutral position. Clin Biomech 1997;12:122–127.

109. McGill S, Childs A, Liebenson C. Endurance times for low back stabilization exercises: clinical targets for testing and training from a normative database. Arch Phys Med Rehabil 1999;80:941–944.

110. McGill SM, Belore M, Crosby I, Russell C. Clinical tools to quantify torso flexion endurance: normative data from student and firefighter populations. Occup Ergon 2010;9: 55–61.

111. Uhl TL, Carver TJ, Mattacola CG, Mair SD, Nitz AJ. Shoulder musculature activation during upper extremity weight-bearing exercise. J Orthop Sports Phys Ther 2003;33:109–117.

112. Liebenson CS, Skaggs C. The role of chiropractic treatment in whiplash injury. In: Malanga G, Nadler S, eds. Whiplash. Philadelphia, PA: Hanley and Belfus; 2002:313–338.

The Magnificent 7

Name _____ Date _____

1. Joint ROM of Chief Complaint (e.g. Lumbar)

ROM	Pass (3) ☐
	Pain (0)
	>50% loss = 1
__/65	Flexion (2)
__/30	Extension (2)
__/25	L Side Bending (2)-no smooth convexity
__/25	R Side Bending (2)-no smooth convexity
	Hypermobility (2)
A S	TOTAL SCORE (0-3)

2. Wall Angel Position

L	R	Pass (3) ☐
		Pain (0)
		Head not vs. wall with horiz eyes-FHP (1)
		All five fingers not touching wall (1)
		↓ Shldr Ex Rot (wrist >1 cm fr wall) (1)
		No ant. rib cage motion with flattening back (1)
		Wrist not flat vs. wall (2)
		T/L lordosis > 1 cm from wall (2)
A S		TOTAL SCORE (0-3)

3. Overhead Squat

L	R	Pass (3) ☐
		Pain (0)
		Arms do not reach vertically OH (1)
		Thighs do not reach past horiz. (1)
		L/S Flexion before thighs horiz. (1)
		Heels raise before thighs horiz. (1)
		L/S Flexion when thighs are horiz. (2)
		Chin poke/Neck not packed in (2)
		Knee Valgus (2)
		Anterior Patellar Shear (2)
		Hyperpronation (2)
A S		TOTAL SCORE (0-3)

4. Single Leg Balance

L	R	Pass (3) ☐
		Pain (0)
		< 10 sec EO on either leg (1)
		< 5 sec EC on either leg (1)
		< 30 sec EC on either leg (2)
		Hyperpronation (2)
		> 1" Pelvic side shift (2)
		Trendelenburg sign (2)
		EC Best Time
A S		TOTAL SCORE (0-3)

5. Single Leg Squat

L	R	Pass (3) ☐
		Pain (0)
		Can't squat to 30 deg. knee flexion (1)
		Knee valgus (medial to Gr Toe) (1)
		L/S Flexion (2)
		Anterior Patellar Shear (2)
		Trendelenburg sign (2)
		Hyperpronation (2)
A S		TOTAL SCORE (0-3)

6. Single Leg Bridge (kicks & up/down)

L	R	Pass (3) ☐
		Pain (0) - Descent/Ascent
		Pelvic drop or rotation (1)
		Can't maintain full hip extension (2)
		Thighs don't remain parallel (2)
A S		TOTAL SCORE (0-3)

7. Respiration/IAP		
	Pass (3) ☐	
	Pain (0)	
	Paradox resp inhale - abdomen in (1) **Ribs ↑ in upright/vert test (1)**	
	IAP-Cued 3 Flxn ↑ ant-inf rib cage (1)	
	Chest breathing predominates on inhal (2)	
	Lower rib cage does not widen laterally (2)	
	IAP-Uncued 3 Flxn ↑ ant-inf rib cage (2)	
	TOTAL SCORE (0-3)	

Scoring (from G Cook (14))

0 Painful
1 Cannot perform
2 Performs w/ compensation
3 Performs w/ out compensation

FHP = forward head posture
OH = overhead
L/S = lumbo-sacral
EO = eyes open
EC = eyes closed
A = asymmetric
S = symmetric

Total Score (max 21)

CHAPTER 7

Craig Liebenson, Jason Brown, and Jeff Cubos

Fundamentals of Training the Locomotor System

THE AIM OF TRAINING

The aim of training is to promote athletic development and durability (e.g., injury prevention) so as to enhance performance (see Chapter 34). Developing the athlete requires an integrated approach focused on the whole person rather than just individual components. Vern Gambetta, a well respected coach has said, "All components of physical performance: strength, power, speed, agility, endurance and flexibility must be developed" (1). Athletic development coaches improve athletic performance by preparing athletes to be adaptable and to handle all demands required to compete (see Chapter 35).

> The *goal of training* is "to cause biologic adaptations in order to improve performance in a specific task." McArdle and Katch (2)

Athletes who avoid injury and/or recover quickly are able to develop their skills faster and to higher levels, thanks to consistent training and practice. In contrast, "injury-prone" athletes are not only frequently unable to participate but also unable to develop the skill sets necessary to subsequently perform at high levels. Previous injury is the most powerful predictor for future injury, suggesting that appropriate rehabilitation is likely a key factor in promoting durability and thus athletic development (3). The challenge in training is finding the right balance between intensity and recovery to build athletes up without inadvertently breaking them down.

High demand combined with a capacity shortfall may lead to injury or pain. The key to increasing an athlete's durability is to increase functional integrity or capacity. Functional capacity must exceed the physiological demands or stress of one's sport or activities (Figure 7.1). The surplus capacity will provide a stability margin of error, therefore reducing injury risk. Functional capacity as a concept is one which is built on a foundation of movement competency (see Chapter 6).

Athletic development is crucial to team success. Significant relationships have been found between team average jump height (countermovement jump and standing jump) and team success (4), as well as inverse relationships among

leg extension power and body composition (% body fat) with total number of injury days per team (4).

Athletic development and increasing durability should incorporate the fundamental ABCs of agility, balance, and coordination (i.e. movement competency) and progress into other athletic traits such as posture, mobility, strength, endurance, power, and speed. The strongest person is not necessarily the best athlete, and strength has not been shown to prevent injury (5,6). Verstegen said, "You can be strong without being powerful (because you can't get that strength into motion quickly), but you can't be powerful without having underlying strength of muscles and muscle groups" (7).

Movement competency to ensure injury prevention is the pre-requisite for embarking on a program to build capacity. When competency is assured then capacity can safely become the focus of training. To build capacity, the individual needs to work at the edge of his/her capabilities (Figures 7.2 and 7.3). Training on the edge of the envelope will promote athletic development and increase durability. Walking this thin line has inherent pitfalls, as building up will always entail a risk of breaking down. The skilled professional will guide the athlete effectively to the appropriate type, intensity, and duration of training. In athletic training, the phrase "no pain no gain" holds only a small degree of truth. While hard work, sweat, and pain will help build the necessary capacity to enhance performance traits, pain attributed to joints must always be distinguished from pain attributed to muscles. For example, knee pain, especially medial or lateral joint line pain, should be seen as a warning sign while quadriceps or gluteal "burn" would be the goal!

> "The objective of injury prevention strategies is to ensure that tissue adaptation stimulated from exposure to load keeps pace with, and ideally exceeds the accumulated tissue damage." McGill (8)

LESSONS FROM CLINICAL REHABILITATION

Rehabilitation of the motor system is a systematic approach to restoring function. The aim is to facilitate recovery from injury, to prevent recurrences, and to enhance performance. Functional rehabilitation is part of the continuum of care bridging the gap between pain management and athletic development.

Continuum of Care

- Pain management/recovery, including diagnostic triage (orthopedic/neurologic/red flags)
- Rehabilitation (competency)
- Athletic development/capacity
- Skill/performance

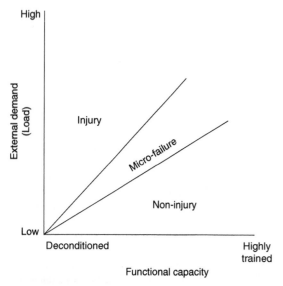

FIGURE 7-1. Relationship between external demand and functional capacity. From Liebenson C, ed. Rehabilitation of the Spine: A Practitioner's Manual. 2nd ed. Philadelphia, PA: Lippincott Williams & Wilkins; 2006.

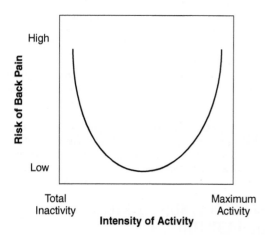

FIGURE 7-2. Too much or too little. From Liebenson C, ed. Rehabilitation of the Spine: A Practitioner's Manual. 2nd ed. Philadelphia, PA: Lippincott Williams & Wilkins; 2006.

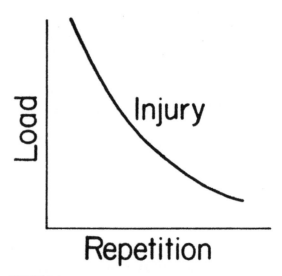

FIGURE 7-3. Excessive load or excessive repetitions. From Liebenson C, ed. Rehabilitation of the Spine: A Practitioner's Manual. 2nd ed. Philadelphia, PA: Lippincott Williams & Wilkins; 2006.

"Too Much, Too Soon"

Middle-aged "weekend warriors" and overly ambitious young athletes commonly have difficulty distinguishing "hurt from harm." They often train too aggressively, with little regard paid to potentially injurious pain sensations or conversely devote much of their awareness to both noxious and non-noxious training stimuli. Stoicism leads many people to ignore "stop rules" (9) in training, consequently leading to a "boom–bust" cycle (Figure 7.4) (10). The "as many as you can" approach leads to persistence until the task is completed and unfortunately frequent painful recurrences (11).

Popular approaches such as CrossFit, P90X, and Insanity workouts are tantalizing with their rapid gains but often foster a boom–bust cycle. These workouts can be risky because the line between building and breaking can become blurred.

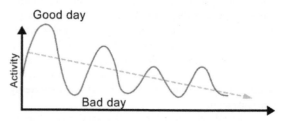

FIGURE 7-4. Boom–bust cycle. Adapted from J Bodywork Movement Ther 2011:1–18. Liebenson, C. Musculoskeletal Myths. J Bodywork Movement Ther 2012;16:165–182.

Pacing

Like rehabilitation, the best approach to training is one that is progressive, planned, and monitored. According to McGill, injury is usually the result of "a history of excessive loading which gradually, but progressively, reduces the tissue failure tolerance" (Figure 7.5) (8). The preferred approach for training therefore incorporates pacing. After exposure to load, in order to build capacity, a period of rest must be implemented to reset the failure tolerance threshold (Figure 7.6) (8). Ironically, this is also true for prolonged static strain such as from sitting where a "microbreak" of movement can reset the failure tolerance threshold (Figure 7.7).

Pacing can also be seen in its cognitive-behavioral context which is "quota-based" or uses "graded exposure" (12–14). "Quota-based" consists of the patient's activity levels being gradually increased, in a stepwise manner limited by quota rather than pain (Figure 7.8). Additionally, periods of rest and recovery must also be built into programs and continuous monitoring must be employed to make necessary adaptations, especially for athletes during competitive seasons and in the presence of recent injury.

Identify Preparedness for Training

Other contemporary methods for monitoring training include measuring load/power output in a specific set (e.g., using a Keiser with power display), monitoring heart rate variability, using a Tendo unit to assess velocity of a loaded movement, or timed set drop offs (15,16). When coaches, trainers, or practitioners see downward deviations in these markers, it can be an early sign that the athlete is overtrained or for some other reason is physiologically compromised. Further exploration will likely reveal other methods of assessing an athlete's readiness for training.

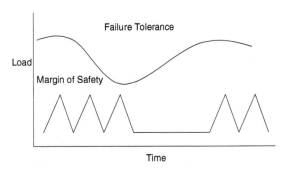

FIGURE 7-6. Failure tolerance restored with pacing. Modified from McGill S. Lower Back Disorders: Evidence-Based Prevention and Rehabilitation. Champaign, IL: Human Kinetics; 2002.

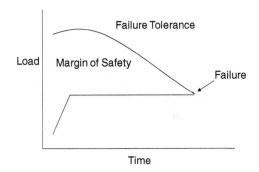

FIGURE 7-7. Failure tolerance decreases with prolonged static strain. Modified from McGill S, Lower Back Disorders: Evidence-Based Prevention and Rehabilitation. Champaign, IL: Human Kinetics; 2002.

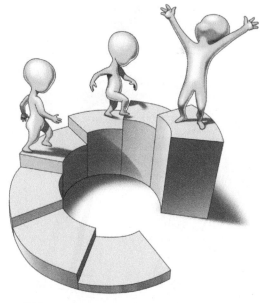

FIGURE 7-8. Paced activity.

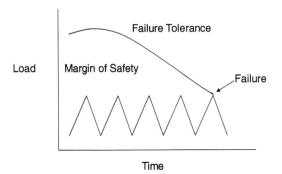

FIGURE 7-5. Failure tolerance decreasing with repetitive strain. Modified from McGill S. Lower Back Disorders: Evidence-Based Prevention and Rehabilitation. Champaign, IL: Human Kinetics; 2002.

Quantity versus Quality

Traditional rehabilitation therapy and fitness training have taught the exercise mantra of "three sets of 10" with little regard paid to specificity of demand. The SAID principle, or Specific Adaptation to Imposed Demands, suggests that the locomotor system adapts to demands placed upon it. Additionally, traditional bodybuilding culture has emphasized isolating individual muscles for hypertrophy while our contemporary understanding of physiology explains, "the brain doesn't think in terms of individual muscles. It thinks in terms of movement." Janda was the first to show that what is important is not how much weight you can lift, but the skill or quality of the movement pattern that is used (17,18). Bigger is not necessarily better, and the strongest athlete in the weight room is rarely the best athlete on the field (Figure 7.9). Thus for athletes, quality of movement is essential, not quantity. Or as Cook says, "Don't build strength on top of dysfunction" (19).

"Too Little, Too Late"

"Let pain be your guide" is a famous adage following acute injury. This is perfectly sensible, especially in the presence of tissue damage (i.e., ligament or tendon), fracture,

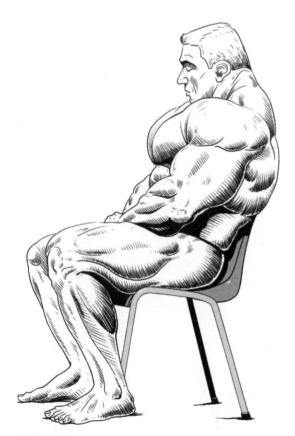

FIGURE 7-9.   "Bigger isn't better."

or similar diagnosis. Unfortunately, many athletes adhere solely to this approach and wait until pain subsides to resume even controlled movement. Such an approach often prolongs recovery and leads to excessive scar tissue buildup and muscle atrophy. Therefore, as swelling subsides early, active mobilization is required to prevent poor resolution and low-quality healing of the injured tissues.

Additionally, in recurrently injured and chronic pain patients, reactivation should be gradual. Individuals who assume "hurt equals harm" follow a "stop rule" called "feel like discontinuing" often leading to early task termination. In such cases, *pain is not a good guide* since appropriate activities may be necessarily uncomfortable. Allowing pain to be a guide leads to activity avoidance and deconditioning.

When training patients or athletes, bear in mind the saying, "the hurt you feel becomes the feeling you hurt" (20). The brain's representation zone for a specific tissue becomes more focused or sensitized. Therefore, in athletes coming off a long-term injury, it is important to realize that what they experience may be influenced by their perceptions.

> Remember, hurt does not equal harm, but people with chronic pain assume it does.

It is important to minimize "labeling" in a clinical setting. This will only validate in the patient's mind that the tissue *site* of symptoms is the key. However, the longer the duration of pain, the greater the likelihood that the issue at hand is really one of pain amplification or processing error. Pain thresholds shift downward in chronic pain so that allodynia (pain felt in response to nonnoxious stimuli) occurs. This is mediated by glial cells undergoing functional and structural changes, a process that amplifies and distorts nociceptive signals (21–23). Melzack has described how neurosignatures are transcribed in the central nervous system (CNS) from perceived threat that outlasts the time it would take for an injured peripheral tissue to heal (24). A famous example in which pain persists without the tissue itself being involved occurs in phantom limb pain in an amputee (Figure 7.10). A novel treatment for phantom limb pain or reflex sympathetic dystrophy, which works on downregulation from the CNS to the periphery, is mirror box therapy (Figure 7.11).

The neurology of pain being in the brain and not the tissue begins with sensitization. Pain markers in the dorsal horn undergo physical change, which results in allodynia and hyperalgesia (exaggerated pain responses). Brain imaging data show that the representation site in the brain that is activated corresponds to the perceived, not the actual, location of stimulation (25).

Therefore, pacing is just as important to the "as many as can" person who falls into the "boom–bust" patterns as to the "feel like discontinuing" person who never achieves his or her full potential due to insufficient conditioning. Adopting a pacing or graduated approach to training that is "quota-based" results in adaptation to necessary

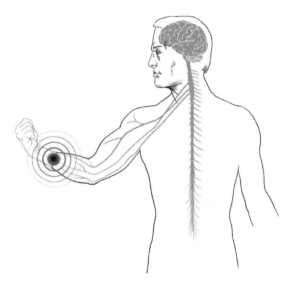

FIGURE 7-10. Phantom limb pain.

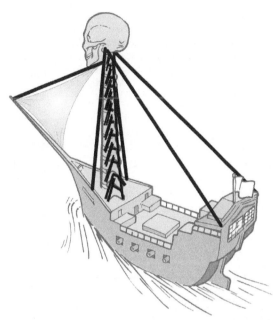

FIGURE 7-12. Antagonist muscle coactivation for spinal stability.

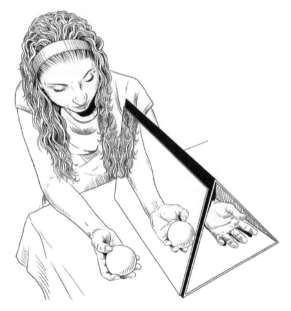

FIGURE 7-11. Mirror box therapy.

applied stress, while simultaneously minimizing the risk of recurrent or new injury.

How Does the Body Resist Injury?

In rehabilitation settings, stability (competency) not strength (capacity) is the objective. The spinal column without muscles buckles at a load of 90 N (20 lb), and according to Panjabi (26), "This large load carrying capacity is achieved by the participation of well-coordinated muscles surrounding the spinal column." Such antagonist muscle coactivation is necessary for aiding ligaments in maintaining

joint stability during loaded tasks (Figure 7.12). Both deep and superficial muscles participate in providing this intermuscular coordination (Figure 7.13). Cocontractions increase spinal compressive load, as much as 12% to 18% or 440 N, but more importantly greatly increase spinal stability by 36% to 64% or 2,925 N (27). They have been shown to occur during most daily activities (28). This mechanism is present to such an extent that without cocontractions the spinal column is unstable even in upright postures! (29). It is the coordinated timing of these muscular contractions that is essential to achieving stability, not merely the force produced by individual muscles.

> At the University of Waterloo, McGill (8) has measured muscle activation versus spine load during a wide variety of different popular and novel exercises (Figure 7.14).
> - Routine activities of daily living (ADLs)—2,000 N
> - National Institute of Occupational Safety and Health limit—6,400 N
> - Acute/subacute low back pain—3,000 N

The **sit-up** is a good example where information about spinal load is necessary for clinicians (8). The traditional sit-up involves 3,350 N of force (Figure 7.15). The clinician dealing with low back pain patients should attempt to cylindrically activate the abdominal wall with minimal load on the lower back. The **McGill curl-up** is an excellent alternative with only 2,000 N of force on the lower back and yet nearly equivalent muscle activation (Figure 7.16). In a society with an 85% lifetime prevalence of low back

FIGURE 7-13. Intermuscular coordination. (A) Deep muscles (diaphragm, transverse abdominis, multifidus, rotators, pelvic floor). (B) Superficial (diaphragm, oblique abdominals, rectus abdominis, quadratus lumborum, erector spinae, pelvic floor). From Liebenson C, ed. Rehabilitation of the Spine: A Practitioner's Manual. 2nd ed. Philadelphia, PA: Lippincott Williams & Wilkins; 2006.

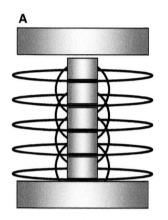
A

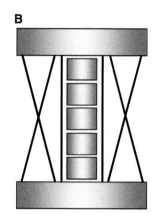
B

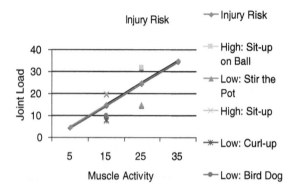

Injury Risk

→ Injury Risk

■ High: Sit-up on Ball

▲ Low: Stir the Pot

✕ High: Sit-up

✳ Low: Curl-up

● Low: Bird Dog

FIGURE 7-14. Injury risk: ratio of muscle challenge to joint load.

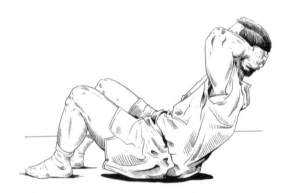

FIGURE 7-15. Sit-up.

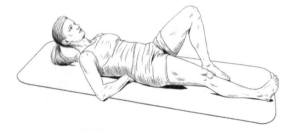

FIGURE 7-16. Curl-up.

pain, perhaps this judicious use of spinal load should be expanded, with everyone considered as potential back pain sufferers and unnecessary training loads avoided.

The **sit-up on the ball** is a more advanced exercise, but the high spinal load to muscle activation ratio makes this a potentially poor training choice for flexion-intolerant low back pain individuals. In contrast, the "**Stir the Pot**" exercise offers an equivalent abdominal challenge with far less spine load (Figure 7.17). Additionally, it will train the spine in its functional role as a "punctum fixum" acting as a strong, stable foundation for the ball and socket joints of the upper and lower extremities to create a pulsed or ballistic force against. When truly stable, the core will facilitate a trampoline-like effect potentiating power production without sacrificing stability.

Trunk extension is another example where spinal load data can influence clinical decisions (8). The **prone superman** involves potentially harmful forces of 4,300 N (Figure 7.18). The quadruped position is a much better choice for spinal extensor training. The **bird-dog** exerts 3,000 N of force on the spine, while the **quadruped leg raise** between 2,000 and 2,300 N of force (Figure 7.19).

Another popular gym exercise that places the spine in a potentially dangerous position is the **leg press machine** (Figure 7.20A). The lumbar spine is placed in kyphosis that adds strain to the posterior portion of the intervertebral disc. One biomechanical modification that will reduce lower back strain is to perform the leg press with one foot on the ground (Figure 7.20B). Another option is to forgo the leg press altogether in favor of more stereotypical human movements. The standing squat (discussed below) places more emphasis on balance and motor control and is more likely going to translate to improved function or athletic performance.

Squats are often performed with excessive weight before form is mastered (Figures 7.21 and 7.22). If the depth is too great given a person's posterior hip capsule flexibility or ankle mobility, a lumbar kyphosis will occur. Many different ways exist to modify the squat so that it can be performed safely. Emphasizing or teaching the "**Hip hinge**" is one such method (Figure 7.23) to

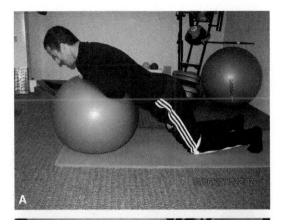

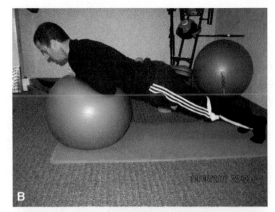

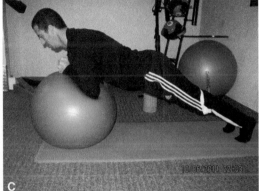

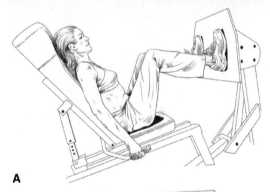

FIGURE 7-17. "Stir the pot."

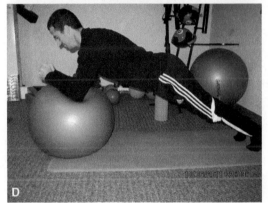

A

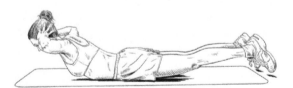

FIGURE 7-18. Prone superman.

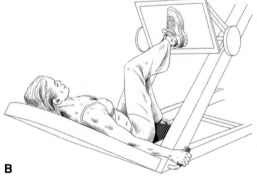

B

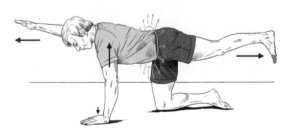

FIGURE 7-19. Bird-dog.

FIGURE 7-20. Leg press. (A) Double leg press (unsafe). (B) Single leg press (safe).

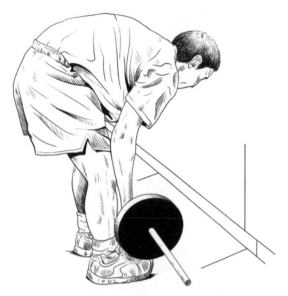

FIGURE 7-21.   Lumbar Hinge—incorrect form.

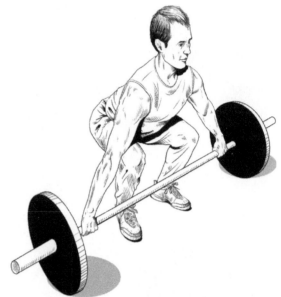

FIGURE 7-22.   Hip hinge—correct form.

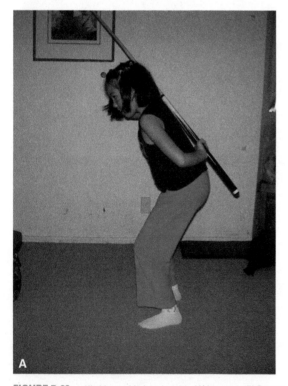

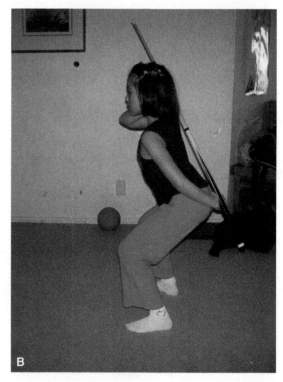

FIGURE 7-23.   Hip hinge with dowel cueing. (A) Incorrect. (B) Correct.

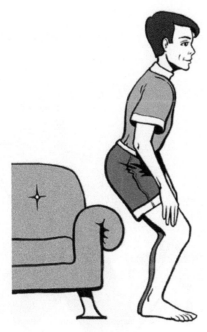

FIGURE 7-24.   Box (arm rest) squat.

promote greater utilization of the acetabulofemoral joint. Performing an arm rest or **box squat** is also an automatic, reflexive method to trigger healthful squat mechanics (Figure 7.24).

   Single leg squats are an example of a challenging exercise, especially for the knee (Figure 7.25), particularly when performed incorrectly. **Rear foot elevated split squats** (popularly known as Bulgarian split squats) are a modification or transitional exercise from two-leg to single leg exercise that facilitates not only better knee stability (Figure 7.26) but also ease of performance.

THE ROLE OF "KEY LINKS" IN NORMALIZING FUNCTION IN THE KINETIC CHAIN

Musculoskeletal problems are often viewed from a narrow perspective. The site of pain and its source are often assumed to be identical, thereby leading many practitioners astray. In clinical rehabilitation, searching for the source of biomechanical overload is of utmost importance when examining a patient (30). The body should be viewed as a kinetic chain involving regional interdependence (31). For example, impairments in the hip may predispose to knee or back injury (Figure 7.27) and loss of thoracic extension mobility can predispose to shoulder

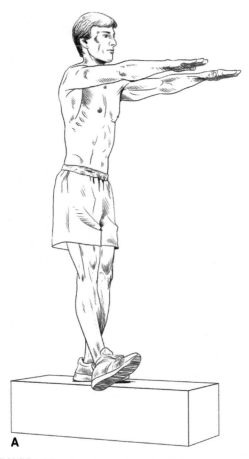

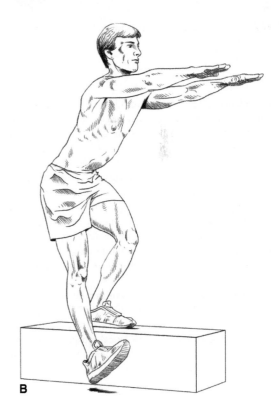

A   **B**

FIGURE 7-25.   Single leg squat. (A) Start. (B) Finish.

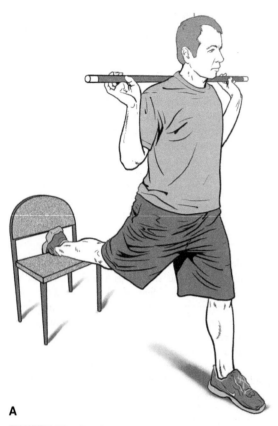
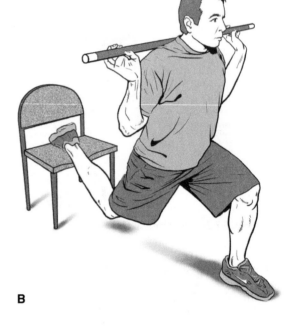

A

B

FIGURE 7-26. Rear foot elevated split squat. (A) Start. (B) Finish.

or neck pain (Figure 7.28). According to Cook, "pain and dysfunction, regardless of their origin, alter motor control. That is why initially we focus on training the most dysfunctional, non-painful pattern" (19). Viewing this in the context of training, impairments in the core may lead to "energy leaks," resulting in decreased force transmission from the lower body to the upper body and vice versa.

The goal of the functional approach is to identify and remediate faulty movement patterns, in both rehab and training settings. Remember, "durability is more important than ability." Loss of force transfer at any link of the kinetic chain may lead to "energy leaks," decreased performance, and resulting injury. Normalizing specific dysfunctions of any movement pattern including the associated joint, muscle, or fascia will likely facilitate improved performance. Mobility deficits of the thoracic spine and hip, and stability deficits of the lateral hip/pelvis and core deserve to be highlighted for their influence throughout the locomotor system.

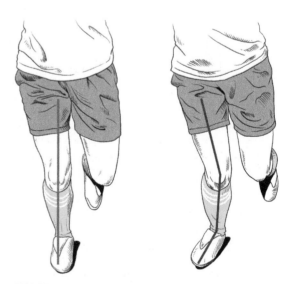

FIGURE 7-27. Single leg squat dysfunction.

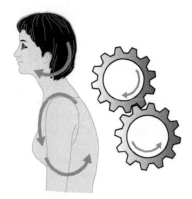

FIGURE 7-28.   Thoracic extension dysfunction.

Thoracic Spine Influences

On the Shoulder

Thoracic spinal manipulation has been shown to be helpful for patients with shoulder impingement syndrome (32–34). In one controlled study, it was shown effective by itself (35).

On the Neck

It has been demonstrated that a significant association exists between decreased mobility of the thoracic spine and the presence of patient-reported complaints associated with neck pain (36). Cleland et al. (37,38) showed that in selected patients, manipulation of the thoracic spine was a successful treatment for patients with neck pain.

Hip Influences

On the Lower Back

Lateral hip instability and posterior hip mobility deficits are functional problems that influence areas above and below it. For example, the active hip abduction test can predict individuals who are at risk for low back pain development during prolonged standing (39).

- Whitman et al. (40) found that treatment of the hip was successful in management of spinal stenosis.
- Cibulka et al. (41) reported that unilateral deficits in hip range of motion were associated with sacroiliac pain syndromes.
- Frost (42) reported that exercise band training designed to facilitate greater gluteal activation did so while sparing the spine.

On the Knee

Cliborne et al. (43) found that hip dysfunction was correlated with knee pain associated with arthritis and that hip mobilization was beneficial in these patients. Improvements in hip flexion strength, combined with increased iliotibial band and iliopsoas flexibility, were associated with excellent results in patients with patellofemoral pain syndrome (44).

Core Influences

On the Knee

Athletes with decreased neuromuscular control of the body's core, measured during sudden force release tasks and trunk repositioning, are at increased risk for knee injury (45,46). Specifically impaired trunk proprioception and deficits in trunk control have been shown to be predictors of knee injury (45,46).

On the Hamstring

A rehabilitation program consisting of progressive agility and trunk stabilization exercises was found to be more effective than a program emphasizing isolated hamstring stretching and strengthening, in promoting return to sports and preventing injury recurrence in athletes suffering an acute hamstring strain (47).

Problems

Any athlete suffering from pain should seek clinical evaluation. However, in order to bridge the gap back to "unstructured movements," he/she must learn the value of maintaining stability in key regions. For example, by way of the hip, the athlete must avoid medial collapse of the knee during single leg training; at the lumbar spine, the athlete should avoid end-range or loaded trunk flexion movements or coupled trunk flexion/rotation; at the shoulder girdle, he/she should avoid shrugging or rounding forward; at the head/neck, the athlete should avoid head forward/chin jut posture; and in all positions must avoid breathing apically.

Clinicians and trainers should also facilitate their athletes to build a "stability margin of error" by not training beyond fatigue and allowing the above form errors. As both Cook and Janda said, "it's not how much weight or how many reps, it's the quality of the movement that is important" (5,19).

FUNCTIONAL TRAINING

To strengthen a muscle requires that the muscle be trained at or near its maximum threshold (see also Chapter 34). Traditional gym exercises achieve this by **isolating individual muscles** and placing the body in an externally stabilized position (e.g., sitting or lying on a bench) to maximize force generation. It is also commonly thought that strength training works best when movement occurs in only one plane and is limited to a single joint.

In contrast, functional training **integrates** many muscle groups by placing the body in the less stable, but more functional positions, often including the performance of multijoint exercises. If the goal is to improve movement patterns that are used in daily life, at work, or in sports or recreational activities, then multijoint training that incorporates movement that is unconstrained and requires multiplanar stability makes sense. Recall that the brain thinks in terms of movement, not muscles. This is of pivotal importance to achieving optimal training results.

Bear in mind that functional training is not mimicry (i.e., sport-specific training) of specific movements carried out in life (see section "Neural Adaptation"). If the goal is to enhance durability and power in sport, then training which enhances these attributes is functional. For instance, an extrinsic cue such as "visualize flying in the air" will enhance performance in a broad jump. This would then be functional. Or, training an individual's dead lift may reduce back pain after a football game. This too would then be functional.

> "Functional training is not sport specific training. It is that which makes a person more functional" Cook (19).

Ironically, in the World's Strongest Man Competition, muscles are rarely activated to their maximum capacity. According to McGill et al., "Training for strongmen events has extended to athletes training for other athletic endeavors that require strength …. Many so-called 'functional' training approaches involved natural constraints on the activation of muscle groups … because joint torques about the three orthopedic axes of each joint must remain in balance to match the task" (48).

In a related study, McGill et al. state "this need for torque balance and functional 'steering' of force through the body linkage creates constraints on activation levels of specific muscles" (49). It is not possible to activate single muscles to 100% of their maximal voluntary contraction (MVC) in functional exercises "because this would upset the balance of moments about the 3 orthopedic axes of the spine, or it would upset the balance of stiffening muscles around the spine required to ensure stability of the spinal column." Muscle activation levels are quite modest even though the tasks are fairly strenuous. He further states, "these constraints are one aspect of what separates 'functional' exercises from muscle isolationist exercises, in which machines create constraints to allow single muscles to activate to very high levels" (49).

It is often taught that to build leaping power strength training of 80% to 95%, one or three to five repetition maximums (RMs) are required (50–54). Sotiropoulos et al. (55) demonstrated that half squats performed as a dynamic warm-up at low to moderate intensity, but maximum velocity improved countermovement jump performance significantly. According to Siff and Verkhoshansky (56) exercises with submaximal loads prepare the nervous systems for explosive activities.

The use of the kettlebell is also a novel way to introduce more functional training since weight distribution of the bell introduces momentum which must be harnessed. Lake and Lauder recently reported that the kettlebell swing was as effective for improving maximal strength and explosive strength (vertical leap) as jump squat power training (57).

Plyometric power in the legs, specifically frontal plane leaping power, has been shown to correlate with throwing velocity in collegiate baseball players (58). Similarly power as demonstrated in an overhead medicine ball toss (greater distance thrown) had a strong direct relationship with throwing velocity in both collegiate baseball and softball players (59). Table 7.1 lists some upright "functional training" exercises.

What typifies these exercises is that the individual is not supported on a bench or chair, not constrained by the exercise machine, and most of the movements are multijoint and multiplanar. They all impose a balance or equilibrium challenge so muscles have to work to maintain stability while at the same time exerting force. Each exercise can be made very strenuous, although initially they should involve controlled resistance only so that the ABCs of agility, balance, and coordination can be programmed.

> "Power is nothing without control"
> Advertising slogan of Pirelli Tyre Company.

When center of mass is dynamically maintained over the body's base, equilibrium is maximized. When key joints are functionally centrated, agonist–antagonist muscles' length–tension relationships are optimized for stability and power.

TABLE 7.1	Examples of Upright "Functional Training" Exercises

Pallof press (anti-rotation press)
Kneeling/standing overhead cable push
Chops/lifts
Medicine ball tosses
Kettlebell swings
Farmers walk
Suitcase/waiter carries
Balance reach
Agility training
Plyometrics

Take Home Points Regarding Functional Training

Upside: Performing strenuous upright tasks automatically creates a stability demand on the individual.
Downside: This stability demand constrains the achievement of individual muscle MVCs.
Note: The constraining of maximum muscle MVCs is not a weakness of "functional training" but more an indication of efficiency of muscle contraction and coordination.

CORTICAL PLASTICITY

When a person is suffering from persistent pain, guarding is an expected yet potentially deleterious response. Janet Travell (White House physician to John F. Kennedy) said, "after an injury tissues heal, but muscles learn, they readily develop habits of guarding that outlast the injury" (60). Similarly, in the sports medicine world, according to Stanley Herring (a team physician for the Seattle Seahawks of the National Football League), "signs and symptoms of injury abate, but these functional deficits persist ... adaptive patterns develop secondary to the remaining functional deficits" (61). Clearly, if guarded movements are programmed and persist even in the absence of pain, then faulty movement patterns will be reinforced over time. As Aristotle said, "Practice doesn't make perfect, it makes permanent."

In ankle sprain patients, a significant delay in onset of activation of the gluteus maximus on the injured side persists post injury. Bullock-Saxton, Janda, and Bullock (62)

Functional training incorporates whole body motor control with particular attention paid to optimal movement quality or competency. Adhering to ideal movement patterns when training the athlete will promote greater movement efficiency and proper energy transfer across contralateral and upper/lower body kinetic linkages and doing so in this manner allows ideal transfer of positive motor learning. By training functionally relevant movement patterns with good motor control as a springboard for the safe development of capacity.

The ideal time to "program" movement skills is before puberty. Both neural myelination and androgenic hormonal influences can be positively influenced by coordination-based training (63). However, proper programming can benefit individuals and athletes at all ages and levels.

Visualization

In 1992, two scientists, Yue and Cole, performed a study to demonstrate the power that the mind has over muscles (64). The study consisted of two groups of people. The first group performed a strength training exercise for the pinky finger, five times per week, for 4 weeks. The second group imagined performing the same exercise for the same frequency

and timeframe. While the subjects that performed the actual strength training improved their strength by 30%, those subjects that simply imagined the strength training exercise improved their strength by 22%.

Neurophysiological research has suggested that, through the use of mental practice, it may be possible to improve muscle strength without actually requiring significant muscle contraction (64,65). Yue, speaking of the plasticity of neural command for MVC ability, asks "Is the command from the brain to muscle for MVC fixed?" If the answer is yes, then only enlarging muscle mass and/or improving muscle coordination results in enhanced muscle strength. If the answer is no, then increasing neural command from the brain through training the neuromuscular system or even the neural system alone leads to improved muscle strength.

Mental practice has similarly been shown to be effective in increasing the force production of the abductor digiti minimi muscle in the hand (66). The improvement in muscle strength for trained groups was accompanied by significant increases in electroencephalogram-derived cortical potential, a measure previously shown to be directly related to control of voluntary muscle contractions. Mental practice also produced strength gains in the larger ankle dorsiflexor muscles, which are important during walking (67). Training of one limb was associated with an increase in the voluntary strength of the contralateral untrained muscles, even though the contralateral muscles remained quiescent during training (68). Mental practice in people without impairments can lead to an increase in torque production similar to that produced by physical practice.

These findings should not be surprising considering that the majority of initial strength gains from resistive exercise are not due to changes in the physiological capacity of the muscle fibers themselves. Muscle hypertrophy resulting from the addition of contractile proteins is a gradual process that takes many weeks to occur (69,70). The ability to increase force production during the initial weeks of training therefore is thought to be the result of neural adaptations (69,71). Possible mechanisms of these neural adaptations include the extent of motor unit activation (72), improved coordination (73), and decreased cocontraction of antagonist muscles (74).

It has been suggested that neuromuscular activity enables the motor cortex to develop motor schema (75) or primes corresponding muscle movement nodes (76). In a more cognitive interpretation, researchers have proposed that mental practice increases performance by improving the preparation and anticipation of movements rather than movement execution (77). Support for this proposal comes from the finding, obtained from positron emission tomography, of increased activity in the medial aspect of the orbitofrontal cortex and decreased activity in the cerebellum following mental practice (77).

Myelination

Coyle explains in his brilliant book, *The Talent Code*, that skill is made not born (78). This is made possible by focused practice. If the student is motivated and has the right teacher, human potential, as Maslow taught, is unlimited (79). Myelination of new neural pathways is a big part of the neuroscience behind such talent development.

- Turn suboptimal movement patterns into optimum movement patterns
- Train the hardest, most functionally relevant movement a person can do well
- "We're built to make things automatic, to stash them in our subconscious mind" (78)

> "The importance of repetition until automaticity occurs cannot be overestimated." Wooden (80)

Myelination is an underappreciated mechanism of activity-dependent nervous system plasticity. One study reported increased myelination associated with extensive piano playing. Practicing piano as a child increased myelination in the posterior limbs of the internal capsule bilaterally, the corpus callosum, and the fiber tracts in the frontal lobe in proportion to the number of hours at the piano. These regions carry sensory-motor information for independent finger movement and cross-connections between auditory regions and premotor cortex coordinating bimanual movement, respectively. In adolescence, increased myelin was seen in interhemispheric fibers from superior temporal and occipital cortical areas, which include auditory and visual processing regions, respectively. Practicing the piano as an adult increased myelination in the arcuate fasciculus, which connects the temporal and frontal regions. The long association fibers of the forebrain, which are increased by adult practicing, continue maturation into at least the third decade of life (81).

Activity-dependent effects on myelination cannot be considered strictly a developmental event (82). Preliminary findings suggest that activity-dependent effects on myelination may not be limited to the visual system or early postnatal development (83).

During motor learning, neural activity in various regions of the brain changes according to the level of the motor skill achieved (84–86). One recent study showed that physical training and mental practice of a motor skill resulted in a similar amount of improvement in performance and a similar pattern of adaptation in the primary motor cortex in human participants (86).

The field of activity-dependent plasticity, historically divided between those favoring a pre- or postsynaptic mechanism as preeminent, is expanding its scope to consider the role of perisynaptic glia in synaptic function and modulation. Now a further expansion may be required to consider a possible role for myelinating glia (Schwann cells and oligodendrocytes) (22,23,87). It has been shown that how a coach or trainer organizes a training or practice session influences the formation of adhesive motor memories, through facilitation of specialized regions in the brain involved in the active preparation and implementation of motor programs (88).

Considering the difficult history of correlating structural changes in synapses with functional plasticity, it is not surprising that activity-dependent plasticity in myelination has become apparent only relatively recently (89). This activity-dependent mechanism promoting myelination could regulate myelination according to functional activity or environmental experience (90).

> "Knowledge is not skill. Knowledge plus ten thousand times is skill." Suzuki (90)

The goal should be to train the nervous system. This is in contrast to training muscles. Whether in sport or in clinical practice, we now know that the human mind is hackable.

> **Steps to Enhance Formation of a New Motor Engram**
> Fire
> Wire
> Seal

NEURAL ADAPTATION

In concert with the SAID principle, the locomotor system will specifically adapt to the type of demand placed upon it. Training effects are known to be velocity (91,92) and position (i.e., joint angle) specific (93,94). Evidence also shows that training leads to length-, task-, and speed-specific changes (93–95). For example, long distance running will improve cardiovascular endurance, but not speed. Also, regular resistance training with near maximum effort and few repetitions will lead to greater gains in strength or power, but little gains in endurance.

Training with slow "negative" work or lengthening under load contractions, for example, increases force output of eccentric contractions without necessarily affecting neuromuscular capacity during concentric contractions. Further, training at a specific joint angle (shortened range of motion, for example) will not or may not influence the force output of the muscle group when the joint is utilized in its full range of motion. Thus, athletic development programs should be specifically adapted to the muscles, joint ranges of motion, and tasks targeted.

While eccentric training may not directly improve concentric strength, it is important in setting the stage for explosive power. Training eccentric control is important for athleticism as dynamic movement involves an eccentric component followed by a momentary isometric state (the amortization phase), and then a concentric contraction. Improved handling of eccentric load will result in higher transitions of kinetic energy into concentric (explosive) contraction. According to Dietz and Peterson, "The key to improved sport performance is producing more force in less time. This results when an athlete can absorb more force eccentrically, allowing him, in turn, to apply higher levels of force concentrically in less time" (96). The concept of Rate of Force (ROF) Development is thus a crucial one which is addressed in Chapters 28 and 34.

Neural adaptation underlying exercise or training effects is often taken lightly. In fact, strength increases can be obtained through modifications at the neural level alone (71). When movement competency and functional capacity are improved such that athletic parameters such as ROF development are emphasized the trainer can predict that residual adaptation will be achieved from the athlete's program (see Chapter 34). When morphologic changes do occur (i.e., increased muscle fiber size), they come into play after the neurophysiological modifications (69,97) measured, for example, through motor unit recruitment frequency or synchronization of motor units. Enoka said, "Although the maximal force which a muscle can exert is directly related to it's cross-sectional area, there is poor correlation between increases in strength and size," "neural changes precede morphological ones" (71).

The more similar the exercise is to the actual activity (e.g., neuromuscular contraction, whole body coordination, speed) the greater the likelihood that improvements in function at home, sports, or work will occur. This is known as the transfer-of-training effect. Therefore, if training programs do not address the specific functional needs of the individual, the goal cannot be achieved.

Controversies in Training

The intent is not to promote "mimicry" of sport during training. Of utmost importance during training is that key dysfunctions are improved. "The goal of training is not to teach perfect patterns but to correct the key fault that is causing the trouble." Lewit (98)

For neural adaptation to occur, it is necessary for training to occur at the limit of one's capability. This is termed the threshold. According to McArdle and Katch, "There exists an appropriate level of stress whereby the system will adapt. Below this level, little or no change will occur." They go on to say, "The intensity must be high enough so that a specific physiologic system is stressed at or near its present maximum capacity in order to cause the system to adapt, thereby improving performance." (2)

LONG-TERM ATHLETIC DEVELOPMENT AND PARTICIPATION

North American society has become ever more sedentary (see also Chapter 34). Americans take approximately 5,000 steps/day while the average in Western Australia or Switzerland is closer to 10,000 and in Japan about 7,000 (99). A study of Amish men (18,000 steps/day) and women (14,000 steps/day) revealed that modern lifestyle has transformed our level of activity (100) and recent data show that

42% of boys and 21% of girls are underactive (101). The result, childhood obesity and diabetes are on the rise.

Early Specialization

Sendentarism notwithstanding, many individuals have fallen into the trap of assuming "more is better." Widespread participation in organized youth sports is occurring at a younger age (National Council of Youth Sport) (102) as young players undertrain and overcompete. Although this early specialization (devoting oneself to a single sport) (103–105) may lead to greater success in the younger years, the opposite seems to be true in the long term. In fact, early specialization and a low training to competition ratio are also correlated with an increased risk of injury (106) and a rise in overuse injuries such as stress fractures and growth plate injuries. Acknowledging the intense draw of athletic success with the potential for college scholarships and professional contracts, parents and youth athletes should be reminded that for lifelong success we must create an athlete that moves exceptionally well, then we can make that athlete excel at a particular sport.

What is becoming more and more prevalent is early sport-specific specialization in late specialization in sports, for example, baseball, Olympic weight lifting, or any sports which we do not see world champions under the age of 18. In the outlier sports, early specialization is required such as gymnastics or figure skating. However, even in these activities caution needs to be applied to avoid overtraining.

Chronological versus Biological Age-Appropriate Training

Skill-appropriate training is necessary because chronological and biological ages are not equivalent. By 7 years of age maturity-related differences in body size are apparent (107). The reasons for participating in a variety of sports at a young age are to promote fundamental movement skills (FMS) as well as develop the mental advantage that comes from learning different strategies (108). It has been shown that preadolescence is the optimal window to develop FMS (63,109,110). In particular, this should occur prior to the period of "peak height velocity" (111). Therefore, children who grow at a younger age should have this coordination-based training initiated earlier. Training should be both challenging and fun—not too easy or too hard, especially in the preadolescent group. This is necessary to keep children engaged and motivated (112,113).

Gender-Appropriate Training

Girls and women have different fitness attributes than their male counterparts. For instance, during puberty boys' vertical jump height increases much more than in girls (114,115). The same is true with respect to hip abduction strength (116,117). Ford identified that pubertal girls have a tendency toward abnormal landing mechanics, which can worsen over time (118,119). Knee injury risk in women (e.g., noncontact anterior cruciate ligament injuries) both in childhood and at the collegiate athletic level is much higher than their male counterparts (120,121). Various contributing risk factors in postpubertal women have been identified and integrative neuromuscular training programs have been shown to improve the faulty biomechanics and reduce injury risk (122–125). When such movement literacy training is added to a traditional conditioning program, improvements in athleticism (balance ability and vertical jump height) have been noted (126).

Neuromuscular Training versus Strength Training

Integrative neuromuscular training is essential for injury prevention. Athletes expose their lower extremity to ground reaction forces up to 5–7 times their body mass in sport (127–129), and integrative neuromuscular training may reduce the injury rate in youth athletics by 15% to 50% (130). Integrative neuromuscular training programs should include *strength and power training* (modified cleans, pulls, presses) and *plyometric exercise* (e.g., single and double leg hops and jumps). Such methods combine resistance and motor control and have been shown to reduce the incidence of sports-related injuries in youth sports (123,131,132) including soccer and football (131,133–135).

Strength development may reduce the risk of injury occurring during sport-related activities (134). Previous weight training has been shown to reduce recovery time from injury although controversy exists regarding the safety of weight training in youth prior to skeletal maturity (136–138). That said, with regard to acquiring necessary movement literacy to perform resistance exercises and lifting techniques with proper coordination and skill, some argue "the younger the better" (112,139,140).

Injury is directly related to the quality of supervision and/or poor technique or both (141). Both in schools and in recreation centers, untrained youth may overestimate their capabilities and increase their risk of injury (141–144). Unsupervised weight lifting, resistance training, or plyometric exercise should not be performed due to enhanced risk of injury (144–146). Two-thirds of all preadolescent (ages 8–13) injuries with weight training are to the hand and foot and related to "dropping" or "pinching" and thus preventable with proper supervision (144).

Other youth injury-related factors include excessive intensity, volume, frequency, or competition or inadequate recovery (147–149). An appropriate injury preventive program must include proper supervision and training. It must also include both resistance and FMS training and must be progressive and varied in volume and intensity over time (i.e., periodization). Training without a plan, especially in younger athletes, results in catastrophe and thus long-term athletic development incorporates stages such as "learning to train" and "training to compete."

Signs and symptoms of overtraining must also be recognized and identified by the supervising professional. These include muscle soreness that lasts greater than 1–2 days, diminished performance, frequent upper respiratory illnesses, sleep or appetite changes, inability to concentrate, mood swings, and so on (111,149,150). It can also include changes in heart rate variability or decline in lifting speed/capacity. Periodic less intense training should therefore be included in a youth athletes' training program (151). Additionally, readiness for sport (preparedness) may also be screened to determine whether baseline movement literacy in the FMS is present before the start of a sport season (111,116,128,141).

Resistance Training in the Elderly

Decreases in muscle strength and mass have been assumed to be an inevitable consequence of aging. Muscle mass decreases by 3% to 6% per decade after the age of 60 (152). However, recent studies suggest that age-related muscle loss—sarcopenia—can to a great extent be prevented with increased activity (153,154). Resistance training of frail men and women in their nineties has been found to be safe and result in significant gains in muscle strength and functional mobility (155). Health care professionals and the public have focused much attention on age-related changes in bone density, but have ignored these muscle changes. Yet, muscle changes are extremely important when one considers risk of falls and fractures and general well-being.

One of the most well-established tests in the strength training field is the 1RM (one repetition maximum) (156). This test is a valuable guide during high-resistance strength training and has been used in people with heart disease as well as in the elderly (157). Elderly individuals exercising at an intensity of at least 80% of 1RM show strength gains and functional improvement (158,159). It has been shown to reduce resting blood pressure in older persons. It has been shown to be safe for older persons both with and without high-risk cardiac conditions (160–162).

According to DiFabio (157), certain prerequisites are necessary for safe 1RM testing in older persons:

- Pain-free range of motion should be measured and the athlete should stay within it.
- Avoidance of the Valsalva maneuver during exertion is required.
- Proper form and slow, controlled movements are necessary.

THE ROLE OF REHABILITATION AND TRAINING

Rehabilitation and training should build the movement competency and functional capacity required to address specific capacity deficits that place the individual at risk for injury or reduced performance. The functional history should identify

TABLE 7.2	Normalization of Faulty Movement Patterns

Mobilize stiff areas

Facilitate "weak" areas

Retrain functional movement patterns on an automatic basis

the individual's activity demands. In particular, what demands are giving them the greatest trouble? Should such demands be limited or disabled in any way, they are termed activity intolerances. For both patients and athletes, the functional examination should also identify their functional capacity deficits. The gap between their capacity and demands is what places them at risk (see Figure 7.1) for injury or decreased performance. The role of rehabilitation and training is to close that gap. Once capacity exceeds demands there is a "stability margin of error" (163). The process of building functional capacity is simple—normalize faulty movement patterns responsible for repetitive strain (Table 7.2).

In the context of pain management and athletic development, the following steps apply:

- Reassurance and recovery: diagnostic triage, threat reduction, palliative care (manual therapy, medication, modalities), inflammation reduction, ergonomic advice (sparing strategies)
- Rehabilitation: functional movement pattern assessment, motor control (stabilization) training, mobilization, cardiovascular training
- Reconditioning: functional capacity assessment, endurance, strength, agility, speed, and power training

Training Methods

It is important to make training safe, effective, and efficient. To do so, it is essential that the focus be on a painless dysfunction (FMS score of 1) that is deemed a source of biomechanical overload in the kinetic chain.

TABLE 7.4	Rehabilitation Tools

Balance boards/pads

Foam roll

Gym balls

Medicine balls

Bands/pulleys

Tubing

Dumbbells

Kettlebells

Bar

Many different exercises can be incorporated in training (Table 7.3). A variety of low-tech tools (Table 7.4) and progressions (Table 7.5) can also be chosen for rehabilitation and training. Training should also occur in a functional training range (FTR) that has been defined by Morgan as "the range which is painless and appropriate for the task at hand". The goal is to expand this FTR until capacity is greater than the demands of one's ADLs or recreational, sport, or work activities, thus ensuring the "stability margin of error". Expanding the FTR "within-session" (see Chapter 5) is the key to the training program enhancing residual adaptation over time (see Chapter 34).

Making this process efficient requires that compliance and motivation are high and that adhesive, transferable results can be reasonably expected in a regular, measurable manner. Avoiding an emphasis on cortical or internal cues and emphasizing facilitatory or external (i.e., target-based) cues is one key element. Goal- or movement-oriented verbal cues instead of explaining muscle contraction or joint position is preferable. "Drive your heels into the floor" is a preferred cue over "contract your glutes" during a hip thrust or glute bridge exercise. As Janda said, "minimize the conscious awareness phase and find something the patient does well automatically as soon as possible" (5).

TABLE 7.3	Types of Exercises

Sensory-motor

Respiration/breathing

Core stabilization/motor control

Thoracic mobilization

Hip mobilization

Bridges

Squats/lunges

Functional reaches

Scapulothoracic facilitation

Dynamic neuromuscular facilitation

Push/pull (horizontal and vertical)

TABLE 7.5	Progressions

Stable to unstable

Single joint to multijoint

Isolated to integrated

Uniplanar to triplanar

Nonweight bearing to weight bearing

Developmentally immature to developmentally mature (higher developmental levels)

Passive modeling to active assistance

Active assisted to active unassisted

Active unassisted to active resisted

"The best resistance is the one that causes the problem to correct itself without verbal or visual feedback." Cook (19)

"First move well, then move often." Cook (19)

CONCLUSIONS

We can see in both the rehabilitation and training fields an evolution toward greater emphasis on motor control with a concurrent lessening of the emphasis on isolation of individual muscles and joints. This new paradigm focuses on promoting activity and sustained athletic participation. It is both patient- and athlete-centered in that it seeks to reduce activity intolerances, enhance performance, return the athlete to play, and prevent injury or recurrence.

There are many sacred cows in both the rehabilitation and strength and conditioning fields. These are the methods of yesteryear that were successful in spite of their flaws. Just like poor quality movements, low-quality training methods must be assessed, improved, and reassessed. While such beliefs or practices are considered by some to be exempt from criticism or questioning despite containing inaccurate dogmas, this book will attempt to expose some of these myths, while proposing alternative, science-based, explanations.

REFERENCES

1. Gambetta V. Athletic Development: The Art & Science of Functional Sports Conditioning. Champaign, IL: Human Kinetics; 2007.
2. McArdle WD, Katch FI, Katch VL. Exercise Physiology, Energy, Nutrition and Human Performance, Chapter 20. 3rd ed. Philadelphia, PA: Lea Febiger; 1991:384–417.
3. Arnason A, Sigurdsson SB, Gudmondsson A, Holme I, Engebretsen L, Bahn R. Risk factors for injuries in soccer. Am J Sports Med 2004;32(1s):5s–16s.
4. Arnason A, Sigurdsoon SB, Gudmonnson A, et al. Physical fitness, injuries, and team performance in soccer. Med Sci Sports Exerc 2004;36(2):278–285.
5. Janda V, Frank C, Liebenson C. Evaluation of muscle imbalance. In: Liebenson C, ed. Rehabilitation of the Spine: A Practitioner's Manual. Philadelphia, PA: Lippincott Williams & Wilkins; 2007:203–225.
6. Biering-Sorensen F. Physical measurements as risk indicators for low back trouble over a one year period. Spine 1984;9:106–119.
7. Verstegen M, Williams P. Core Performance: The Revolutionary Workout Program to Transform your Body and your Life. United States: Rodale; 2004.
8. McGill SM. Low Back Disorders: The Scientific Foundation for Prevention and Rehabilitation. Champaign, IL: Human Kinetics; 2002.
9. Hasenbring M. Attentional control of pain and the process of chronification. In: Sandkuhler J, Bromm B, Gebhart GF, eds. Progress in Brain Research. Volume 129. Amsterdam: Elsevier; 2000:525–534.
10. Butler D, Moseley L. Explain Pain. Adelaide, Australia: Noigroup Publications; 2003.
11. Vlaeyen JWS, Morley S. Active despite pain: the putative role of stop-rules and current mood. Pain 2004;110:512–516.
12. Harding V, Williams AC de C. Extending physiotherapy skills using a psychological approach: cognitive-behavioural management of chronic pain. Physiotherapy 1995;81:681–687.
13. Harding VR, Simmonds MJ, Watson PJ. Physical therapy for chronic pain. Pain—Clin Updates, Int Assoc Study Pain 1998;6:1–4.
14. Linton SJ. Cognitive-Behavioral Therapy in the Early Treatment and Prevention of Chronic Pain: A Therapist's Manual for Groups. Orebro; 2000.
15. Jamieson J. The Ultimate Guide to HRV Training. Seattle, WA: Performance Sports Inc.; 2012:20p.
16. Dietz C, Peterson B. A Systematic Approach to Elite Speed and Explosive Strength Performance: Bye Dietz Sports Enterprise. Hudson, WI; 2012.
17. Janda V. Muscles, central nervous motor regulation and back problem. In: Korr IM, ed. The Neurobiologic Mechanisms of Manipulative Therapy. New York, NY: Plenum Press; 1978:27–41.
18. Janda V. On the concept of postural muscles and posture in man. Aust J Physiother 1983;29:83–84.
19. Cook G. Movement: Functional Movement Systems. Aptos, CA: On Target Publications; 2010.
20. Fisher DD, Worchester TK, Lair J. I Know You Hurt, But There's Nothing to Bandage. Beaverton, OR: Touchstone Press; 1978.
21. Gosselin RD, Suter MR, Ji RR, Decosterd I. Glial cells and chronic pain. Neuroscientist 2010;16(5):519–531.
22. Watkins LR, Maier SF. Beyond neurons: evidence that immune and glial cells contribute to pathological pain states. Physiol Rev 2002;82:981–1011.
23. Watkins LR, Milligan ED, Maier SF. Immune and glial involvement in physiological and pathological exaggerated pain states. In: Dostrovsky JO, Carr DB, Kolzenburg M, eds. Progress in Pain Research and Management. Seattle, WA: IASP Press; 2003:369–386.
24. Melzack R. Pain and the neuromatrix in the brain. J Dental Educ 2001;65:1378–1382.
25. Blankenburg F, Ruff CC, Deichmann R, Rees G, Driver J. The cutaneous rabbit illusion affects human primary sensory cortex somatotopically. PLoS Biol 2006;4:e69.
26. Panjabi MM. The stabilizing system of the spine. Part 1. Function, dysfunction, adaptation, and enhancement. J Spinal Disord 1992;5:383–389.
27. Granata KP, Marras WS. Cost-benefit of muscle cocontraction in protecting against spinal instability. Spine 2000;25:1398–1404.
28. Marras WS, Mirka GA. Muscle activities during asymmetric trunk angular accelerations. J Orthop Res 1990;8: 824–832.
29. Gardner-Morse MG, Stokes IAF. The effects of abdominal muscle coactivation on lumbar spine stability. Spine 1998;23:86–92.

30. Kibler WB. Shoulder rehabilitation: principles and practice. Med Sci Sports Exerc 1998;30(4 Suppl):S40–S50.

31. Wainner RS, Whitman JM, Cleland JA, Flynn TW. Regional interdependence: a musculoskeletal examination model whose time has come. J Orthop Sports Phys Ther 2007;37(11):658–660.

32. Bang MD, Deyle GD. Comparison of supervised exercise with and without manual physical therapy for patients with shoulder impingement syndrome. J Orthop Sports Phys Ther 2000;30:126–137.

33. Bergman GJ, Winters JC, Groenier KH, et al. Manipulative therapy in addition to usual medical care for patients with shoulder dysfunction and pain: a randomized, controlled trial. Ann Intern Med 2004;141:432–439.

34. Muth S, Barbe MF, Lauer R, McClure PW. The effects of thoracic spine manipulation in subjects with signs of rotator cuff tendinopathy. J Orthop Sports Phys Ther 2012;42(12):1005–1016.

35. Boyles RE, Ritland RM, Miracle BM, et al. The short-term effects of thoracic thrust manipulation on patients with shoulder impingement syndrome. Man Ther 2009;14: 375–380.

36. Norlander S, Nordgren B. Clinical symptoms related to musculoskeletal neck-shoulder pain and mobility in the cervico-thoracic spine. Scand J Rehabil Med 1998;30: 243–251.

37. Cleland JA, Childs JD, McRae M, et al. Immediate effects of thoracic manipulation in patients with neck pain: a randomized clinical trial. Man Ther 2005;10:127–135.

38. Cleland JA, Childs JD, Fritz JM, Whitman JM, Eberhart SL. Development of a clinical prediction rule for guiding treatment of a subgroup of patients with neck pain: use of thoracic spine manipulation, exercise, and patient education. Phys Ther 2007;87:9–23.

39. Nelson-Wong E, Flynn T, Callaghan JP. Development of active hip abduction as a screening test of identifying occupational low back pain. J Orthop Sports Phys Ther 2009;39:649–657.

40. Whitman JM, Flynn TW, Childs JD, et al. A comparison between two physical therapy treatment programs for patients with lumbar spinal stenosis: a randomized clinical trial. Spine 2006;31:2541–2549.

41. Cibulka MT, Sinacore DR, Cromer GS, et al. Unilateral hip rotation range of motion asymmetry in patients with sacroiliac joint regional pain. Spine 1998;23:1009–1015.

42. Frost DM, Beach T, Fenwick C, et al. Is there a low-back cost to hip-centric exercise? Quantifying the lumbar spine compression and shear forces during movements used to overload the hips. J Sports Sci 2012;30:859–870.

43. Cliborne AV, Wainner RS, Rhon DI, et al. Clinical hip tests and a functional squat test in patients with knee osteoarthritis: reliability, prevalence of positive test findings, and short-term response to hip mobilization. J Orthop Sports Phys Ther 2004;34:676–685.

44. Tyler TF, Nicholas SJ, Mullaney MJ, et al. The role of hip muscle function in the treatment of patellofemoral pain syndrome. Am J Sports Med 2006;34:630–635.

45. Zazulak BT, Hewett TE, Reeves NP, et al. Deficits in neuromuscular control of the trunk predict knee injury risk: a prospective biomechanical-epidemiologic study. Am J Sports Med 2007;35:1123–1130.

46. Zazulak BT, Hewett TE, Reeves NP, et al. The effects of core proprioception on knee injury: a prospective biomechanical-epidemiological study. Am J Sports Med 2007;35:368–373.

47. Sherry MA, Best TM. A comparison of 2 rehabilitation programs in the treatment of acute hamstring strains. J Orthop Sports Phys Ther 2004;34(3):116–125.

48. McGill SM, McDermott A, Fenwick CMJ. Comparison of different strongman events: trunk muscle activation and lumbar spine motion, load, and stiffness. J Strength Cond Res 2009;23(4):1148–1161.

49. McGill SM, Karpowicz A, Fenwick CMJ, Brown SHM. Exercises for the torso performed in a standing posture: spine and hip motion and motor patterns and spine load. J Strength Cond Res 2009;23(2):455–464.

50. Clark RA, Bryant AL, Reaburn P. The acute effects of a single set of contrast preloading on a loaded countermovement jump training session. J Strength Cond Res 2006;20:162–166.

51. Comyns TM, Harrison AJ, Hennesey LK, Jensen R. The optimal complex training rest interval for athletes from anaerobic sports. J Strength Cond Res 2006;20:471–476.

52. Deutsch M, Lloyd R. Effect of order of exercise on performance during a complex training session in rugby players. J Sports Sci 2008;26(8):803–809.

53. Kilduff LP, Bevan HR, Kingsley MIC, et al. Postactivation potentiation in professional rugby players: optimal recovery. J Strength Cond Res 2007;21:1134–1138.

54. Weber KR, Brown LE, Coburn JW, Zinder SM. Acute effects of heavy-load squats on consecutive squat jump performance. J Strength Cond Res 2008;22(3):726–730.

55. Sotiropoulous K, Smilios I, Christou M, et al. Effect of warm-up on vertical jump performance and muscle electrical activity using half-squats at low and moderate intensity. J Sports Sci Med 2012;9:326–331.

56. Siff MC, Verkhoshansky YV. Supertraining: A Textbook on the Biomechanics and Physiology of Strength Conditioning for all Sport. Pittsburgh, PA: Sports Support Syndicate; 1996.

57. Lake JP, Lauder MA. Kettlebell swing training improves maximal and explosive strength. J Strength Cond Res 2012;26(8):2228–2233.

58. Lehman G, Drinkwater EJ, Behm DG. Correlations of throwing velocity to the results of lower body field tests in male college baseball players. J Strength Cond Res 2013;27(4):902–908.

59. Green CM. The Relationship between Core Stability and Throwing Velocity in Collegiate Baseball and Softball Players. Thesis; 2005.

60. Travell JG. Basic Principles of Myofascial Pain. November 1, 1984. (Presented at the Palm Springs Seminars, Inc., November 2–6, 1984 and to the DC Dental Society, April 16, 1985).

61. Herring SA. Rehabilitation of muscle injuries. Med Sci Sports Exerc 1990;22:453–456.

62. Bullock-Saxton JE, Janda V, Bullock MI. The Influence of Ankle Sprain Injury on Muscle Activation During Hip Extension. Int J Sports Med 1994;15:330–334.

63. Kraemer WJ, Fleck SJ, Callister R, et al. Training responses of plasma beta-endorphin, adrenocorticotropin, and cortisol. Med Sci Sports Exerc 1989;21:146Y53.

64. Yue GH, Cole KJ. Strength increases from the motor program: comparison of training with maximal voluntary and imagined muscle contractions. J Neurophysiol 1992;67:1114–1123.

65. Smith M, Sparkes V, Busse M, Enright, S. Upper and lower trapezius muscle activity in subjects with subacromial impingement symptoms: is there imbalance and can taping change it? Phys Ther Sport 2009;10(2):45–50.

66. Ranganathan VK, Siemionow V, Liu JZ, Sahgal V, Yue GH. From mental power to muscle power – gaining strength by using the mind. Neuropsychologia 2004;42(7):944–956.

67. Sidaway B, Trzaska A. Can mental practice increase ankle dorsiflexion torque? Phys Ther 2005;85(10):1053–1060.

68. Houston ME, Froese EA, Valeriote SP, Green HJ, Ranney DA. Muscle performance, morphology and metabolic capacity during strength training and detraining: a one-leg model. Eur J Appl Physiol 1983;51:25–35.

69. Sale D, MacDougall D. Specificity in strength training: a review for the coach and athlete. Can J Sport Sci 1981;6:87.

70. Moritani T, deVries HA. Neural factors versus hypertrophy in the time course of muscle strength gain. Am J Phys Med 1979;58:115–130.

71. Enoka RM. Neuromechanical Basis of Kinesiology. Champaign, IL: Human Kinetics Books; 1988.

72. Belanger AY, McComas AJ. Extent of motor unit activation during effort. J Appl Physiol 1981;51:1131–1135.

73. Rutherford OM, Jones DA. The role of learning and coordination in strength training. Eur J Appl Physiol Occup Physiol 1986;55:100–105.

74. Carolan B, Cafarelli E. Adaptations in coactivation after isometric resistance training. J Appl Physiol 1992;73: 911–917.

75. Hale BD. The effects of internal and external imagery on muscular and ocular concomitants. J Sports Psychol 1982;4:379–387.

76. MacKay DG. The problem with rehearsal or mental practice. J Mot Behav 1981;13:274–285.

77. Jackson PL, Lafleur MF, Malouin F, et al. Functional cerebral reorganization following motor sequence learning through mental practice with motor imagery. Neuroimage 2003;20:1171–1180.

78. Coyle D. The Talent Code. New York, NY: BantamDell; 2009.

79. Maslow A. Toward a Psychology. New York, NY: Van Nostrand; 1962.

80. Nater S, Gillimore R. You Haven't Taught Until They Have Learned: John Wooden's Teaching Principles and Practices. Fitness Information Technology: West Virginia University, Fitness Info Tech; 2010.

81. Yakovlev PI, Lecours A-R. The myelogenetic cycles of regional maturation of the brain. In: Minkowski A, ed. Regional Development of the Brain in Early Life. Oxford, UK: Blackwell Scientific; 1967:3–70.

82. Fields RD. Myelination: an overlooked mechanism of synaptic plasticity? Neuroscientist 2005;11(6):528–531.

83. Markham J, Greenough WT. Experience-driven brain plasticity: beyond the synapse. Neuron Glia Biol 2004;1(4): 351–363. doi:10.1017/S1740925X05000219.

84. Karni A, Meyer G, Jezzard P, Adams MM, Turner R, Ungerleider LG. Functional MRI evidence for adult motor cortex plasticity during motor skill learning. Nature 1995;337: 155–158.

85. Pascual-Leone A, Grafman J, Hallett M. Modulation of cortical motor output maps during development of implicit and explicit knowledge. Science 1994;263:1287–1289.

86. Pascual-Leone A, Nguyet D, Cohen LG, Brasil-Neto JP, Cammarota A, Hallett M. Modulation of muscle responses evoked by transcranial magnetic stimulation during the acquisition of new fine motor skills. J Neurophysiol 1995;74:1037–1045.

87. Brown J, Cooper-Kuhn CM, Kempermann G, Van Praag H, Winkler J, Gage FH. Enriched environment and physical activity stimulate hippocampal but not olfactory bulb neurogenesis. Eur J Neurosci 2003;17:2042–2046.

88. Wymbs NF, Grafton ST. Neural substrates of practice structure that support future off-line learning. J Neurophysiol 2009;102(4):2462–2476.

89. Ishibashi T, Dakin KA, Stevens B, et al. Astrocytes promote myelination in response to electrical impulses. Neuron 2006;49(6):823–832.

90. Suzuki S. Knowledge Plus Ten Thousand Times is Skill. 2011. www.musicinpractice.com/2011/knowledge-plus-ten-thousand-times-is-skill.

91. Moffried MT, Whipple RH. Specificity of speed exercise. Phys Ther 1970;50:1693.

92. Caizzo VJ, Perine, JJ, Edgerton VR. Training-induced alterations of the in vivo force-velocity relationship of human muscle. J Appl Physiol 1981;51:750.

93. Bender JA, Kaplan HM. The multiple angle testing method for the evaluation of muscle strength. J Bone Joint Surg [Am] 1963;45A:135.

94. Meyers C. Effects of 2 isometric routines on strength, size and endurance of exercised and non-exercised arms. Res Q 1967;38:430.

95. Boucher JP, Cyr A, King MA, et al. Isometric training overflow: determination of a non-specificity window. Med Sci Sports Exerc 1993;25:S134.

96. Dietz C, Peterson B. Triphasic Training: A Systematic Approach to Elite Speed and Explosive Strength Performance [e-book]. 2012.

97. Rutherford OM. Muscular coordination and strength training, implications for injury rehabilitation. Sports Med 1988;5:196.

98. Lewit K. Manipulative Therapy in Rehabilitation of the Locomotor System. 3rd ed. Oxford: Butterworth Heinemann; 1999.

99. Bassett D, Wyatt H, Thompson H, et al. Pedometer-measured physical activity and health behaviors in U.S. adults. Med Sci Sports Exerc 2010;42(10):1819–1825.

100. Bassett D, Schnieder P, Huntington G. Physical activity in an old order Amish community. Med Sci Sports Exerc 2004;36(1):79–85.

101. Tudor-Locke C, Johnson WD, Katzmarzyk PT. Accelerometer-determined steps per day in US children and youth. Med Sci Sports Exerc 2010;42:2244–2250.

102. Hyman M. Until it Hurts: America's Obsession with Youth Sports and How It Harms Our Kids. Boston, MA: Beacon Press; 2009.

103. Bayli, I. Long-Term Athlete Development: Trainability in Childhood and Adolescence. Windows of Opportunity, Optimal Trainability: Sheridan Books, USA; 2003.

104. Bompa T. Total Training for Young Champions: Proven Conditioning Programs for Athletes Ages 6 to 18. Champaign, IL: Human Kinetics; 2000.

105. Abbott A, Collins D. Eliminating the dichotomy between theory and practice in talent identification and development:

considering the role of psychology. J Sports Sci. 2004;22(5): 395–408.

106. Ekstrand J, Gillquist J, Moller M, et al. Incidence of soccer injuries and their relation to training and team success. Am J Sports Med. 1983;11:63–67.

107. Malina RM, Cumming SP, Morano PJ, et al. Maturity status of youth football players: a noninvasive estimate. Med Sci Sports Exerc. 2005;37:1044–1052.

108. Moran, A. Sport and Exercise Psychology Textbook: A Critical Introduction: Routledge; 2003.

109. Gallahue DL, Ozmun JC. Understanding Motor Development: Infants, Children, Adolescents, Adults. Boston, MA: McGraw Hill; 2006.

110. Lubans DR, Morgan PJ, Cliff DP, et al. Fundamental movement skills in children and adolescents: review of associated health benefits. Sports Med 2010;40:1019–1035.

111. Myer GM, Faigenbaum AD, Ford KR, et al. When to initiate integrative neuromuscular training to reduce sports-related injuries and enhance health in youth? Am Coll Sports Med 2011;10:157–166.

112. Faigenbaum AD, Kraemer WJ, Blimkie CJ, et al. Youth resistance training: updated position statement paper from the national strength and conditioning association. J Strength Cond Res 2009;23:S60–S79.

113. Faigenbaum A, Farrell A, Radler T, et al. Plyo Play: a novel program of short bouts of moderate and high intensity exercise improves physical fitness in elementary school children. Phys Educ 2009;69:37–44.

114. Kellis E, Tsitskaris GK, Nikopoulou MD, Moiusikou KC. The evaluation of jumping ability of male and female basketball players according to their chronological age and major leagues. J Strength Cond Res 1999;13:40–46.

115. Quatman CE, Ford KR, Myer GD, Hewett TE. Maturation leads to gender differences in landing force and vertical jump performance: a longitudinal study. Am J Sports Med 2006;34:806–813.

116. Brent JL, Myer GD, Ford KR, Hewett TE. A longitudinal examination of hip abduction strength in adolescent males and females. Med Sci Sports Exerc 2008;40(5):s50-s51.

117. Lloyd DG, Buchanan TS. Strategies of muscular support of varus and valgus isometric loads at the human knee. J Biomech 2001;34:1257–1267.

118. Ford KR, Myer GD, Hewett TE. Valgus knee motion during landing in high school female and male basketball players. Med Sci Sports Exerc 2003;35:1745–1750.

119. Ford KR, Myer GD, Toms HE, Hewett TE. Gender differences in the kinematics of unanticipated cutting in young athletes. Med Sci Sports Exerc 2005;37(1):124–129.

120. Hewett TE, Myer GD, Ford KR, et al. Biomechanical measures of neuromuscular control and valgus loading of the knee predict anterior cruciate ligament injury risk in female athletes: a prospective study. Am J Sports Med 2005;33(4):492–501.

121. Myer GD, Ford KR, Barber Foss KD, et al. The incidence and potential pathomechanics of patellofemoral pain in female athletes. Clin Biomech 2010;25:700–707.

122. Hewett TE, Stroupe AL, Nance TA, Noyes FR. Plyometric training in female athletes. Decreased impact forces and increased hamstring torques. Am J Sports Med 1996;24:765–773.

123. Myer GD, Ford KR, Palumbo JP, Hewett TE. Neuromuscular training improves performance and lower-extremity

biomechanics in female athletes. J Strength Cond Res 2005;19:51–60.

124. Myer GD, Ford KR, McLean SG, Hewett TE. The effects of plyometric versus dynamic stabilization and balance training on lower extremity biomechanics. Am J Sports Med 2006;34:490–498.

125. Myer GD, Ford KR, Brent JL, Hewett TE. Differential neuromuscular training effects on ACL injury risk factors in "high-risk" versus "low- risk" athletes. BMC Musculoskelet Disord 2007;8:1–7.

126. DiStefano LJ, Padua DA, Blackburn JT, et al. Integrated injury prevention program improves balance and vertical jump height in children. J Strength Cond Res 2010;24: 332–342.

127. Dufek JS, Bates BT. The evaluation and prediction of impact forces during landings. Med Sci Sports Exerc 1990;22:370–377.

128. Hewett TE, Myer GD, Ford KR. Anterior cruciate ligament injuries in female athletes: part 1, mechanisms and risk factors. Am J Sports Med 2006;34:299–311.

129. McNitt-Gray JL, Hester DME, Mathiyakom W, Munkasy BA. Mechanical demand on multijoint control during landing depend on orientation of the body segments relative to the reaction force. J Biomech 2001;34:1471–1482.

130. Micheli L. Preventing injuries in team sports: what the team physician needs to know. In: Chan K, Micheli L, Smith A, et al., eds. F.I.M.S. Team Physician Manual. Hong Kong: CD Concepts; 2006:555–572.

131. Hewett TE, Myer GD, Ford KR. Reducing knee and anterior cruciate ligament injuries among female athletes: a systematic review of neuromuscular training interventions. J Knee Surg 2005;18:82–88.

132. Mandelbaum BR, Silvers HJ, Watanabe DS, et al. Effectiveness of a neuromuscular and proprioceptive training program in preventing anterior cruciate ligament injuries in female athletes: 2-year follow-up. Am J Sports Med 2005;33:1003–1010.

133. Lehnhard RA, Lehnhard HR, Young R, Butterfield SA. Monitoring injuries on a college soccer team: the effect of strength training. J Strength Cond Res 1996;10: 115–119.

134. Cahill B, Griffith E. Effect of preseason conditioning on the incidence and severity of high school football knee injuries. Am J Sports Med 1978;6:180–184.

135. Emery CA, Meeuwisse WH. The effectiveness of a neuromuscular prevention strategy to reduce injuries in youth soccer: a cluster-randomised controlled trial. Br J Sports Med 2010;44:555–562.

136. American Academy of Pediatrics. Strength training by children and adolescent. Pediatrics 2008;121:835–840.

137. Miller MG, Cheatham CC, Patel ND. Resistance training for adolescents. Pediatr Clin North Am 2010;57:671–682.

138. Young JL, Herring SA, Press JM, et al. The influence of the spine on the shoulder in the throwing athlete. J Back Musculoskel Rehabil 1996;7:5–17.

139. Behm DG, Faigenbaum AD, Falk B, Klentrou P. Canadian Society for Exercise Physiology position paper: resistance training in children and adolescents. Appl Physiol Nutr Metab 2008;33:547–561.

140. Pierce K, Brewer C, Ramsey M, et al. Youth resistance training. Prof Strength Cond 2008;10:9–23.

141. Faigenbaum AD, Myer GD. Resistance training among young athletes: safety, efficacy and injury prevention effects. Br J Sports Med 2010;44:56–63.

142. Plumert J, Schwebel D. Social and temperamental influences on children's overestimation of their physical abilities: links to accidental injuries. J Exp Child Psychol 1997;67:317–337.

143. Jones C, Christensen C, Young M. Weight training injury trends. Phys Sports Med 2000;28:61–72.

144. Myer GD, Quatman CE, Khoury J, et al. Youth versus adult "weight-lifting" injuries presenting to United States emergency rooms: accidental versus non-accidental injury mechanisms. J Strength Cond Res 2009;23:2054–2060.

145. Brady T, Cahill B, Bodnar L. Weight training related injuries in the high school athlete. Am J Sports Med 1982;10:1–5.

146. Risser WL. Weight-training injuries in children and adolescents. Am Fam Physician 1991;44:2104–2108.

147. Bergeron MF. Youth sports in the heat: recovery and scheduling considerations for tournament play. Sports Med 2009;39:513–522.

148. Bergeron MF, Laird MD, Marinik EL, et al. Repeated-bout exercise in the heat in young athletes: physiological strain and perceptual responses. J Appl Physiol 2009;106:476–485.

149. Brenner JS. Overuse injuries, overtraining, and burnout in child and adolescent athletes. Pediatrics 2007;119:1242–1245.

150. Winsley R, Matos N. Overtraining and elite young athletes. Med Sport Sci 2011;56:97–105.

151. Faigenbaum AD, McFarland J. Make time for less intense training. Strength Cond J 2006;28:77–79.

152. Thompson LV. Aging muscle: characteristics and strength training. Issues Aging 1995;331:821–827.

153. Volpi E, Sheffield-Moore M, Rasmussen BB, et al. Basal muscle amino acid kinetics and protein synthesis in healthy young and older men. JAMA 2001;286(10):1206–1212.

154. Roubenoff R, Cadtaneda C. Sarcopenia—understanding the dynamics of aging muscle. JAMA 2001;286(10):1230–1231.

155. Fiatarone MA, Marks EC, Ryan ND, et al. High-intensity strength training in nonagenarians: effects on skeletal muscle. JAMA 1990;263(22):3029–3034.

156. Carey Smith R, Rutherford OM. The role of metabolites in strength training. I. A comparison of eccentric and concentric contractions. Eur J Appl Physiol 1995;71:332–336.

157. DiFabio RP. One repetition maximum for older persons: is it safe? J Orthop Sports Phys Ther 2001;31:2–3.

158. Morganti CM, Nelson ME, Fiatarone MA, et al. Strength improvements with 1 year of progressive resistance training in older women. Med Sci Sports Exerc 1995;27:906–912.

159. Taaffe DR, Duret C, Wheeler S, Marcus R. Once-weekly resistance exercise improves muscle strength and neuromuscular performance in older adults. J Am Geriatr Soc 1999;47:1208–1214.

160. Barnard KL, Adams KJ, Swank AM, Mann E, Denny DM. Injuries and muscle soreness during the one repetition maximum assessment in a cardiac rehabilitation population. J Cardiopulm Rehabil 1999;19:52–58.

161. Kaelin M, Swant AM, Adams KJ, Barnard KL, Berning JM, Green A. Cardiopulmonary responses, muscle soreness, and injury during the one repetition maximum assessment in pulmonary rehabilitation patients. J Cardiopulm Rehabil 1999;19:366–372.

162. Verrill DE, Bonzheim KA. Injuries and muscle soreness during the one repetition maximum assessment in a cardiac rehabilitation population (letter). J Cardiopulm Rehabil 1999;19:190–192.

163. McGill S. Stability: from biomechanical concept to chiropractic practice. J Can Chiro Assoc 1999;43:75–87.

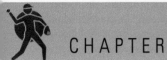
Baseball

Baseball is a popular sport, with an estimated 16 million children playing organized baseball in the United States (1). Little League Baseball alone recorded more than 2.6 million participants in 2007 (2). With the increase in participation, there has also been an increase in the number of injuries. Nationally, an estimated 131,555 high school baseball-related injuries occurred during the 2005–2006 and 2006–2007 academic years, for an injury rate of 1.26 injuries per 1,000 athletic exposures. The most commonly injured body sites were the shoulder (17.6%), ankle (13.6%), head/face (12.3%), hand/finger (8.5%), and thigh/upper leg (8.2%). The most common injury diagnoses were ligament sprains (incomplete tears) (21.0%), muscle strains (incomplete tears) (20.1%), contusions (16.1%), and fractures (14.2%). Although a majority of injuries resulted in a time loss of <7 days, 9.7% resulted in medical disqualification for the season, and 9.4% required surgery (3).

Another prospective cohort study of 298 youth pitchers conducted over two seasons showed that frequency of elbow pain was 26% and of shoulder pain, 32%. Risk factors for elbow pain were increased age, increased weight, decreased height, lifting weights during the season, playing baseball outside the league, decreased self-satisfaction, arm fatigue during the game pitched, and throwing fewer than 300 or more than 600 pitches during the season. Risk factors for shoulder pain included decreased, arm fatigue during the game pitched, throwing more than 75 pitches in a game, and throwing fewer than 300 pitches during the season. In conclusion, arm complaints were common, with nearly half of the subjects reporting pain. The factors associated with elbow and shoulder pain were different, suggesting differing etiologies. Developmental factors may be important in both shoulder and elbow injuries. To lower the risk of pain in both locations, young pitchers probably should not throw more than 75 pitches in a game. Other recommendations are to remove pitchers from the game if they demonstrate arm fatigue and limit pitching in nonleague games (4).

Several authors attribute most shoulder and elbow injuries to overuse which mostly affects pitchers and catchers rather than other positions (4–9). Overuse may occur during a single game or throughout a season or year in the young baseball player. Pitch type and velocity have been associated risk factors in young pitchers (7–11).

With the majority of injuries occurring at the shoulder and elbow, understanding the biomechanics of the throwing motion is necessary to preventing injuries. It is generally understood that the dominant arms of most throwing athletes are subject to significant forces. Improving pitching mechanics has been recommended as a means of improving the performance and possibly the safety of young pitchers (12–16).

The maintenance of shoulder health in adolescent throwers may be achieved by an appropriate stretching and strengthening program as a normal part of their routine. Young pitchers should be coached regarding proper throwing mechanics, which involve the coordination of all muscle groups including the lower extremity and core musculature, to generate the forces required to pitch at high velocities. This coordinated muscle activity protects the involved joints by redistributing the forces to the distal segments. Much of the focus in the latest research has been on the shoulder and elbow, but understanding that throwing requires a transfer of energy up the kinetic chain from the lower body to the upper body may refocus preventative thoughts. Hence, strengthening the core muscles of the thoracic and lumbar spine as well as the lower extremities should be a key component in a thrower's exercise program. A stable shoulder girdle is also critical to proper pitching mechanics, and strengthening the periscapular muscles is as important as strengthening the rotator cuff (17–21).

In an effort to reduce injury in the sport, the fundamentals of throwing must be considered. With proper mechanics, appropriate pitch counts, and a quality exercise program, many throwing injuries may be avoided. While each player has their own unique throwing style, the pitching motion requires timing, and landmarks have been identified to help break the movement into six critical phases:

1. Wind-up
2. Stride
3. Arm cocking
4. Arm acceleration
5. Arm deceleration
6. Follow-through

The pitcher begins in the wind-up phase, providing a good position for a timely progression through the six landmark phases. The wind-up is often referred to as the balance point where the pitcher stands on the rear leg while flexing the lead hip and leg. The stride phase ideally begins as the ball is removed from the glove and the pitcher's center of gravity begins to move toward the plate. The arm cocking phase begins when the front foot strikes and ends when the throwing shoulder reaches maximal external rotation. This phase of the throwing motion is responsible for generating extreme positions and torques. Maximum external rotation ranges from 160° to 185° (11). This extreme position creates the distance that the arm acceleration phase will use to internally rotate the humerus and create velocity. By the end of this phase, the pitcher is almost completely facing the plate. The acceleration phase is marked by the transition from humeral external rotation to forceful internal rotation. It is during this phase that arms of elite pitchers can reach speeds in excess of 6,000 degrees per second, thus placing tremendous forces on the shoulder and elbow (11). Internal rotation of the arm occurs at approximately 90° perpendicular to the torso. Once the ball leaves the fingertips the job description for the shoulder is no longer about creating force. The action about the arm is focused on deceleration and dissipating force. The more efficient the deceleration phase, the more force or velocity a pitcher can generate without injury.

The follow-through phase, the final phase, is probably the single most important factor that can be manipulated to reduce the risk of injury. Although the shoulder is involved in most of this phase, pitching also involves other body parts. Using larger muscle groups like the trunk and hips to help further dissipate the acceleration forces created is an excellent means of injury prevention. It is important to note that once the follow-through phase is over, the pitcher must be ready to field his position.

Function of the shoulder complex in the overhead athlete requires synchrony of multiple neuromuscular components. The precise timing of shoulder neurodynamics, osteodynamics, and neuromuscular dynamics is dependent upon function of the entire kinetic chain. In-depth understanding of how the shoulder complex functions in relationship to the torso and lower extremities (kinetic chain) will allow adequate conditioning in preparation for competitive sport or rehabilitation from injury.

The specific movements of the overhead athlete create multiple adaptations throughout the kinetic chain. Specific exercises to promote healthy adaptation are paramount to the success of any pitching program; moreover, injury prevention is the primary objective with performance enhancement and return from injury being secondary objectives.

KINETIC CHAIN CONCEPTS AND CONNECTION

A baseball player may be required to move or react in various methods to accomplish sports-specific movements. The end result of a perfectly executed movement is the result of several body parts working in synchrony with each other. This synergy is accomplished by function of the neuromuscular system. The movement of the throwing athlete is initiated in the foot, transferred through the torso, and eventually ends with a force being applied by the hand. It is important to understand how function in one part of the neuromuscular system can affect function in others. The function of the entire kinetic chain is paramount to injury prevention, performance enhancement, and return from injury.

If one component of the kinetic chain is dysfunctional then deficiencies should be identified and corrected. This may require specific soft tissue manipulation (flexibility, manual therapy) and activation of specific musculature (strengthening exercises or muscle activation exercises). Isolation for activation of specific musculature should be accomplished prior to sports-specific movements for synchrony. If not, the neuromuscular system will find a means of compensation around the deficient components.

When looking at sports-specific motions, the range of motion, the speed of movement, the muscles activated, and how they are activated (concentrically, eccentrically, isometrically) are all things that must be understood to create an adequate conditioning program. As all movements have an optimal biomechanical position, it is imperative to achieve the best biomechanical efficiency, which eases stress on tissues and improves functional qualities. It is important to emphasize quality of effort and proper intensity to gain optimum results from exercises in any conditioning program.

ADAPTATION

All athletes develop physiological adaptations to their given sports, some more drastically than others. Repetitive stresses, which are all too common in baseball, may be compromising tissues that are shortened and/or weakened from environmental influences. An in-depth understanding of interaction and adaptation from psychosocial, biochemical, and biomechanical demands will allow proper program design. The balancing act of loading the tissue to maximize the training response without overloading the adaptive potentials must be constantly monitored.

Selye (22) offered the Specific Adaptation to Imposed Demand (SAID) principle which describes the changes that occur throughout the body in response to training or athletic demands. Wilk (23) demonstrated that the baseball player has a specific adaptation about the throwing shoulder. As different researchers have tried to determine the exact cause of this adaptation (24–27), it is apparent that each athlete adapts in a similar pattern dependent on their sport and position within the sport. Although similar patterns of adaptation do occur, each player responds in their own unique way. Evaluating each player will allow a path to preventative exercise programs that have a more specific approach.

As adaptation may help the athlete to meet the demands of the game and/or prevent injury, clinicians and sports training professionals must be careful in selection of their therapeutic interventions. A specific look at the overhead throwing athlete shows adaptation occurring throughout the kinetic chain. Scapular, torso, and hip adaptations all appear to play a role in the athlete's success from a performance and well-being standpoint. As more distal adaptation may ultimately affect the shoulder or elbow, it is necessary to look at all aspects of the body. Promoting a healthy adaptation may require one or more of the following: exercise, flexibility, recovery, soft tissue therapy, and proper nutrition.

ASSESSMENT

The idea that connectivity exists between the shoulder and the rest of the kinetic chain requires a look at proper length tension relationships. This will in turn allow the best chance for optimal baseball movement patterns. An evaluation of the entire body is imperative as it may identify and help correct any problems prior to implementing a conditioning program. A misguided program may actually promote dysfunction or necessitate new adaptation patterns, either of which could result in injury. The evaluation should take into account overall gross movement dysfunction, postural abnormalities, mobility, bilateral symmetry, joint and muscle function. This evaluation should give a reasonable picture of a player's current state of function and direction for program design.

It is very common for overhead throwers to develop muscular imbalances. They are often overlooked until the player has an injury. A thorough postural (static, dynamic), muscular tension, and functional movement evaluation will help identify abnormalities, which will allow a corrective exercise strategy that may offset any associated muscular imbalances. The corrective exercise program should strive to obtain optimal posture and alignment, which will lend to functional efficiency.

In the presence of poor posture, dysfunctional muscular patterns may develop. These dysfunctions may be responses to overuse, misuse, abuse, or disuse (28). A normal response of muscle to any stress is to potentially increase tightness. A chain reaction then occurs whereby the stressed muscles tighten and their antagonists weaken, which creates altered movement patterns (29). Many times these chain reactions create predictable patterns of dysfunctions. Vladimir Janda has described them as upper and lower crossed syndromes. It should be noted that these syndromes may have detrimental effects on the shoulder of any thrower.

Sherrington's law of reciprocal innervation indicates that tight muscles act in an inhibitory fashion to their antagonists (30). Therefore, it may be prudent to lengthen the tightened muscles before strengthening the weakened muscles.

In conclusion, it is important to evaluate all baseball players for postural abnormalities, proper length tension relationships, and proper muscular firing patterns. A program to correct flexibility deficits, activate neuromuscular isolation, and integrate exercises may then be developed for each player dependent upon their individual needs.

Stabilization/Neuromuscular Control

Stabilization is a primary fundamental of injury prevention and proper neuromuscular function. Stabilization is the ability of the neuromuscular system to allow antagonist, agonist, synergist, stabilizers, and neutralizers to work synergistically.

The shoulder girdle has very little static or ligamentous stability. Therefore, the stability required is dynamic and requires specific synergism of the neuromuscular system. It is essential to understand the difference between muscles that provide power for shoulder motion (deltoid, latissimus dorsi, and pectoral muscles) and those that provide shoulder stability (subscapularis, infraspinatus, teres minor, and supraspinatus) (31). Shoulder complex stabilization is a critical element to the overall conditioning program as improved stabilization/neuromuscular control and reactivity will enhance performance and injury prevention qualities.

Coordination or Skill Movements

Coordination or skill movements can show how well the neuromuscular firing patterns are working. It also shows motor unit recruitment for force production and timing of movement qualities. In essence, a specific movement with a specific force with the proper timing is the by-product of properly executed skill movements. It is neuromuscular control and proprioception that allow these movements to happen in the most efficient method. To improve all physical conditioning components of the shoulder/scapular complex is very important but ultimately it is the skill movements that are required for success. It must be noted that skill movements should be classified as an exercise in and of their self. For example, a throwing or hitting program must be considered an exercise. Skill movements are normally practiced repetitiously for maximum biomechanical efficiency. With this in mind the importance of the skills coach is vital to the success of any baseball player. A properly designed conditioning program must take into account the volume, frequency, and intensity of skills training and implement the conditioning program around those variables for best results.

Recovery

The most overlooked area of training may be recovery. As in any sport it is not the amount of work the athlete does that determines good health and improved performance, instead it is the recovery that takes place between exercise and game competition. The process of recovery, or more specifically regeneration, is a complex biological reaction influenced by both external and internal environments. Unfortunately, presently there is a greater emphasis on stressing the body than recovery. There are many methods that can be utilized to promote recovery. Proper nutrition/hydration, hot/cold hydrotherapies, sports massage, relaxation techniques, and rest/sleep can be used to aid an athlete's recovery (32). Planning recovery is a critical component to maximizing the overall conditioning effect.

FUNDAMENTAL SKILLS (AGES 7–10)

The following drills and pointers will help young athletes develop fundamentally sound baseball skills regardless of position. For athletes of increasing age, more advanced and specific drills will be discussed.

Catching Fly Balls

The player should have a good athletic stance with feet shoulder width apart when he is under or in the flight of the ball. This may be different for balls that are over the head of or in front of the player which will require running to a specific point to catch the fly ball. The player should have his hands above waist level and thumbs pointing toward each other (see Figure 8.1). The player should be instructed to watch the ball until he feels the impact upon the glove.

Catching Ground Balls

The player should have a good athletic stance prior to recognizing the ground ball. Once he determines that it is a ground ball he must make appropriate movement to get within reach of the ball and preferably have the ball catchable between his feet as this is the only position that will be

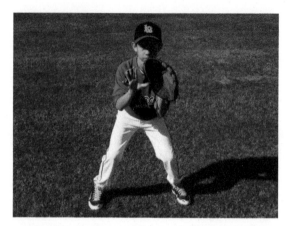

FIGURE 8-1. Proper hand and glove position for catching fly balls.

discussed at this age level. The player must then lower his glove with a combination of his hands dropping but more importantly bending in his hips and secondarily his knees (see Figure 8.2). This will create a good position to see the ball until it impacts the glove. The player must keep his chin in a somewhat tucked position with his throwing hand positioned slightly above glove for a quick removal of the ball prior to the throw.

Throwing with Follow-Through and Balance

It is imperative that a player learns to follow through when throwing a caught baseball. This will allow a decrease in the stresses on the arm and allow for an accurate throw. The player must go from the catching position (ground ball or fly ball position) to a throwing position which means rotating the body 90° to the throwing arm side. In turn, this will position the arm to move to an elevated position prior to the throw. After release of the ball, the player should

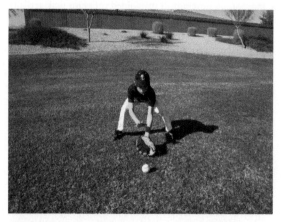

FIGURE 8-2. Proper hand and glove position for catching ground balls.

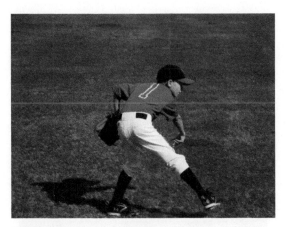

FIGURE 8-3. Proper follow-through after throwing.

focus on flexing torso forward toward target; this will allow deceleration of the arm which is critical for injury prevention (see Figure 8.3).

Hitting with Balanced Stance and Follow-Through

Hitting is another fundamental baseball skill. Although there can be many different styles that are effective, there are basic points that every hitter should be instructed on. Starting with a balanced and athletic stance will allow transfer of body weight and rotation of the torso which will give the hitter a good biomechanical position to hit the ball. In addition, the player should keep eye focus on the ball until it reaches the bat which will create a head down position. At the moment of ball/bat impact the player should be shifting some of his body weight from his back leg to a firm front leg. His back foot should pivot allowing for proper hip turn and an efficient follow-through (see Figure 8.4).

Base Running with Leadoff and Sliding

Base running is often a fundamental that is undervalued as a key fundamental to baseball as most focus is on hitting, throwing, and catching. Base running, like all other baseball skills, can be very complicated depending upon what base the runner is on and what the situation of the game is and demands.

On any base, the runner should start in a good athletic position with feet shoulder width apart, hips flexed, and hands in front of waist. This position will allow an advance to the next base or return to existing base. Thereafter, the focus should be on proper running mechanics until the player moves to next base or is required to slide into base (see Figure 8.5). If sliding is indicated, then tucking one leg under the upper thigh of the opposite leg is the best technique for efficient sliding and injury prevention. Sliding with hands closed and not into the ground is recommended.

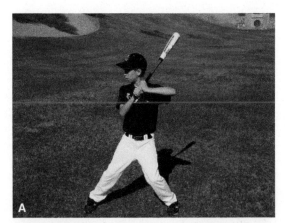

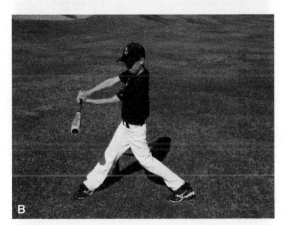

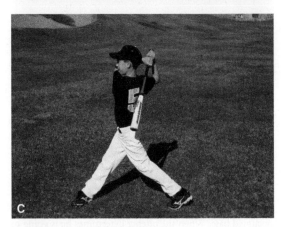

FIGURE 8-4. (A–C) Proper mechanics of hitting.

SPORTS SKILLS (AGES 11–15)

The sports skills build upon the movement patterns and fundamentals already established in younger players. The skills become more position specific and are only a few examples of the many sports skills that are needed to play baseball.

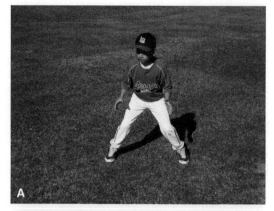

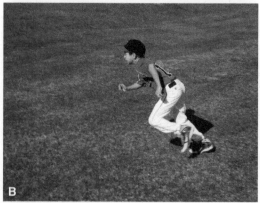

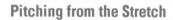

FIGURE 8-5. (A, B) Proper base stealing mechanics.

Pitching from the Stretch

As most pitchers learn to pitch from the wind-up, it is imperative to understand how to pitch out of the stretch to compete in higher levels of baseball. When runners are on base, this is the preferred method for holding base runners close to the base and giving the defense a better opportunity for getting the base runner out. Pitching from the stretch requires the pitcher to have his back foot in contact with rubber on mound; he starts with feet and hands apart while determining which pitch he will throw. He then comes to the set position with hand on the ball in the glove and must stop prior to throwing the ball to home plate or to an occupied base. When the pitcher determines he is going to throw the ball to home plate, he should focus on proper mechanics of throwing which would include using the legs, torso, and upper extremities to deliver an accurate and effective pitch. This should be complemented by a follow-through to dissipate the forces generated from the acceleration phase of throwing (see Figure 8.6).

Position-Specific Throwing

Each position requires unique throwing mechanics, but all have a few commonalities. Using the legs and

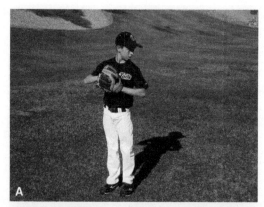

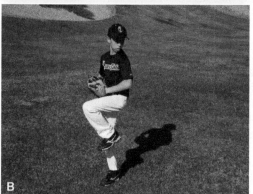

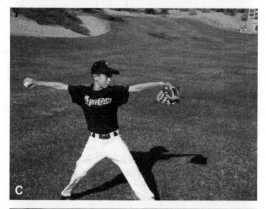

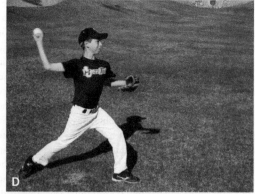

FIGURE 8-6. (A–F) Proper pitching mechanics from the stretch.

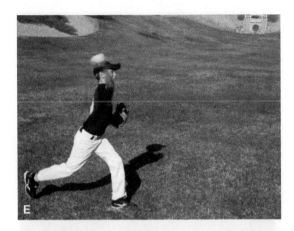

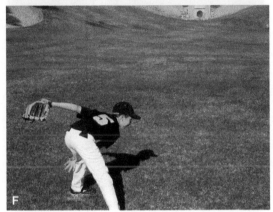

FIGURE 8-6. (Continued)

torso to accelerate the upper extremity is a good general rule—along with an efficient follow-through. Sometimes, unique aspects of the catcher's position may alter throwing mechanics. Many times the catcher must throw the ball very quickly from a fully squatted position as base runners may be unpredictable; this combined with the catcher's protective equipment can inhibit an efficient throw.

Hitting to All Fields with Balance

Hitting the ball to all fields with balance takes advanced hand–eye coordination. The swing is essentially the same as previously discussed, but the hitter must decide where to hit the ball dependent upon what type of pitch and the location of the pitch. If the pitch is outside, then the general rule would be to hit the ball toward the right side of the field, whereas if the pitch is inside, the ball may be "pulled" and hit to the left side of the field for a right-handed hitter. Each swing must have balance, weight shift, and follow-through, and only the location of bat to ball contact changes. This can be done off of a tee to begin with and progress to hitting off of a batting practice thrower.

REFINED SKILLS (AGES 18 TO ELITE)

Refined skills are a further advancement on the sports skills and are done at a very high skill level. Many players become limited by physical potential by the time they reach this level and thus cannot efficiently improve these skills which separates the average player from the elite or professional player. Below are a few drills that can be done.

Hitting Balls to a Specific Area Based on Where the Pitch Is

As a player becomes more skilled with hitting, they learn to hit a specific pitch to a certain location on the field. This skill is highly individual and very dependent upon pitch location, game situation, and quick recognition/reaction to ball speed. If the ball is thrown to the inner side of the plate, the hitter will hit the ball to the left side of the field given he is a right-handed hitter. If the ball is thrown to the outside of the plate, the hitter will hit the ball to the right side of the field given he is a right-handed hitter (see Figure 8.7).

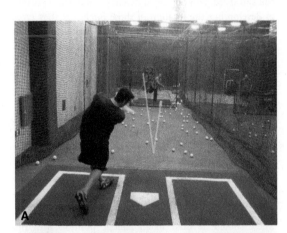

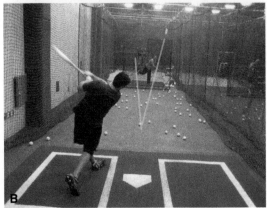

FIGURE 8-7. (A–C) Hitting different pitches to different areas of the field.

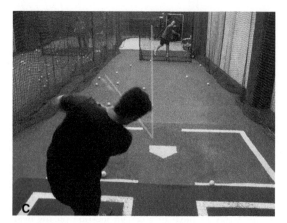

FIGURE 8-7. *(Continued)*

Mastering Off-Speed Pitches

A very critical skill for a pitcher to develop is how to throw different types of pitches to deceive the hitter. Two of the more common pitches are a changeup and a curveball. Both have similar arm action and only differ in the grip on the ball and speed. Not only are different pitch types important to develop but the location of those pitches as they cross the hitting zone is equally as important. Figure 8.8 shows the common grips used to throw a changeup and curveball. Mastering location requires a lot of repetition.

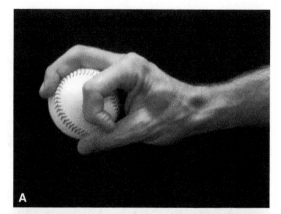

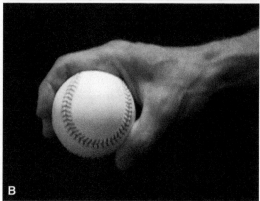

FIGURE 8-8. (A, B) Hand grip for a changeup and curveball.

FUNCTIONAL EXERCISES

The following examples of functional exercises can be done with the corresponding sports skills at various age levels.

Ages 11–15 (Beginner Level)

Sumo Squat

These should be done in an athletic position with the player's bottom as close to the ground as possible (see Figure 8.9). This exercise focuses on hip strength and hip motion during fielding.

Forward Lunge

The player should take one step forward and return to standing (see Figure 8.10). This exercise focuses on leg, hip, and core strength, and balance and control during fielding.

Lateral Lunge

The player should take a large step directly to the side while keeping his landing heel in contact with the ground and move his bottom as close to the ground as possible, then return to standing (see Figure 8.11). This exercise focuses on hip, groin, and leg strength as well as balance and control. These are also fundamentals of fielding.

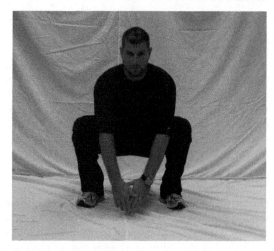

FIGURE 8-9. Sumo squat exercise.

Double Leg Glute Bridge

While lying face up, the player bends the knees and lifts the bottom up from the ground so that the shoulder, hip, and knee are collinear. This exercise focuses on glute and hamstring strength as well as core stability and control.

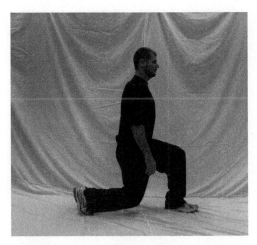

FIGURE 8-10.   Forward lunge exercise.

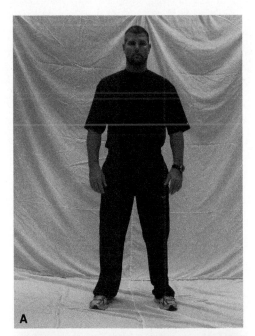

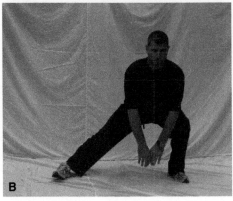

FIGURE 8-11.   (A, B) Lateral lunge exercise.

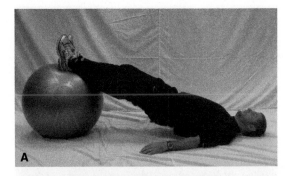

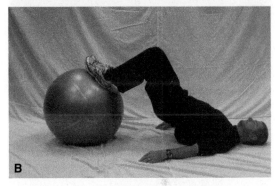

FIGURE 8-12.   (A, B) Double leg physioball hamstring curl exercise.

Stability Ball Hamstring Curl

Lying face up with shoulders and hips on the ground and feet on the stability ball, lift the hips into the air and slowly pull the ball toward the body and then return the ball to the start position (see Figure 8.12). This exercise focuses on hamstring and glute strength to help prevent strength deficits that may lead to injury.

Plank Series

Begin facing floor on forearms and toes. Hold a neutral spine for a predetermined duration. Face left and use single elbow and stack both feet so only one is in contact with the floor. After the predetermined duration, face the opposite direction. Be sure to maintain a straight axis from head through toes in all three positions (see Figure 8.13). These exercises focus on lateral oblique control and strength. This exercise is chosen for its attention to the front and side of the core.

Upper Body Tubing: Single-Arm Row

Standing with tubing resistance securely anchored in front, use one hand to pull the handle toward the body while rotating away from the resistance (see Figure 8.14). Be sure to encourage leg utilization. The focus of this exercise is to integrate hip motion as well as hip/upper body/back and arm strength.

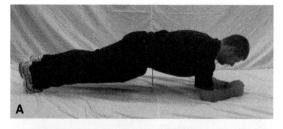

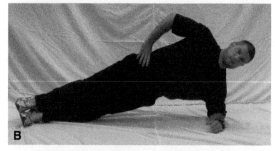

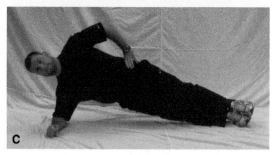

FIGURE 8-13.   (A–C) Front and lateral plank exercise.

Upper Body Tubing: Single-Arm Push

Standing with tubing resistance securely anchored to the rear, use one hand to push the handle away from the body while rotating away from the resistance (see Figure 8.15). Be sure to encourage leg utilization. The focus of this exercise is to integrate hip motion as well as hip/upper body/chest and arm strength.

Bent-Over Pull

Stand with feet shoulder width apart flexed to 90° at the hip and the resistance anchored belt high and in front of the exerciser. Use one or two hands to pull the elbow toward the hip (see Figure 8.16). The focus of this exercise is to increase arm and back strength and motion. This exercise also strengthens the muscles partially responsible for bat speed.

Shoulder T&Ms (Figure 8.17)

- Ts: Standing with resistance securely anchored at chest height, bring both arms with elbows straight away from the resistance at shoulder height.
- Ms: From the same position, extend the shoulders until they are even with the body. Hand position is about 12″ out to the side and away from the body.

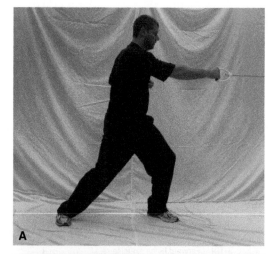

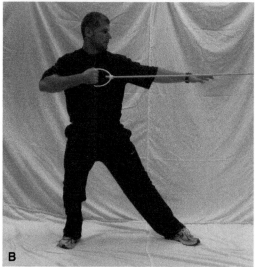

FIGURE 8-14.   (A, B) Single-arm row exercise.

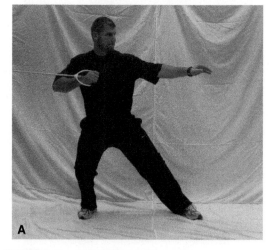

FIGURE 8-15.   (A, B) Single-arm push exercise.

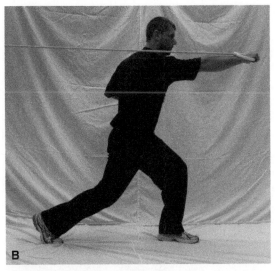

FIGURE 8-15. *(Continued)*

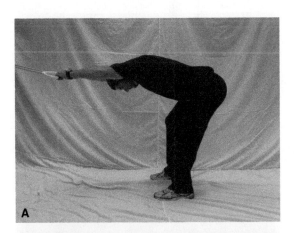

FIGURE 8-16. (A, B) Bent-over pull exercise.

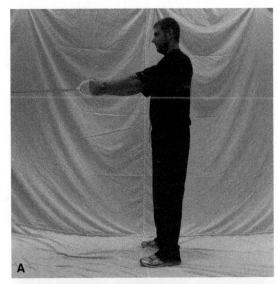

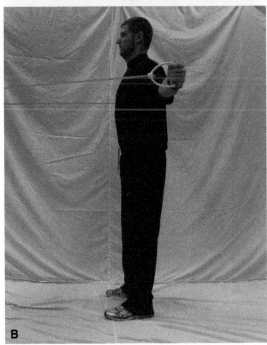

FIGURE 8-17. (A–C) Shoulder/scapular tubing exercises.

The focus of this exercise group is to strengthen the smaller muscle groups that are predominantly used for throwing.

Ages 15–17 (Advanced Level)

Single-Leg Squat

Standing on one leg, the athlete should lower level/even hips as deep as possible. Keep the uninvolved leg off the

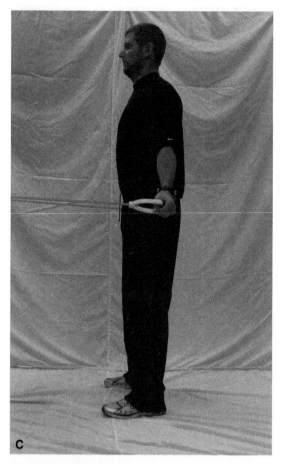

FIGURE 8-17. *(Continued)*

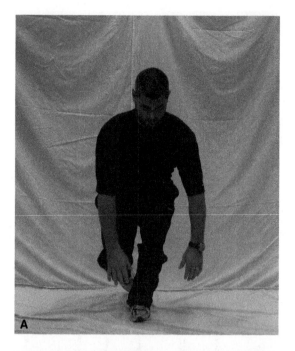

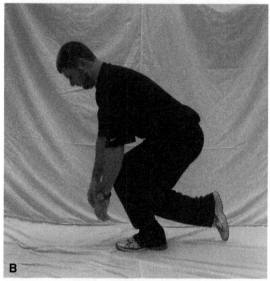

FIGURE 8-18. (A, B) Single-leg squat exercise.

ground. Be sure to keep the hip, knee, and foot collinear and push up through the heel (see Figure 8.18). The focus of this exercise is hip, leg, and ankle strength in addition to balance and control.

Step-Up/Step-Down

Standing on a 12″–24″ step, have the athlete step off and lower the hips as deep as possible or until the foot touches the ground. Be sure to keep the hip, knee, and foot collinear and push down through the step with the heel. Eccentric control of the knee and hip is essential to performing this exercise properly (see Figure 8.19). Eccentric strength is also essential in deceleration during running.

Weighted Lunge

The player may begin with a weighted vest/sandbag/dumbbell/barbell and should take one step forward and return to standing. Variations include walking, lateral, reverse, or multidirectional (see Figure 8.20). This exercise focuses on leg, hip, and core strength, and balance and control. It is important for proper form to be maintained while loading a previously unloaded exercise.

Lateral Skater Lunge

The player jumps at a 45° angle to the right while landing in a controlled fashion on the right foot. Be sure the knee does not rotate medially (twist in) upon foot strike (see Figure 8.21). Be sure to alternate jump direction with each jump (left then right). This exercise focuses on hip/leg strength as well as lower extremity coordination and efficiency.

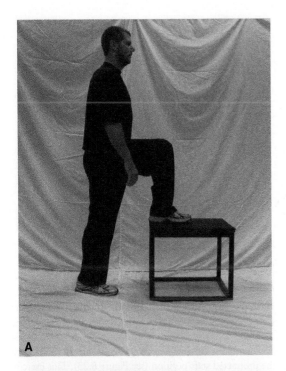

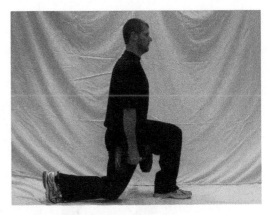

FIGURE 8-20. Weighted forward lunge exercise.

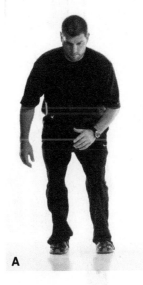

A

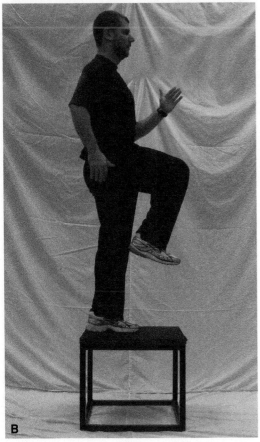

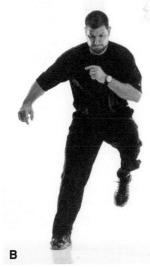

B

FIGURE 8-19. (A, B) Step-up and step-down exercise.

FIGURE 8-21. (A–D) Lateral skater lunge exercise.

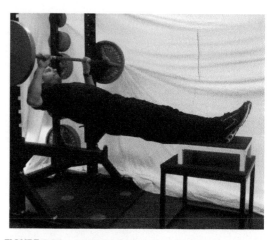

FIGURE 8-22.   Inverted pull-up exercise.

Push-Up with Plus

Have the hands comfortably placed shoulder width apart with only toes and hands in contact with the ground. The shoulder, hip, and ankle are collinear. Protract the scapulae then lower the body to the ground and then return to the protracted start position (see Figure 8.23). This exercise

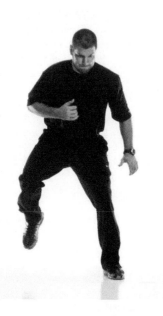

C

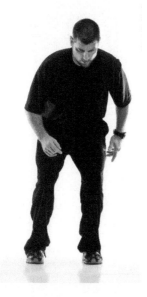

D

FIGURE 8-21.   (*Continued*)

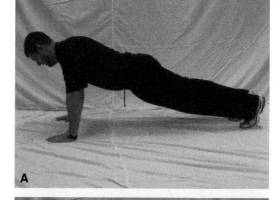

A

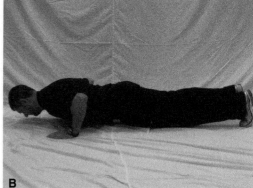

B

FIGURE 8-23.   (A, B) Push-up with plus exercise.

Inverted Pull-Up

From a secure handhold, have the athlete perform a pull-up from a horizontal/face-up position. The feet may be anchored manually or rested on a secure footing. Keep the shoulder, hip, and ankle collinear (see Figure 8.22). This exercise focuses on posture muscles as well as back and arm strength. This exercise also strengthens the rhomboid muscles which are important for throwing.

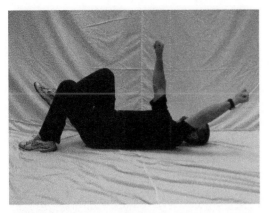

FIGURE 8-24. Dead bug core exercise.

focuses on the chest, core, and serratus anterior. The "plus" part of the motion is the most important as it isolates the serratus anterior which is a very important scapular stabilizer.

Dead Bug March

From a properly inflated, "ribs down" position, instruct the athlete to maintain oblique tension while alternating heel touches. Add in contralateral hand as athlete progresses (see Figure 8.24). This series of exercises focuses on the strength and function of the abdominal muscles.

Shoulder Tubing

These five exercises target the rotator cuff and scapular muscles.

1. "Y"s: Standing with resistance securely anchored at mid-chest height (all exercises), bring the handles away from the resistance over the head up into a Y shape (see Figure 8.25).

2. "T"s: Bring both arms with elbows straight away from the resistance at shoulder height (see Figure 8.26).

3. "M"s: Extend the shoulders down until they are even with the body. The hand position is about 12″ out to the sides away from the body (see Figure 8.27).

4. External rotation at 90°: With shoulders abducted to 90°, also flex the elbow to 90° and externally rotate against resistance (see Figure 8.28).

5. External rotation at 0° abduction: Place a bolster between the upper arm and the thorax. With arm by side flex the elbow to 90° and externally rotate against resistance (see Figure 8.29).

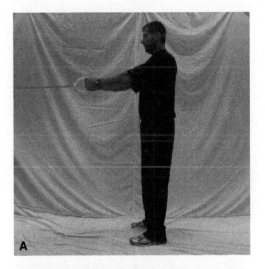

A

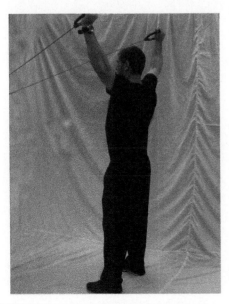

FIGURE 8-25. Standing "Y" shoulder/scapular exercise.

B

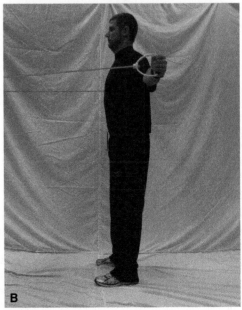

FIGURE 8-26. (A, B) Standing "T" shoulder/scapular exercise.

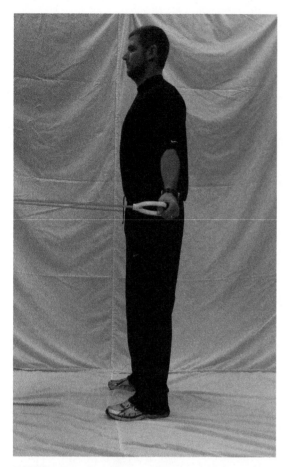

FIGURE 8-27.   Standing "M" shoulder/scapular exercise.

Ages 18 and Up (Refined Level)

Loaded Step-Up

Step onto a 12″–24″ step with a preferred load variation. Be sure to keep the hip, knee, and foot collinear and push up through the step with the heel. Be sure to alternate step-up leg (see Figure 8.30). This exercise focuses on hip, leg, and ankle strength as well as balance and control. The additional load, as long as it does not compromise form, will help elicit muscle growth and strength adaptations.

Romanian Dead Lift

Stand on a slightly bent leg (10°–20° of knee flexion). Flex forward from the hip with the trail leg collinear to hip and shoulder and reach for the ground foot with the opposite hand (see Figure 8.31). This exercise focuses on hamstring and glute strengthening while challenging balance and coordination. This exercise simulates and strengthens the deceleration demands of throwing in the lower extremity.

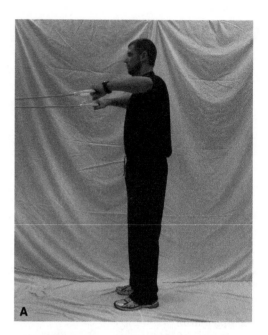

A

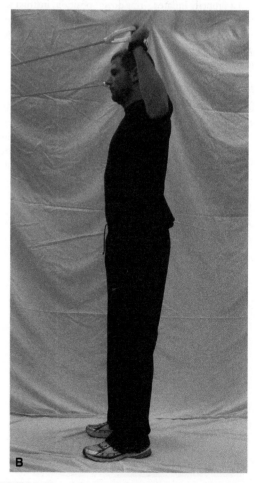

B

FIGURE 8-28.   (A, B) Standing 90°/90° shoulder/scapular exercise.

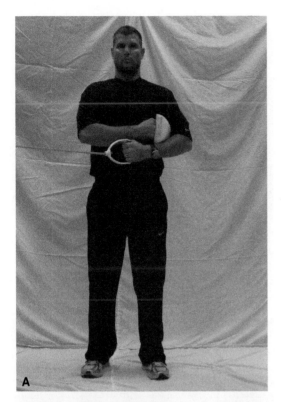

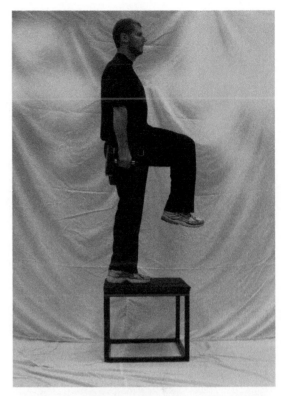

FIGURE 8-30. Weighted step-up with alternate leg lift exercise.

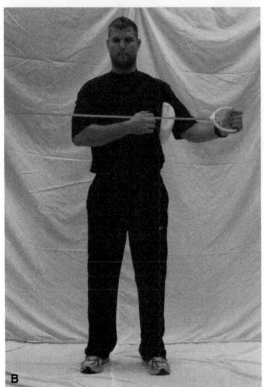

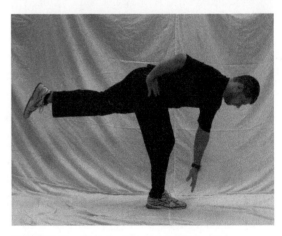

FIGURE 8-31. Single-leg Romanian dead lift exercise.

Single-Arm Cable Pull-and-Push (Loaded)

Standing with chest high cable resistance in front (pull) or behind (push), use one hand to pull/push the handle toward/away from the body while rotating away from the resistance (see Figure 8.32). Be sure to encourage leg utilization. This loaded exercise focuses on hip motion as well as hip and upper body strength in an effort to stimulate growth and strength gains.

FIGURE 8-29. (A, B) Standing external rotation at 0° abduction exercise.

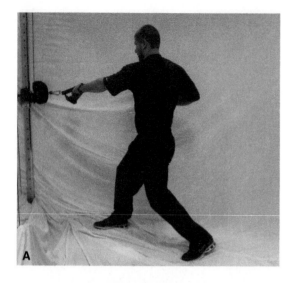

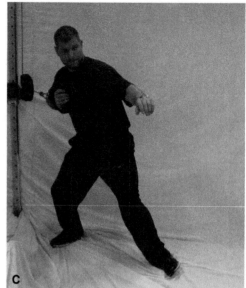

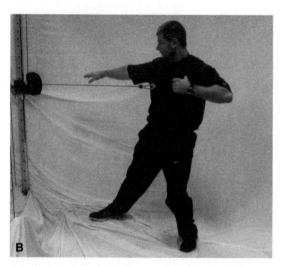

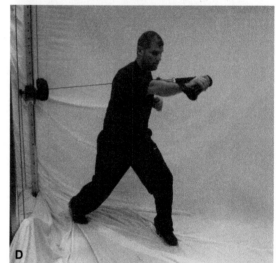

FIGURE 8-32. (A–D) Weighted single-arm pull-and-push exercise.

Diagonal Bar Chop

In a standing lunge position, place the lead leg on the side closest to the pulley. Use standing head height cable resistance and pull down and across the front of the body until the cable side arm is straight. Generate movement from the abdominal area. Avoid torso rotation as much as possible (see Figure 8.33). This series of exercises focuses on total body integration and coordination and abdominal strength.

Dead Bug on a Foam Roll

Lying longitudinally on a foam roll in a "ribs down" position, instruct the athlete to maintain oblique tension while alternating heel touches. Add in contralateral hand as athlete progresses (see Figure 8.34). This series of exercises helps maintain the fundamental strength and function of the abdominal muscles.

Single-Leg Glute Bridge

While lying face up, the player bends the knees and lifts the bottom up from the ground so that the shoulder, hip, and knee are collinear. Once this position has been achieved, the athlete brings one leg pointed to the ceiling and proceeds to lower and raise the hips, using the leg in contact with the ground (see Figure 8.35. This exercise focuses on glute and hamstring strength as well as core stability and control.

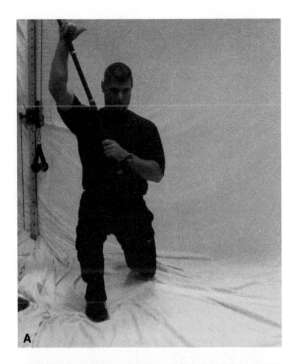

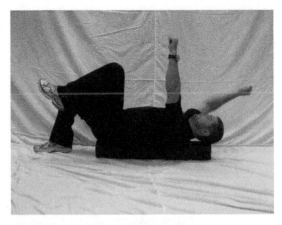

FIGURE 8-34. Dead bug foam roll core exercise.

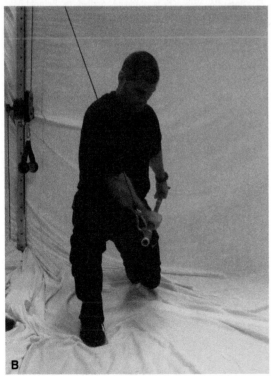

FIGURE 8-33. (A, B) Diagonal bar chop exercise.

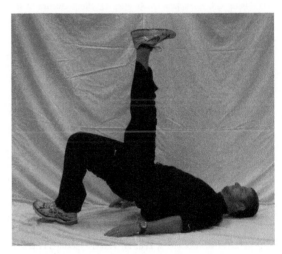

FIGURE 8-35. Single-leg glute bridge exercise.

REFERENCES

1. Yen KL, Metzl JD. Sports-specific concerns in the young athlete: Baseball. Pediatr Emerg Care 2000;16(3):215–220.
2. Taylor DC, Krasinski KL. Adolescent shoulder injuries: consensus and controversies. J Bone Joint Surg Am 2009;91:462–473.
3. Collins CL, Comstock RD. Epidemiological features of high school baseball injuries in the United States, 2005 through 2007. Pediatrics 2008;121:1181–1187.
4. Lyman S, Fleisig GS, Waterbor JW, et al. Longitudinal study of elbow and shoulder pain in youth pitchers. Med Sci Sports Exerc 2001;33(11):1803–1810.

5. Klingele KE, Kocher MS. Little league elbow: valgus overload injury in the paediatric athlete. Sports Med 2002;32(15):1005–1015.

6. Hang DW, Chao CM, Hang YS. A clinical and roentgenographic study of Little League elbow. Am J Sports Med 2004;32(1):79–84.

7. Lyman S, Fleisig GS, Andrews JR, Osinski ED. Effect of pitch type, pitch count, and pitching mechanics on risk of elbow and shoulder pain in youth baseball pitchers. Am J Sports Med 2002;30(4):463–468.

8. Mullaney MJ, McHugh MP, Donofrio TM, Nicholas SJ. Upper and lower extremity muscle fatigue after a baseball pitching performance. Am J Sports Med 2005;33:108–113.

9. Pappas AM. Elbow problems associated with baseball during childhood and adolescence. Clinical Orthop Relat Res 1982;164:30–41.

10. Petty DH, Andrews JR, Fleisig GS, Cain EL. Ulnar collateral ligament reconstruction in high school baseball players. Am J Sports Med 2004;32(5):1158–1164.

11. Fleisig GS, Shouchen D, Kingsley D. Biomechanics of the shoulder during sports. In: Wilk KE, Reinold MM, Andrews JR, eds. The Athlete's Shoulder. Philadelphia, PA: Churchill Livingstone Elsevier; 2009:365–384.

12. Ellis S. The Complete Pitcher Web Site. http://www.thecompletepitcher.com

13. House T. Pitching Mechanics (video). Dallas, TX: Robert Steinfield Productions; 1989.

14. Johnson R, Rosenthal J, Ryan N. Randy Johnson's Power Pitching: The Big Unit's Secrets to Domination, Intimidation, and Winning. New York, NY: Three Rivers Press; 2003.

15. Ryan N, House T, Rosenthal J. Nolan Ryan's Pitcher's Bible: The Ultimate Guide to Power, Precision, and Long-Term Performance. New York, NY: Simon & Schuster; 1991.

16. Davis JT, Limpisvasti O, Fluhme D, et al. The effect of pitching biomechanics on the upper extremity in youth and adolescent baseball pitchers. Am J Sports Med 2009;37(8):1484–1491.

17. Kebaetse M, McClure P, Pratt N. Thoracic position effect on shoulder range of motion, strength, and three-dimensional scapular kinetics. Arch Phys Med Rehabil 1999;80(8):945–950.

18. Alexander CM, Harrison PJ. Reflex connections from forearm and hand afferents to shoulder girdle muscles in humans. Exp Brain Res 2003;148:277–282.

19. Kibler WB, Sciascia A, Dome D. Evaluation of apparent and absolute supraspinatus strength in patients with shoulder injury using the scapular retraction test. Am J Sports Med 2006;34(10):1643–1647.

20. Ebaugh DD, McClure PW, Karduna AR. Scapulothoracic and glenohumeral kinematics following an external rotation fatigue protocol. J Orthop Sports Phys Ther 2006;36(8):557–571.

21. Cools AM, Declercq GA, Cambier DC, Mahieu NN, Witvrouw EE. Trapezius activity and intramuscular balance during isokinetic exercise in overhead athletes with impingement symptoms. Scand J Med Sci Sports 2007;17(1):25–33.

22. Selye H. The Stress of Life. New York, NY: McGraw Hill; 1956.

23. Wilk KE. Rehabilitation Guidelines for the Thrower with Internal Impingement. Presentation, American Sports Medicine Institute Injuries in Baseball Course, January 23, 2004.

24. Crockett HC, Gross LB, Wilk KE, et al. Osseous adaptation and range of motion at the gleno-humeral joint in professional baseball pitchers. Am J Sports Med 2002;30(1):20–26.

25. Reagan KM, Meister K, Horodyski MB, et al. Humeral retroversion and its relationship to gleno-humeral rotation in the shoulder of college baseball players. Am J Sports Med 2002;30(3):354–360.

26. Osbahr DC, Cannon DL, Speer KP. Retroversion of the humerus in the throwing shoulder of college baseball pitchers. Am J Sports Med 2002;30(3):347–353.

27. Borsa PA, Wilk KE, Jacobson JA, Scribek JS, Reinold MM. Correlation of range of motion & glenohumeral translation in professional baseball pitchers. Am J Sports Med 2005;33:1392–1399.

28. Chaitow L. Muscle Energy Techniques. 2nd ed. Edinburgh: Churchill Livingstone; 2001.

29. Janda V. Muscles central nervous regulation and back problems. In: Korr I, ed. Neurobiological Mechanisms in Manipulative Therapy. New York, NY: Plenum Press; 1978.

30. Chaitow L, Delany JW. Clinical Application of Neuromuscular Techniques. Vol 1: The Upper Body. Edinburgh: Churchill Livingstone; 2001.

31. Hammer WI. Functional Soft Tissue Examination and Treatment by Manual Methods: New Perspectives. 2nd ed. Gaithersburg, MD: Aspen Publishers; 1999.

32. Calder A. Recovery: restoration and regeneration as essential components within training programs. Excel 1990;6(3):15–19.

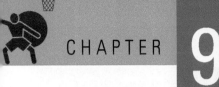

CHAPTER

9

Koichi Sato and Yohei Shimokochi

Basketball

"Moving without the ball" is a key to success in basketball. Players tend to dedicate the majority of their practice time to improving their skills with the ball (i.e., shooting and ball handling). A comparatively smaller amount of time is spent on fundamental movement skills (FMS) without the ball, such as jumping, sliding, running, and crossover step. Just like shooting skills, FMS improve when a movement-specific training program is implemented. This program consists of a series of specifically designed exercises to improve each movement skill. Ultimately, the goal of the program is to develop players' ability to sustain efficient and powerful movement patterns that minimize the risks of injuries and improve performance. The aim of this chapter is to assist rehabilitation and performance professionals in developing a movement-specific training program for players' success.

FUNDAMENTAL MOVEMENT SKILLS IN BASKETBALL

These skills are common to many sports, but basketball places unique demands on each of them.

Jumping

Basketball players perform a variety of jumps frequently during the game as part of other skills such as a jump shot, rebounding the ball, and blocking a shot. In a study of Australian professional basketball games, players jumped an average of 46 times during approximately 36 minutes of live time (the time the ball was in play), and jumping was considered a high-intensity activity in the game (1). Jumping skill training includes both jumping and landing. Mastery of landing skills is the initial priority, because some have suggested that many acute injuries occur during sudden deceleration motions such as landing (2,3). Proper landing skills, therefore, reduce the risk of lower extremity injuries (4–7).

Sliding

Sliding (also known as "cutting" and "shuffling") is often overlooked but is one of the most frequently used skills in basketball. In a study, players spent 31% of live time sliding (shuffling), of which 20% was high-intensity sliding

movements (1). Sliding is a primarily lateral movement skill combined with a crossover step. A few steps of explosive sliding seem to be a key in defense for cutting off the dribble drive and staying in front of opponents with the ball. The frequency of sliding in the game should be reflected in the time allocated for sliding skills in the program.

Running

Acceleration and maneuverability (e.g., agility and deceleration) are central to running in basketball. The duration of continuous running is short in the game. A study found that the average duration of high-intensity running during basketball games is 1.7 seconds, and only 27% of all high-intensity running lasts longer than 2 seconds (1). Powerful acceleration should be the focus of running skill training because players do not have time to build their running speed in such short spurts and are unlikely to achieve maximum running speed. Maneuverability is a player's ability to run tight turns and curves efficiently without losing speed. Players often run nonlinear paths through congested areas, and that should be factored into designing a running skill training program.

Crossover Step

A crossover step occurs when the base leg swings and the lead leg pushes off. An offensive player performs this when performing a crossover dribble during an attempt to break free from a defender. In players without possession of the ball, the crossover step is primarily used as (1) a lateral movement skill together with sliding and (2) a transitional movement from sliding to running. Considering the frequent use of sliding and the frequent changes in movement categories in the game (every 2 seconds on average (1)), the crossover step should be included as a fundamental skill in basketball.

PROGRESSION FOR A MOVEMENT-SPECIFIC TRAINING PROGRAM

Correction of Faulty Movement Patterns

Correcting faulty movement patterns (FMPs) is a keystone of the program and has to be addressed first and monitored continuously through the program. Common FMPs occur when players' body segments are improperly aligned (Figure 9.1) and joint motions follow improper sequences (Figure 9.2). The FMP may cause microtrauma to musculoskeletal tissues and eventually result in musculoskeletal pain syndrome (8,9). If players continue to train and play with the uncorrected FMP, they increase their risk of developing musculoskeletal pain. Therefore, correction is the priority.

Monitoring FMP is useful in guiding exercise progressions. These patterns often manifest as the demand (i.e., speed, load, repetitions, and complexity) of exercise increases. Therefore, exercise progression should be dictated by a player's ability to control movement of the body. If a player is performing an exercise poorly, the exercise should be adjusted accordingly. To maximize the effects of training, exercises should not be too challenging or too easy.

Development of Movement-Specific Endurance and Power

Considering the nature of the game, in which accelerations and decelerations are frequently repeated, power development is essential. Players also need endurance to generate high power output at the end of the game. Endurance is important for reducing the risk of injury because fatigue has been shown to affect lower extremity mechanics in sports-specific activities in both men and women (10–13), and these changes in mechanics have been suggested to increase the risk of injury (14). Exercise parameters such as resistance, sets, repetitions, tempo, and recovery time may be manipulated to gear the program toward movement-specific endurance and power development.

Integrated Movement Drills

The last focus of the program is to improve players' overall ability to move using integrated movement drills. The drills consist of a series of FMS to simulate common movement sequences in the game. Starting with simple and planned activities, the drills are progressed to complex and reactive activities that simulate and sometimes go beyond the demands of a basketball game.

EXERCISE PROGRESSIONS FOR FUNDAMENTAL MOVEMENT SKILLS

Squat Exercise

Mechanics of Squat Exercise

Squats are preparatory exercises for FMS. They involve triple flexion and extension of the legs that require (a) sufficient range of motion (ROM) of the ankle, knee, and hip joints; (b) sufficient lower extremity muscle function

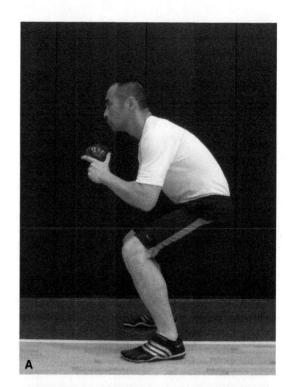

A

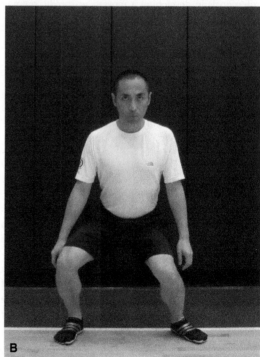

B

FIGURE 9-1. (A) Excessive spinal flexion and forward head position during double leg squat. The proximal segments (i.e., head, spine, scapulae, and pelvis) should be aligned neutral. (B) Femoral adduction and internal rotation and foot abduction in the left leg. The femur and foot should be aligned so that the knee and foot are pointing in the same direction.

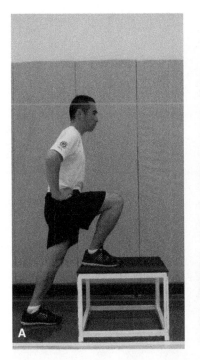
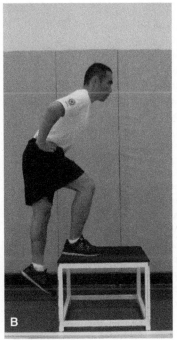
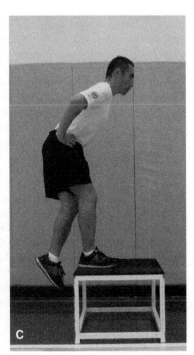
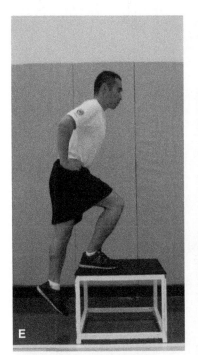
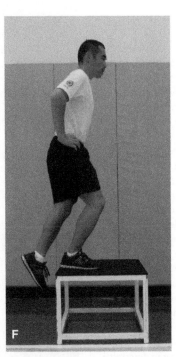
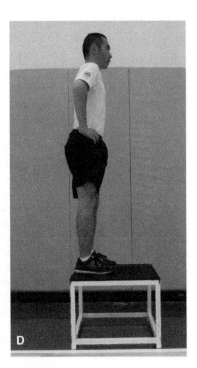

FIGURE 9-2. (A–F) Hamstring dominance in step-up. Dominant hamstring is causing the knee to extend early relative to hip extension, which results in backward movement of the knee (A-B-C-D). An optimal sequence is shown in A-E-F-D.

(i.e., endurance, strength, and power) to generate force for explosive movement and control of joint motions against given loads; (c) optimal motor control to maintain alignment of the joints and sequentially flex and extend them without FMP; (d) sufficient proximal stability to maintain neutral alignment or minimize unnecessary movements of the proximal segments; and (e) sufficient distal stability to maintain proper foot contact with the floor. These requirements are interrelated, and insufficiency in any of them may result in FMP.

Range of Motion

A player should be able to squat until the thighs are parallel to the floor. This provides a foundation for a player to perform the FMS comfortably without FMP. Limited ankle dorsiflexion and hip flexion ROM is a common finding and may be addressed individually (Figures 9.3 and 9.4) and through various squat exercises (Figures 9.5 and 9.6). The active loading exercises force active flexion of the hip(s) (see Figure 9.4) and legs (see Figure 9.5) by applying relatively large resistance against the flexion patterns. The goblet squat (see Figure 9.6) is very useful to improve squat mechanics for basketball players who tend to have long thighs.

Muscle Function

To sustain explosive and efficient movements, players must improve muscle function (i.e., endurance, strength, and power) to control joint movement through the available ROM without FMP.

Motor Control

Motor control is the capacity of the body to coordinate joint movement. FMPs are signs of suboptimal motor control. Players often acquire FMP from posture and movement habits in daily activities. With repetition, FMPs affect joint ROM and muscle function, which further facilitates the patterns, resulting in a vicious cycle and possibly pain and injury. FMP may be corrected with appropriate exercise prescription, feedback, and cueing with repetition (which is also how a player acquires faulty patterns). When limited ROM or muscle function contributes in tandem, they may be addressed individually along with correcting movement patterns to facilitate the process. For example, if ankle dorsiflexion is limited owing to a lack of joint mobility, forcing the dorsiflexion through exercises may be ineffective without mobilizing the ankle joint to create adequate joint mobility. At the same time, addressing limited ROM and muscle function alone may be ineffective without directly correcting movement patterns. A player may not use the improved ROM and muscle function if the movement patterns remain faulty. Rehabilitation and performance professionals should apply clinical reasoning to determine the causes of the FMP and plan effective management strategies.

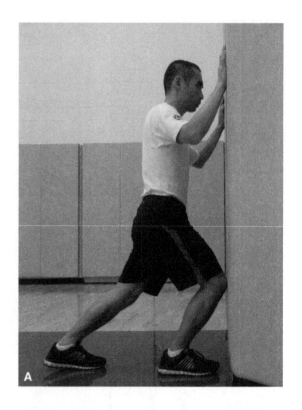

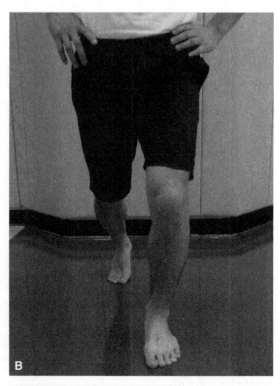

FIGURE 9-3.   (A and B) Wall ankle dorsiflexion. The thigh and foot are aligned.

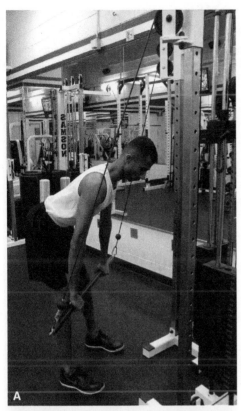

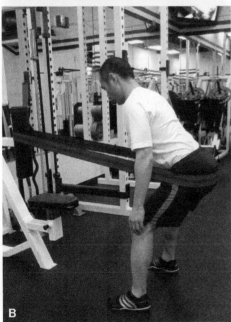

FIGURE 9-4. Deadlift—active loading to improve hip flexion range of motion. The resistance forces a player to flex the hip joints with active flexion of hip, rather falling into the hip flexion. The proximal segments are in neutral alignment. (A) Press down. Pressing the bar down against cable resistance toward ankles. (B) Press back. Stretching the elastic band by shifting the pelvis backward.

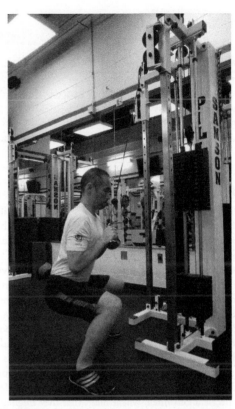

FIGURE 9-5. Double leg squat—active loading. Actively squatting down against cable resistance. Relatively large resistance is applied to facilitate active flexion of the ankles, knees, and hips.

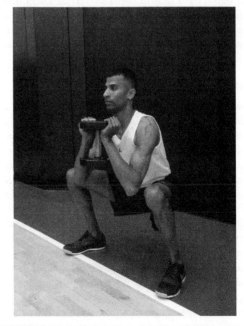

FIGURE 9-6. Goblet squat. The elbows are kept between the knees to facilitate the foot–thigh alignment.

TABLE 9.1	Traditional Internal vs. Modern External Cues	
Internal	**External**	
"Tuck the chin"	"Look at a spot on the ground 6 feet in front of you"	
"Widen your shoulders"	"Get tall with proud chest"	
"Extend the legs"	"Push off the floor"	

Proximal Stability

Preliminary study found a proximal stability ("stiffer torso") as a predictor of future performance in college basketball players (15). Proximal stability refers to the competency of a player to maintain neutral alignment of the proximal segments (i.e., head, spine, scapulae, and pelvis). The neutral alignment may be achieved by appropriate cueing (Table 9.1). (External cues (focus on the movement effect on the environment) are more effective in learning motor skills compared to internal cues (focus on body movements) (16,17).) Movements of the extremities and of the body center of mass (COM) place stability demands on the proximal segments, which increase as speed and complexity increase. In basketball, players repeat accelerations and decelerations often, which mean that they frequently experience large accelerations and decelerations of the body COM and receive large amounts of ground reaction force (GRF). Because the proximal segments constitute the largest mass in the body, each player must have sufficient proximal stability not only to overcome inertial forces during sudden deceleration and acceleration but also to establish a stable foundation on which the extremities can move efficiently and powerfully. For this reason careful monitoring of foundational squat exercises is required.

Distal Stability

Distal stability refers to the competency of the foot and ankle joints to control body COM and maintain proper foot contact with the floor. A proper foot–floor interface is also essential for efficient force exchanges (i.e., push-off and GRF) between the body and the floor for effective movement. Neuromuscular control of the foot and ankle joints plays a crucial role in maintaining optimal distal stability (18). For example, if the body COM moves anteriorly, the ankle joint must produce plantar flexor moment, shifting the center of pressure anteriorly beneath the foot. Then, GRF rotates the body posteriorly to keep the body COM within the foot (base of stance). The adjustments are made reflexively, especially when the foot is making brief contact with the ground during FMS. Single leg emphasis exercises, such as single leg squat, are useful to improve players' awareness of distal stability and neuromuscular control of the foot and ankle joints.

Types of Squat Exercises

Double Leg Squat

The double leg squat (Figure 9.7) is suited for improving ROM as well as learning basic triple flexion and extension patterns.

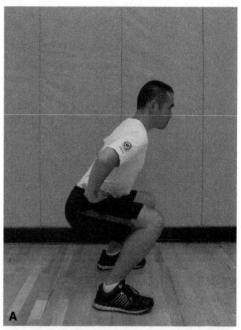

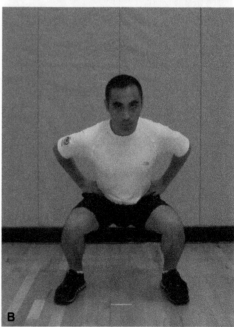

FIGURE 9-7. Double leg squat. (A) The head, knees, and toes are aligned vertically. The thigh is parallel to the floor. The proximal segments are aligned to neutral and approximately parallel to the tibias. (B) The thigh and foot are aligned.

Split Squat

The split squat (Figure 9.8) is an exercise with single leg (front leg) emphasis and increased lateral stability demands. It is useful for improving sagittal plane hip mobility—the front hip flexion and rear hip extension essential for running. The direction of load may be changed to vary the focus.

Lateral Squat

The lateral squat (Figure 9.9) has a single leg emphasis and is useful for improving push-off mechanics for sliding. Resistance is applied laterally through a Rotational Training Strap (Physical Industries), which provides a better feel for push-off in sliding to produce lateral displacement of the body COM.

Rotational Squat

Rotational squat (Figure 9.10) exercise has a single leg emphasis and places rotational demands on the lower extremities.

Single Leg Squat

The single leg squat (Figure 9.11) is the most demanding exercise among all squat exercises because it has the smallest base of support and the largest stability and strength demand. At the same time, it might be the most important exercise because most movement skills are based on a single leg support. Single leg box squat (Figure 9.12) is a good alternative as a progression for single leg squat.

Common Faulty Movement Pattern in Squat Exercises

Hamstring Dominance in Knee Extension during Push-Off (See Figure 9.2)

During the push-off, the knee extends early relative to the extension of the hip, bringing the knee backward toward the body instead of bringing the body up to the knee. The hip remains in a slightly flexed position even after knee extension is completed. Sahrmann (9) explained that the hamstring muscles become dominant in the action of knee extension owing to weakness in the quadriceps muscles, resulting in this FMP. This pattern may be corrected with deadlift (Figure 9.13) to facilitate early hip extension and use of elastic band at the knee (Figure 9.14).

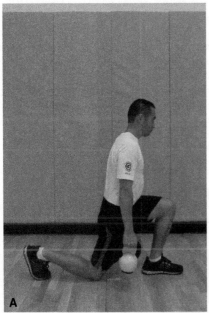

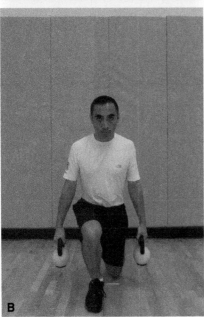

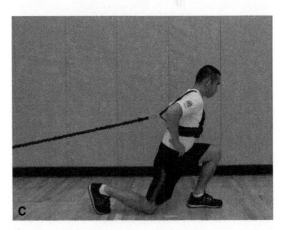

FIGURE 9-8. Split squat. (A) The tibia is vertical and parallel to the proximal segments. The rear hip is in neutral or slightly extended. (B) The feet are aligned along a line that splits the sagittal plane. (C) Load is applied with a shoulder harness through cables to increase demands on proximal stability and facilitate the use of the front leg for push-off to imitate first step mechanics.

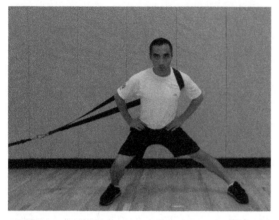

FIGURE 9-9. Lateral squat. The push-off leg is flexed as that for the double leg squat (see Figure 9.7). Avoid shifting the spine over the push-off leg to preserve optimal push-off angle for multidirectional agility (see Sliding section).

Vertical Trunk and Excessive Ankle Dorsiflexion

The trunk remains in vertical alignment and the knees are driven forward excessively. The ankle joint is driven into extreme dorsiflexion (Figure 9.15). This movement pattern may reduce the contribution of the hip extensors during push-off and consequently may increase stress on the knee and ankle joints. Limited hip flexion ROM may facilitate this movement pattern, preventing the hip from flexing. The excessive forward movement of the knees may be corrected by placing an object (e.g., a box) in front of the knee (Figure 9.16). The deadlift (see Figure 9.13) and box squat (Figures 9.12 and 9.17) are both effective to facilitate hip flexion.

Excessive Lumbar Spine Flexion (See Figure 9.1A)

It may reduce the contribution of hip extensions during push-off and increase the risk of lower back injuries. The movement is usually due to insufficient proximal stability or an inability of the hip joint to flex against a given load. For example, a player may be able to maintain the neutral alignment in a double leg squat but not in a single leg squat owing to the increased load. The load may be adjusted to accommodate a player's capacity. Elastic tape may also be applied over the lumbar spine for tactile feedback to facilitate players' awareness (Figure 9.18).

Excessive Spinal Extension

The spine is excessively extended particularly at the neck. This FMP is a sign of poor proximal stability and dysfunction of the deep neck flexors at cervical spine.

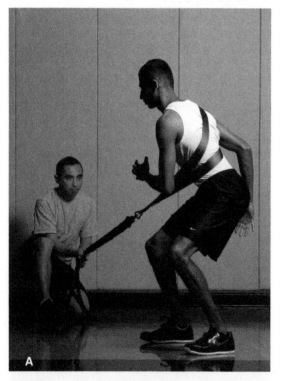

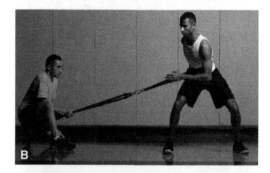

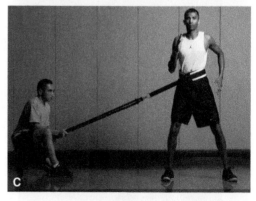

FIGURE 9-10. Rotational squat. The Rotational Training Strap is wrapped around the torso to apply rotational load. The proximal segments remain neutral and are rotated toward the push-off (right) leg (A and B). This anti-rotation maneuver minimizes spine twisting. During push-off with the right leg (C), a "relative" right hip external rotation occurs. Simultaneously, the opposite hip internally rotates and the proximal segments rotate away from the push-off foot.

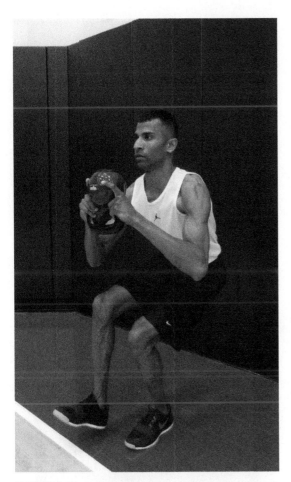

FIGURE 9-11. Single leg squat. The push-off hip is slightly adducted and the ankle is in eversion so that the spine is aligned over the push-off foot.

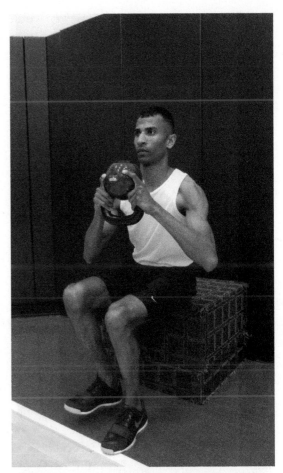

FIGURE 9-12. Single leg box squat. Box height is adjusted so that the thigh is parallel when seated.

Femoral Adduction and Internal Rotation

The femurs are adducted and internally rotated, resulting in valgus angles in the knees (see Figure 9.1B). Research suggests femoral adduction and internal rotation may increase the risk of knee injury (19). Limited ankle dorsiflexion ROM is a common cause of foot abduction. Goblet squat (see Figure 9.6) and the use of elastic band around the knees (Figure 9.19) are reactive exercises to correct this. The medial aspect of the foot (i.e., ball of foot) should stay in contact with the floor to maintain distal stability.

Lateral Weight Shift

A common mistake when correcting medial collapse of the knee (see Figure 9.1B) is to shift weight to the lateral aspect of the foot. Limited ankle eversion ROM may be related to this. Use of elastic band between the ball of foot and floor is effective to prevent lateral weight shift (see Figure 9.19).

Lateral Trunk Tilt

The trunk is tilted (Figure 9.20) toward the weight-bearing leg. Weakness of hip abductors in the weight-bearing leg may be associated with the lateral trunk tilt that is suggested to increase the risk of knee injury in female athletes (19). The use of elastic band to facilitate normal alignment is effective (Figure 9.21).

Exercise Progression in Squat Exercises

Squats may be progressed by manipulating resistance, sets, repetitions, tempo, and recovery time to create a specific focus (i.e., improving ROM, muscle function, and motor control). Triple flexion and extension patterns in the squat exercises should be carried over to the movement-specific exercises for fundamental skills that are presented in the following sections.

Jumping

Among all training for FMS, jumping skill training may be most familiar to players. Height provides a significant

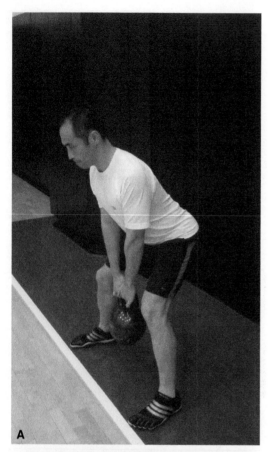

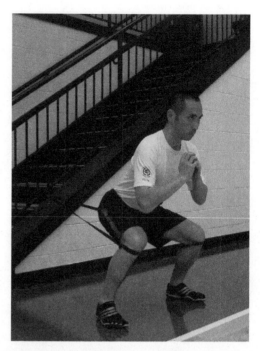

FIGURE 9-14.   Use of elastic band to prevent early knee extension during push-off.

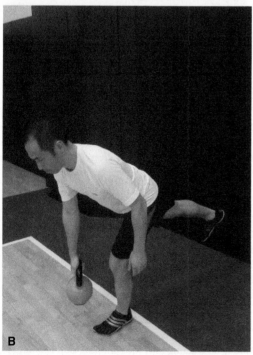

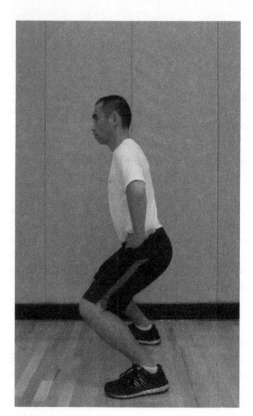

FIGURE 9-13.   Deadlift. (A) Double leg. (B) Single leg.

FIGURE 9-15.   Vertical trunk and excessive ankle dorsiflexion in double leg squat.

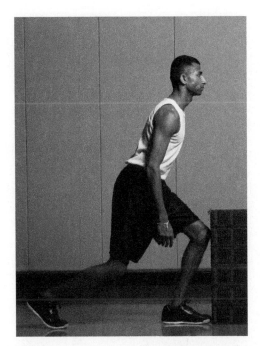

FIGURE 9-16. Use of a box to prevent excessive ankle dorsiflexion.

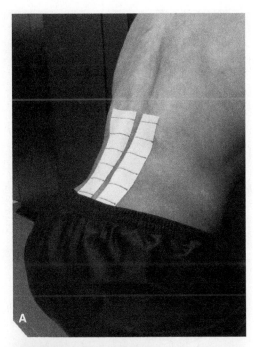

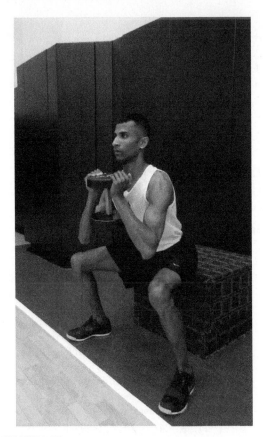

FIGURE 9-17. Double leg box squat.

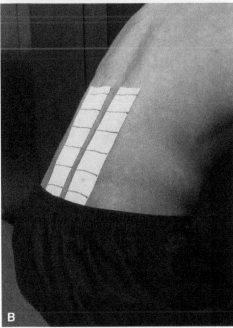

FIGURE 9-18. Elastic tapes are applied over the lumbar spine. (A) Neutral spine is maintained. (B) The tape is stretched due to excessively flexed lumbar spine.

advantage in the game of basketball, and measurements of players' abilities to jump are commonly used to characterize their physical skills. Even though players tend to focus on how high they can jump, the focus of jump skill training is (1) mastery of landing, (2) powerful push-off

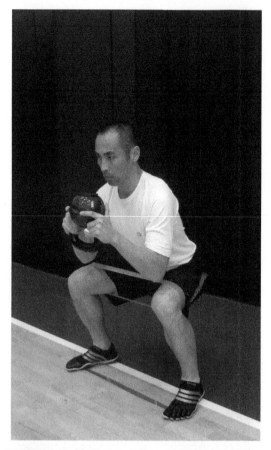

FIGURE 9-19. Elastic band at the knees prevents femoral adduction and internal rotation. Ends of stretched elastic band are placed between ball of foot and the floor to facilitate foot–floor contact.

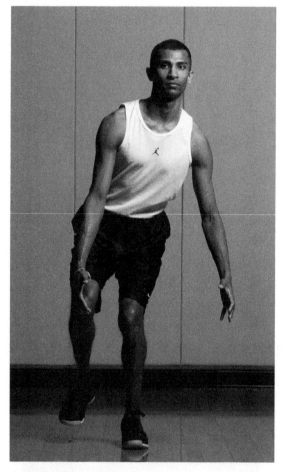

FIGURE 9-20. Lateral trunk tilt.

for jumping, and (3) execution of a variety of jumps and landings, in that order. *Caution:* Jumping is high-intensity activity and stressful to the body. Jump skill training must be prescribed carefully based on players' capacity.

Mechanics of Jumping

Jumping exercises are a direct progression of squat exercises in which the push-off actually lifts the foot off the floor. Thus, the basic mechanics of the triple flexion/extension during the squat exercises apply to the mechanics of jumping. Obviously, more power is generated during push-off than during the squat exercises; consequently, players experience increased demands on their bodies during jumping and landing.

Common Faulty Movement Patterns

The common FMPs in jumping exercises are the same as those that occur with squat exercises.

Exercise Progression in Jumping

Jumping exercises may be progressed by adjusting the following variables.

Base of Support

- Double Leg Support: Double leg jump
- Split Stance Support: Split jump
  - Unilateral. Jumping and landing on the same side (i.e., jumping and landing with a split stance with the right foot forward).
  - Alternate. Jumping on one side and landing on the other (i.e., a stance for jumping with the right foot forward and landing with the left foot forward).
- Single Leg Support
  - Bounding (Figure 9.22). Jumping with one foot and landing with the other foot (i.e., jumping with the right foot and landing with the left foot).
  - Hopping (Figure 9.23). Jumping and landing with the same foot.

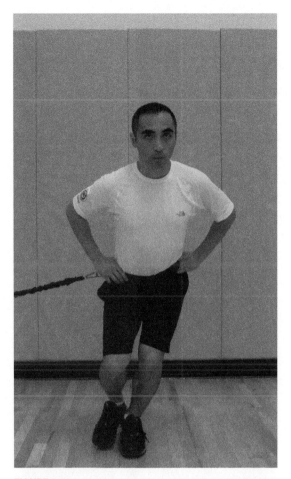

FIGURE 9-21.   Use of elastic band at pelvis to correct the alignment.

Movement Variables

The exercises may be divided into jumping and landing to emphasize each component separately.

- Landing Emphasis. "Soft landing" with triple flexion is a goal for landing. Players should land softly

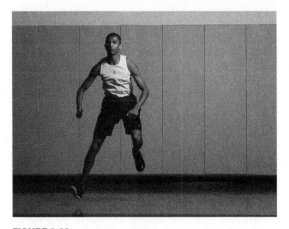

FIGURE 9-22.   Lateral bounding.

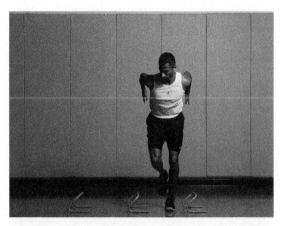

FIGURE 9-23.   Lateral hopping over mini hurdles.

for efficient deceleration such that minimal sound is heard when the foot/feet make a contact with the floor.

- Drop Squat. From standing, a player rapidly drops into the respective beginning of push-off stance (i.e., double leg, split, and single leg). A small lift (jump/hop) of the foot/feet from the floor before the drop may facilitate the action of the drop. A player should experience a "sense of falling" during the drop. Drop squats are useful exercises for mastering landing and quickly getting to the beginning of the push-off position.
- Box Landing. A player steps off from a box and lands on the floor in the respective stance. The height of the box may be adjusted. Box landing allows players to focus on landing mechanics.
- Jumping Emphasis
- Box Jump (Figure 9.24). The box jump allows players to focus on push-off mechanics for jumping. The height of box should be set based on a player's capability. You may progress this by landing on one leg, putting weights in the hands, or adding a weighted vest.

Box Jumps Reduce Injury Risk

The box jump is ideal for building power while reducing injury risk because landing forces are minimized compared with landing on the floor. (But make sure to step off from the box, not jump off after landing on the box!)

- Jumping. A player jumps from and lands on the floor. Both jumping and landing skills are practiced.

Other Variables

Players perform a variety of jumps during the game. The following variables may be adjusted to expose players to various jumping skills and focus specifically on muscle

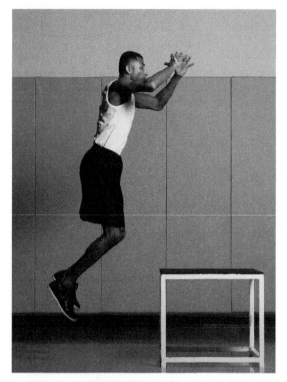

FIGURE 9-24.   Box jump.

- Rotation. Jumping may be performed with rotation to right or left against resistance (Figure 9.25) or to predetermined degrees such as 90° and 180°.
- Tempo. Jumping may be performed repetitively with or without pausing between each jump.
- Resistance, Repetition, Set, and Recovery Time. These parameters may be manipulated to gear the exercise toward specific muscle functions (i.e., endurance, strength, and power).

Sliding

Sliding ("cutting" or "shuffling") is an essential agility skill that is crucial to change of direction ability in sport (See Chapter 23). In this way sliding is a distinguishing feature between a sport like basketball and track (where speed is normally *only* straight ahead).

Mechanics of Sliding

In sliding, a player moves laterally by pushing off with the base leg (i.e., leg away from the direction of sliding). Lateral

functions (i.e., endurance, strength, and power). Rehabilitation and performance professionals have to make sure that players are ready for the adjustments and not challenged too much too soon to avoid potential injury.

- Counter Movement. Countermovement is a triple flexion of the legs immediately before push-off. In jumping with countermovement, a player squats from standing then pushes off to jump without pausing before push-off. Jump heights with countermovement are usually higher than that of jumps without it. Jumping without countermovement occurs when players first assume the beginning of the push-off position and pause before pushing off to jump. A player most commonly uses jumping without countermovement during the jump ball in the game.
- Arm Swings. Arm swings are downswings of the arms with triple flexion and upswings of the arms with the push-off of a jump. Arm swings usually improve vertical jump height.
- Loading Depth. Loading depth may be specified to train specific ROM from shallow to deep triple-flexed positions.
- Horizontal Displacement. Jumping may be performed with horizontal displacements, such as jumping forward and backward or laterally and diagonally.

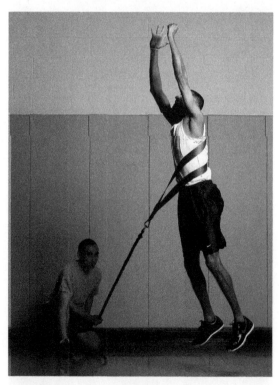

FIGURE 9-25.   Rotational jump against resistance with Rotational Training Strap.

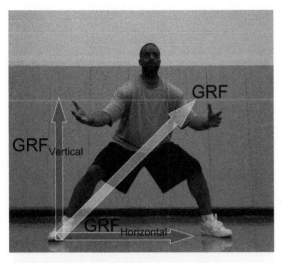

FIGURE 9-26. Vertical and horizontal ground rotation force.

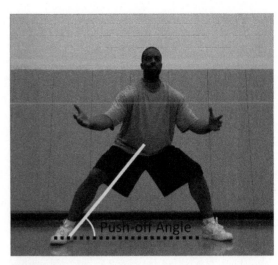

FIGURE 9-27. Push-off angle.

displacement of the body COM is the result of the body receiving a GRF that pushes the body COM horizontally. GRF has two components that should be considered for effective sliding: vertical and horizontal ($GRF_{Vertical}$ and $GRF_{Horizontal}$, respectively; Figure 9.26). If players want to obtain maximum $GRF_{Horizontal}$ to move quickly in a lateral direction, they should push against the floor at the appropriate angle (21).

Hip Extension and Lateral Push-Off

To maximize lateral push-off stay low and push sideways. The lateral push is in reality a sagittal plane hip, knee, and ankle extension (triple extension). A study (21) suggests that a powerful triple extension of the legs and lower COM, not hip abductor functions, is crucial for lateral deceleration–acceleration motion of sliding.

Push-off angle can be evaluated by estimating the direction of GRF acting on the body (Figure 9.27). While the body accelerates in the lateral direction, GRF originates from the center of pressure within the foot pushing the floor and is directed toward the body COM which is approximately located around the player's naval.

Why Aren't the Knee and Foot Stacked Vertically?

Traditional lateral squats are performed with the knee stacked vertically above the ankle. However, to generate first step accelerative power in sliding the knee must be placed medial to the foot so that during push-off the moment of force propels the player laterally. But remember to maintain thigh–foot alignment.

Thus Push-off angles can be estimated by looking at the angle between the floor and the line connecting the base of the push-off foot with the player's naval. A biomechanical study (21) showed that appropriate angles are 45°–50°. To achieve these push-off angles, players should place their feet sufficiently far apart and flex their lower extremity to lower their body COM, which is also essential for effective sliding (21). The speed of sliding is a function of step length and step frequency. To gain speed, a player has to take larger steps, increase the frequency of the steps, decrease ground time, or a combination of these techniques.

Common Faulty Movement Patterns

Excessive External Rotations of the Push-Off Hip and Foot

When the hip and foot joint are excessively externally rotated (i.e., thighs and feet are excessively pointing out), hip extensors and ankle plantar flexors are in disadvantageous positions to produce force for push-off resulting in slow, sluggish sliding motions. Double leg and lateral squat (see Figures 9.7 and 9.9) are appropriate to address this FMP.

Early Lead Leg Reaching

A player is initiating sliding with lead leg reaching by abducting the lead hip toward the direction of sliding. A common misconception is that the reaching is a key to speeding up sliding. Base leg push-off is the key and should initiate the slide. The reaching occurs and is a natural motion during sliding, but the focus should be on the push-off. This FMP may be a naturally acquired movement or a movement that is due to insufficient power or sense of push-off from the base leg. Exercises such as

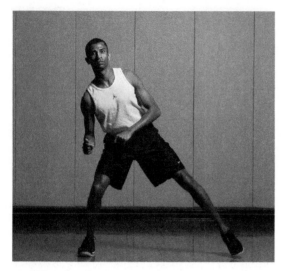

FIGURE 9-28. Lateral trunk tilt.

lateral squat (see Figure 9.9) and resistive slide may be beneficial to improve push-off force and develop a solid sense of push-off.

Closely associated with this is lateral trunk tilt (Figure 9.28). Exercises such as resistive slide with a Rotational Training Strap is effective in preventing lateral trunk tilt.

Exercise Progression for Sliding

Lateral Wall Drill

Lateral wall drill (Figure 9.29) is designed to improve the proximal stability for running, sliding, and crossover step.

Resistive Sliding

Resistive sliding (Figure 9.30) is designed to facilitate a sense of push-off and improve muscle function. Resistance may be applied manually or through cable resistance at the waist or shoulder. Resistance at the shoulder (see Figure 9.9) increases the demand on proximal stability compared to that at the waist (see Figure 9.30). A solid push should occur before or at the same time as the lead leg comes off the floor.

Power Sliding

Power sliding is designed to improve explosiveness in sliding. Players are instructed to take two to three powerful slides against elastic resistance as if they were attempting to cut off a dribble drive by getting in front of an opponent.

Assistive-Resistive Sliding

With assistance, a player is instructed to focus on moving their legs as fast as possible to keep up with the faster movement of the body and consciously push-off even if the elastic cord is assisting the movement. Against resistance, a

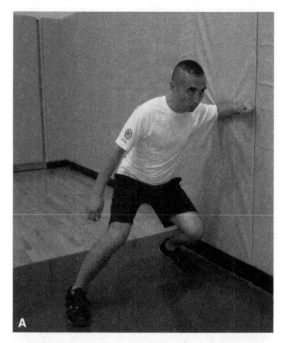

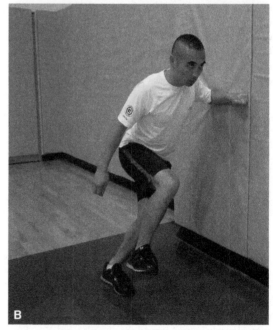

FIGURE 9-29. Lateral wall drill. (A) Outside leg hold. (B) Inside leg hold.

player performs power sliding focusing on powerful push-off (Figure 9.31).

Reactive Sliding

A player is instructed to change the direction of sliding by reacting to cues. The cues could be other players'

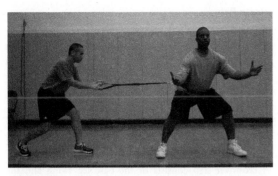

FIGURE 9-30. Resistive slide. Manual resistance with a waist belt and nonelastic strap.

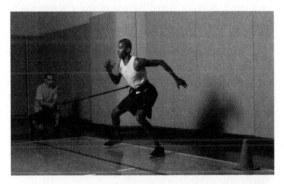

FIGURE 9-31. Assistive-resistive sliding. A player slides against elastic resistance to the cone then slides back with assistance.

movements (Figure 9.32), visual signals (i.e., pointing direction of movement), or audible cues (sounds of a whistle).

Running (See Chapter 23)

Acceleration and maneuverability are the focus of running skill training in basketball. The main skills of training are (1) to accelerate quickly in the first few steps using

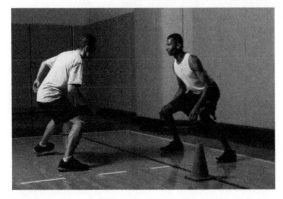

FIGURE 9-32. Reactive sliding. A player is reacting to the other player's movement.

powerful push-offs and (2) to improve the ability to maneuver through tight turns and curves.

Mechanics of Running

The quality and angle of push-off are the primary determinants of the amount of acceleration of the body's COM. During the quick acceleration of running, the body must lean forward and push off the ground powerfully with triple extension of the lower extremities to receive an appropriate amount of $GRF_{Horizontal}$, just as in the case of sliding. The amount of forward lean of the body decreases as running speed approaches its maximum, however, or when no or little acceleration of the body COM is necessary (i.e., constant speed).

In basketball, the functions of the push-off leg to perform triple extensions are extremely important because quick acceleration of the body must be implemented more frequently than constant speed running during the game. The squat exercises, especially split squat, and the running-specific exercises in this section are appropriate for improving the function of the push-off leg.

Upper body functions are also important in the performance of powerful push-offs during running when the law of conservation of angular momentum is considered. As both legs alternately push off the floor and swing forward while running, players constantly create angular momentum on the body in the horizontal plane in both directions alternately. Because the body initially has no angular momentum, the upper body must exert the same amount of angular momentum but in the opposite directions of that of the lower legs to keep the net angular momentum on the body zero. This requirement means that if players want to accelerate the body COM powerfully in running, they must have the ability to rotate the trunk and swing the arms fast enough to counterbalance the angular momentum created by the legs.

Maneuverability requires proper footwork and higher degrees of proximal stability compared to those of linear running (i.e., running straight). Footwork refers to a player's ability to reactively adjust foot placements and step length/frequency to maximize running velocity. Running nonlinear patterns places greater lateral and rotational torque on the body, which requires additional proximal stability compared to that required to run linearly.

Common Faulty Movement Patterns

Common faulty postures and movement patterns are discussed subsequently.

Exercise Progression for Running

Exercise progression starts with the focus of building proximal stability, then moves to more dynamic exercises that involve leg actions and muscle functions. Refer to Chapter 23 for linear wall drills such as Wall Marching and Load and Lift exercises.

Common Faulty Movement Patterns for Linear Wall Drills

The common FMPs (Figure 9.33) are seen when the head-to-heel alignment is not maintained.

Shoulder Harness Drills

Shoulder harness drills (Figure 9.34) are a progression of linear wall drills and are useful in further challenging proximal stability and improving running-specific muscle functions. Single leg hold, march, skip, and other running drills can be performed (see Chapter 23).

Forward Bounding

Forward bounding is part of the jumping/landing skill exercises and is useful for running skill progression as well because it alternates the pushing off and landing of individual legs, similar to the action of running. A key is to land in a single leg base stance with proper alignment and pause each bound. The exercise is progressed by speeding up a tempo of bounding by shortening the pause between landing and push-off.

Linear Acceleration

In split stance acceleration, a player sprints from the split stance (Figure 9.35). The emphasis is on powerful push-off in the first few steps.

Zigzag Run

A player runs a zigzag pattern (Figure 9.36) around the cones. The emphasis is on making a smooth deceleration by lowering the body COM toward each cone to make a turn and quickly accelerate to the next cone.

Crossover Step

Mechanics of the Crossover Step (See Multidirectional Movement in Chapter 23)

A crossover step consists of the base leg swing and the lead leg push-off. The leg swing facilitates the advancement of body COM to create an optimal push-off angle (Figure 9.37) for the lead leg. The base leg swing should be a rapid, laterally aimed leg action and a player has to maintain the lower body COM to create a positive push-off angle with sufficient $GRF_{Horizontal}$.

The crossover action of the legs places greater demand on proximal stability, especially in the frontal and transverse planes. Players must control unnecessary movement of the proximal segments during the crossover step as well as when they return to the base stance to be ready to transition to following action.

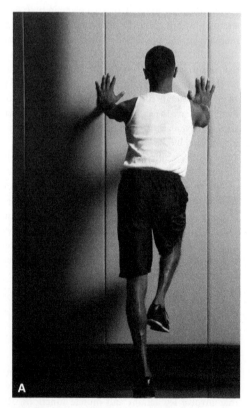 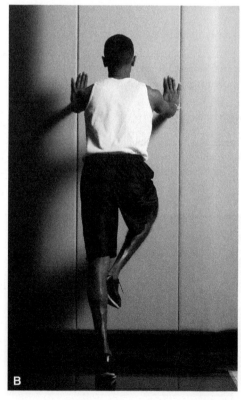

FIGURE 9-33. Common faulty movement patterns for linear wall drills. (A) Laterally shifted pelvis. (B) Abducted hip in nonweight-bearing side. (C) Flexed hip. (D, E) Excessive lumber flexion.

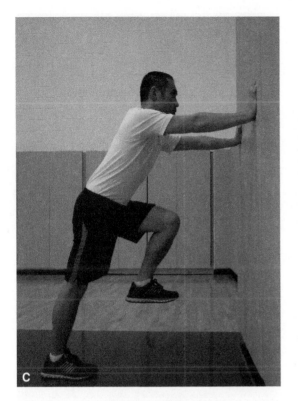

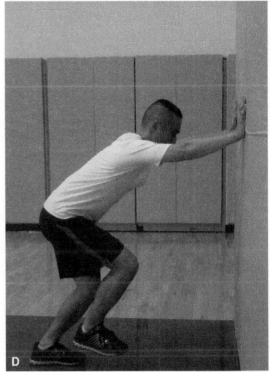

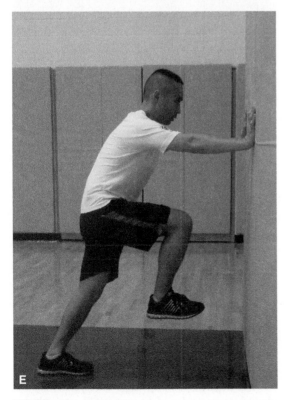

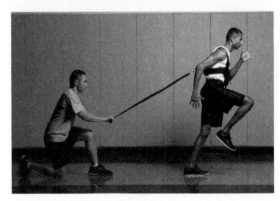

FIGURE 9-34.   Shoulder harness drill.

Common Faulty Movement Patterns

Excessive vertical displacement may occur. Just as in sliding a player has to maintain low body COM and swing the base leg laterally to create the optimal push-off angle for lead leg push-off.

Exercise Progression for the Crossover Step

Crossover Squat

Crossover squat (Figure 9.38) is effective for improving mobility and ROM of the hip joints.

FIGURE 9-33.   (Continued)

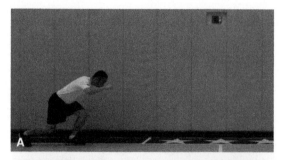

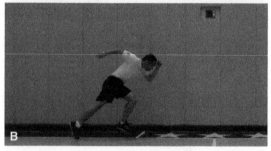

FIGURE 9-35. (A, B) Split stance acceleration.

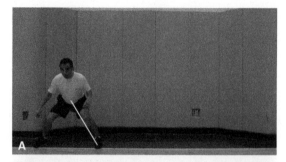

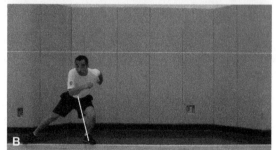

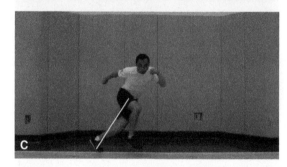

FIGURE 9-37. (A–C) Crossover step. Push-off angle for lead (left) leg changes as the body center of mass (COM) advances in the direction of movement (left). In the base stance, the lead foot is in front of the body COM (A). As the body COM passes the lead foot in the horizontal plane, a positive push-off angle is created (C).

Lateral Wall Drill (See Figure 9.29)

A player holds the stance to maintain low body COM and neutral alignment of the proximal segments.

Base Leg Swing

From the base stance, a player performs the base leg swing (Figure 9.39) and returns to the base stance. The hand is placed in front of the opposite waist as an aim for the knee to facilitate lateral movement of the swing leg. The leg swing should be rapid, and the lead leg should remain flexed to maintain low body COM.

Crossover Step

From the base stance, a player performs one complete crossover step (Figure 9.40). Step length and repetition may be adjusted for progression of the exercise. Shorter step length

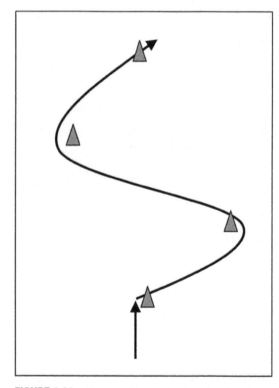

FIGURE 9-36. Zigzag run. Placement and number of cones may be adjusted.

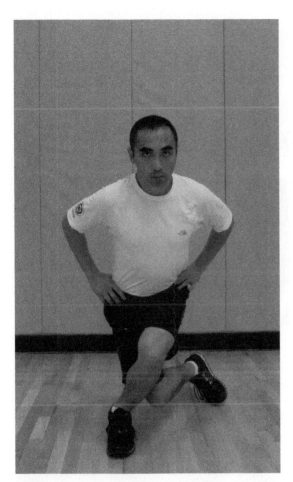

FIGURE 9-38. Crossover squat.

may be used to improve footwork and quick leg exchange in the crossover step. Longer step length may be used to emphasize powerful lead leg push-off to accelerate and gain maximum horizontal displacement. Repetition of the crossover step challenges proximal stability by changing the direction in every step. The crossover step may be repeated two (e.g., crossover step to right then to left) to three times (e.g., crossover step to right, then to left, and to right). Alignment of the proximal segments should be maintained, especially when the direction of movement is changed.

Resistive Crossover Step

A player moves laterally by repeating crossover step (Figure 9.41) in the same direction against resistance, focusing on lead leg push-off.

Resistive-Assistive Crossover Step

A player performs the crossover step with assistance. The focus is on performing the crossover action of the legs quickly so a player is ready for landing. Upon landing, a player should be balanced in the base stance.

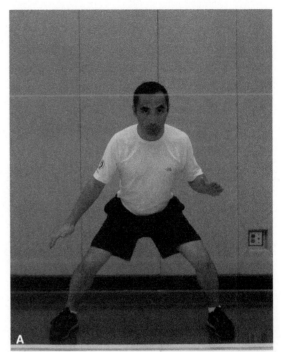

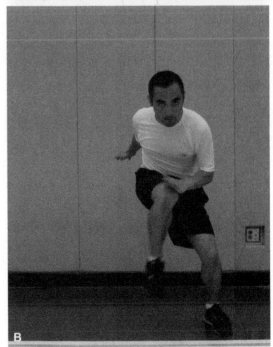

FIGURE 9-39. (A and B) Base leg swing.

Integrated Movement Drills

Integrated movement drills are designed with a series of FMS to improve players' overall ability to move without the ball. The drills are useful as part of a rehabilitation

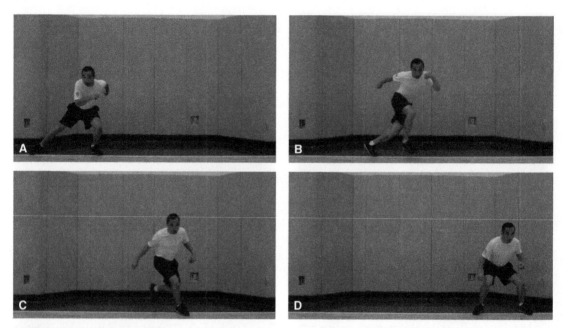

FIGURE 9-40. (A–D) Crossover step.

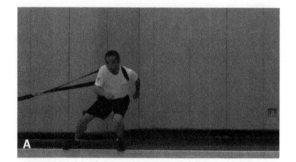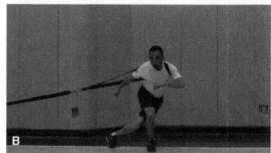

FIGURE 9-41. (A and B) Resistive crossover step.

program before return to play, warm-up before practice, and general fitness/conditioning programs. A study by McInnes et al. (1) found that players spent 75% of live time at a heart rate response greater than 85% of peak heart rate and were engaged in high-intensity activity approximately 15% of live time. Along with the other demands of the basketball game, these physiological requirements of the game should be considered to tailor game-like drills.

The complexity of the drills is progressed by adding more components, such as (1) a higher number of movement skills, (2) greater frequency of direction changes, and (3) more reactive components that reflect the nature of basketball games. As the complexity of the drill progresses, it becomes just like specific basketball drills. The integrated movement drills provide opportunities to emphasize and remind players of the importance of movement without the ball. The focus of the drills should continue to be on players' executions in the FMS, however.

Players will shift their attention to the "outcomes" of play (e.g., making or missing shots) rather than focusing on the "processes" (e.g., how they are getting separation from their defenders to get an open look, keeping up with an opponent defensively).

Slide Crossover-Run

A player slides for a few steps then makes a transition to running using a crossover step.

Slide-Reverse Crossover-Run

A player slides for a few steps then reverses the direction of movement using a crossover step into running.

5-Cone Drill

A player performs a series of FMS using cones (Figure 9.42). The distance between the cones may be adjusted based on step length and size of player.

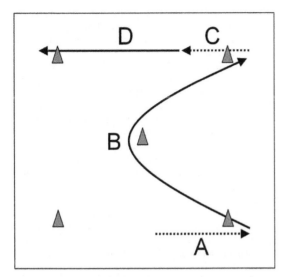

FIGURE 9-42. An example of 5-cone drill. A player starts sliding to right and performs a crossover step into running at the cone (A). A player then runs around the cone (B). Then, a player slides to left for a few steps (C) and performs crossover step into running (D).

DESIGNING AND IMPLEMENTING THE MOVEMENT-SPECIFIC TRAINING PROGRAM

Evaluation

Evaluating players and their limitations is the first step in designing a movement-specific program. Each player presents unique limitations that challenge both the individual and rehabilitation and performance professional. The limitations are usually in ROM, muscle function, motor control, proximal stability, or distal stability. Rehabilitation and performance professionals have to take a comprehensive approach to identify the limitations and recognize their underlying causes to design and set expectations for a player.

Selecting the Primary Focus of the Program

If a player presents with limitations and significant FMP, the initial emphasis should address these issues. Players may start from advanced movement-specific exercises and drills if they present with a minimal amount of FMP. Once the primary focus of program is set, progression should be presented to players so that they understand where they stand in the progression and what the next step is. Clear communication fosters similar expectations about a program for both the rehabilitation and performance professionals and a player.

Exercise Selection and Coaching

Exercise selection and its parameter setting are important to maximize the outcome of the program. Exercises should be challenging but not too easy so that players are able to make and recognize steady progress both quantitatively (i.e., speed, resistance, repetitions, and sets) and qualitatively (i.e., quality of movement patterns). Qualitative progress is not as recognizable as quantitative progress because it is not as measureable. Rehabilitation and performance professionals should make conscious effort to help players "sense improvement in their movement patterns." Visual feedback (pre-post video), reduction in painful movements, clear improvement in movement patterns, muscle strength, and flexibility all help the athlete appreciate the role of movement pattern correction.

Importance of Facilitating and Challenging

Rehabilitation and performance professionals should be facilitators for players' experiences outside their comfort zone. These experiences may be movement patterns, feelings and awareness of movement, resistance to movement, and speed of movement. The program should always challenge and expose players to something that they are not used to. These exposures outside of the game will improve their performance in the game.

ACKNOWLEDGMENTS

The authors would like to thank photographer Ned Dishman as well as models Wes Unseld Jr. and Navin Hettiarachchi, MS, ATC. The authors also appreciate Vasso Chronis and Physical Industries, Inc.

REFERENCES

1. McInnes SE, Carlson JS, Jones CJ, et al. The physiological load imposed on basketball players during competition. J Sports Sci 1995;13:387–397.
2. Ferretti A, Papandrea P, Conteduca F, et al. Knee ligament injuries in volleyball players. Am J Sports Med 1992;20:203–207.
3. Shimokochi Y, Shultz SJ. Mechanisms of noncontact anterior cruciate ligament injury. J Athl Train 2008;43:396–408.
4. Blackburn JT, Padua DA. Influence of trunk flexion on hip and knee joint kinematics during a controlled drop landing. Clin Biomech (Bristol, Avon) 2008;23:313–319.
5. Blackburn JT, Padua DA. Sagittal-plane trunk position, landing forces, and quadriceps electromyographic activity. J Athl Train 2009;44:174–179.
6. Hewett TE, Lindenfeld TN, Riccobene JV, et al. The effect of neuromuscular training on the incidence of knee injury

in female athletes. A prospective study. Am J Sports Med 1999;27:699–706.

7. Shimokochi Y, Yong Lee S, Shultz SJ, et al. The relationships among sagittal-plane lower extremity moments: implications for landing strategy in anterior cruciate ligament injury prevention. J Athl Train 2009;44:33–38.

8. Comerford MJ, Mottram SL. Movement and stability dysfunction—contemporary developments. Man Ther 2001;6:15–26.

9. Sahrmann SA. Diagnosis and Treatment of Movement Impairment Syndromes. St. Louis, MO: Mosby; 2002.

10. Chappell JD, Herman DC, Knight BS, et al. Effect of fatigue on knee kinetics and kinematics in stop-jump tasks. Am J Sports Med 2005;33:1022–1029.

11. Kernozek TW, Torry MR, Iwasaki M. Gender differences in lower extremity landing mechanics caused by neuromuscular fatigue. Am J Sports Med 2008;36:554–565.

12. McLean SG, Fellin RE, Suedekum N, et al. Impact of fatigue on gender-based high-risk landing strategies. Med Sci Sports Exerc 2007;39:502–514.

13. Rozzi SL, Lephart SM, Fu FH. Effects of muscular fatigue on knee joint laxity and neuromuscular characteristics of male and female athletes. J Athl Train 1999;34:106–114.

14. Santamaria LJ, Webster KE. The effect of fatigue on lower-limb biomechanics during single-limb landings: a systematic review. J Orthop Sports Phys Ther 2010;40:464–473.

15. McGill SM, Andersen JT, Horne AD. Predicting performance and injury resilience from movement quality and fitness scores in a basketball team over 2 years. J Strength Cond Res 2012;26:1731–1739.

16. Makaruk H, Porter JM, Czaplicki A, Sadowski J, Sacewicz T. The role of attentional focus in plyometric training. J Sports Med Phys Fitness 2012;52:319–327.

17. Wulf G, McConnel N, Gärtner M, Schwarz A. Enhancing the learning of sport skills through external-focus feedback. J Mot Behav 2002;34:171–182.

18. Winter DA. Biomechanics and Motor Control of Human Movement. 4th ed. New York, NY: Wiley; 2009.

19. Ford KR, Myer GD, Hewett TE. Valgus knee motion during landing in high school female and male basketball players. Med Sci Sports Exerc 2003;35:1745–1750.

20. Hewett TE, Torg JS, Boden BP. Video analysis of trunk and knee motion during non-contact anterior cruciate ligament injury in female athletes: lateral trunk and knee abduction motion are combined components of the injury mechanism. Br J Sports Med 2009;43:417–422.

21. Shimokochi Y, Ide D, Kokubu M, Nakaoji T. Relationships among performance of lateral cutting maneuver from lateral sliding and hip extension and abduction motions, ground reaction force, and body center of mass height. J Strength Cond Res 2013;27:1851–1860.

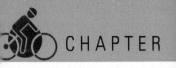
Cycling

COMMON INJURIES

The most common injuries to youth and recreational cyclists are nontraumatic injuries associated with overuse or improper fit of the bicycle. The incidence of these injuries can be as high as 85%. Competitive cyclists are more likely to experience traumatic injuries as a result of collisions and falls associated with the high speeds of racing (1,2).

Nontraumatic

Nontraumatic injuries result from a "combination of inadequate preparation, inappropriate equipment, poor technique and overuse" (3). The asymmetric variants of the human body often collide with the symmetric design of the bicycle, producing high stress loads on the muscles, tendons, and joints (4). Due to the constrained posture of cycling, the knees, cervical spine, scapulothoracic region, hands, gluteal region, and perineum are often the victims of repetitive stress loads (2). Neck and back pain occurs in up to 60% of riders (5). Nontraumatic injuries on the bicycle can be drastically reduced by assiduous attention to the custom design and fit of the bicycle to the athlete. Once the bicycle has been custom-tailored to the athlete, the athlete must then learn to interact with the bike efficiently.

Traumatic

Traumatic injuries are most often the result of forceful ground contact. They account for 500,000 emergency room visits in the United States each year. Contusions, strain/sprain injuries, and fractures are most common to the shoulder, lower arm, hand and wrist, lower leg, and ankle (5).

BIOMECHANICS OF CYCLING

In cycling, the design of the bicycle is critical so as to allow the athlete freedom of movement from a functionally efficient and relaxed posture while fixed at the feet, pelvis, and hands. The femur, tibia, foot, and crank arm of the bike comprise the four-bar system that transfers power from the rider to the bicycle via linkage at the shoe/pedal interface. "This transmission site, by design, can either create smooth transfer of energy or abnormally high repetitive

loads which are potentially injurious to the body" (6). Pedal designs allowing for varying degrees of float to the toe-in/heel-out or heel-in/toe-out movement patterns have helped "enhance power transfer from rider to bike" and have also helped to reduce stress–strain injuries (6).

The pedal cycle, one complete rotation of the crank arm, is divided into two phases: the power phase and the recovery phase. The power phase, starting at 12 o'clock and ending at 6 o'clock, contributes the greatest amount of power to forward movement. The recovery phase, starting at 6 o'clock and ending at 12 o'clock, can actually negate power being produced during the power phase unless the athlete actively pulls up on the pedal. Idleness during the recovery phase wastes energy that could propel the cyclist forward as the weight of the leg on the crank arm must be overcome by the power phase leg. Although primarily fixed in space while the legs move to produce power, the upper body is very much involved in force production. When the athlete is in a neutral spine position with the diaphragm parallel to the pelvic floor and the lumbopelvic stabilizing system is engaged, the trunk becomes a solid functional link between the upper and lower body. This allows the upper body to contribute to the overall power production whether the athlete is in or out of the saddle. During the power phase, the cyclist in the saddle can transfer to the pedal a force equal to approximately half of his or her body weight. When out of the saddle, the cyclist can transfer to the pedal forces up to three times his or her body weight. This additional power can be generated because the cyclist is able to pull up on the handlebars while pushing down on the pedals (7).

Power Phase

As studied by Gregor (8) and Okajima (9), "the force applied to the crank is most effective in converting to a rotational force (torque) when the force is perpendicular to the crank. The force is greatest and closest to being perpendicular to the crank during the middle half of the power phase." At other positions, the forces are slightly less. "Because the direction is more parallel than perpendicular to the crank, little force in the first and last quadrants is translated into rotational force" (7).

Power generation requires a requisite range of motion and can be altered by changing the bicycle geometry. Typically at the top of the power phase, 12 o'clock, the thigh is approximately 10° to 20° below the horizontal plane and the knee is flexed approximately 110° (7). The ankle should be at approximately a 90° angle or dorsiflexed 10° to 15°. A slight dorsiflexion of the ankle will allow the cyclist to achieve a vector of force into the power phase earlier than if the ankle is plantarflexed. The hips travel through a range of motion of approximately 55°; the knees travel through the greatest range of motion of the lower-extremity joints, approximately 75°; and the ankles travel through a range of motion of approximately 25° (7).

The quadriceps push the pedals forward and over top dead center to begin the power phase. The quadriceps muscle then extends the knee and is active during the first half to two-thirds of the power phase. Gluteal muscles assist in extending the hip joint in the first two-thirds of the power phase and contribute more effectively the more the hip is flexed, which is based on saddle height (7). As the gluteal muscles extend the hip, the entire lower limb pushes down on the pedal. When the cyclist's foot is clipped into the pedal, the "downward movement of hip extension translates into knee extension because the limb is forced to travel with the pedal" (7). The hamstring muscles assist in extending the hip and are active during the last three-quarters of the power phase. "The hamstring muscles have the longest activity period of any lower-extremity muscles during cycling. When the hamstring muscles pull posteriorly on the knee, the knee does not flex because the foot is held on the pedal by friction or a cleat. Instead, the posterior pull on the knee extends the knee and creates downward pressure on the pedal" (7). The soleus and gastrocnemius both become active during the middle half of the power phase and provide a significant amount of force to the pedal in the second half of the power phase. Because of the two-joint action of the gastrocnemius, it stays active well into the recovery phase. The single joint soleus however, does not. The calf muscles and their action at the ankle are critical to provide a solid transfer of force into the pedal (10). The calf muscles, when properly used to take advantage of their first-class mechanical leverage, place the foot in a plantar flexed position during the early recovery phase. This greatly improves the efficiency of the hamstring muscles in that phase (11).

Often the cyclist will allow the legs to track with internal hip rotation as the knees brush close to the top tube. This, however, is not an efficient functional pedaling action since the gluteals are neurologically facilitated when the external rotators of the hip are engaged. Ideally, "the flexed knee at top dead center moves away from the bicycle." This occurs primarily because the "posterior surface of the femoral condyles is more nearly symmetrical than the distal surface and because subtalar and mid-tarsal joint resupination externally rotates the leg and tilts the leg away from the bicycle top tube." With medial column dorsiflexion, hamstring activity, and knee extension during the power phase, the knee at bottom dead center moves closer to the bicycle, which increases the functional Q angle (7).

The core stabilization system, which is the foundation from which the cyclist generates power, must engage so the pelvis and lumbar spine can provide a stable origin for the quadriceps, gluteal, and hamstring muscles. Abt et al. concluded that "core fatigue resulted in altered cycling mechanics that might increase the risk of injury because the knee joint is potentially exposed to greater stress. Improved core stability and endurance could promote greater alignment of the lower extremity when riding for extended durations as the core is more resistant to fatigue" (12).

Recovery Phase

"The recovery phase actively realigns the foot and leg for the next power phase, thereby creating a smooth transition from one power phase to the next" (11). It also provides a rest period for the power phase muscles. "During the recovery phase, the weight of the recovering limb always applies some downward force on the pedal. The weight produces a negative torque at the crank, which reduces the effectiveness of the opposite limb's power phase" (11). Active recovery and reduction in negative torque can be achieved by engaging the iliopsoas and rectus femoris muscles to flex the hip and the hamstring muscle to flex the knee. "The gastrocnemius can also assist in knee flexion during the early recovery phase" (7). During the second half of the recovery phase, the anterior tibial muscle begins dorsiflexion of the ankle and the quadriceps muscle begins knee extension and hip flexion (7,13–15). Efficient use of the anterior tibialis to dorsiflex the ankle during the recovery phase allows for an earlier entrance into the next power phase. A dorsiflexed ankle at the top of the pedal stroke creates a forward vector of force entering the power phase. A plantarflexed ankle will create a posterior vector of force at the top of the pedal stroke. This delays entrance into the power phase and results in a loss of power production

BICYCLE FIT

When discussing the biomechanics of cycling, it is necessary to discuss the topic of bicycle fit. "The underlying principle of positioning a cyclist on a bicycle is to remember that the bicycle is adjustable, and the cyclist is adaptable" (16). The cyclist should be both interviewed and evaluated before he or she mounts the bike.

Interview

The interview will determine the cyclist's age, height, weight, and gender; riding goals; type of riding and training engaged in; and history of any injuries or known limitations. The interview will provide the information necessary to custom fit the bike to the rider. For example, a criterium rider will spend most of the race in the drops of the handlebars and will dive into and accelerate out of corners all the while elbow to elbow in a pack of riders. Throughout the race the heart rate dips below the lactate threshold and then elevates above it. The fit must allow the rider to be both metabolically and mechanically efficient in the drops. The bottom bracket of the bike must be high enough to clear the ground with tight sharp turns and the handlebars narrow enough to avoid contact with other riders while in a tight pack yet wide enough to be mechanically efficient for the rider's anatomy. The long-distance triathlete will maintain a constant aerobic workload and must consume fuel during the race to replenish energy. The fit must allow the athlete to be metabolically, mechanically, and aerodynamically efficient. The fit must provide comfort due to prolonged time in the saddle as-well-as good balance to facilitate the cyclist's safe control of the bike with one hand while consuming food or drink.

The riding goals and style will determine both the frame material and geometry. Many materials are used to build frames, from steel and aluminum to titanium and carbon fiber, as well as exotic materials such as bamboo. The materials greatly affect the quality of the ride (how the rider feels on the bike) and the responsiveness of the bike. Most bicycle companies offer stock frame materials and geometries that will meet the average cyclist's needs and goals. Factory standard frames can be fit to the average athlete by choosing the handlebars, stem rise and reach, seat post, saddle, and pedals to position the cyclist correctly. However, cyclists who have functional or structural limitations, are riding at a competitive level, or simply have a passion for the sport of cycling have the option of enjoying a bicycle frame custom designed for them.

Following the interview, the cyclist must be physically evaluated to determine functional and structural barriers. These barriers, once identified, must either be removed or respected so they do not interfere with the cycling activity.

Functional barriers, such as limited hip flexion or deficient stabilization of the core, must be assessed and considered during fitting. Often, the skilled functional rehabilitation specialist can treat and remove these barriers, allowing the athlete to achieve optimal biomechanical and aerodynamic position on the bicycle.

Structural barriers, such as degenerative disc disease, degenerative joint or structural leg length inequality, are barriers that must be respected and "fit around." These limiters may preclude the athlete from attaining the optimal positioning.

Initial Evaluation

Supine

- Ankle dorsiflexion. The cyclist, ideally, should be able to dorsiflex the ankle between 10° and 15°. The cyclist can generate up to 20% of the total positive mechanical work by optimal use of the ankle plantar flexors (17).

- Knee flexion. At the top of the pedal cycle, the knee is flexed approximately 110°. Limited knee flexion may affect the ability to lower the saddle to the ideal height. This will adversely limit hip flexion, thereby affecting maximum effectiveness of the gluteals.
- Hip flexion with the knee in relaxed flexion (measure while cyclist is supine and in neutral spine). Hip flexion is one of the most important measurements taken before the athlete mounts the bike. When the athlete is on the bike, the measurement will be important when determining saddle height and the optimal drop of the handlebars. Handlebars that are too low will force the athlete to expend energy to flex the hip against a functional/structural barrier, thus "leaking energy" that would otherwise contribute to the total positive mechanical work.

Hook Lying

- Pelvic tilt affects the lumbar spine. Optimal power is generated from a position of neutral lumbar spine. The cyclist's ability to maintain pelvic position will largely determine the lumbar spinal position.
- Ability of the cyclist to engage the core. The core stabilization system is the foundation from which the cyclist generates power. An inefficient bracing system will affect the rider's ability to maintain neutral spine and to generate optimal power.

Seated

- Distance between ischial tuberosities. This distance is best measured by having the cyclist sit on a square of pressure-sensitive foam, leaving an indented mark to measure. This will aid in choosing a saddle that will properly support the cyclist's pelvis.
- Shoulder flexion. The shoulder should be flexed to approximately 90° when on the road bike. Cyclists with limited shoulder flexion (e.g., shoulder impingement syndrome) will be compromised in their ability to reach the handlebars. A shorter stem with an increased rise will lift the rider to more of an upright position accommodating for the restricted range of shoulder flexion. This position will be less aerodynamic but functionally more efficient with reduced risk of repetitive strain injury.
- Shoulder width. This distance is measured from the lateral aspect of the acromions. This will determine the appropriate handlebar width in centimeters. It is better to err on the wider side unless the cyclist is racing in a pack of riders as discussed above in the criterium race.

Cleat/Pedal Interface

Once the cyclist has been interviewed and evaluated, the saddle, handlebars, and a shoe/cleat/pedal system must be chosen. First the shoe/cleat/pedal system is aligned, and then the saddle height and saddle fore/aft position are established. After the cyclist is positioned over the crank for the greatest power transfer, the height and reach of the handlebars can be determined.

The cleat should be placed on the shoe so that the first metatarsal head is directly over the pedal spindle. Although there is very little published research regarding pressure distribution in the cycling shoe, Sanderson and Cavanagh (18) observed that the pressure distribution was localized in the forefoot, specifically the first metatarsal head. Therefore, to achieve the most efficient power transfer from cyclist to crank arm, the placement of the cleat is critical.

Evaluation on Bicycle

After the optimal cleat/pedal interface has been achieved, the cyclist will mount the bike that is on a stationary trainer and spin to warm up. He or she should settle into a comfortable relaxed posture, finding the "sweet spot" on the saddle.

To determine the saddle height, the cyclist will "freeze" the leg at the furthest reach of the crank in the crank cycle—approximately 5:30 for the right foot and 6:30 for the left foot. The knee flexion should be between 25° and 35° (Figure 10.1 A). With too little flexion, the hamstring will not engage at the bottom and the foot will not be able to achieve enough dorsiflexion to take advantage of the powerful calf muscles. With too much flexion, the leg will be compressed at the top, muscles will not engage to their optimal potential, and power will be lost.

The fore/aft position of the saddle is determined by having the cyclist "freeze" the leg at the 90° position in the power phase of the crank cycle (3 o'clock for the right foot and 9 o'clock for the left foot). A plumb line, dropped from the tibial tuberosity for the road bicycle and Gerdy's tubercle for the time trial (TT) bicycle (or triathlon bicycle), should bisect the pedal spindle (Figure 10.1 B).

The angle of saddle tilt is very much dependent on the style of saddle and rider personal preference. Usually a 0° to 5° downward tilt is customary. A saddle that is tilted up will often cause soft tissue irritation and a saddle with too much downward tilt will cause the rider to "fall forward," placing too much pressure on the hands.

With the cyclist positioned on the saddle for optimal power transfer to the crank, the position of the handlebars can now be determined. The height of the handlebars is determined by the hip flexion measurement taken during the initial evaluation. The rider should be guided to achieve neutral spine with the hands in the drop position of the road bars and aero position of the TT bars. After a few revolutions of the crank, the cyclist freezes the leg at top dead center of the crank cycle. The hip with the least range of motion is the limiting hip and is the side to measure while determining handlebar height. Hip flexion on the bike cannot be greater than the measurement taken during

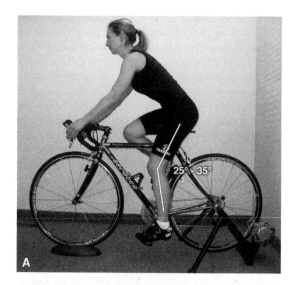

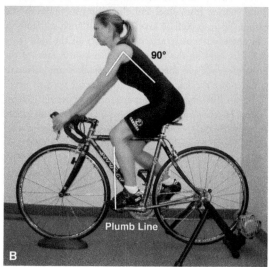

FIGURE 10-1. (A and B) Evaluation after mounting bicycle.

the initial evaluation. Handlebars that are too low cause the drop from saddle to bars to be too great, and the rider will be compressed at the top of the crank cycle resulting in lost power. Handlebars that are too high will create less of an aerodynamic position, and the cyclist will again "leak energy" to overcome air resistance.

The reach to the handlebars on the road bicycle is placed so that the rider has approximately 90° of flexion at the shoulder joint when the spine is in functional neutral and the scapulothoracic connection is centrated (Figure 10.1 B). There should be a relaxed flexion in the elbow joints, and the cyclist should have his or her hands resting comfortably on the hoods of the brake/gear system. The reach to the aero bars on the TT bike is placed so that the rider's elbows are slightly forward of the shoulders in the vertical plane with the proximal aspect of the forearms resting on the pads. When looking at the rider from the front, the arms should fall within the lateral margins of the thighs. If the arms fall outside or inside of the thighs, they will increase the frontal surface area and will decrease the aerodynamic efficiency.

Training Principles

Although cycling is primarily a sagittal plane motion, the cyclist must be trained in triplanar motions so as to train the core to withstand the torsional loads associated with sprinting, out-of-the-saddle climbing, and high-speed racing and cornering. A properly functioning core stabilization system provides a solid platform for prime drive musculature while resisting high-torsion triplanar loads.

While seated in the saddle, multiplanar high torque forces demand that the core engage to stabilize the pelvis. A stable pelvis will provide a solid anchor for the legs to drive the crank arms with symmetry and power. The pelvis, when out of the saddle, is no longer fixed in space. With the pelvis now free of the saddle and only the hands and feet fixed to the bike, the demand on the core to stabilize is greatly increased. The pelvis must continue to provide a solid anchor for the legs to drive the crank arms with symmetry and power.

The function of the shoulder complex in concert with the cervical and thoracic spine is critical for the cyclist. Hours are spent "in the saddle" with the cervical spine in extension. Proper extension mechanics of the head, specifically, extension into the upper thoracic spine as opposed to fulcruming at the mid-cervical spine, helps reduce the stress–strain load to the cervical spine. Centration of both the scapula on the thorax and the glenohumeral joint allows for a relaxed upper body and proper function.

It is essential that a thorough musculoskeletal evaluation and functional capacity evaluation be performed at the start of the athlete's training program. Initial evaluation should identify the problems or limitations and determine if they are symmetrical or asymmetrical; asymmetry is important to address first. Functional training must also take into consideration the closed chain position of the hands on the handlebars, the locked position of the feet in the pedals, and both the defined position of the pelvis on the saddle and the dynamic position of the pelvis when out of the saddle.

Start the training protocols from the lowest developmental postures of hook lying, quadruped, and plank. Progress to the half and tall kneeling chop and lift postures, which serve not only as functional training but also as evaluation tools using the four-quadrant assessment protocol described by Voight, Hoogenboom, and Cook. Finally, transition to the higher level of standing (19). Kneeling, seated, and standing chop and lift multiplanar movement patterns facilitate core muscular recruitment to stabilize the spine through spiral and diagonal challenges. "When the chop and lift patterns are used in conjunction with half and tall kneeling developmental postures, the techniques are an excellent assessment of core stability/instability" (19).

Periodically, reassess during phases of increased volume and intensity and especially in the case of crash-related injuries.

TRAINING FUNDAMENTALS

The functional development of the cyclist is consistent with any other athlete. Attention must be given to develop the fundamentals of proper diaphragmatic activation and stabilization of the core. Only when correct respiration is achieved, through centration and control of the diaphragm, can stabilization of the lumbopelvic region exist. Scapulothoracic and glenohumeral centration is also critical for the stability and function of the cyclist. Since the cycling posture tends to restrict or impinge upon anterior belly breathing, it is critical for the athlete to develop lateral and posterior diaphragmatic activity. This will allow the athlete to ventilate while on the bicycle, especially when in the TT/triathlete aero bar position.

FUNCTIONAL TRAINING PROGRESSIONS: YOUTH, COMPETITIVE, AND ELITE

In each of the following sections, the presentation moves from fundamental to advanced based on current skill level. Basic progressions are appropriate for youth athletes. More advanced progressions appropriate for competitive and elite athletes are identified.

Diaphragm

- Belly breathing in hook lying
- Modified cycling-specific child's pose to facilitate lateral and posterior activity of the diaphragm. The shoulders are at 90°, and the hands are in an aero bar grip (Figure 10.2).

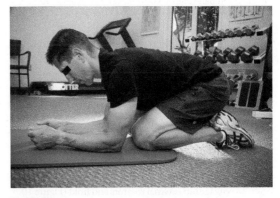

FIGURE 10-2.   Shoulder angle of 90° and aero bar grip.

Lumbopelvic Stability and Shoulder Complex Stability

- Cat/camel for proprioception and spatial awareness of the pelvis, spine, and rib cage
- Sit on ball and develop isolation of pelvic motion under a still torso.
  - Anterior/posterior pelvic tilts, lateral shifts, and rotations
  - Anterior/posterior pelvic tilts, lateral shifts, and rotations balanced on one leg; alternate legs
  - Anterior/posterior pelvic tilts, lateral shifts, and rotations with one eye closed; alternate eyes
- Quadruped track to address the closed chain function of the arms/hands, the extensor system, and the diagonal stability demand, between the upper and lower body, of cycling. When performing this track of exercises, go very slowly so as to feel the internal shift of muscular tension as the diagonal support system engages. Focus on maintaining a stable anchor against which the extremities can move.
  - Hand march
  - Bird dog with opposite arm and leg
  - Bird dog on disc or foam
  - Quadruped track progressed from the bird dog to the bear stance to force the stabilization link between the feet and hands consistent with cycling
    - Hand march with both scapula stabilized in protraction by bending the elbow to lift the mobile arm (competitive).
    - Foot march by way of hip and knee flexion on the mobile leg to mimic the cycling action while bending the elbow to lift the opposite arm (Figure 10.3) (competitive).
- Plank track
  - Knees and palms
  - Toes and palms
  - Knees with elbows on ball, keep toes on ground (competitive)
  - Toes with elbows on ball (elite)
  - Progress to one foot and alternate while elbows are on ball (Figure 10.4) (elite)
- Bridge track in hook lying
  - Two-leg hold
  - Two-leg hold with resistance loop around thighs to engage external hip rotators, hold
  - Two-leg hold with resistance loop around thighs to engage external hip rotators, dip
  - One-leg dips with loop, maintain level pelvis (competitive)
  - One-leg dips with loop, which maintains level pelvis (competitive)
  - Shoulders on ball with feet on floor and knees at 90° and arms in air at 90°. Loop around legs to engage hip external rotators and hold (Figure 10.5) (competitive).

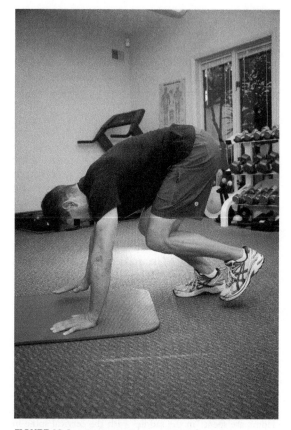

FIGURE 10-3. Bear stance.

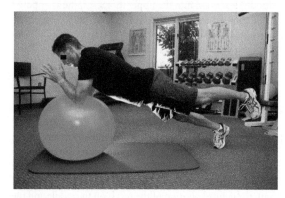

FIGURE 10-4. Plank track.

- Shoulders on ball with one foot on floor; alternate marching (Figure 10.6) (competitive)
- Scissor arm motion (elite)
- Scissor arm motion with weights (Figure 10.7) (elite)
- Scissor arm motion with weights with scapulae and body weight off center on the ball (elite)
- One-leg stance training
  - Floor
  - Rocker board

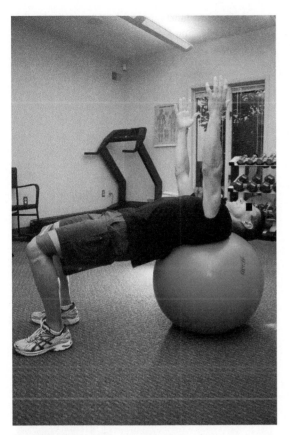

FIGURE 10-5. Bridge track in hook lying with loop.

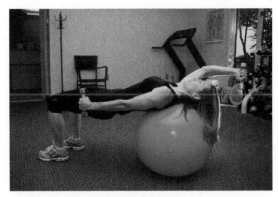

FIGURE 10-7. Scissor arm motion with weights.

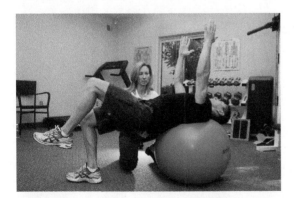

FIGURE 10-6. Shoulders on ball with alternate marching.

- Above with eyes closed
- Foam/disc
- Janda sandals (competitive)
- Repeat one-leg stance training with scapular centration and tubing in both hands, shoulder external rotation (Figure 10.8) (competitive)
- More advanced motions/positions with eyes closed (elite)

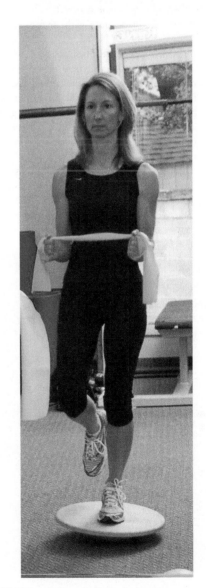

FIGURE 10-8. One-leg stance.

- Modified split squat
  - Begin in athletic pose with neutral spine and approximately 45° squat. Close the stance to pedal width distance. Place one foot behind at a distance equal to pedal circle diameter with full contact on the front foot and the back foot on ball of the foot. Put the hands forward on imaginary hoods with shoulder centration and upper arm torso angle 90° and pelvis back on imaginary saddle. Have the eyes looking "down the road."
  - Squat to functional depth with weight distribution 50/50. Keep front knee behind the toe. Functional depth is defined as the leg position on the bike when the crank is at the 12 o'clock and the 6 o'clock position (Figure 10.9).
- Modified split squat (competitive)
  - Begin in athletic pose with neutral spine and approximately 45° squat. Close the stance to pedal width distance. Place one foot behind at a distance equal to pedal circle diameter with full contact on the front foot and the back foot on ball of the foot. Put hands forward on imaginary hoods, holding tubing, with shoulder centration and upper arm torso angle 90° and pelvis back on imaginary saddle. Have eyes looking "down the road."
  - Squat to functional depth with weight distribution 50/50. Keep front knee behind the toe. Functional depth is defined as the leg position at the 12 o'clock and 6 o'clock crank arm position (competitive).

- Squat to functional depth with weight distribution 80 front foot and 20 rear foot (competitive).
- Squat to functional depth with weight distribution 80/20 on the eccentric or sinking of the squat. On the concentric lift the rear foot off the ground (competitive).
- Stand on box to allow for cycling motion of open chain leg. Use tubing in hands with external rotation to set shoulders. Use tubing anchored under foot to have athlete pull up on while single-leg squatting to mimic the counterpull on the bars (Figure 10.10) (elite).
- Chop and lift track to address the chronic hip flexor and quadriceps tension from hours in the saddle
  - Core stability
    - Seated on stability ball with wand and tubing
    - Cable bar
    - Rope
    - Tall kneeling (Figure 10.11)
    - Half-kneeling (Figure 10.12)
  - Corrective
    - Half-kneeling challenges balance reactions laterally.
    - Tall kneeling challenges balance reactions in anterior/posterior directions.

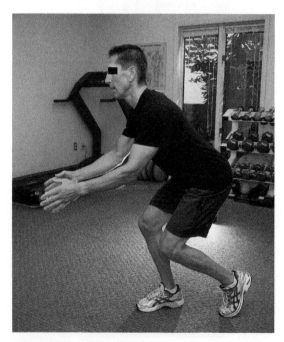

FIGURE 10-9. Modified split squat.

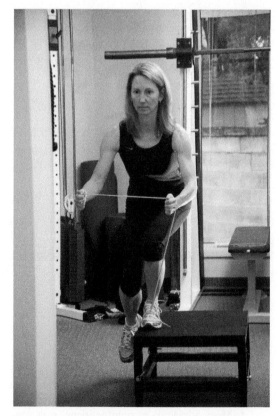

FIGURE 10-10. Modified split squat using box and tubing.

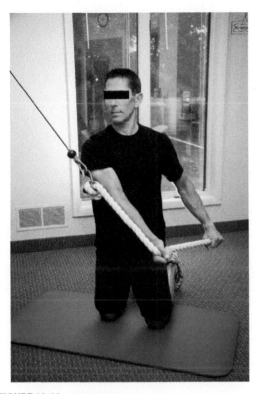

FIGURE 10-11. Tall kneeling.

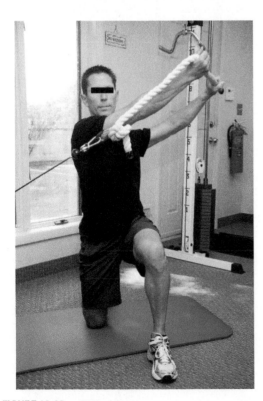

FIGURE 10-12. Half-kneeling.

REFERENCES

1. Cohen GC. Cycling injuries. Can Fam Physician 1993;39:628–632.
2. Dettori NJ, Norvell DC. Non-traumatic bicycle injuries: review of the literature. Sports Med 2006;36:7–18.
3. Wanich T, Hodgkins C, Columbier JA, Muraski E, Kennedy JG. Cycling injuries of the lower extremity. J Am Acad Orthop Surg 2007;15(12):748–756.
4. Holmes JC, Pruitt AL, Whalen NJ. Lower extremity overuse in bicycling. Clin Sports Med 1994;13:187–205.
5. Mellion MB. Common cycling injuries. Management and prevention. Sports Med 1991;11:52–70.
6. Gregor RK, Wheeler JB. Biomechanical factors associated with shoe/pedal interfaces. Implications for injury. Sports Med 1994;17(2):117–131.
7. Sanner WH, O'Halloran WD. The biomechanics, etiology, and treatment of cycling injuries. J Am Podiatr Med Assoc 2000;90(7):354–376.
8. Gregor RJ. A biomechanical analysis of lower limb action during cycling at four different loads [dissertation], Pennsylvania State University, State College, PA; 1976.
9. Okajima S. Designing chain wheels to optimize the human engine. Bike Tech 1983;2:4.
10. Gregor RJ, Cavanagh PR, LaFortune M. Knee flexor moments during propulsion in cycling: a creative solution to Lombard's Paradox. J Biomech 1986;19:523.
11. Daily DJ, Cavanagh PR. Asymmetry in bicycle ergometer pedaling. Med Sci Sports 1976;8:204.
12. Abt JP, Smoliga JM, Brick MJ, Jolly JT, Lephart SM, Fu FH. Relationship between cycling mechanics and core stability. J Strength Cond Res 2007;21(4):1300–1304.
13. Faria FE, Cavanagh PR. The Physiology and Biomechanics of Cycling. New York, NY: Wiley; 1978.
14. Despires M. An electromyographic study of competitive road cycling conditions simulated on a treadmill. In: Nelson RC, Morehouse CA, eds. Biomechanics IV. Baltimore, MD: University Park Press; 1974:349p.
15. Hull ML, Jorge M. A method for biomechanical analysis of bicycle pedaling. J Biomech 1985;18:631.
16. Burke ER. Proper fit of the bicycle. Clin Sports Med 1994;13:1–14.
17. Ericson M. On the biomechanics of cycling. A study of joint and muscle load during exercise on the bicycle ergometer. Scand J Rehabil Med Suppl 1986;16:1–43.
18. Cavanagh PR, Sanderson DJ. The Biomechanics of Cycling: Studies of Pedaling Mechanics of Elite Pursuit Riders. Science Cycling, Ch 5. Champaign, IL: Human Kinetics Books; 1986.
19. Voight ML, Hoogenboom BJ, Cook G. The chop and lift revisited: integrating neuromuscular principles into orthopedic and sports rehabilitation. N Am J Sports Phys Ther 2008;3(3):151–159.

Robert Lardner and Jonathan A. Mackoff

CHAPTER 11

Dance

Dance, as an art, in all its different forms, requires much athleticism to perform the many complicated movement patterns, body positions, and partnering in various choreographic endeavors. The dancers must accomplish this at various tempos, including explosive movements, aerial work, and holding difficult positions for lengths of time.

In training and performing the art of dance, the dancer may risk injury, due to several factors that will be discussed further. Table 11.1 lists representative common injuries found in dance (1–10). A few predisposing factors can increase the likelihood of injury if not addressed or maintained with proper exercises and therapy.

- Genetic factors (e.g., scoliosis, hypermobility syndrome, pes planus, angulation of femoral head, and leg length discrepancy)
- Intrinsic physiological factors (e.g., muscle imbalance, faulty movement patterns, and poor nutrition)
- Extrinsic factors (e.g., duration of training, volume of training, quality of training, training equipment/costumes, floor type, and choreography)

Some biomechanical causes of injuries prevalent among dancers can be due to

- Increased pronatory forces caused by the high degree of turnout demanded in some forms of dance.
- Increased torque in the knee and hip to accommodate the required range of motion utilized in various dance forms, especially with the extremity loaded.
- General increased flexibility among dancers, coupled with the poor intrinsic muscular control and/or fatigue, which may lead to overload of the spinal column. Inadequate flexibility can also be a factor.

Some epidemiological studies for injuries among dancers indicate the following:

1. Back injuries are the most prevalent, ranging from 31% for professional dancers (4) to as high as 82% in surveyed professional ballet dancers (5). In addition, one survey of dancers with scoliosis reported a history of chronic or recurrent low back pain (11).
2. Hip injuries are reported as high as 11% in ballet dancers and 4% in contemporary dancers (6,7).
3. Knee injury prevalence ranged from 9% to 17% (6,8).
4. Foot injury prevalence ranged from 38% to 48.5% in both modern and ballet dancers (9,10).
5. Upper extremity injuries in dancers are poorly reported. However, in break dancers 23% of injuries were to the hand, 9% in the shoulder and 7.5% in the wrist (12).

With proper training and good maintenance of muscle balance and stability, people with these issues can have successful and satisfying dance careers.

As in all sporting activities, a participant must achieve fundamental goals through achieving a series of progressions. Usually this is done through increasing difficulty. Progression can be described in hierarchy of skill levels. There is a need to master or achieve a competency at each level and then be able to integrate those skills/ movements into the next progressive level. Here are some samplings of exercises at the fundamental, sport-specific, and refined/professional levels.

FUNDAMENTAL SKILLS

Bracing (and Breathing with Bracing)

The dancer has to learn at an early point in training about body positioning and finding his or her center and balance under varying circumstances. One of the first steps to accomplish this awareness is to learn how to "connect" the upper body and lower body positioning through rib cage positioning and bracing. The steps to accomplish this are as follows (13–15):

- The dancer takes an inhalation then an exhalation to find the lowered position of the rib cage.
- The dancer then tries to slowly contract the abdominals to push laterally outward (or have the dancer put the thumbs directly above the rim of the pelvic bone and visualize repelling the thumbs gently away from the body).
- The dancer then tries to maintain this rib cage position, as well as the full abdominal brace while breathing in and out (Figure 11.1).
- After this is accomplished in standing position, this should then be practiced in plié, various 1st–5th positions, one-legged balance positions, and relevée.
- The dancer must concentrate and focus internally on the sensations, quality, and feel of the exercise.
- Potential mistakes that may be made include

TABLE 11.1 Representative Common Injuries in Dance

Ankle/Foot	Knee	Hip/Pelvis	Lower Back/Neck	Shoulder
Stress fracture (tarsal, metatarsal, sesamoid)	Anterior cruciate ligament injury	Groin strain	Lumbosacral sprain/strain	Acromioclavicular joint sprain/strain
Posterior ankle impingement/os trigonum syndrome	Medial collateral ligament injury	Piriformis syndrome	Bulge/herniated disc	Rotator cuff injury
		Labral tear	Compression injury	Shoulder dislocation
	Meniscal injury	Osteoarthritis/stress fracture	Nerve compression	Shoulder instability/laxity
Tendonitis/tendinosis	Patellar dislocation	Hamstring strain	Spondylolysis/spondylolisthesis	Biceps tendonitis/tendinosis
Inversion sprain	Patellar femoral pain syndrome	Snapping hip syndrome	Facet syndrome	Impingement
Hallux Valgus/Bunions		Trochanteric bursitis		
Sesamoiditis	Tendonitis/tendinosis	Sacroiliac inflammation/dysfunction		

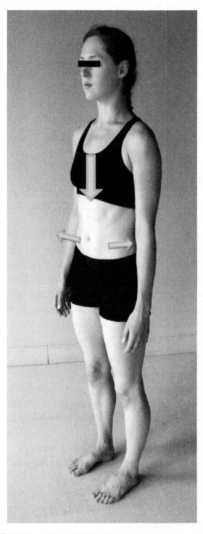

FIGURE 11-1. Abdominal bracing. Correct expiratory rib cage position with pushing abdominal wall laterally.

- Elevated rib cage (this raises a person's center of gravity, overcompresses the spine, and overworks the spinal erector muscles)
- Pulling inward of abdominal muscles, which bypasses the postural function of the diaphragm and inhibits the orchestrated integration of all of the abdominal muscles, pelvic floor muscles, deep back muscles, and the diaphragm working together for core stability
- Posterior pelvic tilts or spinal flexion in an attempt to broaden the posterolateral abdominal wall

Tripod Stance

The dancer needs to learn how to properly balance and to ground, when standing flat-footed and/or when on relevée. The tripod stance helps with the coactivation of the anterior, posterior, medial, and lateral chains of the leg to help support and stabilize the dancer in various standing and balancing positions (16,17):

- In a standing position, the dancer imagines a circle under the 1st metatarsal head, 5th metatarsal head, and middle of their calcaneus (Figure 11.2).
- The dancer then imagines pushing through those points as if they were trying to slowly push through the floor below (Figure 11.2B).
- When done correctly, from the muscle cocontraction, there should be a subtle lengthening of the spine, without a flaring of the rib cage.
- This should be practiced in various positions, as well as one legged and relevée.
- Relevée is slightly different, since the heel is off the ground, the imagined intention of force should be directed 90° from the calcaneal position, to activate the posterior chain of muscles, as well as prevent impingement in the posterior ankle joint (Figure 11.2C).

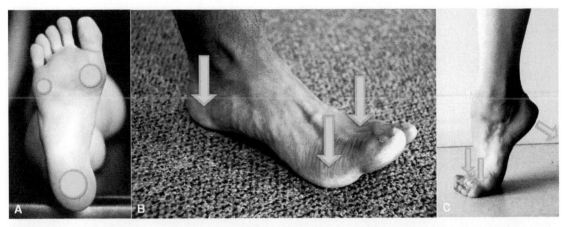

FIGURE 11-2.   Tripod foot. (A) Points of weight-bearing contact. (B) Vector direction for pressure of contact points in standing. (C) In relevée, vector of pressure of contact on 1st and 5th metatarsal heads and intentional pressure through middle calcaneal points.

Balance

Since all positions and movement in dance require balance, in the beginning stages of training, the dancer has to practice balance, with associated body position, in various positions. This should be practiced in various two-legged positions in relevée and on one leg in relevée. In these balance positions, the dancer should maintain the proper bracing technique as well as the relevée tripod position as described above (Figure 11.3).

Scapular Stability

Scapular stability is vital for the maintenance of injury-free loading of the arms and during partnering. The arms are usually active in dance, and therefore, the shoulder girdle must be well stabilized and strong to meet a variety of extreme demands.

The Plank

This exercise can be done either on the forearms and feet or on the forearms and knees (for those who cannot hold proper body posture in the other position). It helps the dancer experience the kinetic chain linking of the arms and scapulae to the stabilization of the lumbopelvic area.

- The dancer is face down, balancing on the forearms, palms down, as well as the feet.
- The dancer initiates a neutral spinal position while initiating an inferior position of the rib cage, as well as initiating an abdominal brace (as described above).
- The dancer should also have the intention of initiating a tripod stance from this position, to activate the cocontraction in the lower extremities (as described above).

- Some mistakes to avoid are scapular "winging," adduction or superior shift, chin protrusion or over-retraction, anterior head carriage, hyperlordosis in their low back, and pelvis pushing up toward the ceiling (Figure 11.4A).

Modified Side Bridge

This exercise is important to incorporate single-arm support and side stability in the training process. As in the plank exercise, it helps the dancer become aware of the kinetic chains involved in anchoring the shoulder girdle to the rest of the torso (14,15).

- The dancer is on his or her side, balancing on the forearm, with the bottom leg straight and the top leg in front in a stepping position.
- The dancer initiates the proper rib cage position while performing an abdominal brace.
- The dancer must actively elongate the thoracic spine without compensating through shoulder adduction and neglecting the scapular stabilizers.
- While maintaining the brace and breathing in a relaxed manner, the dancer pushes through the forearm and the tripod points of the stepping foot and raises himself or herself off the floor in proper spinal alignment (Figure 11.4B).

RECREATIONAL-LEVEL SPORT SKILLS

Two-Person Balance Rotation on Single Leg with Exercise Band

The goal of this exercise is to strengthen and emphasize the hip rotators and the role of the abdominal muscles in

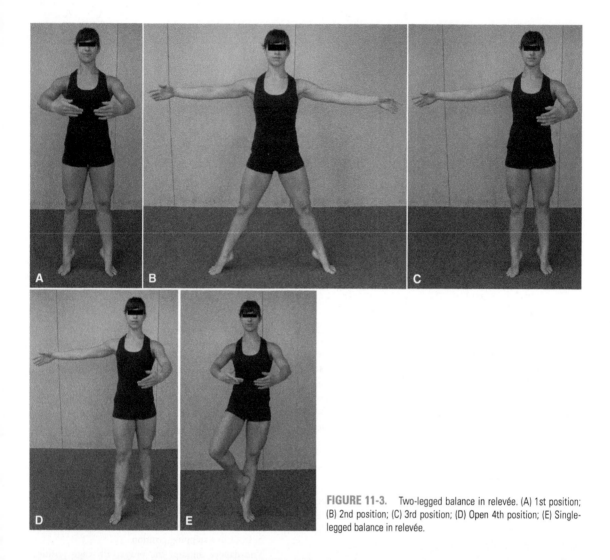

FIGURE 11-3. Two-legged balance in relevée. (A) 1st position; (B) 2nd position; (C) 3rd position; (D) Open 4th position; (E) Single-legged balance in relevée.

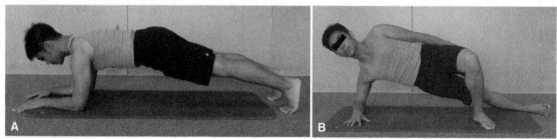

FIGURE 11-4. (A) Modified plank. (B) Modified side bridge.

providing impetus and maintaining the turnout and stability during turns.

- The dancer begins with having an exercise band wrapped flatly 1½ times around the abdominal area.
- The training partner/trainer/therapist holds the other ends of the exercise bands.

- The dancer then starts in a preparatory turn position.
- From the turn preparation the dancer turns to a passé position (Figure 11.5).
- Resistance is applied unilaterally through the band, as decided by the assistant.
- This can be done from both the front and back.

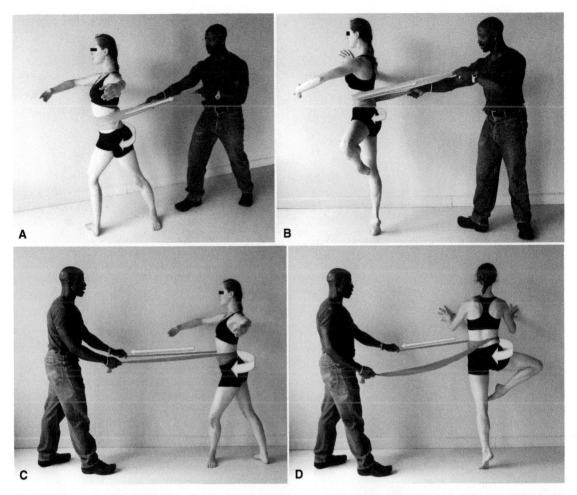

FIGURE 11-5. Preparation for pirouette and progression to assisted balance, with therapist providing resistance to the dynamic activity of pelvis and hip from behind. (A and B) en dedans: Two-person balance rotation on single leg with exercise band. (C and D) en dehors: Two-person balance rotation on single leg with exercise band.

Clock Lunge with Various Arm Positions

The dancer, in class and especially in various choreography, has to be able to lunge, land, and push off from various positions. In addition, he or she must know how to line up the joints for optimal force distribution, optimal potential push-off ability, and optimal body awareness to be able to land and push off with the least stress on the joints and ligaments. It is essential to be able to reach the required "line" of the pose and not sacrifice maintenance of a flexible and dynamic abdominal brace. Performing a lunge in various directions is a progression in accomplishing this.

- A lunge can be done at either a long stride or a short stride. The most important aspect is to maintain proper body and arm positioning while stepping forward, have proper knee tracking over the 1st and 2nd toe, have adequate hip hinge (hip flexion), have very little impact on landing and placement by utilizing good eccentric control, and then push back to the original starting position (maintaining proper body position).

- The dancer imagines himself/herself standing in the middle of a clock face and can now perform the following lunges with bracing, breathing, and proper control of their body alignment. This can be performed in an infinite amount of positions. Some examples are as follows (18):
  - Forward lunge (12 o'clock) (Figure 11.6A)
  - Backward lunge (6 o'clock) (Figure 11.6B)
  - Lateral lunge (3 and 9 o'clock) (Figure 11.6C)
  - Diagonal forward lunge (10:30 and 1:30 o'clock) (Figure 11.6D)
  - Diagonal backward lunge (4:30 and 7:30 o'clock) (see Figure 11.6D)

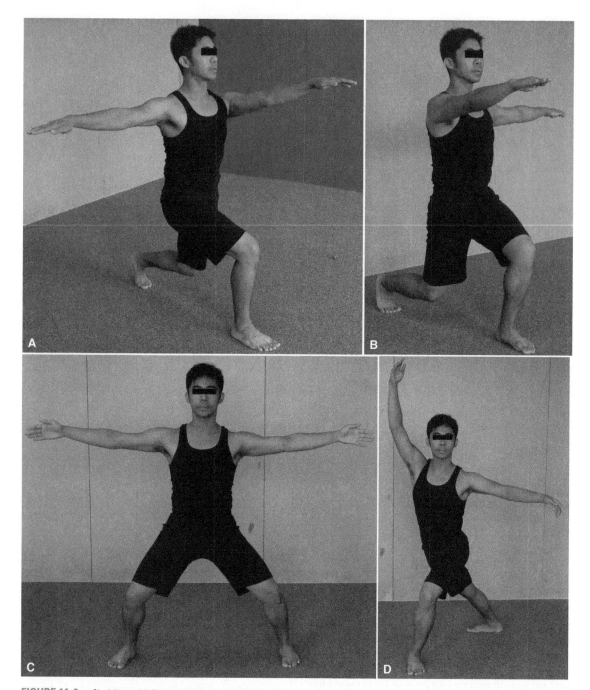

FIGURE 11-6. Clock lunge. (A) Forward; (B) Backward; (C) Side; (D) Diagonal forward (clock position, 1:30) and backward (clock position, 7:30).

Overhead Press/Lift with Exercise Band

The dancer utilizes the Bruegger wrap for resistance as shown in Figure 11.7A–F (19).

- The preparatory plié to press overhead can then be performed, while paying attention to coordination, scapular stability, and lower extremity alignment.

- The ability to control the abdominal brace throughout the movement, while breathing normally, is very important.
- Different stance positions may be used, and the band can augment actual lifting of partners (Figure 11.8A–C).

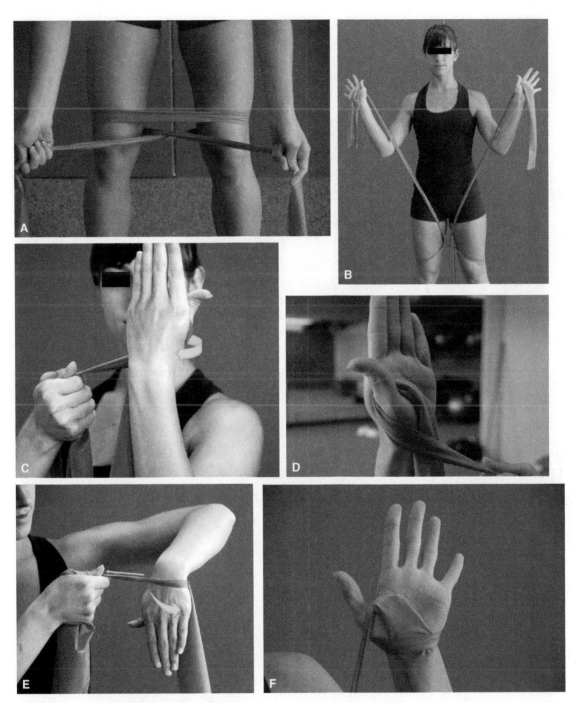

FIGURE 11-7. (A–F) Bruegger wrapping technique.

Jump Preparation and Landing Training with Bruegger Wrap

Using the same wrapping technique as above, the dancer can facilitate correct alignment and control of take-off and landing during jumping exercises. Axial skeletal and scapular control are also challenged by the resistance band. Different preparatory positions may be used such as parallel (see Figures 11.8A and 11A) or turned out (see Figure 11.9B and C). Training these helps establish various motor patterns within the dancer's repertoire.

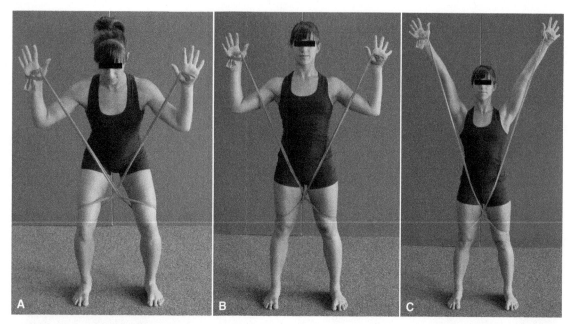

FIGURE 11-8. (A–C) Overhead press with Bruegger wrap.

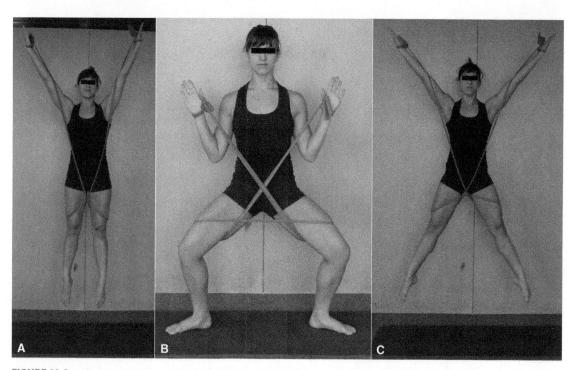

FIGURE 11-9. (A) Jump preparation and landing training in parallel. (B–C) Jump preparation and landing training in turn out.

Exercise Band Kicks (En Croix) Training Balancing Leg and Kicking Leg

With the simple wrap to the active leg, which is then anchored to the stance leg and the barre, kicks in several vectors can be performed at varying heights and speeds, as required (Figure 11.10). It is possible to perform these:

- Forward (Figure 11.11A)
- Side (see Figure 11.11B)
- Back

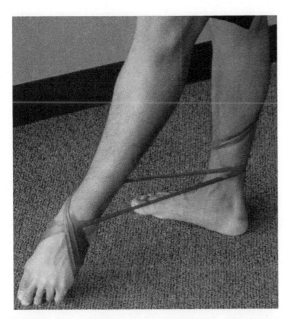

FIGURE 11-10. Close-up of wrapping technique for exercise band kick (en croix) training.

REFINED-LEVEL SPORTS SKILLS (ELITE, PROFESSIONAL LEVEL)

Upper Quarter Ballistic Movements

Ballistic movements (also known as plyometrics) should be trained to improve acceleration–amortization–deceleration function in fast movements. Ballistic control is important for injury prevention. This can be performed with ball tosses (Figure 11.12). Also, the dancer may perform a plyo-metric push-up with a clap on a soft mat (Figure 11.13A and B). The degree of scapular and spinal control will determine the suitability of the exercise level, which can be peeled back to no clap push-up, or advanced to support on the feet (i.e., full push-up position).

Lower Quarter Ballistic Movements

For lower quarter training, quick two-legged or one-legged jumps can be used in varying directions with emphasis on speed and recoil during the contact phase with the floor. These exercises help train the dancer's ability to absorb

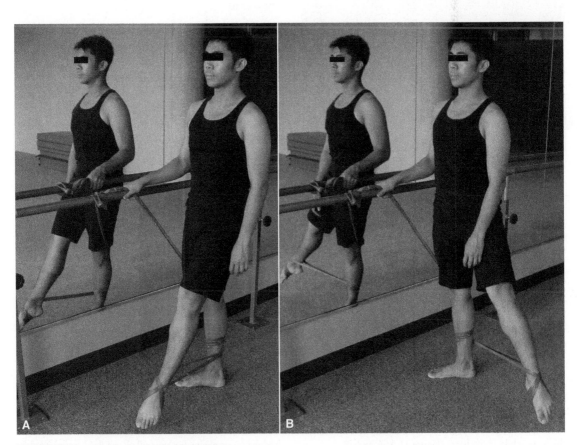

FIGURE 11-11. Kicks (en croix). (A) Forward; (B) Side.

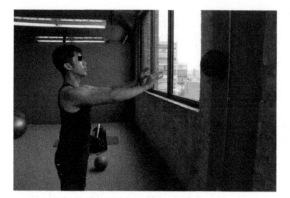

FIGURE 11-12. Plyometric upper extremity ball throw.

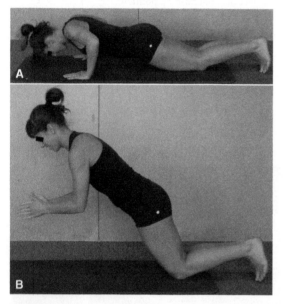

FIGURE 11-13. (A and B) Plyometric upper extremity push-ups with clap.

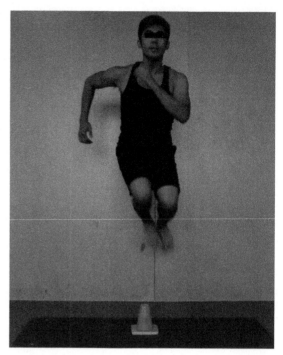

FIGURE 11-14. Plyometric lower extremity alternating two-legged lateral jumps.

shock and change vectors rapidly, allowing the quick load of ligaments and tendons, which should strengthen them and aid in injury prevention. This type of exercise also challenges the dancer's sense of position of space and time. One example is alternating lateral jumps, both two legged and one legged (Figures 11.14 and 11.15A and B).

Two-Person Resisted Turning Initiation with Exercise Band

The dancer's awareness of control of turning, utilizing the core and hip muscles during the initiation of turns, can be enhanced by resistance to the planned movement. The resistance can be applied from the dancer's preparation position through the final balance position at the start of the turn, while at the barre (Figure 11.16A and B).

CONCLUSIONS

In the art of dance, the initial three levels of training, in general, are universal to the various forms of dance. Among most dance genres, a variety of knee bends (plié), turning, jumping and arm movements, and so on, are required. The latter three levels, as described here, are more appropriate for ballet and those dance forms that are rooted in the balletic technique.

The fundamental exercises were chosen to help provide the starting, intermediate, and professional dancer with the ability to help stabilize and evenly distribute forces throughout their body and grounding evenly through their feet (R>L, A>P, and connect their upper and lower extremities through their trunk and pelvis) as well as connecting to a low center of gravity to help them find their center for balance (one legged or two legged).

The intermediate exercises were chosen to help the developing dancer train multiplane movement patterns and how to absorb shock from landing and hopefully prevent injury with this awareness. Also, these exercises are made to help with learning proper technique, body posture, and positioning for jumping, landing, lifting (for partnering), and turning.

The advanced exercises were chosen to help train explosive movements (from upper body to lower body or lower body to upper body), as well as turning. This attempts to utilize the dancer's body awareness and ability to connect the body's kinetic chains for controlled and fluid movement.

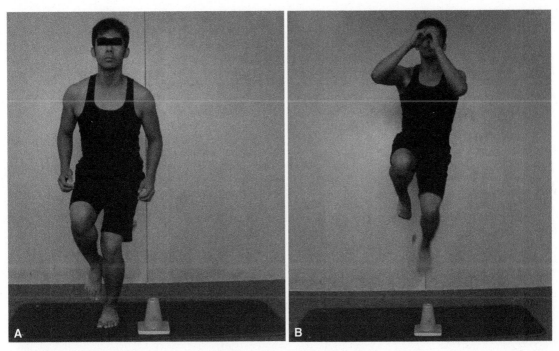

FIGURE 11-15.   (A and B) Plyometric lower extremity alternating one-legged lateral jumps.

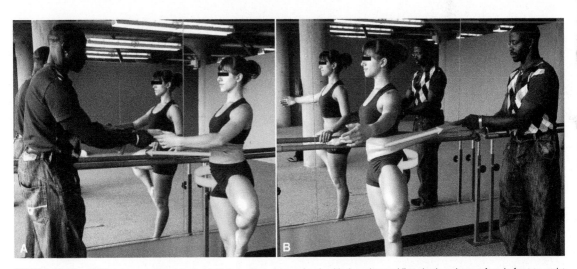

FIGURE 11-16.   (A) Two-person resisted turning initiation with resistance band, with therapist providing elastic resistance from in front to assist dancer in experiencing kinetic chain control hip and pelvis turn out on stance leg, en dehors. (B) Two-person resisted turning initiation with resistance band, with therapist providing resistance from behind to assist dancer in experiencing kinetic chain control of hip and pelvis turn out on stance leg, en dedans.

REFERENCES

1. Bowling A. Injuries to dancers: prevalence, treatment and perceptions of causes. Br Med J 1989;298:731–734.
2. Gamboa JM, Roberts LA, Maring J, Fergus A. Injury patterns in elite preprofessional ballet dancers and the utility of screening programs to identify risk characteristics. J Orthop Sports Phys Ther 2008;38(3):126–136.
3. Solomon R, Solomon J, Minton SC, eds. Preventing Dance Injuries. 2nd ed. Champaign, IL: Human Kinetics; 2005.
4. Garrick J, Requa R. Ballet injuries: an analysis of epidemiology and financial outcome. Am J Sports Med 1993;21(4):586–590.
5. Ramel E, Moritz U, Jarnlo G. Recurrent musculoskeletal pain in professional ballet dancers in Sweden: a six-year follow up. J Dance Med Sci 1999;3(3):93–101.

6. Quirk R. Ballet injuries: the Australian experience. Clin Sports Med 1983;2(3):507–514.

7. Schafle M, Requa R, Garrick J. A comparison of patterns of injury in ballet, modern and aerobic dance. In: Solomon R, Minton SC, Solomon J, eds. Preventing Dance Injuries: An Interdisciplinary Perspective. Reston, VA: American Alliance for Health, Physical Education, Recreation and Dance; 1990:1–14.

8. Rothenberger LA, Chang JI, Cable TA. Prevalence and types of injuries in aerobic dancers. Am J Sports Med 1988;16(4):403–407.

9. Garrick J, Requa R. The epidemiology of foot and ankle injuries in sports. Clin Sports Med 1988;7(1):29–36.

10. Garrick J. Early identification of musculoskeletal complaints and injuries among female ballet students. J Dance Med Sci 1999;3(2):80–83.

11. Liederbach M, Spivak J, Rose D. Scoliosis in dancers: a method of assessment in quick-screen settings. J Dance Med Sci 1997;1(3):107–112.

12. Washington E. A medical and sociological consideration of break dancers and pop-lockers. In: Ryan A, Stephens R, eds. Dance Medicine: A Comprehensive Guide. Chicago, IL: Pluribus Press; 1987:281–293.

13. Kolar P. Manual Medicine and Developmental-Sports Kinesiology Course a Prague. Czech Republic; 2005.

14. Kolar P, Liebenson C. Exercise & the Athlete: Reflexive, Rudimentary and Fundamental Strategies Course. Chicago, IL; 2009.

15. McGill S. Ultimate Back Performance. Waterloo, ON: Wabuno Publishers; 2004.

16. Cumpilik J. Advanced Yoga Stabilization Techniques Course. Chicago, IL; 2005.

17. Kapandji IA. The Physiology of the Joints, Volume 2: Lower Limb. 5th ed. Edinburgh: Churchill-Livingstone; 1987.

18. Gray G. Lower Extremity Functional Profile. Adrian, MI: Wynn Marketing; 1995.

19. Förster J. The Brügger Concept, Diagnosis and Treatment of Motor System Dysfunction. Seminar, New Orleans; 2008.

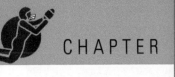
Football

The skills of American football resemble many other sports. Blocking is found in basketball and hockey; tackling is in judo and wrestling; and throwing and catching are similar to baseball and water polo. Upon greater analysis, skill assessment for the game of football becomes a complex endeavor due to the inherent strategy of the game and the collision nature of the sport. Player positions differ greatly from one another, with a player's individual attributes of size, strength, weight, speed, agility, coordination, and explosiveness all being a factor in determining position selection for optimal performance. Uniquely, practice primarily involves drills rather than actual game play. This contrasts with sports such as basketball and wrestling where preparation often involves playing the actual sport. Before one can assess the skills of football, it is important to understand that it is a game of deception, match-ups and adjustments. Offensive strategy is dictated by the defensive formation, personnel, field position, and down count. The defense adjusts according to the presenting scheme of the offense, field position, and down count (1). Slight changes in a player's stance and alignment may offer an advantage to outmaneuver or outleverage the opponent. We will provide several examples of basic progressions of skill development beginning with "FUNdamental skills" (2). These drills should be fun, low intensity, and cultivate ideal and symmetrical motor patterns. Sport-specific exercises then build upon the established fundamental skills and can be further isolated to position-specific skills. Refined exercises further hone the position skills typically at the elite or professional level of play (3).

As football is a collision sport, injuries are common even with proper technique. Key biomechanical consideration should focus on good posture when initiating and receiving contact. While evading opponents requires relaxed posture to yield quick and efficient movement, achieving whole-body stiffness at the ideal moment is critical to transfer or absorb force (4). Protective padding is designed to distribute these forces through larger areas, and similarly, the athlete's ability to brace, absorb, and transfer force through a well-functioning musculoskeletal system deflects damage.

According to USA Football, there are currently more than 3 million participants in youth football leagues (5). While other sports may have a greater overall number of participants and injuries, football has a greater rate of injury when compared with other sports (5). Estimates of injury rates have been as high as 5% in youth football (6).

Increased risk variables were determined to be greater in the older age divisions, with game injury rates being greatest on game days (6,7). Table 12.1 lists some common injuries.

There has been increased attention to the development and reduction of sports concussion (8,9). Experts differ in determining concussion risk at different levels of play (9–12). Sports concussion represents the majority of brain injuries occurring in the United States with estimates between 1.6 and 3.8 million cases annually (8). There seems to be consensus that skilled position players such as quarterbacks, wide receivers, and defensive secondary players are at greater risk for sustaining a concussion (11). Recent findings suggest that prevalence of football concussion correlates with players who sustain more head impacts, with peak linear acceleration impact of the helmet representing the greatest predictor of concussion (13).

USA Football has taken a proactive step in their "Heads Up" campaign to teach proper biomechanics with tackling to minimize the chance of concussion onset in players (5). These same biomechanical fundamentals are depicted in the following contact drills.

FUNDAMENTAL SKILLS/POP WARNER (AGES 7–10)

Ordinarily simple movements may initially feel awkward to the child due to the new experience of wearing protective padding. The following brief sampling of drills serves as a rudimentary base for the fundamentals of movement. Regardless of the position, movements are developed to react to play dynamics while maintaining good posture and body control (14).

Ball Flow Drills

Initially, the players take a shoulder-width stance with 2/3 hip and 1/3 knee flexion, maintaining a straight low back and head in neutral spine position. The center of gravity is through the rear hips to allow the players to step forward, step left or right, run laterally down the line, or step backward into pass protection. They may assume a two-point or four-point (bear crawl) stance maintaining a head up/bottom down position with neutral spine (see Figure 12.1). The coach points various directions with the football, and the players run or crawl

TABLE 12.1	Common Injuries in Football			
Ankle/Foot	**Knee**	**Hip**	**Back/Shoulder**	**Head/Neck**
Ankle sprain	Meniscus injury	Hamstring strain	Muscle strain	Cervical muscle strain
Achilles tendonitis	Anterior cruciate ligament injury	Groin strain	Herniated disk	Pinched nerve/stinger
Turf toe/shin splints	Medial knee ligament injury	Hip contusion	Shoulder separation/ dislocation/fracture	Concussion

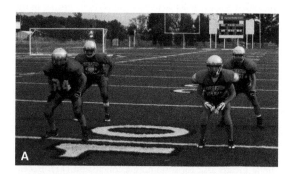

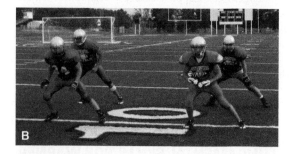

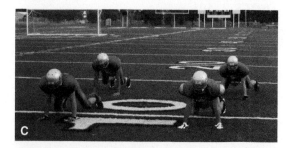

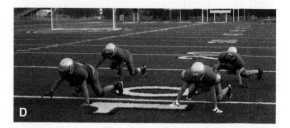

FIGURE 12-1. (A) Four players, ready position. (B) Four players, angle step. (C) Four players, on all-fours. (D) Four players, bear crawl.

toward that direction. The coach then hits the ball with his hand, and the players sprint forward ten yards. Good posture with multidimensional movement is monitored and corrected.

Functional exercises include

- Angle lunges
- Squat
- Bird dog
- Commando crawl
- "Stir the pot" (15,16)

Hand-Off Drill

This running back football skill drill trains technique in receiving, securing, carrying, and handing off the football without a fumble. Proper stance, footwork, and ball control are monitored and corrected.

Functional exercises include

- Lunges
- Squats
- One-legged squats (15)

Lateral Running/The Ladder

Initially, the players face the coach and run laterally along a ladder. The players try to place each foot in each box while keeping their knees high, chest up looking forward at the coach (see Figure 12.2). Note that the coach should be able to see the athlete's eyes and numbers on the jersey.

Functional exercises include

- Matrix angle lunges
- One-legged squats
- One-legged balance
- Running man
- Airplane (15,16)

RECREATIONAL-LEVEL SPORTS SKILLS (MIDDLE SCHOOL–HIGH SCHOOL)

With regard to Gambetta's model, sport-specific skills build upon the movement patterns already established in the athlete. In football, sport-specific skills become more position specific (3). Following are a few examples of recreational-level sports skills.

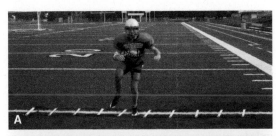

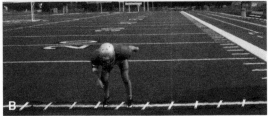

FIGURE 12-2. (A) Single player, running the ladder, with knees high and head up. (B) Single player, running the ladder, with head and chest down and hips high (poor form).

Receiver/Defensive Back Drill

Receivers and defensive backs have to quickly stop and change direction, and controlling center of gravity is an essential skill for these positions. The players should have good control with stopping and changing direction, lowering the hips to absorb momentum, and maintaining good low back posture with the head up. The players should then break on the football, focusing on hip and opposite arm extension. For the defensive player the most important element is the initial athletic posture with hip hinge (Figure 12.3).

Functional exercises include

- Squats
- One-legged balance
- Lunges

- Running man
- Farmer's walk
- Suitcase kettlebell carry (15,16)

Form Tackling

A rudimentary base for this exercise is the neutral spine hip/hinge or squat.

Stance

Linebackers and defensive backs must quickly react to the offensive play and so take a balanced, neutral stance. There is slight hip and knee flexion to give them the ability to quickly move in any direction. They assume a straight low back (neutral spine) with shoulder and head elevated, hands hanging at their side.

Exercise: Form Tackling (Full Pads)

This drill teaches proper tackling technique using three stages: fit, fit and lift, and form tackle.

Fit

On command by the coach, the tacklers walk up to their partner and fit into tackling position. The tacklers hold that position for correction. Attention is placed on having a shoulder-width stance, wide arm wrap under his partner's buttocks, lowered hips, flexed knees, straight low back, chest and head up at the partner's waist level (see Figure 12.4).

Fit and Lift

Upon command by the coach, the tacklers assume fit position and stop. At second command the tacklers roll the hips up while extending the legs. The partners may assist the lift with a small jump. Attention is placed on maintaining a neutral spine with power generated through the hips (see Figure 12.5).

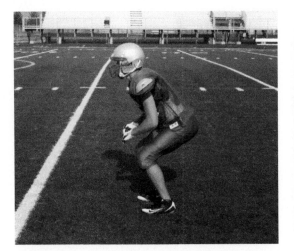

FIGURE 12-3. Defensive athletic posture with hip hinge.

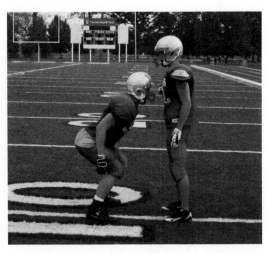

FIGURE 12-4. Two players, fit tackle.

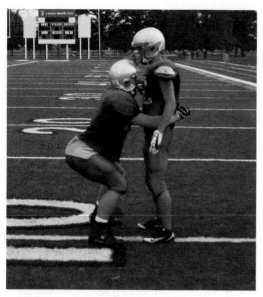

FIGURE 12-5. Two players, fit and lift.

Form Tackle

This is a fluid progression of the fit and lift. The drill is performed at half speed. The tackle should be performed in one fluid motion. The partners are not to change direction or resist and are not to be taken to the ground. Attention is placed on wide arm wrap, lifting from the hips, straight back, and head up at the partner's chest level. Functional exercises include

- Squat
- Overhead squat
- Side planks
- Neck retraction
- Slamball pulses
- Kettlebell swings (15,16)

REFINED-LEVEL SPORTS SKILLS (ELITE LEVEL, PROFESSIONAL)

Stripping the Football

This defensive football drill builds upon the skill of tackling. As the player is making the tackle, he focuses on hitting the football, breaking the runner's grasp. Functional exercises include

- Pulley punches
- Pulley chops (16)

Feet In-Bounds

This receiver-specific drill improves ability to touch two feet in-bounds when catching the ball at the out-of-bounds line. The receivers begin by running an out route toward the out of bounds, catch the ball, and maintain two feet in-bounds before they step out. This drill focuses on balance, footwork, and body awareness. Functional exercises include

- Matrix lunges
- Balance training (15)

Sticky Hands–Staying on the Block

This advanced drill for linemen trains sensitivity, whole-body stiffness, and body control. Two players face one another and hold a firm blocking shield. The players are allowed to press against the pad with open hands but not grasp it or move their feet. The players then move the pad left, right, up, and down reacting to the other player's energy without taking a step or letting the pad drop (see Figure 12.6).

Attention is focused on maintaining proper posture for hip and thorax reactivity. Check for failure to maintain

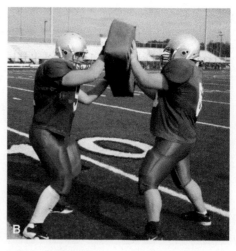

FIGURE 12-6. (A) Two players, hands on pad, chest level. (B) Two players, hands on pad, head level.

| | **Fundamental Skill** | | |
Player Position	**(Functional Exercise)**	**Sports Skill**	**Refined Skill**
Offensive linemen	Diagonal step (angle lunges)	Reach block	Staying on the block, chip block
Wide receivers	Catching and securing the football (overhead ball toss)	Route running with catch	Dragging toes after catch
Quarterbacks	Throwing (cable punch)	Throwing with pump fake	Looking off a defender, quick release of the ball
Linebackers/defensive backs	Form tackling (hip hinge)	Open-field tackling	Stripping football while tackling, intercepting the pass

TABLE 12.2   Skill Set Progression Examples by Player Position

slight low back extension and inability to react to gross movement variations. Functional exercises include

- Warrior stick
- Slamball pulses
- Kettlebell swings into braced plank position (16)

SUMMARY

These are but a few examples of fundamental, sports-specific, and position skills in the game of football. It is noteworthy that while the fundamental skills of tackling, throwing, and catching are found in many sports, each naturally becomes more specific to the game of football and set the foundation for the more position-specific sports skills (Table 12.2). These fundamental skills can be reduced to functional exercises which groove the appropriate motor pattern (3). Sports skills can then serve as a foundation to refine skills such as stripping the football from a ball carrier or dragging the toes in-bounds once a catch has been made.

REFERENCES

1. American Football Coaches Association. Football Coaching Strategies. Champaign, IL: Human Kinetics; 1995.
2. Canadian Sport for Life. Long-term Athletic Development. Canadian Sport Centres; 2007.
3. Gambetta V. Athletic Development: The Arts and Science of Functional Sports Conditioning. Champaign, IL: Human Kinetics; 2007.
4. McGill S. Core training: evidence translating to better performance and injury prevention. Strength Cond J 2010;32(3): 33–46.
5. Rizzone K, Diamond A, Gregory A. Sideline coverage of youth football. Curr Sports Med Rep 2013;12(3): 143–149.
6. Goldberg B, Rosenthal PP, Robertson LS, Nicholas JA. Injuries in youth football. Pediatrics 1998;81(2):255–261.
7. Malina R, Morano PJ, Barron M, Miller SJ, Cumming SP, Kontos AP. Incidence and player risk factors for injury in youth football. Clin J Sport Med 2006;16(3):214–222.
8. Broglio SP, Schnebel B, Sosnoff JJ, et al. The biomechanical properties of concussions in high school football. Med Sci Sports Exerc 2010;42(11): 2064-2071.
9. Halstead ME, Walter KD. American Academy of Pediatrics. Clinical report—sport-related concussion in children and adolescents. Council on Sports Medicine and Fitness. Pediatrics 2010;126(3):597–615.
10. Solomon GS, Ott SD, Lovell MR. Long-term neurocognitive dysfunction in sports: what is the evidence? Clin Sports Med 2011;30(1):165–177.
11. Schnebel B, Gwin JT, Anderson S, Gatlin R. In vivo study of head impacts in football: a comparison of National Collegiate Athletic Association Division I versus high school sports. Neurosurgery 2007;60(3):490–495.
12. Pellman EJ, Powell JW, Viano DC, et al. Concussion in professional football: epidemiological features of game injuries and review of the literature—part 3. Neurosurgery 2004;54(1):81–94.
13. Beckwith J, Greenwald RM, Chu JJ, et al. Head impact exposure sustained by football players on days of diagnosed concussion. J Am Coll Sports Med 2013;45(4):737-746.
14. Elphinston J. Stability Sport and Performance Movement, Great Technique Without Injury. Apple Tree Cottage, Chicester, UK: Lotus Publishing; 2008.
15. Liebenson C. Rehabilitation of the Spine. 2nd ed. Philadelphia, PA: Lippincott Williams and Wilkins; 2007.
16. McGill, S. Ultimate Back Fitness and Performance. Waterloo, ON: Wabuno Publishers; 2004.

13

Greg Rose

Golf

INTRODUCTION: LONG-TERM ATHLETIC DEVELOPMENT

Junior golf development has undergone a huge transformation over the past 7 years. Much of the change comes from the overwhelming amount of experimentation and research being done in the field of long-term athlete development (LTAD). The Titleist Performance Institute (TPI) has spearheaded this change by beginning to unravel the mysteries of why some junior golf programs excel at creating major champions and why many others fall short.

Some of this research comes from retrospective studies where Professional Golfers' Association (PGA) and Ladies Professional Golf Association (LPGA) golfers were asked how they became so talented. Questions included:

- How old were you when you began to play golf?
- What other activities or sports did you play when you were young?
- When you started competing, what type of lessons did you receive?

After reviewing such studies and looking for any common pathways, one key trend began to emerge. Almost all of these elite athletes were involved in an LTAD program, whether or not they knew it.

LTAD describes the life-long athletic development model first coined by Hungarian scientist Istvan Balyi in 1990 (1). LTAD is a detailed curriculum that outlines each step in an athlete's yearly development. Balyi showed that an LTAD model can help coaches and athletic directors design effective training programs for each phase of development. LTAD is a form of periodization of athletic training that spans an athlete's entire career.

The TPI model is designed to honor each golfer's developmental age. The model is not focused on chronological age (the amount of time the athlete has been on Earth) like most athletic development programs. Instead, each golfer is evaluated and placed into developmentally appropriate activities that allow maximum athletic skill improvement. The athlete's program progressively becomes more complex and more specialized as the golfer reaches new development phases.

As all parents with multiple children know, young people never develop at the same rate. LTAD breaks the mold of simply teaching all children of the same chronological age the same way.

Remember, chronological age simply means the number of years and days since birth—the age that increases at a steady rate and is the same for all of us. This is not the same as developmental age, which involves physical, mental, cognitive, and emotional maturity and measures how close the child is to becoming an adult. To truly measure a child's developmental age, one has to look at skeletal development, sexual development, brain development, and motor skill development. A child's body does not need to have signs of height growth or weight growth to mature.

Most LTAD models use growth velocity to predict developmental age. Growth velocity is the rate (cm/year) at which a child is growing. We can predict a child's developmental age by determining where the child is on a growth velocity curve (Figure 13.1) (2).

The TPI junior LTAD program divides golfers into multiple phases similar to the belt system used in many martial arts programs. This division enables the coaches to focus on skills and drills that are appropriate for each player's developmental age. TPI's junior program, which spans from birth to college, uses a simplified model to Balyi's original eight phases of development (3):

1. Active Start (for developmental ages 0 to 5 for boys and 0 to 4 for girls)
2. Fundamentals (for developmental ages 6 to 8 for boys and 5 to 7 for girls)
3. Play (for developmental ages 9 to 11 for boys and 8 to 10 for girls)
4. Train (for developmental ages 12 to 14 for boys and 11 to 13 for girls)
5. Elite (for developmental ages 15 to 18 for boys and 14 to 17 for girls)

Another important concept to discuss in all LTAD programs is the new science of windows of trainability. Many experts believe there are sensitive periods or critical times in every child's life where certain skills can be learned at an accelerated rate. Most coaches have noticed these windows through experience, but no one has really defined these periods until now.

As stated by Bouchard, "trainability refers to the responsiveness of children and adolescents at different stages of growth and maturity to a training stimulus" (4). LTAD

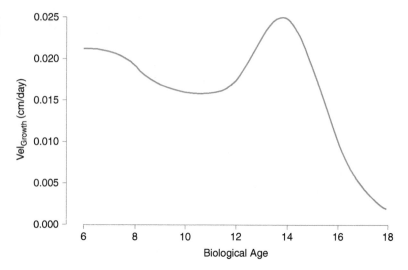

FIGURE 13-1. A typical growth velocity curve used to predict developmental age (2).

programs use the word "trainability." Many factors can influence trainability including age, sex, growth velocity, maturity, genotype, preinstruction, hormonal influence, strength development, nervous system development, and muscle fiber type differentiation.

Even though training can be variable, there does seem to be critical times in every child's development when the body is more responsive to certain skills due to their changing maturity.

Balyi and Way in 1995 described five primary windows of optimal training (5). We now suspect that up to 13 windows should be addressed (Table 13.1). As you can see from the diagram in Figure 13.2, you can think of these windows as building a skyscraper. Fundamentals and Learn to Play phase windows help build the foundation of the athlete. The main floors are built during the Train to Play phase and the top floors are finished during the Elite phases.

This chapter will serve as a highlight of TPI's LTAD program, and it will also discuss many of the key factors that make up any successful LTAD program. We will begin in the Fundamentals phase, skip to the Train phase, briefly describe our Elite phase, and finish talking about adults and senior golfers.

FUNDAMENTALS PHASE

The Fundamentals phase is all about helping a child move confidently and efficiently in a wide range of physical activities. It is easier to build elite golfers from children who already have a solid base of athletic skills. That base begins with a basic physical fitness foundation. TPI develops that base by focusing on creating solid Fundamental Movement Skills (FMS) first. FMS are best defined as the basic building blocks of athleticism. TPI's LTAD model is designed to make all players proficient in their FMS before they enter the Learn to Play phase. This is radically different from programs that focus solely on golf-specific skills.

FMS can be broken into four categories (6):
1. Locomotive skills (running, jumping, dodging, skipping, hopping, bounding, sprinting)
2. Stability skills (ABCs of athleticism—agility, balance, coordination, speed, change of direction, disassociation)
3. Manipulative/object control skills (ABCs of athletics—throwing, kicking, striking, catching, dribbling, dodging)
4. Awareness skills—spatial awareness, kinesthetic awareness, body awareness, rules

TPI's programming makes this phase easy for children to learn and simple for coaches to organize by structuring the class into a program called the fundamental "cyclone." The cyclone focuses on developing all of the FMS and consists of 6 to 12 stations laid out in a circular fashion (Figure 13.3). Some favorite cyclone stations are described here.

TABLE 13.1	Training Window to Address
1. First Suppleness Window (Mobility)	
2. First Speed Window	
3. Functional Stability	
4. First Skill Window	
5. Second Suppleness Window	
6. Functional Strength	
7. Second Speed Window	
8. 3D Integration Window	
9. First Stamina Window	
10. Olympic Strength Window	
11. Second Skill Window	
12. Power Window	
13. Second Stamina Window	

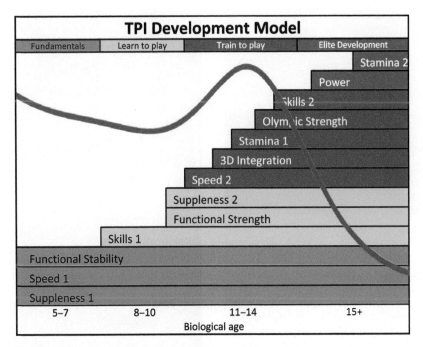

FIGURE 13-2.   Junior athlete development model.

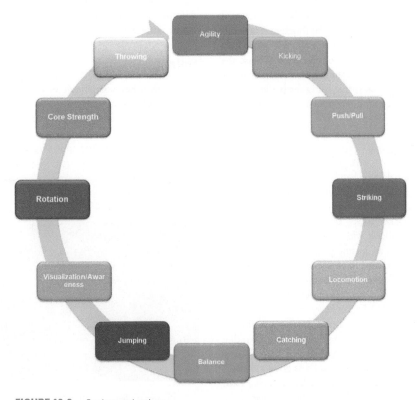

FIGURE 13-3.   Fundamental cyclone.

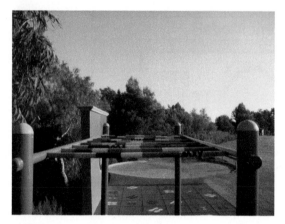

FIGURE 13-4.   Push–pull station.

Push/Pull Station

This station focuses on developing upper body strength and stability. Activities like monkey bar races, pull-ups with power bands (Figure 13.4), tug-of-war competitions, push-ups on stability balls, and sumo wrestling are all class favorites. Body weight strength activities are important to add in this phase. Even though children still lack the hormonal development to build true muscular hypertrophy, they can dramatically improve their neurological recruitment of muscle fibers.

The monkey bars are a key piece of equipment that is always an instant hit in any junior golf program. Have different color athletic tape wrapped around each bar to help children create fun games while on the bars. We use the colors to create progressions from hard to easy, red stripes being the easiest and black stripes being the hardest. Hand placement gradually gets farther and wider apart with each different color.

Striking Station

These activities help develop hand–eye coordination, rotary speed, spatial awareness, weight shift, and upper and lower body speed and balance. Hitting golf balls with golf clubs, slap shots with hockey sticks, striking with field hockey sticks, and playing cricket with a bat are all great ways to introduce striking on an incline plane. You can alternate which activities to practice in this station each time. Tee ball batting, ground strokes with a tennis racquet, and table tennis are all great activities to help children practice horizontal striking (Figure 13.5A,B). Have them focus on hitting it as hard as possible. Make sure you use a stationary ball at first and progress to moving balls. For all striking activities beginners should use large ball sizes, large hitting areas, and large target zones, and speed is always encouraged. For advanced strikers use smaller balls, smaller bats, smaller target zones, start tracking distance and carry, use

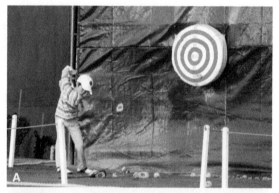

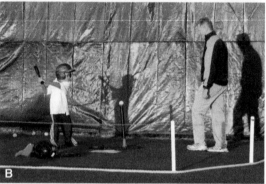

FIGURE 13-5.   (A, B) Striking station.

multiple grip styles, and single hand and single leg striking can be introduced.

Balance Station

Balance is a key component to any athletic movement. Children can rapidly improve their feel and balance by challenging their stability. We have a multifaceted obstacle course that we set up for the kids to try to maneuver around in the shortest amount of time (Figure 13.6). The course

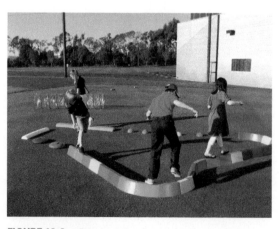

FIGURE 13-6.   Balance station.

includes a multicolor balance beam, balance pods, foam cushions, and air-filled discs. Children can call out colors and their partners need to avoid or touch the color named. They can try different types of walking patterns as well, forward, backward, and side to side.

Throwing Station

Have you ever noticed how good major league baseball pitchers are at golf? They are usually very talented when they pick up the game. This is not a fluke. It is due to the similarity of throwing to the motion of the golf swing. There is a backswing load, hip and shoulder separation, weight shift toward the target, and transfer of energy from the ground to the implement (ball versus club). For this reason, we encourage lots of throwing activities with our junior golfers. Children will throw different objects and throw for distance and accuracy. We use catchtail balls, footballs, baseballs, Frisbees, and bean bags (Figure 13.7).

Visualization (Green Reading) Station

This is another favorite of the children and it is focused on learning how to visualize slope. One of the hardest skills for a child to learn is how to read a green. Not only is practicing putting boring for most children, but their visual system is still not fully developed. We use fun games such as bowling and billiards on a large sloping green to teach these skills in a fun way. Actually, most of the children have no idea they are actually learning how to read a green. They just like to make strikes (Figure 13.8).

Many experts believe that it takes a minimum of 10 years and at least 10,000 hours of training for an athlete to reach elite levels. Herbert Simon, a 1978 Nobel Prize winner, was one of the first to study the role of knowledge in expertise. He has said that to become an expert it required 10 years of experience or roughly an accumulation of 50,000 chunks of information. Many years later, in Gibbons and Forster's landmark

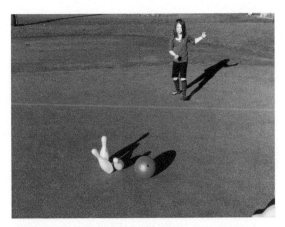

FIGURE 13-8. Visualization station.

study "The Path to Excellence," they found most Olympians reported a 12- to 13-year period of talent development from their sport introduction to making an Olympic team (7). A 10-year rule has been shown to apply to the development of expertise in most fields, including music (8).

On the other hand, the 10,000-hour rule is still highly debatable in research (some say 4,000 hours—some argue 6,000 hours), but all studies suggest a significant investment in time is required. Much of the debate about how many hours are required is due to the lack of agreement between experts on what they consider practice. There are two main forms of training that are used in LTAD programs, deliberate play and deliberate practice.

Deliberate Play

This is defined as any activity that has minimal rules, is enjoyable for the participants, and resembles a primary sporting activity. An example would be the basketball game "horse." This is a game using a basketball, basketball hoop, and as much fun and creativity from the children participating. In this game, children try to make difficult shots from anywhere on the court and their playing partners have to try and duplicate the shot or get eliminated.

Deliberate play activities are those designed to maximize enjoyment. Deliberate play activities have simple sporting rules that are enforced by the children or an adult involved in the activity. The big question among researchers is, "Do these types of activities add to the athlete's 10,000 hours of expertise and count as practice?" This is a great question, which has not been answered yet.

Côté and Hay emphasized the importance of "deliberate play" (as opposed to deliberate practice) in the early years (9). This view is shared by many other researchers. The cyclone is an example of well-organized deliberate play stations.

Deliberate Practice

This is defined as any activity that has been designed by a coach to directly improve the skills of a student. It is

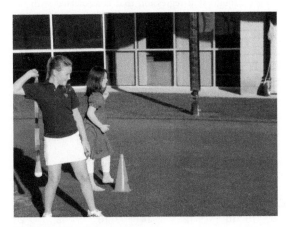

FIGURE 13-7. Throwing station.

not really enjoyable for most students, it usually does not show immediate results, and the only reason or motivation to perform deliberate practice is to improve your skills. A child practicing musical scales on a guitar would be an example of deliberate practice.

In 1991, Anders Ericsson, a psychologist investigating the role of natural talent among elite violinists at the Music Academy of West Berlin, made an incredible discovery. After hours of interviews, Ericsson and his team found only one difference between the best international soloists and the rest of the violinists at the academy, the number of hours they spent in deliberate practice. Ericsson was one of the first to challenge the thought that talent was something you were just born with. Instead he felt it was something that was developed through 10,000 hours of deliberate practice (10).

We do know that long hours of both play and practice are crucial for all LTAD programs. Most LTAD programs have fundamental phase athletes focus on deliberate play activities (the Cyclone) and then progress them to deliberate practice in later phases.

The important concept here is the progression of developing FMS before fundamental sport skills (FSS) are introduced. Children should progress from basic FMS to FSS in that order. This is the natural progression from simple tasks to more complex movements. Skipping over the movement skills and jumping into sport skills too early can be disastrous for the child.

Overview of All Fundamentals Phase Concepts

- Make sure all FMS are mastered—locomotion, stability, object control, and awareness skills. FMS acquisition should make up 75% of the program.
- Perform fundamental screen periodically to monitor progress in FMS development.
- Utilize games to capitalize on the first speed window by encouraging agility, quickness, and change in direction activities.

- Appropriate weight and length of golf clubs is paramount in this phase. Too often the clubs are too heavy and too long.
- Physical fitness should be 25% of the program and focus on body weight exercises for stability and overall mobility.
- One to nine holes a week of on-course activities that simulate golf, but keep it fun.
- One to two 90-minute sessions going through the Fundamental Cyclone per week.
- Concepts of grip, posture, alignment, ball position, balance, and weight shift may be introduced.
- Ratio of competition to training should be 10% competition and 90% training.
- Introduction to rules, safety issues on the course, and etiquette should be introduced.

TRAIN TO PLAY PHASE

We will skip the Play phase and jump ahead to the Train phase, where children begin their pubertal growth spurt. This is a very challenging time for the young adolescent and the coach. Hormones are all spiking, social and emotional interactions change, coaches can be challenged by the athlete, and growth occurs at an accelerated rate.

If you look at the growth velocity curve, you can see the rapid increase in growth over 2 to 4 years. The point at which growth velocity starts to decline (green star) is called peak height velocity (PHV) (Figure 13.9).

From most of the studies that have been performed on juniors, the growth spurt occurs at around ages 9 to 10 for girls and at ages 11 to 12 for boys. Girls usually start about 2 years earlier than the boys. PHV has an average age of 11.8 for girls and 14 for boys (10).

Once the growth spurt begins, we need to start to minimize skill acquisition and begin to focus on skill maintenance and on-course tactics. This will allow the player to go through skill regression that is associated with the

FIGURE 13-9. Growth velocity curve with peak height velocity point marked.

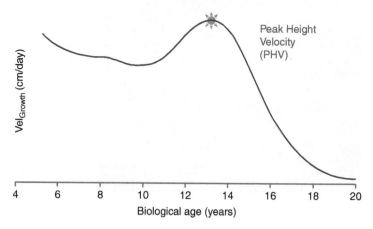

growth spurt, but still shoot lower scores due to improved scoring abilities.

We enter children into a new training circuit called "The Wave." We call it the Wave since there is an up and down growth velocity during this time frame. There are nine stations in the Wave. They include speed, mobility, stamina, three deliberate practice stations, stability/strength, and 3D integration. We recommend setting up six stations at a time, but include all three practice stations each time. Each station should be at least 10 minutes long, with a 10-minute warm-up and cooldown.

Some of our favorite Wave stations are described in the following sections.

Strength Station

Once puberty hits, children will get a surge in all sexual hormones. Boys get a large surge in testosterone, while girls get a spike in estrogen (5). This difference in circulating hormone levels can make strength training a challenge for the girls. The high testosterone levels in boys will promote a rapid increase in their muscle size with hypertrophy (enlargement of muscle fibers). Girls on the other hand do not get the benefit of testosterone so their strength gains will not be as noticeable. Before puberty, most of the strength gains were neural based (better recruitment of muscle fibers and better coordination of muscle firing patterns).

We begin the strength training phase for girls immediately following PHV. Since the growth plates are still fusing, and boys mature later than girls, we advise the next phase of weightlifting to begin 12 to 18 months after PHV for the boys.

The goal here is to begin to build a good base of strength. We introduce them to resistance training using free weights, like dumbbells or small kettlebells, and go through the same movements that were learned in the previous phase. Introduce them to an unloaded barbell and go through the same movements again.

Start to add weights to the barbell slowly. You are in no hurry to develop large force. Just keep building slowly over a 3- to 10-year period.

Some of our favorite strength activities are discussed here.

Barbell (Body Bar) Resistance

We like to begin adding resistance using medicine balls and body bars. Standard Olympic lifting movements are performed (Figure 13.10).

Turkish Get-Up

Turkish get-ups hit everything. There is thoracic flexion and extension, ankle dorsiflexion, hip flexion and extension, and shoulder flexion, extension, and stabilization (Figure 13.11). There is abdominal strength and stabilization, glute, quadriceps, and calf strength, too. If there are only three exercises a teen golfer does, the Turkish get-up should be one of them.

3D Integration Station

3D integration is vital. We know today that proprioception (knowing where their body parts are in space) goes haywire during puberty. This is the reason why teenagers rely so much on vision when it comes to orientation in space. For golf, we have to deal with rapidly elongating limbs and insufficient proprioception and kinesthesia. At PHV, juniors experience themselves as adults and have to cope with ever-increasing challenges in sports and academics.

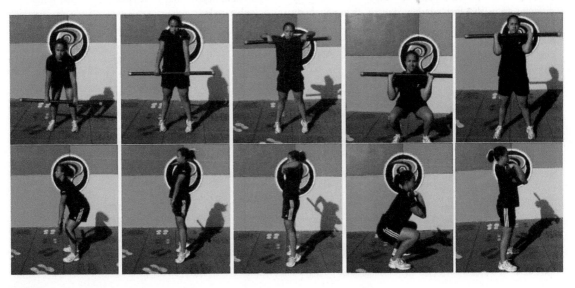

FIGURE 13-10.   Barbell (body bar) resistance.

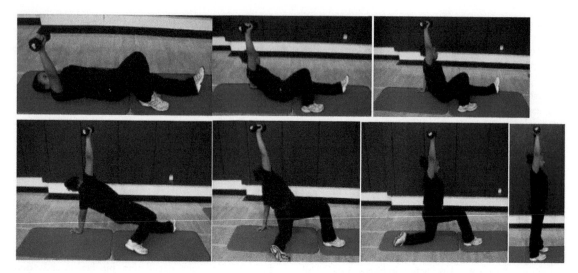

FIGURE 13-11.   Turkish get-up.

This is the time we have to do 3D integration. Challenging them in three dimensions is fun and develops an aspect that they are not aware of.

This station includes all nongolf swing activities that challenge their kinesthetic and spatial awareness. Activities like ropes courses, trampolines, climbing activities, and gymnastics can all serve this purpose (Figure 13.12A,B). Simple tumbling activities like cartwheels, front somersaults, backward rolls, and handstands are all forms of 3D integration as well.

Speed II Station

This is our second chance to develop more speed in our junior golfers. The focus on speed window two is slightly different from the first window due to changing body chemistry. Once puberty hits and the gonadal hormones increase, the cardiovascular and respiratory systems go into overdrive. For this reason, we can begin to develop anaerobic power and speed. Activities such as sprinting, jumping, throwing, and overspeed training are always included. Some of our favorite speed activities are listed here.

Plyometrics

These exercise train the central nervous system to produce rapid and powerful movements. Plyometrics help athletes hit harder, run faster, jump higher, and throw farther.

There are hundreds of plyometric exercises available to the junior golfer. There are low-grade plyometrics such as jumping rope and highly intense plyometrics such as a handstand depth jump or scissored split squat jumps with a double cycle.

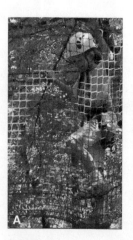
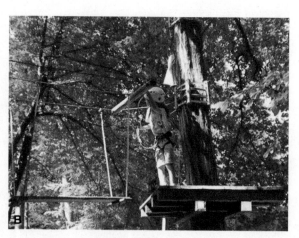

FIGURE 13-12.   (A, B) 3D integration station.

Stamina Station

Stamina window one is the first time a young athlete has the physical readiness to begin endurance training. Their cardiovascular system is improving for endurance training. This occurs at or around the onset of PHV. For example, a 16-year-old boy has three times greater maximal oxygen uptake (VO_2 max) than he had when he was 5 (11).

Most children can improve their VO_2 max the most during their growth spurt. Before puberty, VO_2 max increases at approximately the same rate for boys and girls. Once puberty and the growth spurt hits, boys start to improve at a much higher rate. This is due to high levels of testosterone allowing boys to increase their muscle mass, while girls increase estrogen production which increases their body fat instead. Therefore, boys will have higher levels of aerobic capacity, larger cardiac outputs, and increased pulmonary capacity. Even though girls may lag behind the boys in this phase, it is still the best phase to train endurance for girls.

Endurance training at this phase also has two additional benefits:

- The better their endurance, the more they can cope with high levels of training hours and sessions in the future.
- Improved endurance helps players recover faster between shots and rounds.

There is a debate among most experts on how to train endurance. Some believe that long-duration "cardio" training is the most effective, while others say high-intensity short-duration training is the best (12). To make this debate a nonissue, we encourage both forms.

Some of our favorite stamina activities include:

- Jumping rope. This low-grade plyometric exercise provides an excellent platform for gaining stamina. It is an exercise that does not require a golf fitness professional's constant monitoring, yet it helps develop coordination, balance, stamina, and muscular endurance.
- Speed golf. Hit and run has never been so much fun—at least for some. This brand of golf requires and helps improve both golf skill and physical stamina.
- High-intensity interval training (HIIT) cycle. This can be any form of HIIT (e.g., stepper, spin bike, jumping jacks, sprinting) that can be performed for 20 to 30 seconds followed by 20 seconds of rest. Then repeat this cycle up to four times.

Mobility Station

One of the most important aspects to focus on during the Train phase is mobility. Both boys and girls go through big changes that may affect their mobility for the rest of their lives during puberty. Their entire stature changes during the growth spurt due to multiple factors:

- Long bones grow first—the long bones of the body, like the femur, grow first. And they don't grow at the same time or with the same velocity. This can be very problematic for children, not only for mobility but for coordination as well.
- Muscles are set on tension—since the bones are growing faster than the muscles, muscle tension increases. This can lead to all kinds of muscle injuries if mobility is not slowly and safely improved.
- Muscle mass increases—due to hormonal changes (like testosterone and growth hormone) muscle hypertrophy begins (which means the actual size of the muscle fiber finally begins to enlarge). In previous phases, children were actually learning how to use the muscles more efficiently and how to neurologically fire more of the muscle. Now, the muscle begins to grow in size. This phase is great for strength, but can be a nightmare for flexibility.
- Growth plates get thinner—since the size of the growth plate begins to shrink, they become more vulnerable at this phase. Poor mobility can lead to growth plate injuries.

Primary areas that need to be targeted include the thoracic spine, hips, hamstrings, and lower back. Below are some of our favorite mobility exercises for this phase.

Mobility Warm-Up

We like to incorporate any mobility exercise that includes movement throughout end ranges of motion. These are not static exercises. They are exercises that force the body to stabilize one part while moving others. The exercises shown in Figure 13.13 are a sample of the various mobility exercises that can be performed during this phase.

Deliberate Practice Stations/Skill II Station

As stated earlier, from the onset of the growth spurt through to PHV, improving mechanics will typically be more difficult. In fact, many juniors may suffer a drop off in skill level as they struggle to cope with the changes occurring in their rapidly growing body. As a result, in the first stage of Train Phase, we shift our focus away from improving mechanics and onto improving shot-making and course skills.

This focus does not mean we entirely abandon swing mechanics. In fact it is critical that we continue working on them. The focus of mechanics, however, will be on maintaining what has already been learned. In a weird way, they will be learning the same skills again for the first time using an entirely different body. Longer levers and bigger muscles need to be retrained.

Taking all of the above into account, the golf stations in The Wave up to PHV are dedicated to maintaining swing

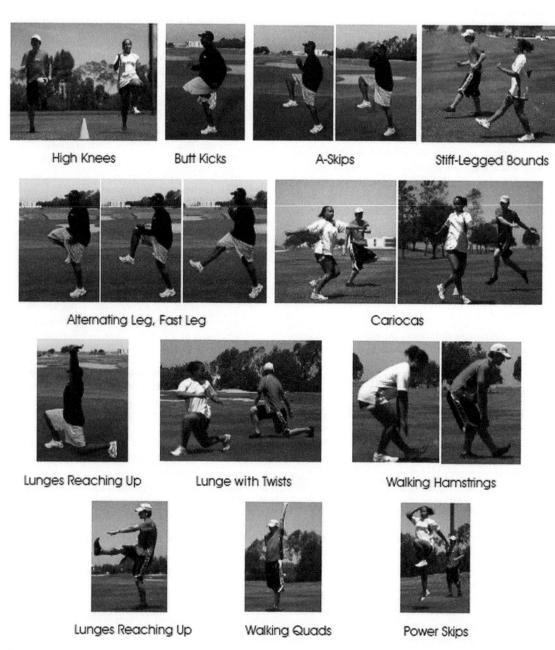

FIGURE 13-13. Mobility warm-up.

mechanics, improving shot-making skills, refining the process of shot making (i.e., developing preshot routines), and creating a competitive practice environment in which to test it all.

From PHV onward the rate of growth is slowing down. With the growth spurt coming to an end, the second skill window is opening. Alter the Wave to reflect this by adding

stations that dedicate time to refining swing mechanics, introducing the techniques required to hit shots required to play at elite level.

Practice stations should include putting, chipping, pitching, full swing, and game simulations. A variety of games during practice can be introduced to reduce the boredom of deliberate practice.

Overview of All Train Phase Concepts

- Children should be physically literate (FMS plus FSS) by this phase.
- They should excel at the Learn to Play screen but should be monitored for regression.
- They usually go through a growth spurt in this phase. So look for poor coordination or skill regression.
- They fall into the second speed window. Focus on speed, power, and strength.
- Physical fitness should be 40% of the program. All aspects of conditioning should be introduced. Activation, body prep, mobility, stability/strength, cardiovascular conditioning, and recovery techniques should be covered.
- Should play 36 to 54 holes a week and practice two to three times per week.
- Practice should be 10% to 20% block practice and 80% to 90% random per session.
- They should be hitting around 1,000 balls per week—including putts and chips.
- They should be practicing golf skills 20 to 40 hours per week (including time on the course).
- Plus, they should own a full set of custom-fit clubs.
- Ratio of competition to training should be around 40% competition and 60% training.
- They should have a USGA handicap and compete on courses that are at least 6,000 yards for men and 5,400 yards for women in 10 to 12 competitions per year.
- They should know the rules of golf and have good control of their own game while playing (knowing their distances with each club, shot tendencies, and risk-reward decision making).
- Limit other sport participation to two sports.

ELITE PHASE

At the beginning of the Elite phase we ask the athletes to decide what they want to be when they grow up. They need to decide what pathway they would like to follow: Elite Development Program (EDP) for a potential professional career in golf or college golf scholarship, or the Golf 4 Life Program (G4LP) to become a high-level amateur player who loves the game. Based on that decision, we move athletes from the Wave to one of two different training programs.

The Elite Development Program

This program is designed to develop the adolescent into an elite competitive player. All aspects of tournament golf will be covered. Pre- and postgame workouts, effective practice sessions, advanced shot-making skills, yearlong periodization programs, sports nutrition, recovery basics, statistical tracking, media and publicity training, and college recruiting protocols will all be covered. Athletes are encouraged to attend the EDP group practice sessions three times a week, play three times a week, and practice 4 to 5 days a week.

The following is an overview of all Elite concepts for adolescents in EDP:

- Adult physical screening can now be utilized to monitor progress.
- Make sure to start full strength development 18 months after PHV.
- Advance biomechanics testing and adult club fitting should be introduced. Clubs should be checked once or twice a year.
- Physical fitness should still be 40% of the program. All aspects of conditioning should continue with a high focus on strength and power development.
- Should play 36 to 72 holes a week and practice three to four times per week.
- Practice should be 5% to 10% block practice and 90% to 95% random.
- Ratio of competition to training should be around 40% competition and 60% training.
- There should be practice and competition on regulation length courses: 15 to 25 competitions per year.
- Preround preparation and practice-day routines should be introduced.
- Nutrition and recovery techniques should be stressed.
- Limit all other competitive sport participation.

The Golf 4 Life Program

This program is designed to develop the best skills needed for high-level amateur golf. Pre- and postgame workouts, effective practice sessions, advanced shot-making skills, sports nutrition, and statistical tracking will all be covered. Athletes are encouraged to attend G4LP sessions one to two times a week, play one to two times a week, and practice 1 to 2 days a week.

ADULT GOLFERS

Let us now shift our attention to recreational adult golfers, ages 25 to 55. As a player ages, new demands and obstacles present themselves along the way. For most adults, the ever-demanding world of poor prolonged posture and reduced physical activity takes a toll on their body.

The number one challenge for the adult recreational golfer is to maintain proper mobility and stability to perform the proper golf swing. We all accumulate physical limitation with age and injuries. This can make it impossible to swing the way we learned to swing or prevent us from swinging the way our coach is telling us to swing.

Either way, we need to address these physical limitations or suffer the consequences.

Proper mobility is imperative for proper mechanics to prevent injury and includes a combination of normal joint range of motion and muscular flexibility. Mobility allows the body to move in all six degrees of motion, therefore giving the ability to perform any motion—without having to sacrifice stability. Mobility also allows the generation of elastic energy, and therefore establishes a base for efficient power production.

Stability is the ability of any system to remain unchanged or aligned in the presence of change from outside forces. Stability is created by combining three things:

1. Balance
2. Strength
3. Muscular endurance

If you want to keep the bow of a bow and arrow stable as you pull the string back, you must have good balance, strength, and muscular endurance. This is the same principle involved in creating a powerful golf swing. The ability to keep one part of the body secure, while stretching and contracting adjacent segments, allows us to generate speed and maintain a consistent posture throughout the golf swing. That is stability.

Since we know both mobility and stability are required for proper swing mechanics, it is important for the adult golfer to address both areas. A very simplistic way to look at the relationship of mobility and stability was recently described by Boyle (13). He showed that the body works in an alternating pattern of stability and mobility from the foot up (Figure 13.14). In other words, the feet require stability, ankles require mobility, knees require stability, hips require mobility, core requires stability, thoracic spine requires mobility, scapulas require stability, shoulders require mobility, elbows require stability, and wrists require mobility. It is important to recognize this pattern.

This alternating pattern of mobility and stability can help describe how injuries occur. If you take lower back pain as an example, you will often find that if the hip joints and thoracic spine are limited in mobility, the lumbar spine will sacrifice stability to obtain more motion. This abnormal motion in the lumbar spine can be one of the primary reasons for disc and facet injuries in the lower back. Unfortunately, limited thoracic spine and hip mobility are two of the most common findings in male adult golfers. This finding may explain why lower back injuries are so common in adult golfers.

When it comes to the LTAD guidelines for adult golfers, we focus primarily on maintaining or restoring back the normal mobility and stability pattern. Physical screening should be used at least once a quarter to determine if the pattern is altered. Tests for ankle, hip, thoracic spine, upper cervical, shoulder, and wrist mobility can easily be performed. Tests for knee, core, scapular, lower cervical, and elbow stability can also be administered.

FIGURE 13-14.   Stability/mobility.

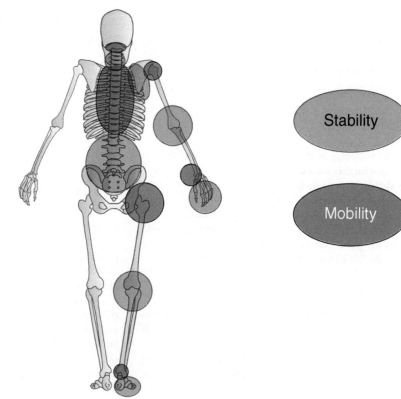

Stability

Mobility

Adults are advised to perform at least some sort of sporting activity two times a week and 30 minutes of regular exercise daily. Exercises should be focused on maintaining the body's pattern of mobility and stability. For golf, we recommend playing at least once a week and practicing one to two times per week.

Mobility

The following are two of our favorite mobility activities for adult golfers.

Starfish Pattern (Hip)

This exercise improves overall lower extremity rotation. It is actually a Proprioceptive Neuromuscular Facilitation (PNF) pattern of the hip combined with resistance. Attach one long piece of tubing from the golfers' right foot to the left foot (Figure 13.15). Then have them lie on their back and grab the middle of the tubing with both hands, extending their arms over their head. Slowly try to flex, abduct, and externally rotate the left leg without moving the rest of the body. Then extend, adduct, and internally rotate the leg again without moving the rest of the body. This maneuver teaches the hip how to move through a full range of motion without using the lumbar spine or pelvis to assist the motion.

Open Books Rib Cage (Thoracic Spine)

This is a great exercise to differentiate thoracic mobility from scapular and lumbar spine compensations. Lie down sideways and bend both knees (Figure 13.16). Take the downside hand and place it on top of the top knee—use the hand to keep the knees from rotating. Now take the top hand and reach under the downside rib cage and grab the ribs. Slowly rotate the chest toward the sky using the top hand to help and the bottom hand to resist lower body rotation. Hold for two slow breaths and repeat in both directions.

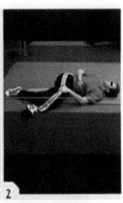

FIGURE 13-16.   Open books rib cage (thoracic spine).

Stability

These are two of our favorite stability activities for adult golfers.

Bridge Progression (Core)

This is a great exercise to build stability in the glutes and abdominals which make up the majority of the core. It also helps regain good hip extension. Lie supine with the knees bent, pelvis in a neutral tilt position, and the feet flat on the ground (Figure 13.17). Place arms out to side and lift the pelvis off the ground. The contraction should be in the glutes. Try to minimize hamstring contractions. Repeat the movement with the arms extended up to minimize support. Extend the left leg straight and lift the hips off the ground using the right glute. Repeat on the other side. They should be able to hold the single leg bridge position for a minimum of 10 seconds without feeling like their back or hamstring is going to cramp.

Box Presses (Scapular)

This is an exercise developed by Dr. Tom House, pitching coach at the University of Southern California. It is fantastic at developing proper stability back in the scapulas and elbows. Hold the right arm out by the side 90° from the shoulder with a 90° bend in the elbow (Figure 13.18). Place the left hand underneath the right wrist for resistance and try to push down the right hand. Push for 3 seconds and resist any motion with the left hand. Try this in three hand positions, thumb up, palm down, and thumb down. Repeat with

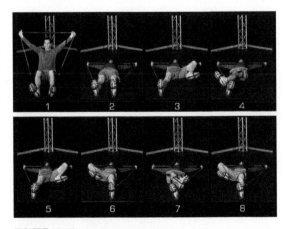

FIGURE 13-15.   Starfish pattern (hip).

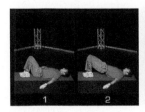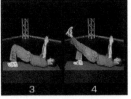

FIGURE 13-17.   Bridge progression.

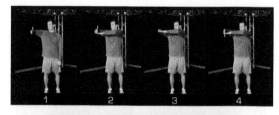

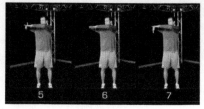

FIGURE 13-18.   Box presses (scapular).

the right hand underneath the left hand and try to push up this time in all three hand positions. Repeat on the other side.

Overview of LTAD for Adult Golfers

- Continue to get screened or assessed for loss of mobility and stability.
- Try to stay physically active as much as possible.
- Should play 18 holes a week and practice once per week.
- Practice should be 5% to 10% block practice and 90% to 95% random.
- Preround preparation and practice-day routines should be introduced.
- Nutrition and recovery techniques should be stressed.

REFERENCES

1. Balyi I. Quadrennial and Double-Quadrennial Planning of Athletic Training. Victoria, BC, Canada: Canadian Coaches' Association; 1990. www.ltad.ca
2. Zwick E. Growth Velocity. Growmetry.com; 2009.
3. Balyi I. Phases of Long Term Athlete Development. ltad.ca.
4. Malina R, Bouchard C, Bar-Or O. Growth, Maturation, and Physical Activity. 2nd ed. Champaign, IL: Human Kinetics; 2003.
5. Balyi I, Way R. Long-term planning of athlete development. The training to train phase. B.C. Coach (Canada) 1995(1); 2–10.
6. Seefeldt V. Longitudinal Study of Physical Growth ... Skills Program (1968–1998) Developmental Sequences of 10 FMS. Michigan State University.
7. Gibbons T, Hill R, McConnell A, Forster T, Moore J. The Path to Excellence: A Comprehensive View of Development of U.S. Olympians Who Competed from 1984–1998. United States Olympic Committee, 2002.
8. Ericsson KA, Krampe RT, Tesch-Romer C. The role of deliberate practice in the acquisition of expert performance. Psychol Rev 1993;100:363–406.
9. Côté J, Hay J. Children's involvement in sport: a developmental perspective. In: J. Silva, D. Stevens, eds. Psychological Foundations of Sport. Boston, MA: Allyn and Bacon; 2002:484–502.
10. Malina R, Bouchard C, Bar-Or O. Growth, Maturation, and Physical Activity. 2nd ed. Champaign, IL: Human Kinetics; 2003.
11. Rowland TW. Children's Exercise Physiology. 2nd ed. Champaign, IL: Human Kinetics; 2004.
12. Smith M. Sprint Interval Training. June 2007. http://www.mytpi.com
13. Boyle M. A Joint-by-Joint Approach to Training. June 20, 2007. http://www.T-nation.com

14

James W. George, Stéphane Cazeault, and Clayton D. Skaggs

Hockey

Ice hockey is a popular sport played throughout the world. Injuries are common in hockey due to the physical nature of the sport as well as the movements and skills associated with skating and shooting. Skating in ice hockey involves rapid acceleration and deceleration movements that require strong contractions of the leg muscles and stress on the hips, knees, and ankles. During shots and especially slap shots, the shoulder is put under tremendous stress, and players need adequate strength in the muscles of their hips, trunk, shoulders, and arms to deliver a forceful shot. Players who lack proper technique, have poor hockey-specific coordination, or lack adequate strength are less likely to perform at a high level and more likely to suffer an injury.

One of the most common injuries suffered in hockey are pulled groins or more technically, adductor strains (1). The adductors are a group of muscles in the inside part of the thigh that help bring the leg inward, a motion that is heavily utilized in skating. How common is this injury? For elite Finnish hockey players, approximately 43% of their muscle strains involved the groin (2). Although these injuries can occur to anyone during anytime of the season, they most often happen in the preseason and to individuals with previous groin strains.

Why are there so many groin strains in hockey? Most authorities believe it has to do with the stress put on the groin muscles during skating as well as a lack of strength in the hip muscles. Skating requires a significant amount of eccentric contraction of the groin muscles. This means the muscles have to contract as they lengthen. The adductors or groin muscles are important for decelerating or controlling the leg during the skating stride. When the player lacks strength in the posterior hip muscles and/or stability in the lower back, the adductor muscles take on more contraction than they are designed and are predisposed to injury. Studies have shown that when players do not have proper strength in their hips, they are more likely to suffer a groin injury (3).

Another common injury seen in hockey players involves the shoulder. Shoulder injuries tend to become more common as the skill level and intensity of the sport increase (4). Most often these injuries are due to players colliding during a check or falling on their outstretched arm. Common injuries include shoulder separations

as well as injuries to the rotator cuff. Properly giving and taking a check can help reduce these types of injuries; however, a variable that is often overlooked is the importance of the stability of the shoulder, mid-back, and trunk. Strength training that misses structural weakness in the rotator cuff or mid-back decreases the athlete's ability to take hits to the shoulder. Once shoulder injury has occurred it is vital to rehabilitate and strengthen the shoulder functionally in consideration of the kinetic links to the mid-back, trunk, and low back.

Other common injuries seen in hockey players include knee sprains, ankle sprains, and muscle strains of the neck and low back (5). These injuries can also be attributed to the physical nature of the sport as well as the demands placed on these joints during the quick stopping and starting movements that players use to maneuver on the ice.

Although injuries are common in hockey, proper physical evaluation and sport-specific training can help players reduce their chance of injury and improve performance. Players should ideally begin this training during their youth period. Youth exercises are fundamental activities that will help train basic movement patterns and skills the athlete will use as they begin to learn the foundational movements of hockey. As the athlete moves to the intermediate level and competition improves, these fundamental exercises are progressed to an exercise set that focuses on improving strength and stability throughout the body. Finally, at the professional level, the exercise program will be focused on sport-specific movements and high-level strength and conditioning exercises. Through all these phases, the evaluation of the individual athletes' needs is paramount to the success of the training program.

YOUTH LEVEL

The training goal of this stage starts by emphasizing fundamental movement patterns and skills. The exercises that follow show the beginning of the general physical preparedness (GPP) of the youth athlete. During this initial strengthening stage, proper skill involving both intramuscular and intermuscular coordination will be emphasized to ensure proper muscle balance and range of motion.

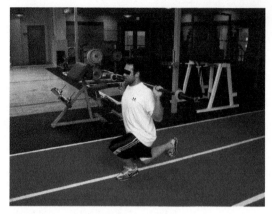

FIGURE 14-1. Barbell split squat exercise.

Split Squat

This exercise helps strengthen the quadriceps and improves knee tracking and stability by increasing the strength of the vastus medialis oblique (Figure 14.1). The athlete should take the following steps:

- Position barbell on back of shoulders and grasp barbell to sides.
- Stand with feet far apart; one foot forward and other foot behind.
- Squat down by flexing knee and hip of front leg until knee of rear leg is almost in contact with floor.
- Return to original standing position by extending hip and knee of forward leg.
- Repeat. Continue with same leg until all reps are completed.

Step Up

This exercise helps strengthen the quadriceps and hip extensors and improves balance and strength of the hip flexors for a faster skating stride (Figure 14.2). The athlete should take the following steps:

- Stand facing platform.
- Position bar on back of shoulders and grasp barbell to sides.
- Place foot of first leg on platform.
- Stand on platform by extending hip and knee of first leg.
- Step down with second leg by flexing hip and knee of first leg.
- Repeat first step with same leg until all repeats are completed.

Chin Up

This exercise will strengthen the upper back and is a good overall upper body exercise for strength development (Figure 14.3). The athlete should take the following steps:

- Step up and grasp bar with underhand shoulder width grip.
- Pull body up until chin is just above bar.
- Lower body until arms and shoulders are fully extended.
- Repeat.

Push-Up

This exercise helps strengthen the chest, shoulders, and triceps and is a good overall upper body exercise (Figure 14.4). The athlete should take the following steps:

- Lie prone on floor with hands slightly wider than shoulder width.
- Raise body up off floor by extending arms with body straight.
- Keeping body straight, lower body to floor by bending arms.
- Push body up until arms are extended.
- Repeat.

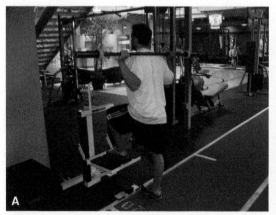
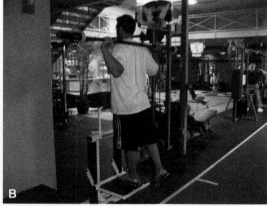

FIGURE 14-2. Step up exercise. (A) Starting position. (B) Ending position.

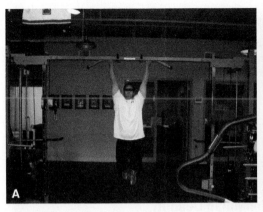
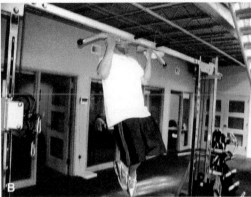

FIGURE 14-3.   Chin up exercise. (A) Starting position. (B) Ending position.

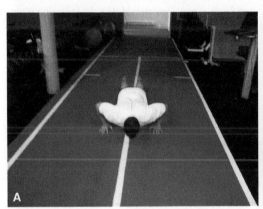
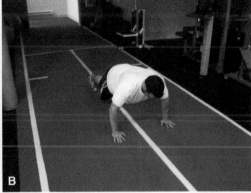

FIGURE 14-4.   Push-up exercise. (A) Starting position. (B) Ending position.

Penta Jump

This exercise is good for coordination and power development (Figure 14.5). The athlete should take the following steps:

- Stand feet shoulder width on a start line.
- Jump feet together 5 times in a row in a continuous fashion.

Sideway Sled Drag

This exercise improves strength in the groin area. Muscles here are highly recruited while skating (Figure 14.6). The athlete should take the following steps:

- Hold straps in each hand.
- Move sideways by abducting the working leg and adducting the trailing leg.

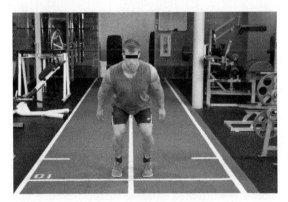

FIGURE 14-5.   Penta jump exercise: starting position. From this position the athlete completes five continuos forward jumps.

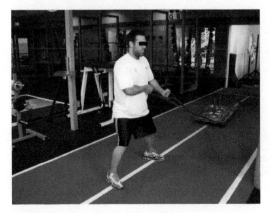

FIGURE 14-6.   Sideway sled drag exercise.

- Complete the desired distance on one side.
- Repeat with opposite leg.

COMPETITIVE LEVEL

In this phase, more emphasis will be on strength and muscle mass development as GPP progresses.

Squat

This exercise strengthens the quadriceps and develops strength and mass through a full range of motion (Figure 14.7). The athlete should take the following steps:

- From rack with barbell upper chest height, position barbell on back of shoulders and grasp bar to sides.
- Dismount bar from rack.
- Bend knees forward while allowing hips to bend back behind, keeping back straight and knees pointed the same direction as feet.
- Descend until knees and hips are fully bent.
- Extend knees and hips until legs are straight.
- Return and repeat.

Lying Leg Curl

This exercise will strengthen the hamstrings. Having strong knee flexors improves knee stability (Figure 14.8). The athlete should take the following steps:

- Lie prone on bench with knees just beyond edge of bench and lower legs under lever pads.
- Grasp handles.
- Raise lever pads to back of thighs by flexing knees.
- Lower lever pads until knees are straight.
- Repeat.

Romanian Deadlift

This exercise strengthens the hip extensors and lower back (Figure 14.9). The athlete should take the following steps:

- Stand shoulder width with feet flat beneath bar.
- Bend knees and bend over with lower back straight.
- Grasp barbell with shoulder width overhand grip.
- Lift weight to standing position.
- With knees bent 15 to 20 degrees, lower bar toward top of feet by bending hips.

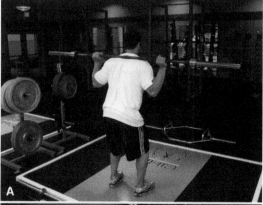

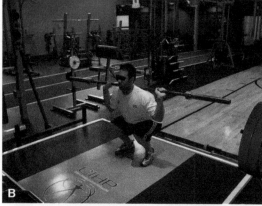

FIGURE 14-7. Barbell squat exercise. (A) Starting position. (B) Fully descended position.

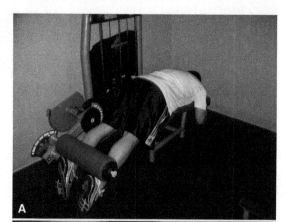

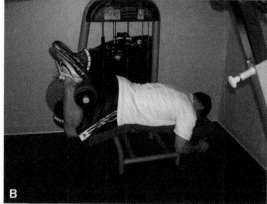

FIGURE 14-8. Lying leg curl exercise. (A) Starting position. (B) Fully flexed position.

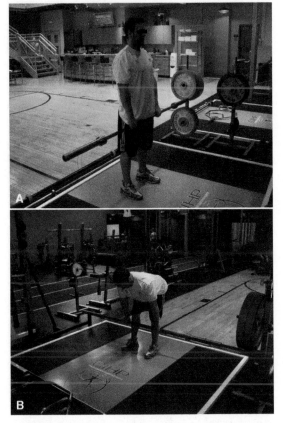

FIGURE 14-9. Romanian deadlift exercise. (A) Starting position. (B) Bottom position.

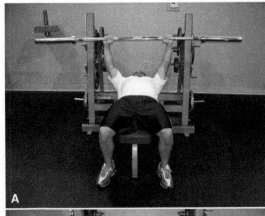

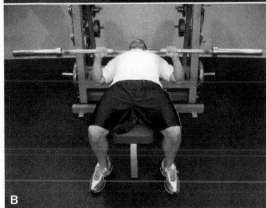

FIGURE 14-10. Barbell bench press exercise. (A) Starting position. (B) Bottom position.

- After hips can no longer flex, lift bar by extending waist and hip until standing upright.
- Repeat.

Barbell Bench Press

This exercise improves strength of the chest, shoulders, and triceps and is a good overall upper body exercise for strength and mass (Figure 14.10). The athlete should take the following steps:

- Lie supine on bench.
- Dismount barbell from rack over chest using wider than shoulder overhand grip.
- Lower weight to chest.
- Press bar until arms are extended.
- Repeat.

Backward Sled Drag

This is a great functional exercise for lower body, upper back, and grip development (Figure 14.11). The athlete should take the following steps:

- Hold straps in each hand while facing the sled.

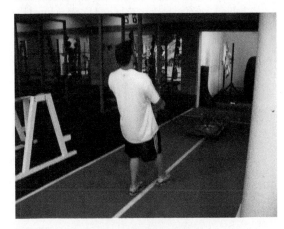

FIGURE 14-11. Backward sled drag exercise.

- Step backward by keeping torso slightly leaning back and by flexing at the knee.
- When toes are in contact with ground, forcefully extend the knee.
- Repeat on opposite leg until the desired distance is covered.

Unilateral Farmers Walk

This exercise improves ankle, knee, and torso stability (Figure 14.12). The athlete should take the following steps:

- Hold the apparatus to the side in one hand.
- Walk forward at a brisk pace while maintaining stability at the torso.
- Hold the nonworking arm abducted and parallel to the ground.
- Repeat until desired distance is completed.

ELITE LEVEL

For the elite athlete, the focus is on sport-specific movements, speed, and power.

Inertia Top Half Squat with Ankle Extension

This exercise helps strengthen the quadriceps and increases explosive power of the lower body (Figure 14.13). The athlete should take the following steps:

- From power rack, adjust side pins to half squat level.
- Barbell resting on side pins, position barbell on back of shoulders and grasp bar to sides.
- Extend knees and hips until legs are straight and simultaneously extend calf on top of movement.
- Bend knees forward while allowing hips to bend back behind, keeping back straight and knees pointed the same direction as feet.
- Descend until barbell goes to a complete stop on side pins.
- Repeat.

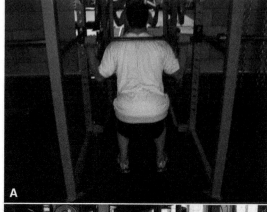
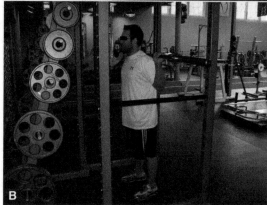

FIGURE 14-13.   Top half squat exercise. (A) Starting position with barbell resting on pins. (B) Top position with knees extended.

Glute-Ham Raise

This exercise improves strength of the entire posterior chain, which is a key factor for speed (Figure 14.14). The athlete should take the following steps:

- Position thighs prone on padded hump.
- Place lower legs between padded braces and feet against platform.
- Cross arms over chest.
- Lower torso by flexing hips.
- Extend hips until torso is parallel to legs.
- Raise body by flexing knees.
- Keep hip straight.
- Lower body until horizontal by straightening knees.
- Lower torso by flexing hips.
- Repeat.

Barbell Standing Good Morning

This exercise improves strength of the lower back and hip extensors (Figure 14.15). The athlete should take the following steps:

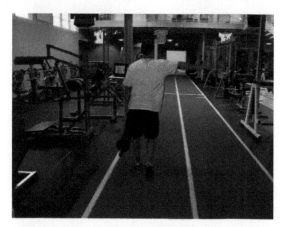

FIGURE 14-12.   Unilateral farmers walk exercise.

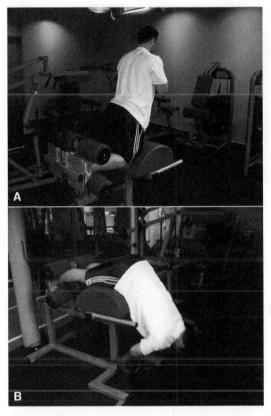

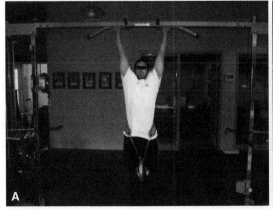

FIGURE 14-14. Glute-ham raise exercise. (A) Starting position. (B) Fully lowered position. From this position the athlete flexes the knees and returns to the starting position.

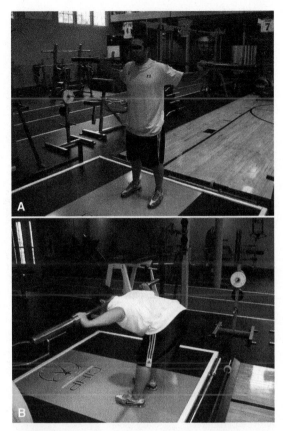

FIGURE 14-15. Good morning exercise. (A) Starting position. (B) Fully lowered position.

Weighted Chin Up

This exercise helps strengthen the upper back (Figure 14.16). The athlete should take the following steps:

- Position barbell on back of shoulders and grasp bar to sides.
- Keeping back straight, bend hips to lower torso forward until parallel to floor.
- Raise torso until hips are extended.
- Repeat.

- Attach weight to a chin/dip belt around waist.
- Step up and grasp bar with underhand shoulder width grip.

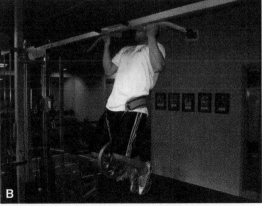

FIGURE 14-16 Weighted chin up exercise. (A) Starting position. (B) Ending position.

- Pull body up until chin is just above bar.
- Lower body until arms and shoulders are fully extended.
- Repeat.

Incline Barbell Bench Press with Chain

This exercise strengthens the chest, shoulders, and triceps. The chains will put emphasis on acceleration of the barbell (Figure 14.17). The athlete should take the following steps:

- Set a pair of chains outside of the weights on both end of the barbell.
- Lie supine on incline bench.
- Dismount barbell from rack over chest using wider than shoulder overhand grip.
- Lower weight to chest.
- Press bar until arms are extended.
- Repeat.

Super Yolk

This is a good functional exercise for ankle, knee, hips, and torso stability (Figure 14.18).

- Position apparatus on back of shoulders and grasp bar to sides.
- Extend knees and hips until legs are straight.

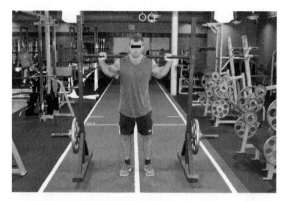

FIGURE 14-18.   Super yolk exercise.

- Walk forward at a brisk pace while stabilizing the apparatus with torso.
- Repeat until desired distance is completed.

REFERENCES

1. Nicholas SJ, Tyler TF. Adductor muscles strains in sport. Sports Med 2002;32:339–344.
2. Molsa J, Airaksinen O, Nasman O, Torstila I. Ice hockey injuries in Finland: a prospective epidemiologic study. Am J Sports Med 1997;25:495–499.
3. Tyler TF, Nicholas SJ, Campbell RJ, McHugh MP. The association of hip strength and flexibility on the incidence of adductor strains in professional ice hockey players. Am J Sports Med 2001;29:124–128.
4. Finke RC, Gerberich, SG, Madden M, et al. Shoulder injuries in ice hockey. J Orthop Sports Phys Ther 1988;10:54–58.
5. Emery CA, Meeuwisse WH. Injury rates, risk factors, and mechanisms of injury in minor hockey. Am J Sports Med 2006;34:1960–1969.

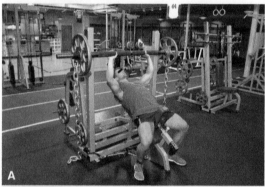

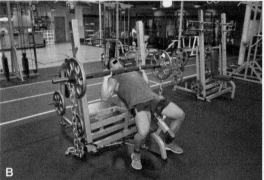

FIGURE 14-17.   Incline bench press exercise with chains. (A) Starting position. (B) Fully lowered position.

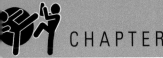
Mixed Martial Arts

The sport of mixed martial arts (MMA) has gained popularity by both participants and spectators in recent years. Competition in MMA has allowed for differing martial art styles to compete against another under regulated conditions (1). Common martial arts represented in MMA events include Brazilian jujitsu, boxing, freestyle, Greco-Roman and shoot wrestling, Muay Thai kickboxing, full-contact karate, Sambo, and Judo with many participants applying attributes of several styles to maximize competitive effectiveness. With the evolution of the sport, rule changes have taken place to help minimize injuries and maintain a reasonable level of safety (2). Sport MMA allows the use of striking and grappling techniques both in standing and on the ground. Sanctioning of the sport brought the establishment of weight classes, round time limits, the requirement of gloves, and the elimination of headbutts, elbow strikes, and knees to a downed opponent (3).

The injury rate within martial arts increases in correlation with the athlete's age and experience level and is particularly safe at young and intermediate levels of training (2,4). Within population-based studies, the injury rate for traditional martial arts training for both men and women was found to be between 0.3% and 1.2% of participation, with fractures being the most common injury at 20% (5). Although the injury rate for MMA has been reduced with sport rules and regulation, it is still high by other noncontact sport standards (2). A 5-year retrospective cohort study from all regulated MMA competitions in Nevada between March 2002 and September 2007 revealed an injury rate for MMA athletes of 23.6 for every 100 fight participants (6). The severe concussion rate was 3% of all matches. No deaths or sports-related critical injuries were reported in the regulated matches during the study period (see Table 15.1 for details concerning injuries in MMA)(6).

While competitive MMA is a highly refined skill set, we wish to briefly discuss some fundamental and recreation/sports-level skills that serve as a foundation for the elite/professional MMA athlete (7). Although many young martial artists may never desire to train for MMA competition, the functional skill progression sets the stage for sport skill training and ongoing refined/competition training (7,8).

It is important to note that many martial arts would never train in specific mechanics as depicted in some of the following examples (e.g., chambering a punch at the hip versus the chin). These examples illustrate the sequence of breaking down common movement patterns into more universal primitive patterns in an effort to reach common ground with various martial art disciplines.

FUNDAMENTAL SKILLS (AGES 7–10)

Knee Taps

This exercise trains balance, coordination and reaction time. The athlete pairs off with good posture of slightly arched back (not rounded), bent knees, relaxed shoulders, and head upright in a bear crawl stance (see Figure 15.1A). The object is to touch the partner's knees while avoiding being touched. Focus is placed on good posture, keeping the bottom down, low back slightly arched, and head up while alternating support from the reaching hands and supporting legs. The drill is performed for 30 seconds.

In Figure 15.1B, note how the athlete on the right correctly maintains a straight back as compared to the athlete on the left. This eases strain on low back tissues, minimizing chance of injury.

Functional exercises include:

- Bird dog
- "Stir the pot"(9,10)

Punch with Brace

This exercise trains whole-body stiffness. The athlete performs alternating punches while stiffening or bracing the stabilizing muscles. The athlete should practice relaxing the muscles between punches as not to stay rigid. Once the athlete becomes aware of bracing when punching, it is necessary to speed up the punches while staying relaxed and then generating whole-body stiffness at end-range. The drill is performed for 30 seconds. The exercise can be made more difficult with another individual adding destabilizing pushes to the shoulders and hips (see Figure 15.2). The athlete must maintain whole-body stiffness to maximize power transfer at striking impact.

Functional exercises include:

- Short foot training
- Punch/pull with band or pulley
- Balance training
- Slamball pulses (9–11)

TABLE 15.1	Frequencies and Rates of Mixed Martial Arts Injuries to Professional Competitors, September 2001 to December 2004 in Nevada[a]	
Injury Site	**Number (%)**	**Injury Rate Per 100 Competitors**
Facial Lacerations	46 (47.9)	13.45
Hand	13 (13.5)	3.80
Nose	10 (10.4)	2.92
Eye	8 (8.3)	2.34
Shoulder	5 (5.2)	1.46

[a]At greater than 5% frequency.

Source: Ngai KM, Levy F, Hsu EB. Injury trends in sanctioned mixed martial arts competition: a 5-year review from 2002 to 2007. Br J Sports Med 2008;42(8):686–689.

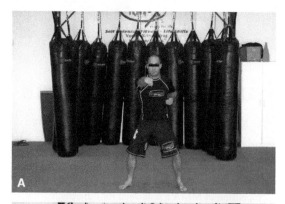

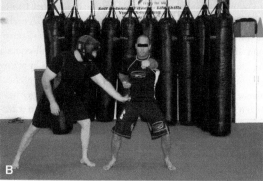

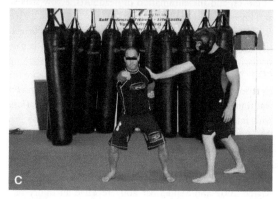

FIGURE 15-2. (A) Punch with brace. (B) Punch with brace, good posture. (C) Punch with brace, altered posture.

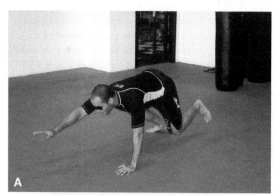

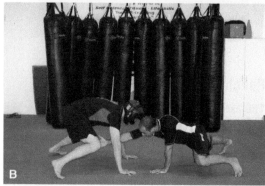

FIGURE 15-1. (A) Bear crawl, ready position. (B) Bear crawl position, reaching for opponent's knee.

One-Legged Stance with Bracing

This exercise prepares athletes for kicking and leg defenses using whole-body stability (see Figure 15.3). The exercise can be made more difficult by adding push resistance. The drill is performed for 30 seconds.

Functional exercises include:

- Short foot
- Balance training
- Single-leg squat
- Running man
- Kettlebell suitcase carry (9–11)

Hip Bridge

The athlete lies on his or her back, braces the core, and raises the hips. Attention is paid to rising through the gluteus and not raising from the back or hamstrings (see Figure 15.4). The athlete performs 10 slow repetitions using good form.

In the squat modification, note that the athlete's hips extend away from his feet while keeping a slightly arched low back and stable center of gravity.

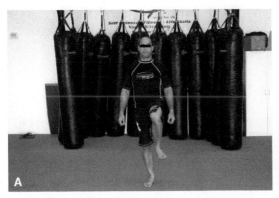

FIGURE 15-3. One-legged stance. (A) With bracing. (B) With push.

Functional training includes:

* Kneeling hip hinge
* Kneeling side bridge
* Kettlebell swing (10,12)

RECREATIONAL/SPORTS-LEVEL SKILLS (MIDDLE SCHOOL–HIGH SCHOOL)

At this level the athlete begins to learn how to prepare for competition (7,8). A fundamental movement base should have been established to address asymmetries in motion (11). This level of the athlete's training emphasizes technique. Economy of motion is discussed as avoiding wasted expenditure of energy while performing the desired task (13). Thus, the athlete is learning how to stay relaxed and apply the appropriate amount of stiffness and force at the appropriate time.

Pummeling

This is a common drill in wrestling and jujitsu that trains sensitivity and fluidity with grappling while trying to achieve an under-hook of the arms on the opponent. The athlete assumes a stance using good posture as mentioned in a squat movement pattern. The athlete takes an under-hook contact and opposite side over-arm contact with an opponent. The side which is the over-arm contact is the side where the athlete places the head. Both athletes then alternate finding a slow rhythm building in speed to each other's energy level (see Figure 15.5). The drill is performed for 30 seconds.

Note that the athlete maintains a slight arched low back with hips extending behind the feet. This offers a stable center of gravity to better react to initiate or counter a throw or takedown.

Functional exercises include:

* Squats
* Overhead squats
* Warrior stick
* Kettlebell swing to braced plank (9,10,12)

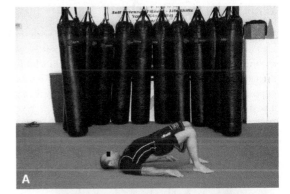

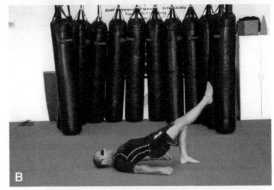

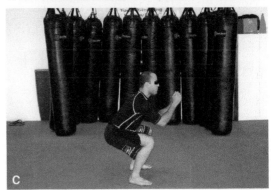

FIGURE 15-4. (A) Bridge. (B) One-legged bridge progression. (C) Squat modification.

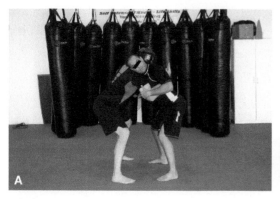
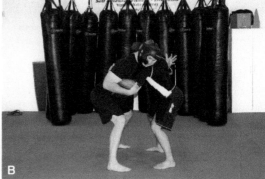

FIGURE 15-5. Pummeling. (A) Over-arm contact. (B) Under-arm contact.

Walking Lunges/Duck Walk

Walking lunges train the ability to "change levels" with the hips of an athlete driving through the opponent as he or she shoots in for a takedown. This athlete performs a lunge then rolls the supporting knee to the mat, dragging the opposite leg to lunge forward and repeat (see Figure 15.6). The drill is continued across the mat.

Functional exercises include:

- Lunge
- Reverse lunge (9)

Paper Punch

This is a modification of Bruce Lee's classic exercise designed to improve punching power using leg and hip rotation (14). The athlete stands parallel to a piece of paper hanging at head level. The athlete turns his hips to face the paper while delivering a punch to the paper. The athlete may first practice with their elbows until they develop rhythm and coordination, moving then to full punching (see Figure 15.7). The drill is to be performed for 10–20 times before alternating hands and position. With practice, the athlete will

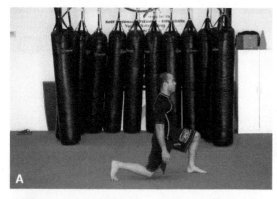
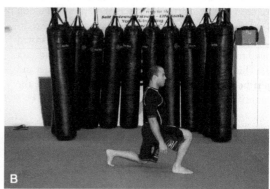

FIGURE 15-6. Walking lunge. (A) Left knee forward. (B) Right knee forward.

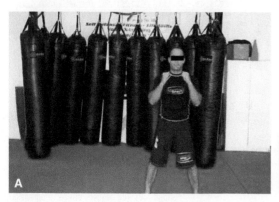
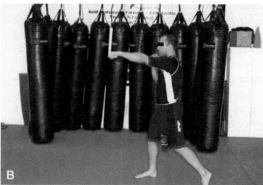

FIGURE 15-7. Paper drill. (A) Start position. (B) Finish position.

notice increased power with their straight-on punching by integrating their legs and hips into the punch.

Functional exercises include:

- Push/pull with band/pulley
- Punch with step and trunk twist (9,10)

REFINED-LEVEL SPORTS SKILLS (ELITE LEVEL, PROFESSIONAL)

Upa Escape

This technique trains escape from an opponent mounted in the high position. It is a progression of a body roll and one-legged bridge. The athlete grabs and secures the opponent's arm and hooks the opponent's same-side ankle in the direction he or she is to roll. The athlete then bridges the hips up hard and rolls to the side while holding the opponent's arm to disrupt support (see Figure 15.8). The athlete rolls the opponent onto his or her back.

It is important to note the control of the opponent's hand and ankle to the rolling side. The athlete's hip drive is fluid and continuous.

Functional exercises include:

- Bridge
- One-leg bridge

- Side bridge
- Turkish get-up
- Functional movement systems rolling (9,10,12,15)

Knee from the Clinch Position

This drill improves the ability to control an opponent from the clinch and deliver a knee strike. The opponent begins in the clinch position, with a stable base and hands fastened behind the neck. The athlete then turns from the hips and pulls with the back muscles (see Figure 15.9). This portion may be repeated several times before the athlete drives his or her knee up to the body of the opponent.

To control the clinch, the athlete clamps with the forearms, squeezing the head and turning the opponent's head. This exercise builds upon skills of pummeling such as whole-body stiffness and hip turning using both power and sensitivity.

Functional exercises include:

- Two-handed cable chop
- Pulley push/pull
- Kettlebell swing to braced plank (9,10,12)

Punch/Kick with Resistance

This exercise is a progression of punching and kicking mechanics. Both whole-body stiffness and hip and leg

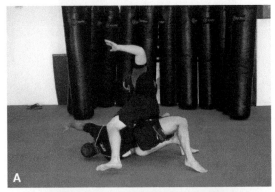

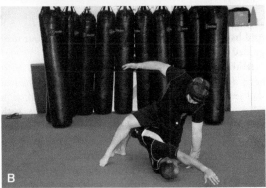

FIGURE 15-8. Upa escape. (A) Side view. (B) Front view.

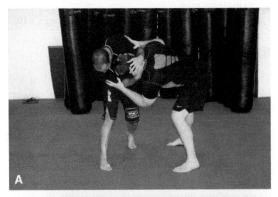

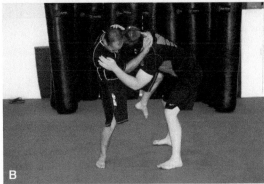

FIGURE 15-9. Clinch position. (A) Head pull. (B) Knee.

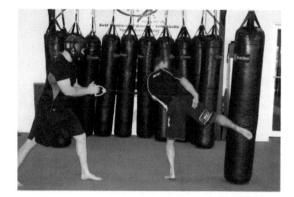

FIGURE 15-10. Kicking with resistance.

rotation are emphasized. The athlete's hips are attached to an elastic Theraband or Gi belt which provides additional resistance while the athlete punches or kicks a heavy bag (see Figure 15.10). Emphasis is placed on proper mechanics, hip power, and maintaining whole-body stiffness. A partner can modify the tension on the band or the vector of resistance to challenge the athlete's posture. The drill is performed for 30 seconds to avoid patterning fatigue-induced, poor striking technique.

Functional exercises include:

* Pulley push/punch
* One-legged balance with angle reaches
* Running man
* Pulsed bracing with overhead slamball swing (9,10)

Shooting

This drill trains the takedown common in wrestling and MMA completion. The athlete "shoots" his leg into a lunge position between the opponent's legs while changing the level of the hips to that of the opponent's knees. The lead knee then rolls down to the mat, past the opponent's feet. The athlete wraps both arms under and around the opponent's hips or upper legs while keeping his or her own head and torso up (see Figure 15.11). The drill is performed slowly, working on technique of either lifting the opponent up, or trapping the leg and tackling the opponent to the mat.

Functional exercises include:

* Lunges
* Walking lunges/duck walk (9)

SUMMARY

"Fighting, is not a matter of petty technique. It is not a question of developing what has already been developed, but of recovering what has been left behind. These things have always been with us...in us...all the time.

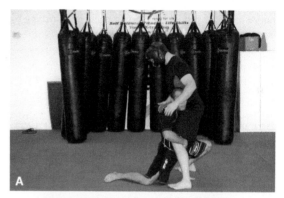

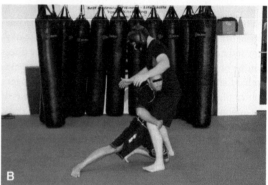

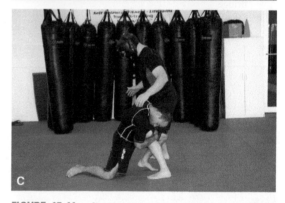

FIGURE 15-11. Shooting. (A) Left leg. (B) Rolling left knee to ground. (C) Poor form; note that the athlete's head is down and his lower back is flexed.

And have never been lost or distorted except by our misguided manipulation of them." Bruce Lee (13)

Although many children and recreational martial artists never desire to compete at the professional level, the refined skill set required at the elite level of training is based, as in other sports, on basic movement patterns. Attributes such as speed and quickness, footwork, power, spatial relationship, reactivity, sensitivity, and economy of motion build upon these basic movement patterns and are crucial to success in MMA competition (13). Sports-level skills further hone and condition these attributes which serve as the core for the elite MMA fighter.

REFERENCES

1. Scoggin JF 3rd, Brusovanik G, Pi M, Izuka B, Tokumura S, Scuderi G. Assessment of injuries sustained in mixed martial arts competition. Am J Orthop 2010;39(5):247–251.
2. Zetaruk MN, Violan MA, Zurakowski D, Micheli LJ. Injuries in martial arts: a comparison of five styles. Br J Sports Med 2005;39(1):29–33.
3. Nishime RS. Martial arts sports medicine: current issues and competition event coverage. Curr Sports Med Rep 2007;6(3):162–169.
4. Bledsoe GH, Hsu EB, Grabowski JG, Brill JD, Li G. Incidence of injury in professional mixed martial arts competitions. J Sports Sci Med 2006;CSSI:136–142.
5. McPherson M, Pickett W. Characteristics of martial art injuries in a defined Canadian population: a descriptive epidemiological study. BMC Public Health 2010;10:795.
6. Ngai KM, Levy F, Hsu EB. Injury trends in sanctioned mixed martial arts competition: a 5-year review from 2002 to 2007. Br J Sports Med 2008;42(8):686–689.
7. Canadian Sport for Life. Long-term Athletic Development. Ottawa, ON: Canadian Sport Centres; 2007.
8. Gambetta V. Athletic Development "The Arts and Science of Functional Sports Conditioning." Champaign, IL: Human Kinetics; 2007.
9. Liebenson C. Rehabilitation of the Spine. 2nd ed. Philadelphia, PA: Lippincott Williams & Wilkins; 2007.
10. McGill S. Ultimate Back Fitness and Performance. Waterloo, ON: Wabuno Publishers; 2004.
11. Elphinston J. Stability Sport and Performance Movement: Great Technique without Injury. Chichester, UK: Lotus Publishing; 2009.
12. Tsatsouline P, John D. Easy Strength. St Paul, MN: Dragon Door Publications; 2011.
13. Lee B. Tao of Jeet Kune Do. Burbank, CA: Ohara Publications; 1975.
14. Lee B, Uyehara M. Fighting Method, Basic Training. Burbank, CA: Ohara Publications; 1977.
15. Cook G. Movement: Functional Movement Systems. Chichester, UK: Lotus Publishing; 2011.

CHAPTER 16

Stuart McGill and John Gray

Olympic Weight Lifting

INTRODUCTION

Olympic weight lifting is a very unique sport for many reasons. The approach for selecting and developing young Olympic lifters is different than approaches used for most other sports and athletic skills. Other chapters in this book have described the typical staged approach for skill progression based on age and development. But developing the Olympic lifter for competition, or to simply use the lifts for athletic development, needs some further consideration. In addition, virtually any developing athlete could play recreational basketball with relative safety, for example, but many would be exposed to substantial risk of injury attempting Olympic weight lifting. Without specific anatomical and biomechanical attributes together with proper coaching, the lifting form needed to minimize injury risk is not possible. The range of motion needed at the hips and shoulders is at the extreme end of that found within the population (Figure 16.1). Without this ball-and-socket joint mobility, the athlete would be forced to create the motion in the spine. The spine is better able to safely support the load when it is not moving (i.e., with good lifting form the motion is at the hip joints, not the spine). In other words, spine motion creates stresses that cause tissues like the discs to damage at much lower loads. If lifting is used as a training tool rather than for preparation to compete, several adaptations in approach and form can be made to enhance athleticism in a safer way.

Having stated these special cautions, training the Olympic lifts offers several special opportunities. As we have found during testing and screening, the great athletes are usually more explosive because they are able to contract and relax muscle faster than their colleagues (1). Olympic lifts train the speed of contraction during initiation of the movement but then also train the rate of relaxation to be faster. Consider the special case of the snatch: the lifter must quickly drop their entire body to snap under the bar. The bar during this phase of the lift is not being lifted, rather it is dropping down at the rate of 1G. Here the body must drop under the bar faster than the bar descending at a 1G rate. Residual muscle tension in the lifter would result in stiffness, slowing their movement causing a failed lift. Relaxation is absolutely necessary to drop into position to receive or "catch" the bar weight. The mental discipline to relax knowing there is substantial load overhead and to accomplish this with speed is one of the unique opportunities in training the Olympic lifts.

This chapter discusses several issues: developing movement and essential athletic competency; selecting young athletes for the Olympic lifts; whether Olympic lifting is the best choice to achieve goals; and thoughts and techniques on training progressions.

SELECTION OF THE ATHLETE

In Olympic lifting not only does the athlete choose the sport but the sport must choose the athlete. By this we mean that first, the athlete must possess hips capable of extraordinary flexion. It is interesting that those countries/cultures that have high rates of hip dysplasia produce good lifters. They tend to have shallow hip sockets and the ability to squat more deeply. This is a hereditary trait that cannot be trained. For example, this trait is common among Eastern European and Western Russian haplogroups—the highest rate of hip dysplasia being Poland (2) (not coincidentally, one of the best Olympic lifting nations in the world). The link between dysplasia and a shallow acetabulum (hip socket) with higher joint laxity has been established for years (3). Differences in the collagen 111/1 ratio of hip capsular ligaments have also been proposed as a link between hip motion and dysplasia (4,5). The other side of the issue is that those with deep hip sockets tend to develop femoral impingement syndrome, and these are more common in the Western European haplogroups (6). The deep hip sockets cause the femur to collide with the anterior labrum of the hip joint when squatting deeply. What this means is that genetics plays a role in the ability to thrive when in deep squat movements under heavy loads. Thus, potential lifters need to be screened for appropriateness to perform the Olympic lifts.

Many other variables influence athlete selection. The second mobility requirement is that the shoulders must be capable of extraordinary overhead abduction and external rotation with simultaneous external rotation. Another consideration is that body segment proportions also influence leverage throughout the linkage such that a relatively shorter femur allows the lifter to pull around the knees with

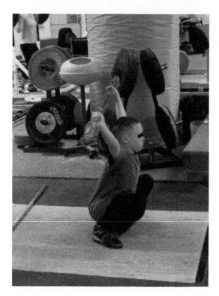

FIGURE 16-1.   Substantial range of motion is required at the hips and shoulders to facilitate the spine locked in a neutral posture. The flexion motion is about the hips, not the spine. This requires a shallow hip socket. Establishing excellent form first, prior to adding load, is essential for performance, enhancing athleticism, and injury avoidance.

such as the back to injury as well. Those with existing neck injury will have difficulty with Olympic lifts. The pulling musculature attaches to the skull from which the shoulder suspension musculature hangs. In addition to skull connections, more of the shrug musculature and connective tissue suspension system connects to the cervical spine. The cervical spine experiences substantial compression during a lift and must have sufficient pain-free tolerance. Existing low back problems are particularly problematic. Intolerance to compressive or shear load, or flexion bending motion will prevent effective training with Olympic lifts unless the hips possess extreme flexion ability.

Research on the predictive ability of certain fitness or exercise scores for weight lifting performance is quite poor, so initial tests of absolute strength or muscle endurance are of questionable value for these athletes. Thus, movement screens appear to have the greatest potential to assist in lifter selection and/or correction of movement flaws. In the tradition of Russian Olympic lifting training, potential athletes are selected first for their range of motion in the shoulders and hips (it must be large) and in explosive contraction/relaxation for muscle power production (the athlete must be quick). Strength and muscle hypertrophy are secondary and are developed later.

more hip power and less spine load. Those who lift closer to world record have less back load than their competitors (but higher hip load) at least in powerlifters (7). The ability to create a very high rate of muscle contraction is important. This is the "pulse." The ability to relax muscle at a high rate is equally as important. This is the "antipulse." The relaxing antipulse is needed to obtain the speed necessary to "catch" the bar. Without these mostly hereditary gifts, the lifter will sacrifice the lifting form needed to reduce the risk of injury. A good coach will see immediately if a young lifter has a chance to lift competitively or will simply break their body. Thus, selection of the mobile, "elastic-power" Olympic lifter is essential for both performance and injury avoidance.

While the requirements listed in the previous paragraph are needed for competitive Olympic lifting, many individuals find that this lifting is still helpful as a conditioning tool for other sports, even those with long limbs and levers who are not ideally suited to higher levels of the Olympic lifting sport. Thus, using Olympic lifting as a training method is a different issue from training to compete. Obviously their lifts will not be to competitive levels, and they may be better advised to incorporate Olympic lifting assistance exercises (power and/or hang variations) instead of the competition lifts to overcome their deficiencies.

The following addresses a few concerns of those with existing injury. Obviously injury to the hip or shoulder that compromises mobility or produces pain will lead to adaptations in lifting form that will predispose other joints

SPECIFIC MOVEMENT SCREENS AND QUALIFICATION TESTS

Assessing movement usually has the dual objectives of determining if a person is capable of a movement and if injury mechanisms are observable. For weight lifting, joints of concern for mobility are the shoulders, hips, knees, and ankles. Areas of concern for stability are the core. Primary injury candidates are the shoulders, knees, back, and hips. Performance variables such as the speed of muscle onset and relaxation, and grip strength athleticism, are also essential. While a more comprehensive discussion of the topic can be found in McGill (8), a brief overview of some movement assessments and qualification tests are as follows:

- Passive hip range of motion (Figure 16.2):
  - The source of any restriction is identified. For example, joint capsule end range of motion is partitioned from hamstring, fascia, ligament, and nerve tensions.
  - Optimal knee width (and foot placement width) is determined for depth of squat by scouring the femur around the acetabulum and finding the deepest depth.
  - Pain may be provoked. If so, follow up with more provocation of the capsule, labrum, muscle, and connective tissues to determine the cause of the pain trigger.
  - Look for left/right symmetry as those with asymmetric hips will usually succumb to injury sooner.

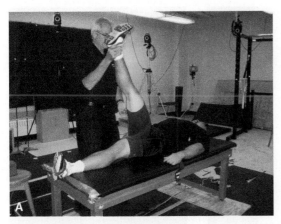
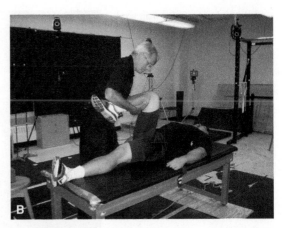

FIGURE 16-2.   (A) Hip range of motion is determined first with the leg raise test to assess muscle and passive tissue tensions. (B) The femur is scoured around the acetabulum to assess the acetabulum shape and depth, to determine the ideal knee width for the squat phase of the lift, and the squat depth potential. If the knee cannot be brought close to the chest without flexing the spine and pelvis, then the lifter will need to limit the depth of the squat and/or will not progress as an Olympic lifter.

- Passive shoulder impingement and range of motion (Figure 16.3):
  - Look for right/left symmetry.
  - Note pain or impingement at the acromioclavicular joint.
  - Also test glenohumeral translation (anterior displacement of the humeral head in the glenoid). This is usually associated with a very tight posterior capsule so that when the athlete performs internal rotation of the glenohumeral joint, the humerus glides forward and places increased stress

on the anterior capsule and long biceps tendon, contributing to the impingement.

- Front squat (Figure 16.4A and B):
  - Observe if a neutral spine posture is lost.
  - Are the hips able to go below knees with the heels on the ground? You may vary the sole of the lifting shoe.
  - Chest up and forward.
  - For the front squat the shoulders are forward to stop the bar from pressing on the trachea.
  - Knee hinge is aligned with ankle hinge.
  - Note that here the wrists are too extended as an accommodation for the hypertrophied bulk around the elbow impeding elbow flexion. This lifter would have more leverage by reducing this elbow flexor bulk.
- Overhead snatch squat (Figure 16.5):
As above, plus
  - Able to maintain straight arms.
  - Minimal loss of natural spine curves.
  - Bar/dowel over shoulders.
  - Junior lifters may use a calibrated dowel (Figure 16.6) to determine grip width and the effects on mechanics throughout the linkage such as shoulder and spine alignment, neck postures for example.
- Forward/backward lunge (with arm straight overhead):
  - Begin lunge (Figure16.7A) then rotate pelvis about the hip joints (Figure 16.7B). The knee does not "dive in" relative to foot (indicative of unwanted hip internal rotation).
  - Able to drive off of front heel in returning to standing/starting position.
  - A variation of the lunge also assesses the hip flexor tightness; in this case a focus is directed toward

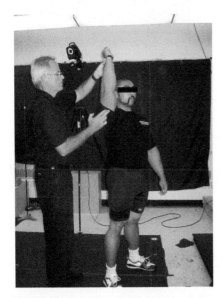

FIGURE 16-3.   The shoulder is assessed for impingement potential through the lifting motion in extension combined with internal/external rotation. Translations may also be probed.

FIGURE 16-4. (A, B) The front squat reveals mechanics when under load, some of which may require correcting with cues and technique. Other anatomically based flaws may restrict qualification to lift Olympic style.

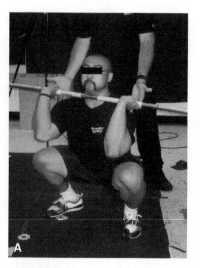
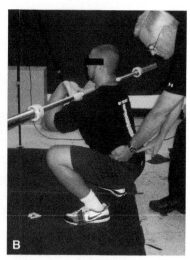

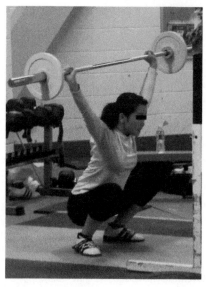

FIGURE 16-5. The overhead snatch squat is practiced to maintain the bar over the shoulders and feet with neutral spine curves.

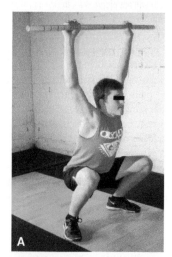

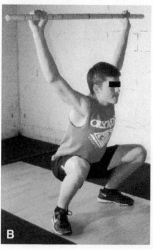

psoas with the arm push overhead elongating psoas up the lumbar spine. Hip internal/external rotational status may also be observed.

- Side lunge (Figure 16.8):
  - As for lunges, plus
  - Able to maintain straight trailing leg without rolling onto the inside of ankle
- Standing shoulder flexion (Figure 16.9):
  - Test uses a dowel with markings starting at 0 in the center, then measuring outward to the ends in inches. For example, a 6 foot dowel would have 0 in the middle, and read 36 inches at each end, with increments each ½ to 1 inch.

FIGURE 16-6. Using a calibrated dowel, grip width is determined that allows the bar to be supported overhead with its gravitational vector projecting down into the feet. (A) Narrow grip. (B) Wide grip.

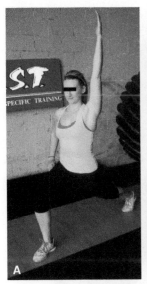 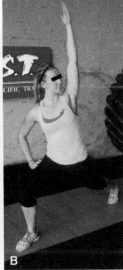

FIGURE 16-7. The forward lunge allows assessment of balance and range of motion. (A) The torso is squared while (B) the torso is rotated about the hips. Also note that this "test" will be used as a psoas muscle stretch later. Traditional hip flexor stretches usually focus on iliacus and ignore that psoas travels laterally alongside the lumbar spine. It is not stretched until the arm is pushed overhead.

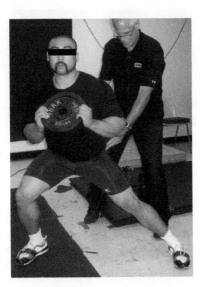

FIGURE 16-8. The side lunge is used to assess hip and ankle mobility. Knee motions are assessed, cued, and corrected.

- Athlete stands holding dowel using wide grip (as in snatch lift). He then raises the arms over the head keeping the elbows straight.
- If the athlete is able to do this without arching the low back, narrow the grip and repeat until the narrowest grip is found that will not cause the low back to arch/extend.

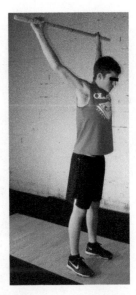

FIGURE 16-9. Standing shoulder flexion. Note in this case the grip is too narrow causing unwanted compensation with head poking and back arching.

- Box jumps (see Figure 16.10):
  - Stand in front of a box that is about the height of the lower sternum.
  - With a small countermovement, leap onto the box. Look for hip mobility and the ability to minimize spine motion.
  - Land trying to make a noise on impact—this will give some indication on pulse production.
  - Next, try and land with no noise—the quality of the soft landing will indicate the relaxation ability (antipulse).
- Assessing grip strength:
  - Have the athlete squeeze your hand and assess the force from each finger. Note that some will have the majority of the force from the first and second fingers.
  - Corrective exercises include training hand grip skill using all fingers and the "lobster grip" through the hand (see Figure 16.11A and B). Then focus on wrapping the bar with strength from each finger (Figure 16.11C).

STARTING JUNIOR WEIGHT LIFTERS AND A SCORING METHOD FOR FORM

Historically, training Olympic lifting in children has been discouraged in North American culture which has impacted development of the sport. For example, in the early eighties the American Academy of Pediatrics issued a position statement discouraging preadolescent participation suggesting

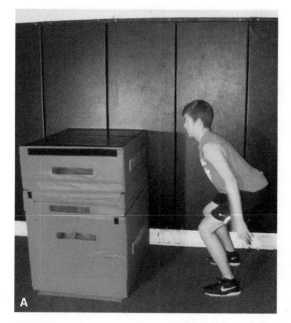
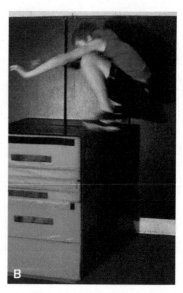

FIGURE 16-10. (A, B) Box jumps. Box height is increased as the athlete learns to maintain good landing form (or weight catch form). Here, the height limit has been found at this skill level given the full flexion seen in the hips and spine. The height should be lowered back to where good form was maintained and practiced.

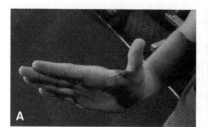
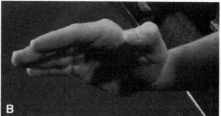
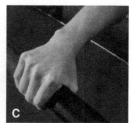

FIGURE 16-11. Grip strength technique. (A and B) The athlete is taught the "lobster claw" which is the greatest strength through the hand. (C) Then finger flexion strength is added with a focus on each of the four fingers wrapping on a bar. A "fat bar" is used in this training situation.

a potential for injury. From the reference material of the National Coaching Certification Program Club Coach (9), it is recommended that weight lifting competitions be organized only for athletes 15 years of age and older. Obviously this age is arbitrary as maturation will vary between the ages of 12 to 15 years. Since junior athletes are almost universally limited by technique, rather than strength, it is helpful to develop an objective scoring method to rate the quality of each lift. In this way athletes learn the proper technical aspects of lifting performance.

This scoring method for determining lifting success renders the typical established percentage schemes used by adults irrelevant. The learning curve is based on movement control, not outright power or strength. Pushing a junior athlete (under 15 years of age) to 1 repetition maximum (RM) is strongly discouraged as injuries to the joints can be much more debilitating than for adults. Testing for

explosive lifts should be done using the scoring scheme while any physical testing (e.g., front or back squats for athletes with at least a year of conditioning experience) should be kept to approximately 5 RM. Note that this should not be performed more than once in each 4- to 6-week training cycle. Since performance is limited by technique in junior athletes, a maximal lift does not imply the athlete is stressing the system maximally, only that the weight lifted is the highest that can be accomplished with appropriate technique and speed. Thus, in training using weight lifting methods, perfect form is the objective. There should be no issue lifting to the highest possible (perfect technique) weight on a repeated basis as skill improvement will be much more relevant to eventual success than physical conditioning. An often-used scoring/evaluation scheme is to let the junior athlete start with 10 points, then subtract a point for each technical error. Scores below an arbitrary number are considered unsuccessful. The arbitrary number is usually adjusted for the skill level of the lifter but always increased as weight increases. For example, a complete beginner working with a very light weight (e.g., broomstick) may only wish to work on getting basic techniques sound (e.g., front squat, overhead squat). The goal may be to improve each component of the weight lifting exercise to a perfect level before combining them into a complete movement, especially with a weighted bar. A fail grade might be 5 to 6 out of 10 as the athlete may be using the exercise to build appropriate mobility and coordination. In contrast, more advanced juniors lifting some load will have a higher risk of injury to, for example, the shoulders, if technique is not maintained. Here, a failing grade may be chosen as 8 out of 10. Some coaches use foam-covered "body bars" (of sufficient length) in these early stages as they increase in 3 lb increments from 9 to about 24 lb, well into the range of "technique bars" (which are approximately 5 or 10 kg but are more expensive and less readily available than body bars). Actual Olympic bars are used later in the athlete development.

CORE TRAINING AND PROXIMAL STIFFNESS—A NONNEGOTIABLE PREREQUISITE TO TRAINING

Discussion of training progressions should start logically with a discussion on core training. Dedicated core training, and the resulting skill to enhance torso stiffness, is essential for injury prevention and performance enhancement.

A discussion of the core requires a three-dimensional perspective. First the issue of injury resilience will be addressed followed by the issue of performance enhancement. The spine is a stack of vertebrae that is called upon to bear loads, yet it is flexible. A design engineer will describe how they are not able to design a structure to be good at both. A steel beam that is straight and stands on its end is stiff and can bear loads that try to compress, shear, and twist it. Thus, the beam can bear load but it cannot move. A flexible rod that allows movement will bend and buckle under load. But the spine is a unique structure that is flexible and allows flowing movement; however, it requires a three-dimensional guy wire system to stiffen and stabilize it when it is required to bear loads. Analysis of the muscular system, together with its associated fascia sheets, reveals a clever guy wire system that creates balanced stiffness eliminating the possibility of buckling and injury (10,11).

The greater the load that is placed down the spine, the greater the need for the musculature to stiffen the spine. How can this be? When muscles contract they do two things: they create force and they create stiffness (12,13). Stiffness is always stabilizing to a joint. Thus, stiffness prepares the joint to bear load without buckling. Failure to appropriately stiffen the core is a major cause of lifting injury, although not the only cause.

On the performance side of the discussion, "core stiffness" is mandatory. It is absolutely essential to carry heavy loads, run fast and change direction quickly, and perform competent Olympic lifts. It determines the rate of speed for movement of the arms and legs. There are those people who state they do not need dedicated core training because they lift and squat. Yet when assessed, many are unable to translate their strength to under-the-bar performance. How does core stiffness enhance limb speed and strength? Consider the pectoralis major muscle for a single joint example—it attaches the rib cage at its proximal end, crosses the shoulder joint, and attaches to the humerus of the upper arm at its distal end. When muscles contract they try to shorten. Consider the specific action in this example—the arm flexes around the shoulder joint moving the arm from muscle shortening at the distal end. But the same shortening also bends the rib cage toward the arm at the proximal end of the muscle. Thus, simply using the pectoralis muscle would not result in a fast or forceful punch. In contrast, if the proximal end of the pectoralis muscle attachment is anchored—meaning stiffen the core, the rib cage could not move. This proximal anchor directs 100% of the pectoralis muscle shortening to its distal end, producing fast and forceful motion only in the arm. In the same way a stiffened core locks down the proximal ends of the hip muscles by fixing the pelvis producing more power to the thighs. Thus, a universal law of human movement is illustrated—"proximal stiffness enhances distal mobility and athleticism."

This discussion now provides context to the question—what is the core? Proximal stiffness occurs between the ball-and-socket joints—that is, the hips and shoulders. The concept incorporates all of the muscles in the torso. They function primarily to stop motion. They should be trained this way. The core also involves the muscles that cross the ball-and-socket joints that have distal connections—psoas, the gluteals, latissimus dorsi, etc. There are many ways to train these in progression to enhance performance and injury resilience, which is out of the scope of this chapter. (The interested reader is directed to reference (8).)

IMPORTANT CORE TRAINING EXERCISES

The importance of core training for lifting was addressed above. Younger athletes can begin core training with exercises, including the plank (Figure 16.12), stir the pot (Figure 16.13), side bridge (Figure 16.14), bird dog (Figure 16.15), push-ups, lunges integrating the shoulders pushing upward and back, to train the supporting guy wire system. When seriously training, exercises including stiffening and breathing exercises, rapid muscle activation and relaxation exercises (see (8) for several training progressions) are integrated in the progressions.

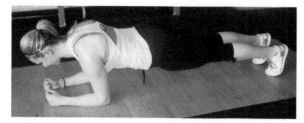

FIGURE 16-12. The front plank, a core exercise. Here, the body maintains alignment. The "hard style" plank developed by Pavel Tsatsouline requires conscious stiffness throughout the linkage. Emphasis is directed toward activating and squeezing the gluteal muscles and the abdominal wall while the latissimus muscles attempt to draw the elbows toward the feet (no motion takes place). Junior lifters begin with repetitions of 10 second holds and typically perform three sets.

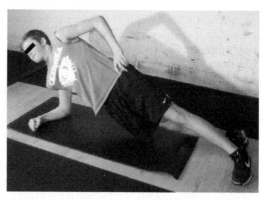

FIGURE 16-14. The side bridge, a core exercise. This form of exercise is usually prescribed with a 10-second hold on one side, then a roll to the plank with no motion in the torso allowed—the rib cage is locked to the pelvis. The plank is held a couple of seconds, then the athlete performs the stiffened role to the other side which is held 10 seconds. This cycle constitutes 1 repetition.

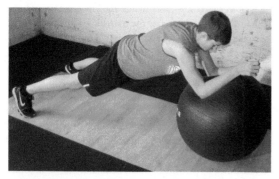

FIGURE 16-13. Stir the pot, a core exercise. Focus is on motion only in the shoulder joints as the ball is stirred with the elbows. The torso does not flex, bend, or twist.

SPECIFIC TRAINING PROGRESSIONS

Form in lifting style is essential for both performance enhancement and injury avoidance. To guide training progressions, think of Olympic lifting as vertical jump training with components that include shrugs, bar clean, hang clean, hip hinge, etc., then moving to speed jumps onto a box.

In the dominant lifting countries athletes are encouraged to develop general athleticism until they are skeletally mature. Many will spend years lifting "broomsticks" to perfect the form, and then form with speed. Then, specific drills to develop stiffness in the starting position, that is, "The lifters wedge," are usually incorporated together with drills to enhance the rate of muscle force development together with faster rates of muscle relaxation. Weight on a bar is introduced but this component of training forms a very low volume in terms of total training. Restorative activity is also much more emphasized in the countries with a developed lifting culture. Olympic lifting training simply cannot be performed every day without breaking the body down, although supplemental exercises may be performed. Specific technique enhancement is then encoded into the lifting motion and motor patterns—creating the perfect engram of the lift.

While coaching specific lifting form is outside of the scope of this chapter, the following discussion of general

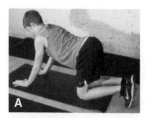
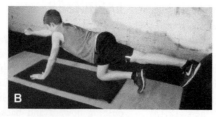
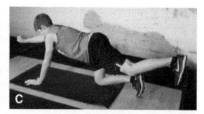

FIGURE 16-15. (A, B) The bird dog, core exercise. These are usually held for 10 seconds, then the athlete "sweeps the floor" with the hand and knee with motion only occurring about the shoulder and hip. Then another 10-second hold forms the next rep. Note the cues to enhance activation of hamstrings, gluteals, and back muscles—the heel is pushed away rather than focusing on the leg lift, and the fist squeeze radiates activation into the upper back on the opposite side. (C) Poor starting posture—this reduces the capacity to train and reach ultimate performance.

form principles may provide insight into the nuances of successful and skilled development for lifting.

Setting Up the Pull

The perfect pull technique "depends on the person." All lifters have a different injury history influencing which tissues may need sparing, different body segment length ratios affecting leverage advantages, different hip socket depths that determine the depth of the squat before the pelvis tucks stressing the lumbar discs, etc. What is best for one lifter will not be best for another. This is a drill we use that will help all lifters set up their pulls, despite their individual differences. It is called the *short stop squat* after a common outfielder posture from American baseball.

Begin with the feet apart. Try a few knee bends and adjust the internal/external rotation of the hip, to get perfect knee and ankle hinge tracking. Observe the turn-out angle of the feet. Remember this angle and start in this position. To begin the drill, stand tall and place the hands on the top of the front of the thighs. Make a "V" between the thumbs and the finger. Keeping the arms straight, slide the hands down the thighs, only hinging about the hips—do not allow the spine to bend. Stop as the hands reach just above the knee cap and robustly grab around the knee. This is the short stop posture (see Figure 16.16).

Observe the position of the knee. A vertical line down from the knee should fall between the balls of the feet and the heels. This ensures that the hips are well behind. Adjust balance to feel the center of pressure from the ground in the middle of the feet. "Carry" the weight of the upper body down the arms and onto the thighs. Focus on the curves in the torso—adjust them until they are the same as when the athlete was standing. If not, cue and adjust them back to the natural curves.

When lifting from this position, many will shrug too soon. Avoid this. Coach the "antishrug" by compressing the shoulders down into the torso with cocontraction of the pectoral and latissimus dorsi muscles. This stiffens the torso with the normal curves intact.

To begin the pull, the novice lifter should be coached to think differently. The tendency is to pull with the back,

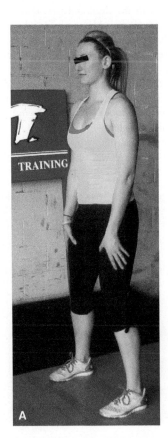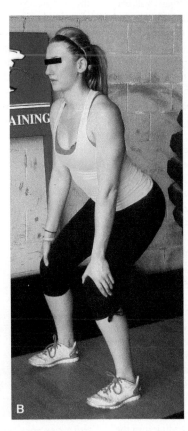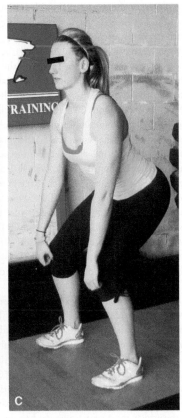

FIGURE 16-16. Short stop squat, a core exercise. This drill is used to perfect the hip hinging mechanics for greater power production. (A) The hands are placed on the thighs. (B) The hands slide down the thighs with the hips translating back rather than the knees forward. Here, the weight is carried down the arms as the body is stiffened and compressed with neutral spine curves. (C) Maintaining this compression, the hands slide lower to grip the bar.

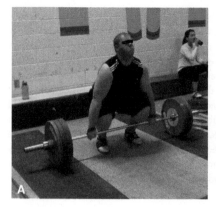
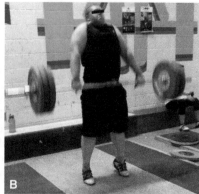
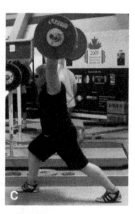

FIGURE 16-17. (A) The clean and jerk begins with the pull. (B) The shrug. (C) The catch prior to the final press overhead.

but instead think about stiffening the back and torso and initiating the rising motion by simply pulling the hips forward as the athlete slides the hands up their thighs. This cue is then adjusted to the lifter: those with proportionally longer thighs will be better to emphasize pulling the hips forward; those with proportionally shorter thighs will better rise from the squat with the legs. This stiffening and motion sequence is practiced progressing the reach lower until the bar is reached.

Now the athlete is ready to pull the bar. Adopt the short stop position with the hands on the thighs. Grip the ground with the toes and heels. Now grab the bar with a double overhand grip, the width being adjusted for the type of lift. Inhale to about 60% to 70% of full tide breath and close the glottis building intra-abdominal pressure. Begin the antishrug further compressing the torso. Try and bend the bar with external shoulder rotation feeling the latissimus dorsi stiffening the back over its length down to its origin on the sacrum. Coach the athlete to image "gathering" the back adding to the stiffness. Squeeze the bar harder thinking about force in all fingers—just not the first and second. Add some more effort to "spread the floor" through the hips activating the gluteal muscles. With torso stiffness now approaching optimal the grip is tightened and the hips are pulled forward. The load rises from the floor and is accelerated.

The strategy changes for the next phase of the lift—the *shrug* and *jump*. A second pulse is now focused to drive downward with the thighs and hips and simultaneously shrug the shoulders. At the end of the pulse the ankles are plantarflexed. Some elite lifters will leave the ground at this stage (in the clean and jerk—see Figure 16.17) illustrating the projection of force to execute a powerful *vertical jump*. In the snatch lift (see Figure 16.18), the pattern is cut short as the athlete must snap under the bar, descending into the deep squat to catch the bar overhead. As previously mentioned, this requires the critical relaxation phase to ensure a quick move to descend faster.

A note on breathing fits here. Once the breath is inhaled, and the glottis is closed during the setup to pull the bar, no further breathing occurs, at least in the traditional sense. Torso stiffness with the breath held maintains the stiffened guy wire system allowing the torso to withstand the compressive loading. In the clean and jerk, once the clean has been accomplished, the athlete may "sip" the air, with very short and shallow breaths never expelling much air. During this moment, the flexural bar stiffness is felt to assist the athlete in timing the pulse of the bar with a previous pulse to that the bending bar recoil is timed with the next pulse driving the bar vertically. Then, the athlete drops under the bar with the lunge split. Walking to the symmetric stand completes the lift.

This description is provided simply to introduce some elements that can be addressed with supplemental and

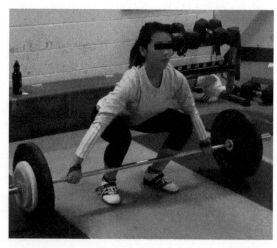

FIGURE 16-18. The snatch begins with a pull, and the bar is held in the catch (see Figure 16.5). Figures of these movements cannot capture the complex and beauty of the events; readers are encouraged to view films of champion lifters.

corrective exercises. The preceding description is not complete nor would every lifter follow these descriptors exactly for the reasons stated at the beginning of this section—the role of the coach is to adjust and fine-tune supplemental exercises to the lifter.

CORRECTIVE EXERCISES

Technique can be enhanced with some corrective exercises. While the causes of movement flaws are endless and often complex, here are a few that may be considered with the caveat that their appropriateness would need to be confirmed with a thorough assessment.

Goblet squat (see Figure 16.19). The goblet squat (popularized by our colleague Dan John) can assist those who need to achieve more depth in their squat by focusing on hip mobility rather than spine flexion. The lifter holds a kettlebell by the horn, or a plate, and descends into a squat. Focus is on achieving depth without allowing any spine motion. Shifting side to side can enhance the exercise. Care is taken not to overload the labrum of the hip creating femoral impingement. Here, gluteal dominant hip extensor patterns (14) will help reduce the labrum load (15).

Thoracic mobility (see Figure 16.20). Some shoulder mobility problems are exacerbated by restricted thoracic extension or may be misdiagnosed as the primary problem when thoracic restriction exists. Furthermore, some cervical spine pain and poor mechanics stem from insufficient thoracic extension or thoracic kyphosis. This thoracic

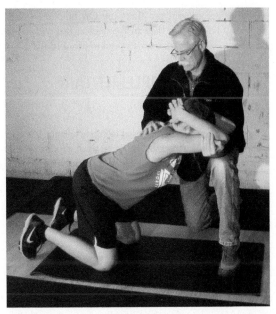

FIGURE 16-20. Thoracic mobility. Many lifters become more competitive and achieve better form with some thoracic spine extension. This wonderful stretch exercise developed by Karol Levit begins as the lifter kneels, the hands are clasped behind the head and the elbows placed on the thigh of a clinician. Light pressure is exerted through the elbows for 5 seconds (the command may be to "push down with your elbows 5 pounds"). This is released and the clinician "draws" the athlete forward focusing on extension of the thoracic spine. This is repeated two to four times. The athlete then stands and should notice better form with overhead extension.

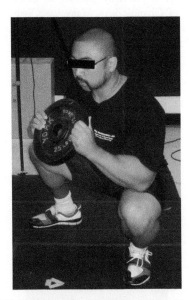

FIGURE 16-19. The goblet squat is used to assist in creating a deeper squat. The pelvis is shifted from side to side with focus on the hip flexors to assist more hip flexion—not spine flexion. Attention is focused on the anterior labrum of the hip and constant monitoring continues to ensure that the tissue is not becoming stressed and painful.

extension stretch facilitates several benefits: the bar may be carried more posteriorly for a more upright posture, the shoulders need not extend to full range enhancing their power production and decreasing joint stress, and the cervical spine is better positioned toward neutral and less stress.

The psoas stretch (see Figure 16.7). The ability to explosively lunge during the clean and jerk is influenced by the mobility of the hips. While some coaches have drills to mobilize the "iliopsoas" or hip flexors, there actually is no such muscle either anatomically or functionally. The iliacus and the psoas muscles are two distinct muscles. With both crossing the hip, only the psoas courses laterally up the lumbar spine connecting each lumbar vertebra. Its role to create hip flexor torque is accompanied with its role to stiffen the lumbar spine onto the pelvis. This is essential for proximal stiffness and therefore hip speed and also for injury resilience to accomplish locking the spine to the pelvis avoiding lumbosacral joint strain. The stretch is accomplished by adopting a lunge then descending deeper while pushing the ipsilateral arm rigorously straight overhead.

Caution is advised for incorporating other forms of corrective exercise that do not specifically address range of motion. For example, some suggest deadlifting to perfect the hip hinge movement. Many top Olympic lifting athletes would discourage such an approach as they would not lift slowly. They always train at speed to lift quickly.

IMPORTANT SUPPLEMENTARY EXERCISES

Supplementary exercises are used to create balance between mobility, stability, strength, and speed throughout the body linkage. They are also usually less demanding than a complete Olympic lift, thus preserving some of the total available training volume.

- Overhead medicine ball throws (Figure 16.21): This progression begins with free explosive jump throws into the air. Then the athlete progresses by standing approximately 5 to 10 feet away with back to a tall wall, and attempts to improve the direction of force production by making contact with the highest point on the wall possible.
- Various jumping exercises—Box jumps have already been introduced to teach explosiveness as well as the quick recovery of legs under the hips necessary for the

"pull under the bar" in weight lifting. The additional benefit of jumping up onto a box is reduced patello-femoral stresses compared to performing drop jumps (e.g., from a box onto the floor, then spring back up). Jump squats (using dowel/broomstick, body bar, or weight) may be added to the progression—we will do this in a squat cage and string a Thera-tube around the front and back uprights of the frame so that the tubing is oriented in a forward/backward direction and is approximately 8 to 12 inches above shoulder height. As the athlete does the jump squats, the intent is to create a vertical target and contact the bar/dowel with the tubing for each rep, while ensuring quality of movement.
- Other auxiliary strength exercises include sled drags and suitcase carries which provide unique opportunities to challenge the lateral torso strength needed for jerking (16,17) (see Figure 16.22).
- Hand over hand rope pull to build hand grip and pulling strength (see Figure 16.23).
- Hip thrusts may be worked to enhance "pulling the hips through" for young lifters prior to speed training (see Figure 16.24).
- Kettlebell swings produce pulsing activation through the hips and torso, while focusing motion at the hips, making them an ideal auxiliary strength exercise (18).

FINAL THOUGHTS

This chapter is primarily focused on developing performance of Olympic lifts. Many use Olympic lifts in training for other athletic pursuits hoping that there is

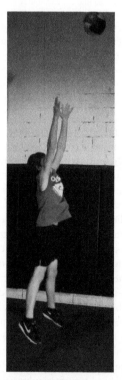

FIGURE 16-21. Overhead medicine ball throws. This progression begins with throws and jumps to get some timing of vertical pulse production—shown here. This is progressed to throws for height with more directed force production up and back over the lifters head.

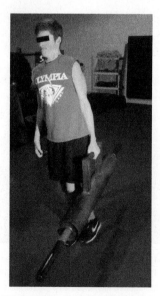

FIGURE 16-22. Suitcase carries provides lateral strength needed for crisp split clean and jerks.

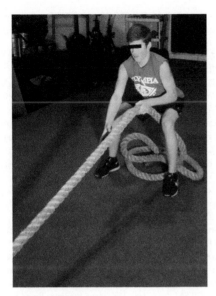

FIGURE 16-23. Hand over hand rope pulling adds more grip strength to the pulling athleticism.

which requires only a few lifts over a day of competition. Explosive vertically projected power in other sports may be needed repeatedly over a match lasting a few hours. Thus, Olympic lifting training for preparation in such a sport would require much lower loads and appropriate set/rep intervals. However, having stated this some very successful Russian athletes have used Olympic lifting as part of power endurance development. Following a few explosive Olympic lifts they may perform a few maximum effort short sprints. They claimed enhanced performance results. But once again, the volume of training with the Olympic lifts is relatively low.

Train when fresh. One of the gifts of Olympic lifting is to develop speed of muscle activation and relaxation. This skill is only enhanced when the athlete is fresh. A fatigued athlete must stop training the Olympic lifts—they only become slow and injury prone. There is a trend on the Internet of performing Olympic lifts for repetitions and to exhaustion. This is problematic for three reasons. First, with repetition and fatigue the athlete breaks form which greatly increases the risk of injury and decreases performance.

Second, performing for repetition means the athlete is lifting at a small percentage of maximum inhibiting athletic development. Third, very few of these participants would qualify to perform Olympic lifts as they lack the rare but necessary joint mobility and speed to execute the lifts without creating injurious tissue stresses. These "games" do not produce performance athletes.

Finally, pulling a bar from the floor requires a special ability that is absolutely necessary for an Olympic lifter but may not be necessary for a National Football League lineman, for example. For these sorts of athletes who may

a skill and athleticism transfer. This may be the case in some athletes but not in others. Olympic lifting is about vertical projection of force. Many sports have more horizontal projections of force and may disappoint those expecting more performance transference. Also many sports require power development with an endurance component as the athletes need to maintain perfect form throughout a match. Typical Olympic lifting training is designed to enhance lifting performance

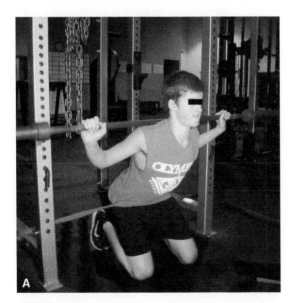
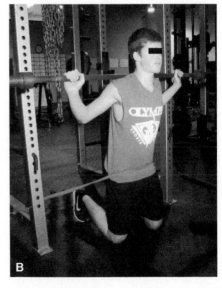

FIGURE 16-24. (A, B) Hip thrusts, with a resistance band across the waist, are used to add more hip extensor power. Used together with kettlebell swings, they may be used either to correct form or to enhance hip extensor pulsing strength.

benefit from Olympic lifting training and the explosive vertical projection of force, there is little need to pull the bar from the floor. Rather set the bar on blocks to eliminate the most demanding loads on the lumbar spine and anterior hip capsule. If an athlete cannot pass the mobility screens shown earlier, they may be well advised to pass on Olympic lift training and utilize another more suitable task.

Development using weight lifting methods will improve first step quickness, flexibility, coordination, balance, and strength endurance, as well as many psychological variables that are important for success in sports. It is hoped that the thoughts contained in this chapter may assist the process with young athletes.

REFERENCES

1. McGill SM, Chaimberg J, Frost D, Fenwick C. The double peak: how elite MMA fighters develop speed and strike force. J Strength Cond Res 2010;24(2):348–357.
2. Loder RT, Skopelja EN. The epidemiology and demographics of hip dysplasia. Orthopedics 2011;Article ID 238607:46pp. doi:10.5402/2011/238607.
3. Czéizel A, Tusnády G, Vaczó G, Vozkelety T. The mechanism of genetic prediposition in congenital dislocation of the hip. J Med Genet 1975;12:121–124.
4. Oda H, Igarashi M, Hayashi Y, et al. Soft tissue collagen in congenital dislocation of the hip—biochemical studies of the ligamentum teres of the femur and hip joint capsule. J Jpn Orthop Assoc 1984;58:331–338.
5. Skirving AP, Sims TJ, Bailey AJ. Congenital dislocation of the hip: a possible inborn error of collagen metabolism. J Inherit Metabol Dis 1984;7:27–31.
6. Inoue K, Wicart P, Kawasaki T, et al. Prevalence of hip osteo-arthritis and acetabular dysplasia in French and Japanese adults. Rheumatology 2000;39(7):745–748.
7. Cholewicki J, McGill SM, Norman RW. Lumbar spine loads during lifting extremely heavy weights. Med Sci Sports Exerc 1991;23(10):1179–1186.
8. McGill SM. Ultimate Back Fitness and Performance. 5th ed., 2014. www.backfitpro.com, Waterloo, Canada.
9. National Coaching Certification Program. Weightlifting Competition Introduction Reference Manual & Coaches Workbook. Canadian Weightlifting Association Halterophilie Canadienne & Coaching Association of Canada; 2008.
10. Kavcic N, Grenier SG, McGill SM. Quantifying tissue loads and spine stability while performing commonly pre-scribed low back stabilization exercises. Spine 2004;29(20): 2319–2329.
11. McGill SM, Grenier S, Kavcic N, Cholewicki J. Coordina-tion of muscle activity to assure stability of the lumbar spine. J Electromyogr Kinesiol 2003;13:353–359.
12. Brown SH, McGill SM. Muscle force-stiffness characteristics influence joint stability. Clin Biomech 2005;20(9):917–922.
13. Brown S, McGill SM. How the inherent stiffness of the in-vivo human trunk varies with changing magnitude of muscular activation. Clin Biomech 2008;23(1):15–22.
14. McGill SM. Low Back Disorders: Evidence Based Prevention and Rehabilitation. 2nd ed. Champaign, IL: Human Kinetics Publishers; 2007.
15. Lewis C, Sahrmann SA, Moran DW. Anterior hip joint force increases with hip extension, decreased gluteal force, or decreased iliopsoas force. J Biomech 2007;40(16): 3725–3731.
16. McGill SM, McDermott A, Fenwick C. Comparison of different strongman events: trunk muscle activation and lumbar spine motion, load and stiffness. J Strength Cond Res 2008;23(4):1148–1161.
17. McGill SM, Marshall L, Andersen J. Low back loads while walking and carrying: comparing the load carried in one hand or in both hands. Ergonomics 2013;56(2):293-302. doi:10.1 080/00140139.2012.752528
18. McGill SM, Marshall L. Kettlebell swing snatch and bottoms-up carry: back and hip muscle activation, motion, and low back loads. J Strength Cond Res 2012;26(1):16–27.

Skiing

ALPINE SKIING

Alpine skiing is the sport of sliding down snow-covered hills on skis with fixed-heel bindings. In competitive alpine skiing, there are four disciplines: slalom, giant slalom, super giant slalom, and downhill. Slalom ski races have courses that require short tight turns, whereas giant slalom races have courses which are set with more widely spaced turns. Super giant slalom and downhill have few turns, with gates spaced widely apart, and skiers often reach speeds of more than 100 km/h.

Alpine skiing can be contrasted with skiing using free-heel bindings (e.g., ski mountaineering and Nordic skiing—cross country, ski jumping, and Telemark). The sport is popular wherever the combination of snow, mountain slopes, and a sufficient tourist infrastructure can be built up, including parts of Europe, North America, Australia and New Zealand, the South American Andes, and eastern Asia (1).

There are four different ways to move downhill: Sliding, slipping, skidding, and carving.

- Sliding: When the skis move downhill in the direction they are pointed. This can be in a straight run down the hill or a traverse across the hill.
- Slipping: When the skis move sideways down the hill at an angle relative to the long axes of the skis. The direction of travel is perpendicular to the skis.
- Skidding: A combination of sliding and slipping as the skis move through the turn. The tails of the skis are making a wider path than the tips. Most turns involve some amount of skidding.
- Carving: When tips and tails travel through the same arched bends created on the snow.

TYPES OF MOVEMENTS

The skier can make four basic kinds of movements:

- Balancing movements: Maintaining body balance when skiing down the hill.
- Edging movements: Adjusting the edge angle of the skis in relation to the snow-surfaced hill inclination.
- Rotary movements: Turning and guiding the skis into desired directions.
- Pressure control movements: Creating pressure variations between the skis and the snow surface.

Dynamic balance is a key factor in downhill skiing technique. Movements that may affect balance include:

- The width of the skier's stance
- The degree and ability of flexion and extension of the ankles, knees, hips, and spine
- The shifting of the center of body mass by forward, backward, and lateral leaning movements
- The movement of the arms and the head
- The ability to rapidly adjust and coordinate muscle tension

Edging movements are created from the center of mass of the skier's body. They are developed by combining two mechanisms: (1) Inclination or tipping of the whole body and (2) Angulations. Angulations involve forming angles between body segments divided into

- Feet and ankles
- Lower legs and knees
- Thighs and hips
- The low back
- The whole body

Edging movements allow the skier to

- Change directions
- Control speed
- Change the shape and size of turns
- Slip, skid, and carve

Angulating different parts of the body throughout the turn allows the skier to

- Change the amount of edge angle of the ski without changing the inclination of the body
- Maintain balance
- Resist g-forces
- Manage the pressure of the skis/parts of the skis against the snow surface
- Regulate speed of foot movements
- Alter the shape of the turns
- Adapt to changing terrain and snow conditions

Most turns in alpine skiing involve both angulations and inclination. Combined angulations take place in the hips, knees, and ankles. The hips and lower back create the biggest changes in edge angle, whereas the knees and ankles are more into fine-tuning the edge angle.

Rotary movements involve turning some parts of the body relative to another part of the body, and in alpine skiing, combining rotary, edging, and pressure-controlled movements allow skiers to initiate turns and direct the skis through the turns. Creating and managing resistive forces between skis and snow marks one of the major achievements in alpine skiing as forces increase dramatically with speed. The major types of rotary movements in alpine skiing are upper body rotation, counter rotation, and leg rotation.

Pressure-controlled movements are often described as the most difficult skills to master. Effective pressure control requires the constant action of muscles and use of specific movements to moderate forces from one foot to the other, along the entire length of the skis, and between the skis and the snow. The amount of pressure that is applied to the skis can be controlled by changing the radius and angle of the turns; speed; amount of flexion of the ankles, knees, hip joints, and lower back; edge angle of the skis; and body weight distribution (2).

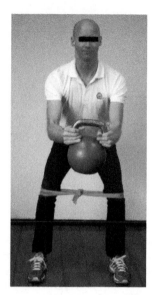

FIGURE 17-1. Goblet squat with Thera-band.

INCIDENCE OF ALPINE SKIING ACCIDENTS

A recording of alpine skiing incidents admitted to the Trondheim Regional and University Hospital during 1 year was completed during the winter season in 1989. Of the 339 injured, 67% were men and 33% were women. Eighty-seven percent were outpatients, and 13% were hospitalized. Of the injuries, falling accidents caused 67%, followed by collision accidents, which caused 17%. The injuries in the lower extremities were caused by falling, and the head injuries were mostly caused by collisions. Knee ligament strains were the most common injuries, and 17% of these patients were hospitalized and required operative treatment. Of the minor knee strains, all 44% were not fully recovered after two and a half years. Seventeen patients sustained tibial fractures, 11 of them spiral fractures and 6 transverse fractures. The patients with spiral fractures were younger than the patients with transverse fractures. Head injuries were the most severe injuries, with 11 concussions and 2 epidural hematomas (3).

Sahlin (3) suggests that injury prevention through specific exercise programs will have its greatest effect on knee injuries. Anterior cruciate ligament injuries are the most common injuries of the elite athletes of alpine skiing according to Bere (4). Bere categorizes three injury mechanisms as a result of numerous hours of video analyses of injury situations (5,6):
1. The "slip-catch" injury
2. The "landing back-weighted"
3. The "dynamic snowplow"
Bere states, "This situation is characterized by a common pattern in which the inside edge of the outer ski catches the snow surface while turning, forcing the knee into valgus

and tibial internal rotation." She concludes, "knee compression and knee internal rotation and abduction torque are important components of the injury mechanism in a 'slip-catch' situation." In terms of clinical relevance, "Prevention efforts should focus on avoiding a forceful tibial internal rotation in combination with knee valgus" (7).

Suggested exercises for prevention of the most common injury mechanisms and for enhanced sports performance in alpine skiing include:

- Goblet squat with a Thera-band around the knees (Figure 17.1)
- Plank with feet on a Swiss ball (Figure 17.2)
- Balance exercises on Bosu in hockey position on two legs. Challenge may be progressed by doing the exercise on one leg
- Balance exercise on a Swiss ball with knees on the ball
Exercises on ice hockey skates for training include:

- Body weight transfer (Figure 17.3)
- Curve balance and pressure control of movement (Figure 17.4)

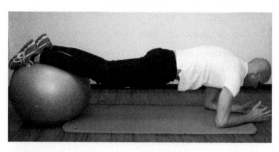

FIGURE 17-2. Plank with feet on ball.

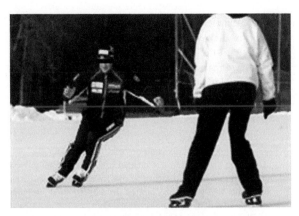

FIGURE 17-3.   Body weight transfer.

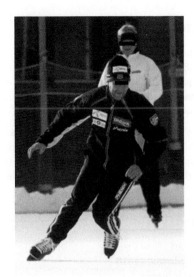

FIGURE 17-5.   Aerobic/anaerobic capacity training.

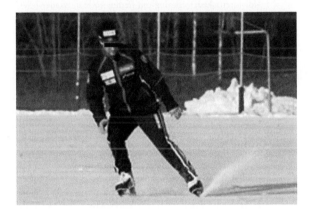

FIGURE 17-4.   Curve balance and pressure control of movement.

- Aerobic/anaerobic capacity (Figure 17.5). Perform a figure-of-eight for 90 seconds at high speeds. Vary between short pauses and longer pauses. Perform four times.
- Hip positioning (Figure 17.6). This exercise utilizes the hockey position while skiing through sharp bends. By holding the hands up toward or on the head it reactively "tweaks" maintenance of the upright lumbar posture when sliding left and right at high speeds.

CROSS COUNTRY SKIING

Exercise List for Cross Country Skiing

Cross country skiing is probably **the** kind of sport that demands strength and endurance in both the upper and lower halves of the body in equally strong demands. Elite cross country ski racers have some of the highest aerobic power values reported for endurance athletes, and aerobic capacity as well as onset of blood lactate accumulation can

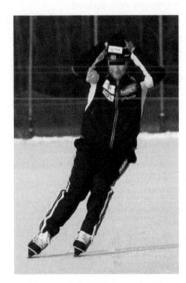

FIGURE 17-6.   Hip positioning. Notice that holding the hands high up towards the level of the head or actually on the head itself will facilitate the use of core muscles to stabilize and maintain the neutral lordosis of the lumbar spine.

be used to predict success in this group of skiers. Cross country skiers are lean, like distance runners, and successful ski racers have high percentage of slow twitch muscle fibers and high anaerobic thresholds (8–11).

There are **two main styles** of cross country skiing (12–14):
1. **The classic techniques** or the diagonal stride
2. **The free technique** or the skating technique
The classic, diagonal stride is the one used most often by recreational athletes for "hiking", as well as in cross country sport for high speed. This technique is used on the plain course, in slightly undulating terrain and moderate inclines.

Functional exercises

* **Running man**
* **Angle lunges**
* **Squat**
* **One-legged squats**
* **Bird dog**

The free technique—skate stride or skating,facilitates a higher skiing speed than the classic style. The skier pushes off vigorously with the one ski that is turned out to an angle to the direction of the skiing track, and most often in conjunction with vigorous double poling.

Functional exercises

* **Squats**
* **One-legged squats**
* **Angle lunges**

Key words for basic cross country skiing skills: Balance, coordination, weight shift, kick off.

Good balance is crucial for coordination and minimal excessive muscle tension, complete weight transmission, and a focused, determined kick off.

5- to 10-Year Olds

Suggested exercises for general development of coordination, balance, agility and strength:

Trampoline, rudimentary walking and running on uneven surface, preferably on forest ground, soccer play, athletics/gymnastics, ice skating, roller skating, swimming.

Exercises for endurance: Running/jogging, bicycling, roller-skating with poles, swimming.

10- to 15-Year-Olds/Weekend Warrior Adults

For neurodynamic consciousness: One leg squat facing wall, star reaches.

For stabilization: Side bridges, "plank," "plank" w turns.

For dynamic strength: Bird dog, bird dog on Swiss ball, oblique abdominals from below, chins, squats.

Forendurance (preferably according to the 4 × 4 principles according to Hoff & Helgerud (15)): Skiing, running, roller-skiing, roller skating w sticks, forest bicycling, swimming.

Elite Performance Athletes

For neurodynamics: Pelvic tilts on one leg, running man.

For stabilization: "Plank" w alternating arms to the side, alternating leg to the side progressing to unsteady surface, squats on unsteady surface, the "stir pot" abdominal exercise.

For dynamic strength: Overhead cable pulls, medicine ball tossing supine over a Swiss ball, "curl-up" back extension exercise, rowing, squats w 4 max reps according to the principles of 4×4 of Hoff and Helgerud (16).

REFERENCES

1. Alpine Skiing. en.wikipedia.org/wiki/Alpine_skiing
2. Leonid Feldman. Core Concepts of Downhill Skiing.www.youcanski.com/en/instruction/core_concepts.htm
3. Sahlin Y. Alpine skiing injuries. Br J Sports Med 1989;23: 241–244. doi:10.1136/bjsm.23.4.241
4. Bere T. How Do ACL Injuries Happen in World Cup Alpine Skiing? http://www.klokeavskade.no/no/Nyhetsarkiv/Nyhetsariv-2013/Vridde-knar--vonde-vinkler-Ny-doktorgrad-fra-Senter-for-idrettsskadeforskning-om-fremre-korsbandskader-i-WC-alpint/
5. Bere T, Flørenes TW, Krosshaug T, et al. A systematic video analysis of 69 injury cases in World Cup alpine skiing. Scand J Med Sci Sports 2013. [Epub ahead of print] Jan 10. doi:10.1111/sms.12038.
6. Bere T, Flørenes TW, Krosshaug T, Nordsletten L, Bahr R. Events leading to anterior cruciate ligament injury in World Cup Alpine Skiing: a systematic video analysis of 20 cases. Br J Sports Med 2011;45:1294–1302.
7. Bere T, Mok K-M, Koga H, Krosshaug T, Nordsletten L, Bahr R. Kinematics of Anterior Cruciate Ligament Ruptures in World Cup Alpine Skiing. Two case reports of the slip-catch mechanism. Investigation performed at the Oslo Sports Trauma Research Center, Department of Sports Medicine, Norwegian School of Sport Sciences, Oslo, Norway. AJSM PreView, published on February 28, 2013.
8. Eisenman PA, Johnson SC, Bainbridge CN, Zupan MF. Applied physiology of cross-country skiing.Sports Med 1989;8(2):67–79.
9. Larsson P, Olofsson P, Jakobsson E, Burlin L, Henriksson-Larsen K. Physiological predictors of performance in cross-country skiing from treadmill tests in male and female subjects. Scand J Med Sci Sports 2002;12(6):347–353.
10. Rusko HK. Development of aerobic power in relation to age and training in cross-country skiers. Med Sci Sports Exerc 1992;24(9):1040–1047.
11. Ingjer F. Development of maximal oxygen uptake in young elite male cross-country skiers: a longitudinal study. J Sports Sci 1992;10(1):49–63.
12. Dybendahl Hartz T. Større Skiglede med bedre Teknikk. Kagge Forlag, 2007.
13. Lovett R, Petersen P. The Essential Cross-Country Skier. Ragged Mountain Press. A division of The McGraw-Hill Companies. USA, 1999.
14. Barth K, Bruhl H. Training Cross-country. SkiingTraining. Meyer & Meyer Sport, 2007.
15. Hoff J, Helgerud J, Wisloff U. Maximal strength training improves work economy in trained female cross-country skiers. Med Sci Sports Exerc 1999 Jun;31(6):870–877.
16. Hoff J, Helgerud J. Endurance and strength training for soccer players. Physiological Considerations. Sports Med 2004:34(3):165–180.

Soccer

Soccer is the most popular team sport in the world. There are more than 265 million registered players; the number of participants is continuing to grow, and the number of women players is particularly increasing (1). Playing soccer, however, entails a big risk of injury. Studies on elite and nonelite male and female soccer players have reported equal rates of injury. Many of these injuries should have been avoided. Statistics shows that at elite level one player injures himself to the extent that he is not able to train or play the next day in every match (2) (Figure 18.1).

Regardless of age and level, the legs are the most vulnerable to injury. Muscle strains in the thigh and groin and ligament injuries in the ankle and knee are the most common. Such injuries could prevent the player from participating in sporting activities for up to a month. Head injuries are less common but warrent concern as repeated concussions having potentially damaging effects to the central nervous system over time (2,3).

Girls are more prone to knee and ankle injuries than boys—particularly injuries to the anterior cruciate ligament. The rate of anterior cruciate ligament injuries is three to five times higher for girls than for boys. Such injuries quite often require a year of rehabilitation and greatly increase the risk of premature gonarthrosis (arthrosis of the knee joint) 15 to 20 years later, even after careful "by the book" surgical treatment and rehabilitation. Therefore, these types of injuries should have the highest focus for prevention by adequate exercise programs (2,4–7).

With boys, muscular pulls in the thigh and groin are more frequent than with girls. Even though such injuries rarely develop into chronic injuries, they are often the cause of long absence from training and matches. They also impose a risk of reinjuring the same area, and many soccer players have had their careers ruined by injuries which at first appeared to be an uncomplicated muscle strain (2).

Soccer differs from many other team sports due to much higher likelihood of direct contact to the lower extremities. Nevertheless, the mechanisms for serious knee injuries seem to result from pivoting and landing movements, being comparable with many other sports, including noncontact sports (4).

Injuries can be prevented by the right kind of training and exercises. Many of these injuries may be avoided by incorporating specific exercise programs into the warming-up regimen, training balance, agility, and strength (2,7,8). Serious knee injuries usually occur in situations of quick changes of direction, for instance during tackling, or when landing after headings and jumps. The players must be taught proper running techniques, keeping the hip, knee, and ankle in alignment and proper thrust- and landing technique by practising landing on two legs while controlling knee over big toe position (2,8,9).

The following combinations of exercises are recommended (2,10):

- Passing the ball precisely from the inside of the foot to coplayer, using light running steps sideways.
- Passing the ball back to coplayer on straight dorsum of foot, using light running steps.
- Doing half-volleys with both inside and straight dorsum of foot, precisely passing the ball to each other.
- Dampening the ball on the thigh, volley-pass ball back to coplayer using alternating legs.
- Dampening ball on chest, then half-volley return to coplayer.
- Heading while on one leg. Remember knee over toe-ankle stability position!
- Heading with high jumps. Note adequate flexion of hips and knees while landing on parallel legs.
- "Sprunglauf" agility exercise, with high jumps and soft landings while maintaining knee over toe-ankle stabilization and knee position (Figure 18.2).

A good start before any exercise program for soccer play is to perform the "fall and jump test"(2) (Figure 18.3A). This screening picks out the players that require special attention with particular emphasis on balance, agility, and coordination for the prevention of injuries to the ankle and knees during standing, running, planting, cutting, jumping, and landing (2,9,11).

In the "fall and jump test," the player will "fall" by jumping down from an elevated level, then immediately jump up as if catching a ball in the air. The examiner notices the positions of the knees during both the first and second landing. The knee should not misalign inward toward the midline into valgus position, and a pelvic tilt should be avoided (see Figure 18.3B, C). It should be possible to draw a straight line from the hip through the knee to the foot, i.e., "knee over toe." Players who are not able to keep "the knee over toe" during landing may be particularly prone to serious knee injury. By improving awareness and neuromuscular control by training core stability for hip

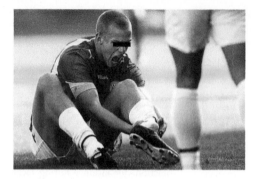

FIGURE 18-1. An injured soccer player who played with the Danish soccer team Viborg. From the Swedish newspaper Aftonbladet (July 12, 2007).

and ankle stability and proper knee alignment during both static and dynamic movements (2,9). By specific training to avoid injury patterns, the risk can be halved even at top-level soccer. This training should consist of balance exercises and exercises designed to enhance awareness of knee positions in different situations during soccer play (2,7–10) (Figures 18.4–18.7).

Stronger hamstring muscles may prevent injuries to the anterior cruciate ligament because the muscles can act as agonists to the ligament during stop and jump tasks, at least at knee flexion angles above 30°. The "Nordic hamstring lower" (glute-ham raise) exercise has been shown to increase eccentric hamstring muscle strength. This has also been shown to decrease the rate of hamstring strain injuries (2,12,13) (Figure 18.8).

A muscle strain in the groin area may cause long-standing pain and frequent reinjuries of the same area, and exercises to strengthen the "core" musculature (i.e., side plank, front plank, stir the pot) are important preventative measures (2,4,14) (Figure 18.9). Hamstring curls on ball challenge abdominal "core" musculature while strengthening the hamstring musculature for this purpose (Figure 18.10).

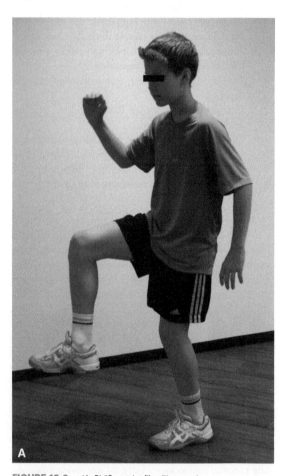

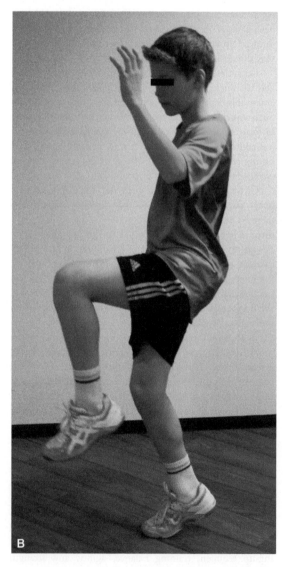

FIGURE 18-2. (A, B) "Sprunglauf" agility exercise.

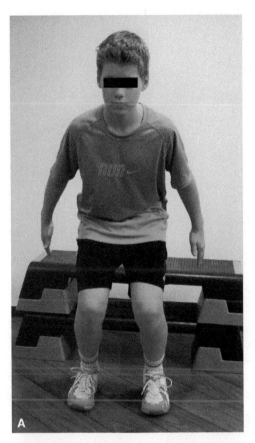

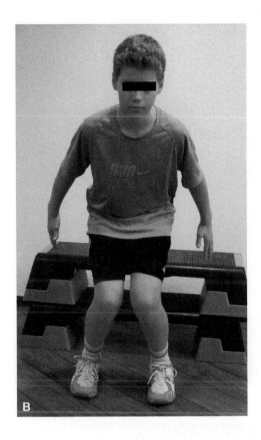

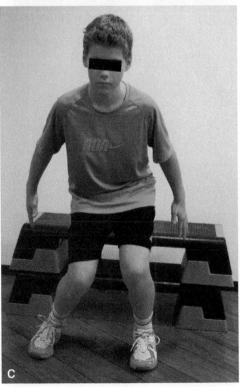

FIGURE 18-3. Fall and jump test. (A) Correct landing. (B) Faulty knee positions. (C) Faulty knee position—right knee.

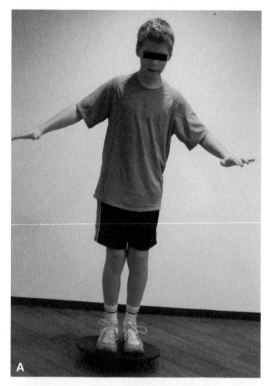
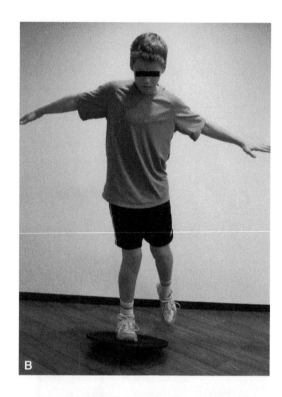

FIGURE 18-4.   Suggested exercises for ankles and knees: (A) Two-legged balance on wobble board. (B) One-legged balance on wobble board.

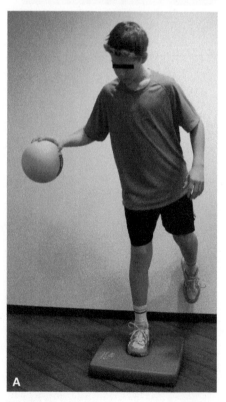
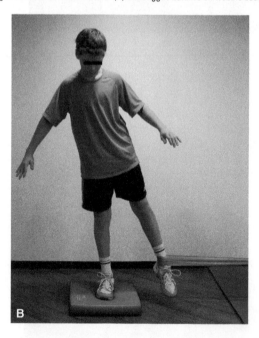

FIGURE 18-5.   Suggested exercises for ankles and knees: (A) One-legged balance on mat, tossing ball. (B) One-legged balance with resistive tubing.

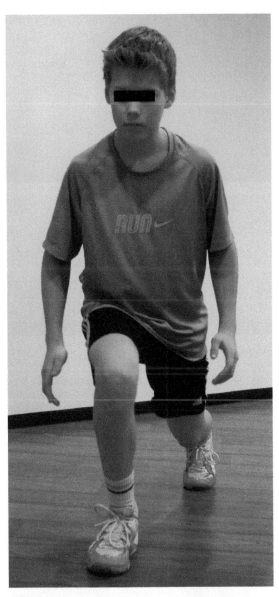

FIGURE 18-6. Suggested exercise for ankles and knees: lunge.

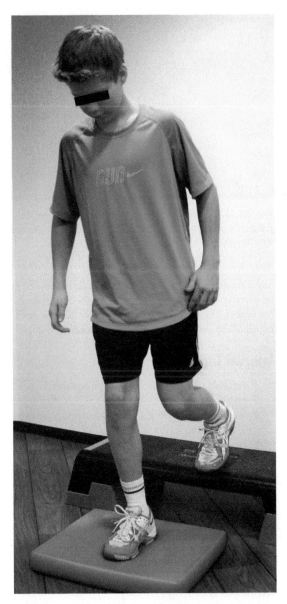

FIGURE 18-7. Suggested exercise for ankles and knees: step down on unsteady surface.

MUSCLE FLEXIBILITY AND STRETCHING

Good flexibility of the hip flexor muscles, particularly the iliopsoas, is important for the prevention of groin pains, and also for proper functioning of the back extensor musculature (2,14) (Figure 18.11). Other important muscle groups that should be stretched regularly are

* the gluteal muscles (in both internal and external hip rotation)
* the quadriceps
* the hamstrings
* the calf muscles

ENDURANCE AND STRENGTH TRAINING FOR SOCCER PLAYERS

New developments in understanding adaptive processes to the circulatory system and endurance performance as well as nerve and muscle adaptations to training and performance have given rise to more effective training interventions (15). Endurance interval training using an intensity at 90% to 95% of maximal heart rate in bouts of 3 to 8 minutes has proved to be effective in the development of endurance and performance improvements in soccer play. Strength training using high loads, few repetitions, and maximal

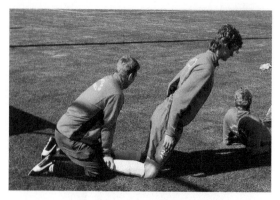

FIGURE 18-8. "Nordic hamstring lower." Keeping the upper body straight, the player falls slowly forward while resisting the movement with the hamstring muscles.

mobilization of force in the concentric mode has proven to be effective in the development of strength. The challenge both for coaches and players is to act upon the new developments and change existing training practice (15,16).

Interval Training (15,16)

- Interval training once a week maintains level of endurance
- Interval training twice a week increases O₂ uptake by 1% per week
- Four-minute intervals are twice as effective compared to other forms of training of the same magnitude.
- Sixteen interval training sessions give an increase by 3 to 5 mL which implies
  - an increase in running distance of 1.5 to 2 km per soccer match
  - twice as many sprints
  - 30% increased involvement with the ball
  - however, no influence on speed, strength, or agility

Strength Training (15–17)

- Strength training once a week maintains level of strength

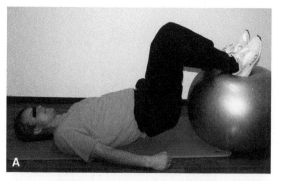

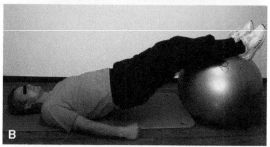

FIGURE 18-10. (A, B) Hamstring curls on ball.

- Strength training twice a week increases strength by 2% to 4% per week
- Sixteen strength training sessions increase strength by 30% to 60%, or 30 to 50 kg in squats, which implies
  - 1 m quicker per 10 m running
  - 3 to 5 cm higher jump
  - 1 km increased running distance capability per match because increased strength enhances energy economy during running

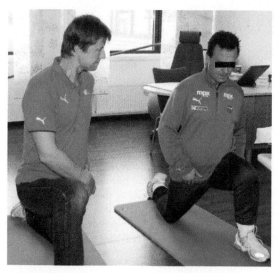

FIGURE 18-11. The coach and the team chiropractor discussing stretching techniques for the hip flexor muscles.

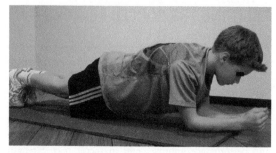

FIGURE 18-9. "Plank" exercise.

Endurance Training in Soccer

Soccer players need technical, tactical, and physical skills to succeed. The physical performance of strength and power and their derivatives; acceleration, sprinting, and jumping are as important as endurance of the soccer performance (15).

Intermittent exercise at 90% to 95% of HRmax for 3 to 8 minutes involves a major load on the oxygen transporting organs. When training at this intensity, the improvement in VO_2 max ranges from 10% to 30% within an 8- to 10-week training period, with individual variations due to initial level of fitness and duration and frequency of training (15,16).

Ideally, endurance training for soccer players should be carried out using the ball which enhances player motivation during training. The players might then additionally develop technical and tactical skills as well as perform agility training. Hoff et al. showed that specifically designed soccer training fulfils the criteria for aerobic interval training, and heart rate monitoring is a valid measurement for actual exercise intensity in this type of training mode (Figure 18.12). They also showed that higher exercise intensity is most easily achieved on a soccer-specific "dribbling track"(16).

Practical Training for Endurance for Soccer Players

The purpose of the training is to maintain or increase the maximal O_2 uptake, which then determines running capacity during the game.

- 6 minutes of warming up, or directly after playing soccer
- 4 × 4 minutes interval and 3 minutes break
- Running on treadmill with 5% inclination, or in dribbling track with ball

Strength and Strength Derivatives: Acceleration, Jump, Sprints

In the aerobic context of a soccer match, the most interesting events during a match are represented by high-intensity

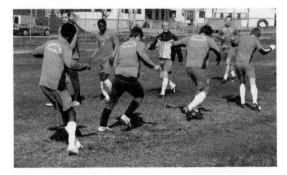

FIGURE 18.12. Elite soccer players of the Sandefjord Football team (Norway).

work, such as sprints, tackles, and shots. A sprint occurs every 90 seconds, lasting 2 to 4 seconds. Sprinting constitutes 1% to 11% of the total match distance, corresponding to 0.5% to 3% of effective play time. A professional player performs about 50 turns sustaining forceful contractions to maintain balance and control of the ball against defensive pressure during a game (16).

A variety of training methods are used in an effort to increase strength and power, mostly in sports demanding acceleration and explosive force development such as sprinting and jumping. *Strength* is defined as the integrated result of several force-producing muscles performing maximally, either isometrically or dynamically during a single voluntary effort of a defined task. *Power* is a product of force and the inverse of time, that is, the ability to produce as much force as possible in the shortest possible time (16,17).

A muscle's ability to develop force is dependent on many different factors. The most common are initial position, speed of lengthening, speed of shortening, eccentric initial phase, types of muscle fibers, number of motor units active at the same time, cross-sectional area of the muscle, impulse frequency, and substrate available for the muscle exercise (16).

The two main basic mechanisms for the development of muscular strength are muscular hypertrophy and neural adaptations.

Muscular hypertrophy is an effect of strength training, and there is a relationship between the cross-sectional area of the muscle and its potential for force development. This increase is associated with a large relative increase in the myofibril content of the fibers. During systematic strength training over time however, there will be hypertrophy of all types of muscle fibers. Several studies show that the fast twitch fibers have the greatest hypertrophy (16,17).

Neural adaptations is a broad description encompassing a number of factors, such as selective activation of motor units, synchronization, selective activation of muscles, ballistic contractions, increased frequency increased reflex potential, increased recruitment of motor units, and increased cocontraction of antagonists. A significant part of the improvement in the ability to lift weights is due to an increased ability to coordinate other muscle groups involved in the movement, such as the core muscles (16,17).

Two major principles for maximal neural adaptation are as follows:

- To train the fastest motor units. These develop the greatest force. One has to work against high loads— 85% to 95% of 1 RM—which ensures maximal voluntary contraction.
- Maximal advantage is gained if the movements are trained with a rapid action in addition to the high resistance. Dynamic explosive movements with few repetitions (3–7) and resistance should range from 85% to 100% of 1 RM, and may result in neuromuscular adaptation with minimal hypertrophy (16,17).

Practical Training for Strength and Speed

To be strong and quick without increasing muscle mass (16), players should adhere to the following instructions:

- Do squats with free weights or knee press progressing until 90° of flexion of the knees (Figure 18.13).
- Do slow descent—short stop—maximal mobilization of force on ascending, complete motion up on toes.
- If training in knee press, also train back and abdominal muscles accordingly.
- Do 4 × 4 repetitions, so heavy that the player cannot manage any more repetitions.
- Add 5 kg each time the player manages 4 × 4 repetitions.
- May receive training in conjunction with endurance training sessions or with soccer training.

Nondominant Leg Training to Improve Bilateral Motor Performance of Soccer Players

The aim of the experiment was to evaluate bilateral motor performance effects from training the nondominant leg of competitive players. The training intervention consisted of the experimental group participating in all parts of their training except full play, using the nondominant leg for 8 weeks. Statistical analysis for soccer-specific tests revealed that the experimental group improved significantly as compared to the control group from the pretest to the posttest period in their use of the trained nondominant leg. Additionally, and somewhat unexpectedly, they also found that the experimental group also improved significantly in the tests that made use of the dominant side. The results might be explained by improved generalized motor programs, or from a Dynamic Systems Approach, indicating that the actual training relates to the handling of all the information available to the subject in the situation, and that the body self-organizes the motor performance. This cross-educational effect implies strong performance effects of using the nondominant leg in training, and also that training the other side of the body during a period of injury or disease might have a substantial effect. The practical applications are obvious: soccer players and coaches should put more emphasis on training the "wrong" leg in order to improve their soccer skills with both the right and left leg (18).

General Stabilization and Functional Exercises

McGill's Big 3 (13)

- Hardest version of the dead bug track: hamstring curl on Swiss ball
- Three versions of the side bridge track:
  - Side bridge
  - The "plank" exercise with turns
  - The hip hinge—the squats with maximum load 4 × 4 as described above. According to Dr Jan Hoff, this is also the most effective stabilizing exercise for soccer players (personal communication).
- The bird dog
- "Nordic hamstring lower" (see Figure 18.8)
- Side-lying hip adduction in sling

EXERCISE LISTS FOR SOCCER

5- to 10-Year-Olds

- Rudimentary exercise activities for development of endurance: Running/jogging, bicycling, roller skating, skiing, skating, swimming
- Exercises for development of coordination, balance, agility, and strength: Trampoline, barefoot running on uneven surface, soccerplay

10- to 15-Year-Olds/Weekend Warrior Adults

- For neurodynamic consciousness: Balance training on wooden bar, lunges, ice skating, roller skating

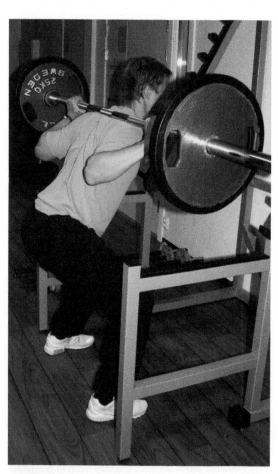

FIGURE 18-13.   Squat training.

- For core stabilization: Dead bug, side bridges, "plank," "plank w turns," single-leg bridges
- For dynamic strength: Squats, hamstring curls on Swiss ball
- For endurance: Running according to the 4 × 4 principles of Hoff and Helgerud, preferably on a "dribble track"(16)

Elite Performance and Professional Athletes

- For neurodynamics: Lunges with weights on unstable surface, running man
- For stabilization: "Plank" with turns, "plank" with alternating arms to the side, alternating leg to the side, then progressing to unsteady surface; oblique abdominals from below; hamstring curl on Swiss ball; one-leg curl on Swiss ball
- For strength: Squats 4 × 4 max according to the principles of Hoff and Helgerud and "Nordic hamstring" lower exercise
- For endurance: Running according to the 4 × 4 principles of Hoff and Helgerud, preferably on a "dribble track"

REFERENCES

1. FIFA. FIFA big count 2006: 270 million people active in football. www.fifa.com/aboutfifa/media/newsid=529882.html
2. www.klokavskade.no/skadefri/fotball
3. Andersen TE, Árnason A, Engebretsen L, Bahr R. Mechanisms of head injuries in elite football. Br J Sports Med 2004;38:690–696.
4. Engström B, Johansson C, Törnkvist H. Soccer injuries among elite female players. Am J Sports Med 1991;19: 372–375.
5. Bjordal JM, Arnly F, Hannestad B, Strand T. Epidemiology of anterior cruciate ligament injuries in soccer. Am J Sports Med 1997;25:341–345.
6. Lohmander LS, Östenberg A, Englund M, Roos H. High prevalence of knee osteoarthritis, pain, and functional limitations in female soccer players twelve years after anterior cruciate ligament injury. Arthritis Rheum 2004;50:3145–3152.
7. Mandelbaum BR, Silvers HJ, Watanabe DS, et al. Effectiveness of a neuromuscular and proprioceptive training program in preventing anterior cruciate ligament injuries in female athletes: 2-year follow-up. Am J Sports Med 2005;33: 1003–1010.
8. Hewett TE, Lindenfeld TN, Riccobene JV, Noyes FR. The effect of neuromuscular training on the incidence of knee injury in female athletes. A prospective study. Am J Sports Med 1999;27:699–706.
9. Hewett TE, Myer GD, Ford KR, et al. Biomechanical measures of neuromuscular control and valgus loading of the knee predict anterior cruciate ligament injury risk in female athletes: a prospective study. Am J Sports Med 2005;33: 492–501.
10. Soligard T, Myklebust G, Steffen K, et al. Comprehensive warm-up programme to prevent injuries in young female footballers: cluster randomised controlled trial. BMJ 2008;337:a2469.
11. Andersen TE, Floerenes TW, Arnason A, Bahr R. Video analysis of the mechanisms for ankle injuries in football. Am J Sports Med 2004;32:69S-79S.
12. Arnason A, Andersen TE, Holme I, Engebretsen L, Bahr R. Prevention of hamstring strains in elite soccer: an intervention study. Scand J Med Sci Sports 2008;18:40–48.
13. Hewett TE, Stroupe AL, Nance TA, Noyes FR. Plyometric training in female athletes. Decreased impact forces and increased hamstring torques. Am J Sports Med 1996;24: 765–773.
14. McGill S. Ultimate Back Performance. Waterloo, ON: Wabuno Publishers; 2004.
15. Hoff J, Helgerud J, Wisloff U. Maximal strength training improves work economy in trained female cross-country skier. Med Sci Sports Exerc 1999;31(6):870–877.
16. Hoff J, Helgerud J. Endurance and strength training for soccer players. Physiological considerations. Sports Med 2004;34(3):165–180.
17. Wisløff U, Castagna C, Helgerud J, Jones R, Hoff J. Strong correlation of maximal squat strength with sprint performance and vertical jump height in elite soccer players. Br J Sports Med 2004;38:285–288.
18. Haaland E, Hoff J. Non-dominant leg training improves the bilateral motor performance of soccerplayers. Scand J Med Sci Sports 2003;13:1–6.

Swimming

OVERVIEW: DEMOGRAPHICS OF COMPETITIVE AGE-GROUP SWIMMERS

Competitive age-group swimming is a highly skilled sport. It requires attention to steady motor development from entry into the sport (in early childhood), through adolescence, and into later levels of elite competition. There are four different strokes, used at varying distances, which correspond to developmental age. These range from short sprints in younger age groups to short, middle, and long-distance events as swimmers mature. Individual medley (all four strokes swam in succession) as well as short and long relays are also part of competitive swimming.

In competitive swimming, age groups range from "6 and under" to "19 and over" for both male and female athletes. There are 286,095 competitive swimmers registered with USA Swimming, which is the major governing body for swimming in the United States (1). This figure does not include collegiate swimmers, senior swimmers, masters swimmers, and age-group swimmers in recreational swim leagues, as these are all non-USA swimming programs.

Younger age children (under 10) make up nearly 100,000 swimmers. This number tapers to approximately 8,000 swimmers by the age of 19. This dramatic difference in participation is often related to burnout and injuries during the swimmers' development in the swimming program (see Table 19.1).

Competitive swimming is performed in several different pool sizes. It is broken into short- and long-course seasons, with short course referring to a 25-yard pool and long course referring to a 50-m, or Olympic-sized, pool. The short-course season generally runs from fall through the spring. Age group, high school, and collegiate-level swimmers compete in the shorter pool. The long-course season typically begins after the completion of the short-course national championship and concludes at the end of long-course nationals, usually toward the end of the summer.

Training between the two seasons may be affected by differences in pool lengths between the short and long courses, technical changes in strokes, number of strokes taken per length, and program design related to strength and conditioning. For example, in short-course swimming there are more turns, which require technique work on turn mechanics, power training of the legs for push phase from the walls, core training for the undulations, and pull-outs and breath-holding for the duration. In contrast, long-course swimming requires conditioning parameters that are directly related to the strokes (length, rate, rhythm) and metabolic aspects of training because there are fewer turns.

Swimming has some contrasts in the requirements on the body from other land-based sports. The water does not allow swimmers to stabilize their bodies against an immovable object, like the ground, as occurs in running and jumping. Stability of the body in the water comes from correctly activating core muscles to reinforce head and trunk alignment as well as body balance in the water. The core must also control the reactive forces of limbs against the water during limb movements. As a result, swimmers must begin to develop control of their bodies at a young age and continue to refine body control as they grow. Throughout the adolescent period, swimmers must increase endurance and strength and continue to build upon this foundation as they progress through the sport at elite levels.

"FUNDAMENTAL" STAGE (6- TO 9-YEAR-OLDS)

In competitive swimming, children under age 6 represent entry-level participants in the sport. Their global development of movement skills is easily addressed through both land- and water-based instruction, in contrast to specific technical instruction on stroke development. To facilitate learning, games and activities that captivate these young people can readily help develop agility, balance, coordination, and speed.

Competitive swim strokes are broken down into two categories, based on the distinct types of trunk and limb movement patterns used. Freestyle and backstroke are long-axis strokes, where the extremities move in opposition to each other, and the trunk rotates around the longitudinal axis of the body. In contrast, breaststroke and butterfly are short-axis strokes because the extremities work in synchronized movement around the coronal axis of the body.

In the fundamental stages of development (ages 6 and under), young swimmers typically learn the long-axis strokes of freestyle and backstroke first. Then, they progress to the short-axis strokes of breaststroke and butterfly.

TABLE 19.1	Registered Swimmers in the United States in 2009*: Breakdown in Numbers by Age										
8 and Under	9	10	11	12	13	14	15	16	17	18	19 and Over
37,514	27,623	31,802	33,645	31,326	28,671	25,830	20,271	17,182	14,457	9,899	7,875

*286,095.

Source: USA Swimming, Inc. 2009. http://www.usaswimming.org.

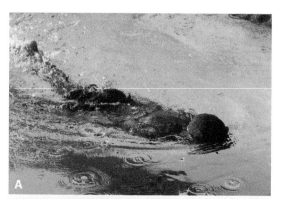

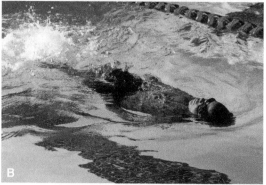

FIGURE 19-1. (A, B) Swimmers in fundamental stage learning to maintain body alignment and balance of the body in prone position.

A major skill that young swimmers must acquire is being balanced in the water (Figure 19.1A,B). Drills and activities that teach correct body position in the prone and supine positions are essential for continued stroke development and aquatic capabilities.

Dry land training in the fundamental stage should focus on general locomotor abilities, including trunk stability, locomotion, and fine manipulation skills. Coaches should be aware of a window of adaptation for speed development during this stage; for girls this occurs between the ages of 6 and 8, and for boys this occurs between ages 7 and 9. Coaches should use body awareness skills that incorporate balance, accompanied by common arm and leg positions in the four strokes of competitive swimming. Examples of these skills include single-leg stance, arms overhead in streamline position, and swing leg in slight extension and/or flexion (Figure 19.2).

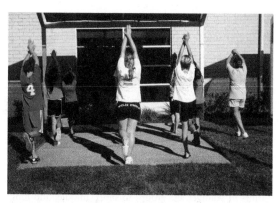

FIGURE 19-2. Swimmers of all ages need to master and improve the ability to assume the streamline body position which is used in all swim strokes to transition from the start and turns into the swimming stroke.

Mixing in games and activities that are fun and dynamic challenges young swimmers' locomotor systems. Examples of such activities include the games leapfrog, rabbits and spiders (2), red light–green light, and dodge ball. The following games help build age-appropriate stability as well as locomotor and manipulative skills:

- Squat, crouch, plank, crawl, jump, throw, kick, skip, run, and sprint (Figure 19.3)
- Leapfrog, spiders, and rabbits

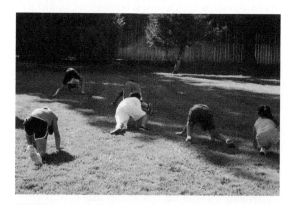

FIGURE 19-3. Playing a game utilizing duckwalks in a "catcher's squat" and jumps alternating between vertical jumps and forward broad jumps. The use of crawling exercises and games to challenge both dynamic stability and coordination of the limbs in a cross-crawl pattern of movement is essential for the athletic development and injury prevention of swimmers.

- Jump rope with single hops, double hops, and jumps. This activity is useful for swimmers of all ages in training rhythm, coordination, and lower extremity kick patterns, as well as endurance, speed, and power development in the older swimmers.
- Ladder agility drills
- Hopscotch (game with rules)
- Red light, green light (game with rules)
- Simon says (game with rules)

The following are examples of basic swimming skills for 6- to 9-year-olds:

Long-axis strokes (freestyle and backstroke):

- Body alignment and buoyancy control in the water
- Using a streamline arm and body position
- Kicking from hips with correct knee bend and flexible ankles
- Alignment of arms in front of shoulders on hand entry
- Body rotation and timing of breath
- Starts, turns, and finishes (Figure 19.4A, B)

Short-axis strokes (breaststroke and butterfly):

- Begin learning correct execution of breaststroke pull-out

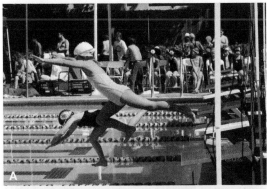
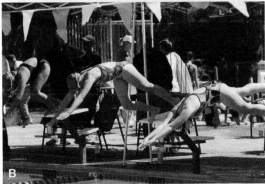

FIGURE 19-4. (A, B) Start, turn, and finish are key technical and tactical components of all levels of competitive swimming. Swimmers in the fundamental stage often have a fear of diving from the blocks; however, a successful start is a requisite for early and late success in swimming.

- Learn a correct pull and kick pattern for breaststroke
- Learn the timing between arm stroke and kick
- Learn a two-hand touch
- Begin to learn a double-arm, fly-pull pattern, and dolphin kick for butterfly
- Learn to undulate the whole body in the water and breathe
- Learn the timing between arm cycles, breaths, and kicks

During this early stage of swimming development, coaches should instruct swimmers and parents on the basic rules and guidelines for each stroke, as well as distances and relay particulars for competition. For example, 6-year-old children who are learning the backstroke should be instructed on the backstroke start, which is unique. They must be taught to stay on their backs during the entire race and not roll over, which would lead to disqualification. Swimmers in relays should be taught how to time the start to avoid false starts and excessive delays on the blocks.

Toward the end of the fundamental stage of development, coaches should pay attention to the aerobic development of 9- and 10-year-old athletes. Because of the aerobic sensitivity, increasing the yardage swim may be wise in order to build a better aerobic base of conditioning, which will benefit the athlete in both the short and long term (3).

REFINED STAGE (10- TO 15-YEAR-OLDS)

As young adolescent athletes progress, they learn to swim longer distances and different strokes. They need more instruction on technique to refine swimming efficiency and to learn to observe technical factors influencing their stroke counts and distance per stroke. Athletes should begin adapting to race pace conditioning and refining technical aspects of their race such as starts, turns, and finishes.

During the adolescent phase, coaches and parents should pay close attention to the sensitive periods of development for both girls and boys. A physical marker related to this phase is termed peak height velocity (PHV), or onset of vertical height growth, and is associated with the pubertal growth spurt. Increases in both aerobic and strength development occur during the PHV period. However, in girls, both aerobic and strength development occur simultaneously around age 11. In boys, PHV occurs later, closer to ages 13 to 14, and correlates to a window of adaptation to aerobic and strength development, but their strength development does not begin until a year after the onset of PHV (4,5).

Coaches should be ready to modify training to take advantage of this window of positive adaptation in both the nervous and energy systems. For example, training should include increases in swimming volume emphasizing aerobic development plus integration of new and more advanced swim drills to take advantage of developing body coordination.

The addition of both technical and tactical training techniques for breath control during starts and strokes into and out of turns is recommended.

During this phase of growth, young athletes can often experience awkwardness or difficulty with simple movement tasks that were perhaps once mastered (e.g., push-ups or squats). A thorough explanation about the biological changes taking place should help to keep the young athlete motivated and inspired to continue through this period of development and training. Refined-stage swimmers are learning to build a bigger engine to optimize performance. Their training program should include a well-rounded conditioning program that does not focus just on sports-specific movements but also on body weight drills, medicine balls, gym balls, and resistance tubing (6). Examples of exercises include

- Squats, single-leg squats, and jump squats
- Multidirectional lunge
- Crawl, plank, and push-up progressions
- Medicine ball use, with whole-body movements
- Tube, pulling in symmetrical and oppositional arm movement patterns

Dry land skills should focus on flexibility, motor control, refinement of kinesthetic awareness of the trunk and limbs during arm recovery, and arm alignment during hand entry (Figure 19.5). An example exercise that focuses on these skills is the "mitt's drill," where the swimmer refines the accuracy of hand position during entry by trying to touch another person's hand held at shoulder width (perform with eyes open and closed).

There is a high incidence of noncontact shoulder, back, and knee injuries in swimmers, which result from faulty movement patterns and overtraining (7). A basic functional assessment at this and following stages of development, followed up with proper exercise instruction and training strategies, can help prevent injuries. Functional assessment of swimmers should include the following:

- Postural assessment to note degree of lordosis, kyphosis, scoliosis, and valgosity of knees
- Functional movement screens, specifically emphasizing kinematics of the shoulder, spine, and knee (e.g., overhead reach and push-up screen to assess thoracic spine and shoulder mobility and stability)

FIGURE 19-5. (A–D) The use of kinesthetic or body awareness training can help swimmers improve accuracy of limb movement and positioning for improved swimming performance and to reduce the risk of injury.

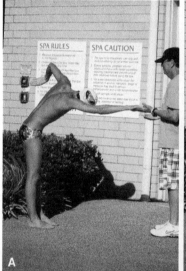
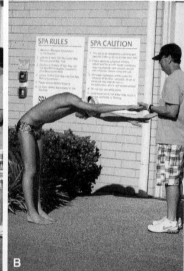
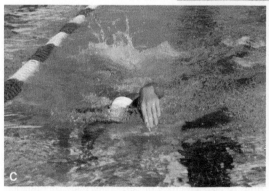
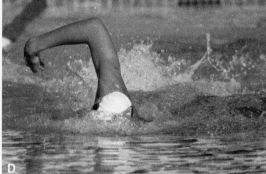

- Ankle, knee, and hip assessment (e.g., squat, single-leg squat, lunge screen)
- Core stability (sport-specific screen)

To perform a sport-specific assessment for core stability, have the swimmer lie down on two raised surfaces (e.g., Bosu and balance discs or pads), with his or her shoulders on one surface and feet on the other (Figure 19.6A). Then, have the swimmer raise his or her hips to a position aligning the head, trunk, hips, and feet (8). Finally, have the swimmer roll gently forward and backward, holding the aligned position.

Another assessment method places the swimmer supine, with one bench supporting the head and shoulders, a middle bench supporting the pelvis, and a third bench supporting the feet at the heels (9). The swimmer should brace the abdominals to stabilize the core, then remove the middle bench and assess the ability to maintain a stable body position head, shoulders, hips, and feet (see Figure 19.6B, C). If there is any fault in performance of this screen, further attention to basic core stabilization exercises and repeated testing are needed before moving the athlete on to more demanding types of training.

ELITE STAGE (16+ YEAR-OLDS)

Elite swimmers typically have progressed to a more superior style of stroke technique than is seen in the two previous stages of development. Therefore, athletes at this stage may benefit from more objective measurements, such as underwater video and biomechanical analysis, distance-per-stroke measurements, and stroke counts.

Coaches should focus on building the athlete's overall endurance, strength, and power with a well-designed periodization program (10). This can be accomplished by a well-supervised resistance training program in the weight room, tethered swims against resistance in the pool (e.g., rubber tubing), and swim sets using fins and snorkels. Examples of useful assessment tests at this stage include squat test (qualitative and quantitative), vertical leap test, push-up test, and plank and side-plank-hold endurance tests. Some examples of exercises for strength training include

- Resisted squats, resisted single-leg squats, plyometric jump squats (Figure 19.7)
- Multidirectional lunges with medicine balls, kettlebells (Figure 19.8)
- Suspension training with webbing, chains, or rings (whole-body exercises)
- Crawl, plank, and push-up progression(s)
- Medicine ball tosses and passes
- Vertical, horizontal, and diagonal tube or pulley training in symmetrical and oppositional arm patterns (vertical pulling on swivel disc; diagonal high to low and low to high, e.g., "wood-choppers"; horizontal or transverse rotational movements) (Figure 19.9)

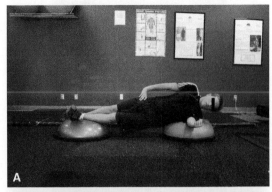

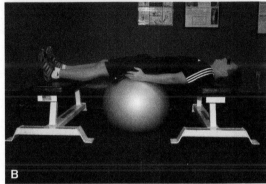

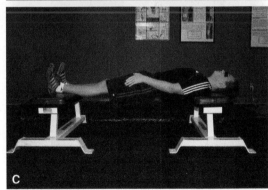

FIGURE 19-6. (A–C) As swimmers progress into the refined stage, assessment of flexibility and core muscle function is necessary to address limiting factors affecting athletic performance and increasing the risk of injury (e.g., modified side-plank-hold test and supine plank test).

An example of sport-specific resistance training is the use of vertical pulling with a swimmer balancing on a Bosu or pad, which is placed on top of a platform that swivels (Figure 19.10). This requires the swimmer to use core muscles to stabilize his or her shoulders, trunk, and pelvis against the reactive forces imposed by the pulling arm motion. Resistance tubing can be used around the feet and ankles to provide resistance against the intended direction of lower limb movement. This training exercise helps balance the long chains of muscles used to generate rotational movements during freestyle swimming.

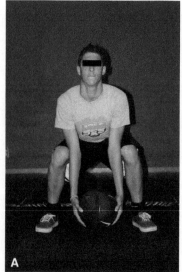

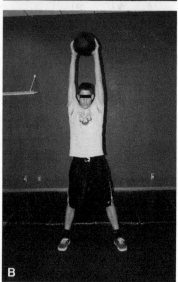

FIGURE 19-7. (A, B) Squat to overhead, an essential functional exercise to develop whole-body fitness and sports-specific aspects of swimming toward the end of refined stage and overlapping into the elite stage of development.

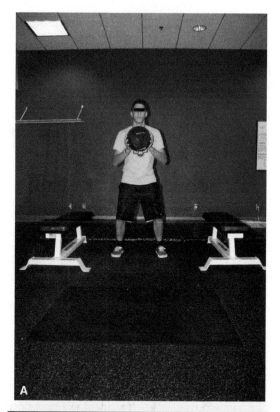

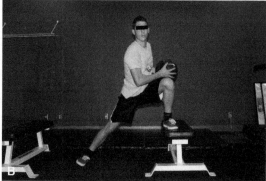

FIGURE 19-8. (A, B) Example of lateral lunge with trunk rotation onto a bench with a medicine ball.

BIOMECHANICS OF SHOULDER INJURY (SWIMMER'S SHOULDER)

Young athletes are still growing. Structural changes to bones, joints, and soft tissues are occurring based on the demands of movements in sport and daily living. Functional stability of the shoulder is a developmental concern that can be addressed by balancing the training loads to meet specific, biological needs. Musculoskeletal injuries in swimmers are most commonly caused by the demands of high training volumes, accompanied by poor or flawed swimming technique (11). High training volumes and early maturation have been linked to top 100 ranked young swimmers abandoning the sport by the ages of 17 to 19 (12). The reason associated with the drop-off is that early success is linked to early maturation and, at the other end, early exposure to high training volumes, which can lead to performance plateau, burnout, or injury. Another example of this type of attrition rate occurs in young freshman swimmers who transition into a year-round collegiate swim program and experience a sudden jump in training volume in and out of the pool. Sudden increase in training is correlated with a high

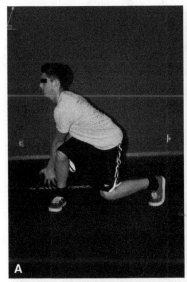
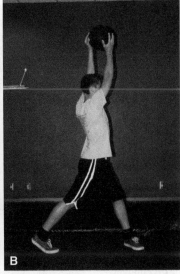

FIGURE 19-9. (A, B) Training of whole-body movement patterns such as rotational low to high and high to low is beneficial at the elite stage.

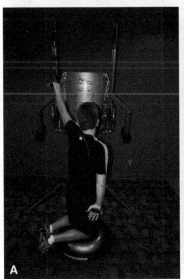
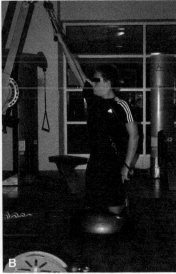

FIGURE 19-10. (A, B) Sports-specific exercises are beneficial for developing key movement patterns associated with a particular stroke (e.g., vertical training on pulley system with a Bosu stacked on a swivel disc).

rate of shoulder injuries (13,14). Training more than four times a week is correlated with a twofold increase in knee injuries and a fourfold increase in shoulder injuries (15).

The most common area of injury in a competitive swimmer is the shoulder region; such injuries are commonly referred to as "swimmer's shoulder" (1,7,16–18). Injuries are defined as an area of complaint that requires any contact with a trainer or physician for diagnosis and treatment (7). There are 2.12 injuries per 1,000 exposures per swimmer (see Table 19.2 for more details about injury rates in swimming). Swimmer's shoulder results from volume of training the freestyle stroke. It is not uncommon for a refined- or elite-level athlete to swim 10,000 to 14,000 m/day; and 80% of time training in the pool is spent swimming freestyle (19).

TABLE 19.2	Injury Rates in Swimming
Injury Rate and Area of Injury	**Related to**
44%	Swimming
44%	Cross-training
11%	Unrelated to athletics
Lower extremity (LE) injury	Cross-training
Upper extremity (UE) injury	Swimming
Ratio of UE to LE injury	Swimming 3:1 to cross-training 1:4

Source: McFarland EG, Wasik M. Injuries in female collegiate swimmers due to swimming and cross-training. Clin J Sports Med 1996;6:178–182.

This translates into roughly 1.2 to 2 million arm strokes per year (20,21). Medial knee pain or "breaststroker's knee" is the most common lower extremity injury, followed by spine-related injuries to the neck and back (22).

Out-of-pool conditioning activities, such as dry land, resistance training, and cross-training programs, are also contributing factors to musculoskeletal injury. The rate of injury for these activities is close to that of swimming (7). Recovery is an important part of the long-term athletic development of swimmers. Unfortunately, the over-emphasis on year-round swimming by coaches, parents, and swimmers competes with the necessary benefits of a recovery period.

In freestyle swimming, the most common stroke flaws that contribute to swimmer's shoulder are inefficient body rotation with arm recovery, dropped elbow position, poor head positioning, and crossing over midline with the trajectory arm after hand entry. The optimal position of arm entry is in line with shoulder and not crossing over midline. In the short-axis strokes, excessive breaststroke competition, kicking and training sets are linked to lower extremity injury also known as "breaststroker's knee."

COMMON SHOULDER INJURIES

The following are some common diagnoses that indicate swimmer's shoulder:

- Biceps tendonitis
- Subacromial bursitis
- Rotator-cuff tendonitis (supraspinatus)
- Myofascial pain syndrome (periscapular muscle groups)
- Anterior subluxation
- Coracoligament injury
- Capsular superior labral tear from anterior to posterior lesion
- Multidirectional instability

Other injuries reported in swimming include

- Breaststroker's knee
- Neck pain
- Low back pain

INEFFICIENT BODY ROTATION IN FREESTYLE SWIMMING

Compromise in performance, as well as shoulder pain in swimmers, can result from inadequate body rotation and/or asymmetrical trunk rotation. This can lead to overuse of the elevators of the shoulder blade during the recovery phase of freestyle. Inadequate body rotation contributes to an altered path of arm motion during recovery, which affects the limb alignment from the hand entry to the catch-and-pull portion of the stroke (Figure 19.11).

As younger swimmers begin to increase training volumes and repetition of arm movements, faulty movement patterns can lead to the development of trigger points and myofascial pain in the periscapular muscles. This can further alter the scapulohumeral rhythm during the arm reach and recovery phase of the stroke (Figure 19.12).

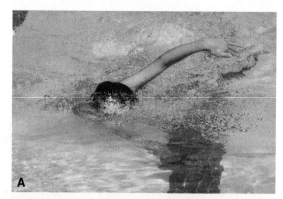

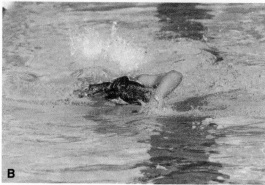

FIGURE 19-11. (A) Example of a swimmer in the refined phase with a significant fault in arm recovery, entry, and mid-pull phase (across midline of the body). (B) Example of a swimmer in the mid-to-late stage of refined phase with a slight fault in arm-hand entry to the inside and legs slightly too wide on the kick.

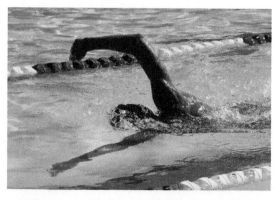

FIGURE 19-12. Example of an early-stage elite swimmer with a high arm recovery that could lead to a shoulder injury in a high yardage and intensity training program.

CONTRIBUTING FACTORS TO MUSCULOSKELETAL PAIN IN SWIMMERS

Poor or faulty posture is a major contributing factor in the development of swimming-related injuries. Postural problems result in the potential for injuries to the shoulder, spine, and knee because they confound proper training techniques in the pool and during dry land conditioning sessions (23). Forward-drawn posture and increased kyphosis have been shown to alter the position and activation of scapular stabilizers (24). This contributes to shoulder impingement and further instability of the glenohumeral joint.

Improper use of both resistance training methods and certain types of shoulder stretches can contribute to further shoulder pain and injury in swimmers. However, the proper use of stretching exercises can reduce the risk of knee injury (25).

REFERENCES

1. USA Swimming, Inc. 2009 Statistics. http://www. USAswimming.com. Accessed October 20, 2009.
2. Elphinston J. Stability, Sport and Performance Movement: Great Technique without Injury. Islands Road, Chichester: Lotus Publishing; 2008:289.
3. Drabik J. Children & Sports Training. How Your Future Champions Should Exercise to Healthy, Fit and Happy. Island Pond, VT: Stadion Publishing; 1996:100.
4. Drabik J. Children & Sports Training. How Your Future Champions Should Exercise to Healthy, Fit and Happy. Island Pond, VT: Stadion Publishing; 1996:19–23.
5. Balyi I, Way R. The Role of Monitoring Growth in Long-Term Athletic Development. Canadian Sports for Life-Supplement 2009. http: //www.canadiansportforlife.ca.pdf.
6. Salo D, Riewald S. Complete conditioning for swimming. Hum Kinet 2008;38–40.
7. McFarland EG, Wasik M. Injuries in collegiate swimmers due to swimming and cross training. Clin J Sports Med 1996;6(3):178–182.
8. Kagan T. Dry Land Training for Swimmers [DVD]. Ultimate Athlete; 2007.
9. Sweentenham B, Atkinson J. Championship swim training. Hum Kinet 2003:263.
10. Salo D, Riewald S. Complete conditioning for swimming. Hum Kinet 2008:185–195.
11. Souza TA, The shoulder in swimming. In: Sports Injuries of the Shoulder: Conservative Management. New York, NY: Churchill Livingstone; 1994:107–124.
12. Costa M, Marinho D, Reis V, et al. Tracking the performance of world ranked swimmers. J Sports Sci Med 2010; 9(3):411–417.   http://www.jssm.org/vol9/n3/9/v9n3-9text .php. Accessed October 14, 2010.
13. Wolf BR, Ebinger AE, Lawler MP, et al. Injury patterns in division 1 collegiate swimming. Am J Sports Med 2009;10(10):1–6.
14. Sallis RE, Jones K, Sunshine S, et al. Comparing sports injuries in men and women. Int J Sports Med 2001;22(6): 420–423.
15. Knobloch K, Yoon U, Kraemer R, et al. 200-400m breastroke events dominate among knee overuse injuries in elite swimming athletes. Sportverletz, Sportschaden 2008;22(4): 213–219.
16. Wolf BR, Ebinger AE, Lawler MP, et al. Injury patterns in division 1 collegiate swimming. Am J Sports Med 2009;10(10):2037–2042.
17. Edelman GT. An Active Shoulder Warm-Up for the Competitive Swimmer [Edelman Spine and Orthopaedic Physical Therapy web site]. 2009. http://www.esopt.com/site/1/docs/ Active_Warm_Up_040809.pdf. Accessed October 14, 2010.
18. Kenal KA, Knapp LD. Rehabilitation of injuries in competitive swimmers. Sports Med 1996;22(5):337–347.
19. Ruwe P, Pink M, Jobe F, et al. The normal and the painful shoulders during breaststroke. Am J Sports Med 1994;22(6):789–796.
20. Allegrucci M, Whitney S, Irrgang J. Clinical implications of secondary impingement of the shoulder in freestyle swimmers. J Sports Phys Ther 1994;20:307–317.
21. Bak K. The practical management of swimmer's shoulder: etiology, diagnosis, and treatment. Clin J Sports Med 2010;20(5):386–390.
22. Wei F. Swimming injuries: diagnosis, treatment & rehabilitation. In: Sports Medicine and Rehabilitation, A Sport-Specific Approach. Philadelphia, PA: Hanley and Belfus; 1994:67–94.
23. O'Donnell CJ, Bowen J, Fossati J. Identifying and managing shoulder pain in competitive swimmers. Phys Sports Med 2000;33(9):3. www. chiro.org/.../Identifying_and_Managing _Shoulder_Pain_in_Competitive_Swimmers.pdf
24. Thigpen CA, Padua DA, Michener LA, et al. Head and shoulder posture affect scapular mechanics and muscle activity in overhead tasks. J Electromyogr Kinesiol 2010;20(40):701–709.
25. Rodeo S. USA Swimming and the Network Task Force on Injury Prevention. USA Swimming, April 2002. http:// www.usaswimming.org/ViewMiscArticle.aspx?TabId=1645& Alias=Rainbow&Lang=en&mid=702&ItemId=700. Accessed September 04, 2009.

Surfing

Surfing has grown to become a global sport, with an estimated 35 million active surfers and 60 countries participating annually in the International Surfing Association world championships. Mendez-Villanueva and Bishop note that surfing is an intermittent sport whose participants tend to be shorter, to be more muscular, and have a lower body mass than other matched-level aquatic athletes (1). The authors also note that 50% of the time surfing is spent paddling, 40% stationary, and only 4% to 5% actually riding a wave; during these high-intensity aerobic and anaerobic periods, surfers have comparable VO$_2$ peak values to other upper-body endurance athletes.

Considered an early development sport, surfing requires a highly evolved sensorimotor skill set similar to snow and skateboarding. According to Treleaven, this sensorimotor control can be functionally enhanced through the introduction of a coordinated joint position, oculomotor and postural stability exercise program (2). These programs can be introduced early and modified to the individual surfer's specific right or left foot forward stance position and to suit the anticipated wave direction, size, and type.

The requirement for prolonged paddling while lying prone braced on a board and duck-diving under waves creates biomechanical stress similar to those seen in swimmers and challenges the surfers' breath-holding capacity and shoulder complex flexibility, coupling patterns of upper and lower cross-dynamic support systems.

Surfing further requires the athlete to perform high-speed, end-range, explosive, and technically difficult water- and aerial-based maneuvers on an unstable surface that is constantly moving three dimensionally. Biomechanical stress in an asymmetrical stance position requires the surfer to be flexible and powerful throughout a combination of complex planned and spontaneous movement patterns.

Brown and Prosser note that elite male surfers presented 50% more often for an ankle and twice as often for a knee injury than their female counterparts and that front foot hip injuries were between 25% and five times more likely than back foot hip injuries in both groups (3). Nathanson et al. observed a higher proportion of soft tissue knee injuries among competitive surfers compared with their recreational counterparts and accounted for this due to the aggressive and acrobatic maneuvers performed in competition (4).

The sport's unique three dimensionally changing and moving waveforms require not only axial and peripheral strength for functional stability to withstand spontaneous deceleration and acceleration impacts but also an acutely sensitive vestibular, visual, and proprioceptive system for accurate timing and skill performance.

Varied wave speed, shape, size, and type of sea floor require location-specific training, skill preparation, and refined adjustment to technique and equipment selection to maximize performance and safety. Nathanson et al. note that the risk of injury although low is more than doubled when surfing large waves or over hard sea floor and that on average 13 acute injuries occur per 1,000 hours of competitive surfing (4).

"FUNDAMENTAL" SURFING DEVELOPMENT (AGES 5 TO 10)

Rudimentary development of timing, coordination, and balance to paddle, catch a wave, and stand up are key and are introduced at this stage on top of a "FUNdamental" broad base of athleticism, aerobic fitness, flexibility, and efficient primal movement patterns. Stance-specific asymmetrical motor learning and symmetrical agility and balance on both stable and dynamic, undulating surfaces is introduced through low-impact, safe barefoot play in and out of the water.

Surfing-specific prehabilitation is introduced at this and the recreational stage. Butel et al. found elite surfer findings of poor performance in coupled shoulder abduction and internal rotation flexibility as well as hip extension (front leg dominant), internal rotation, and short abduction flexibility (5). Poor neck and cervicocranial flexion coordination, lower abdominal stability, and coordination were also noted and should be addressed through the introduction of prehabilitation at this and the recreational stage.

Aerobic capacity/flexibility/stability/athleticism/balance/coordination (ABC) is the goal of this "FUNdamental" stage with a primary focus on functional diaphragm breathing and functional recruitment of deep neck flexors throughout the individual short sets which can start at a 3-breath duration and progress to 6-9-12-breath durations with short rest periods between sets of less than 30 seconds.

Foam Roller Shoulder/Hip Flexibility

- Initial: The surfer lies down supine on the foam roller symmetrically lengthwise with a neutral spine and is taught to functionally breathe with the diaphragm through the nose while maintaining a neutral head and neck position.
- Progression: The surfer engages bracing pattern while unilateral or bilateral arms are taken through abduction or flexion and unilateral hips through flexion; this is coupled and alternated together for cross-patterning, balance, and transverse plane stability training (Figure 20.1). Patterns are held for up to three breath cycles and repeated 3 to 12 times.

Swiss Ball Shoulder/Hip Flexibility

- Initial: The surfer lies supine over height-sized Swiss ball keeping head supported (Figure 20.2A) and is taught to functionally breathe through the nose while maintaining neck in chin tuck/neutral position with arms bilaterally abducted to sides or flexed.
- Progression: The surfer side lies and stretches over ball repeating on both sides while maintaining the sagittal plane spinal neutral (see Figure 20.2B) and is taught lateral diaphragm breathing; all stretches are held for three breath cycles, progressing to up to 12 with use of height-suitable-diameter Swiss balls.

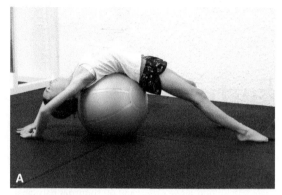
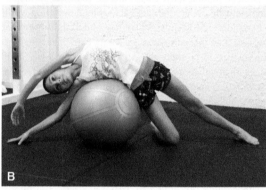

FIGURE 20.2. (A and B) Swiss ball shoulder/hip flexibility.

Swiss Ball Superman

- Initial: The surfer lies prone in a 4-point position over a height-sized Swiss ball and is taught to keep shoulders and neck in neutral while laterally breathing and bracing to stabilize as one arm or leg or both are raised off the ground progressing to a 3, 2, or 1 point position.
- Progression: The prone superman 0 point position is held for a 3 to 12 counts and repeated 3 to 12 times (Figure 20.3).

Swiss Ball Squat

- Initial: The surfer symmetrically stands leaning back toward wall against ball with feet shoulder width apart in foot arch neutral and arm neutral or flexed position (Figure 20.4A) and is taught how to stabilize foot intrinsics (short foot), breathe, brace, and hip hinge squat to 90° or to stable range.
- Progression: This involves a single-leg squat (see Figure 20.4B) with exercises held for 3 to 5 breaths and repeated 3 to 5 times.

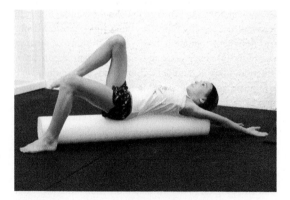

FIGURE 20-1.   Foam roller shoulder/hip flexibility.

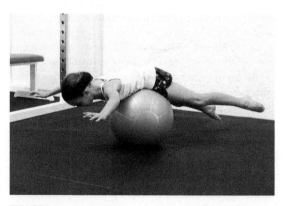

FIGURE 20-3.   Swiss ball superman.

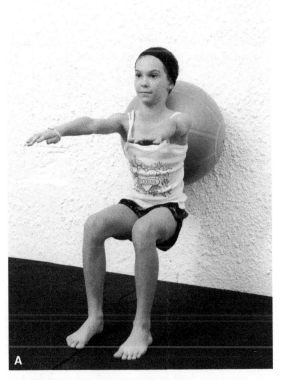
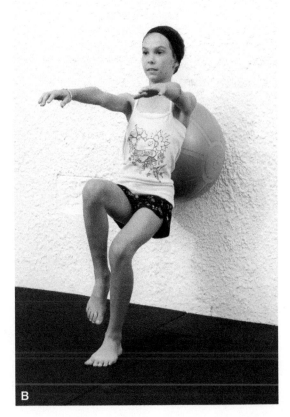

FIGURE 20-4.   (A and B) Swiss ball squat.

Eyes Open/Eyes Closed Balance Plus Coordination

- Initial: The surfer balances on one foot in coronal neutral standing position and holds for 3 to 12 breaths progressing to eyes closed and alternates sides.
- Progression: The surfer develops sensorimotor skills while balancing on one foot going through rainbow and transverse plane rotation (Figure 20.5A), alternating catching and throwing (see Figure 20.5B), and the Hacky Sack warm-up (see Figure 20.5C).

RECREATIONAL SURFING DEVELOPMENT (AGES 10 TO 16)

The athlete's surfing-specific skills are developed at this stage through fun time in the water—surfing—as well as with the introduction of land-based complex, faster paced, multidimensional planes of movement drills on stable and unstable surfaces. Efficient agility and timing to spontaneously adjust body weight and position to optimize surfboard speed and maneuverability is developed through play.

This progression specifically harnesses the skills, strength, and bracing stability required to safely cope with the physical, physiological, and psychological demands of surfing. Larger, more high-performance waves are commonly encountered throughout this stage.

Strength/stability/skills/ABC are the goals of this recreational surfing development stage and are added onto a sound base of the "FUNdamentals" developed functional diaphragm breathing and functional recruitment patterns. Exercise sets progress in length and vary in intensity and recovery time within the set to mimic the base physiological requirements of a 30 to 45 minute competitive heat with explosive wave catching/wipeout/paddling/recovery waiting periods. Individual sets can start at breath durations and progress to repetition sets with short rest periods of less than 30 seconds progressing to 60 to 90 second rest periods.

Forward Ball Roll to Stir the Pot

- Initial: The surfer kneels with forearms resting on Swiss ball in a braced neutral sagittal spine position and shoulders/hips at 90° (Figure 20.6). The ball is then rolled away while maintaining scapular alignment, a neutral spine, and controlled hip

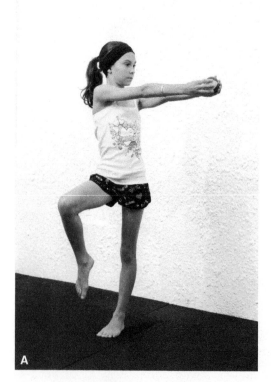

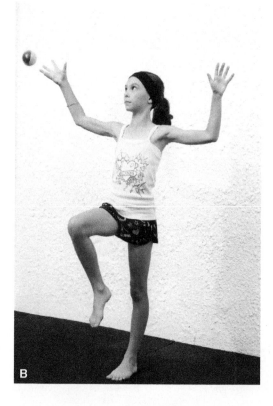

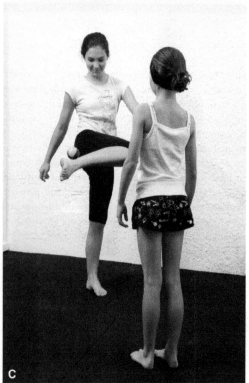

FIGURE 20-5. (A–C) Eyes open/eyes closed balance plus coordination.

extension, holding at functional end range for 3 to 5 diaphragm breaths and repeated.

- Progression: The surfer moves the Swiss ball into clockwise and counterclockwise progressive diameter functional range circles for 3 to 15 sets.

Ball Push-Up to Prone Jack Knife

- Initial: The surfer places hands shoulder width apart on the ground and lies with knees or feet on Swiss ball in a braced neutral spine plank position, performing push-ups.

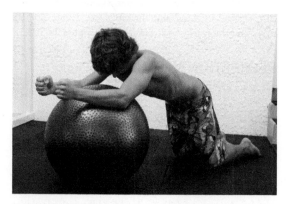

FIGURE 20-6. Forward ball roll to stir the pot.

- Progression: The push-up is repeated with one foot on Swiss ball or the push-up progresses into double-legged or single-legged prone jack knife where the surfer brings knees symmetrically toward chest (Figure 20.7) while maintaining neutral sagittal spine, progressing to single-leg jack knife where the surfer elevates unsupported leg while maintaining transverse plane pelvic stability.

Upper Russian Twist

- Initial: The surfer lies supine over a Swiss ball in a neutral spine plank position with head and shoulders (flexed to 90°) resting on ball, hips in neutral, knees at 90°, and feet hip width apart on ground. While maintaining a spinal sagittal and hip neutral position, slow functional range rotational movements are made bilaterally by rolling the ball under the thoracic spine in a controlled rhythmic side-to-side motion.
- Progression: As the surfer becomes more functionally skilled the range and speed of movement are increased until high-speed ballistic medicine ball catch and throw (Figure 20.8) patterns are practiced bilaterally.

Multidirectional Clock Lunges

- Initial: The surfer stands in the center of a drawn or imaginary clock and develops forward 12 o'clock and backward 6 o'clock functional lunge patterns bilaterally, returning to center and repeating. An upright spinal neutral position is maintained throughout the sequence in a forward facing open shoulder posture with the front ankle in neutral.
- Progression: Multidirectional individual leg sequences or alternating lunge sequences are carried out from the center of the clock to all time points in both clockwise and anticlockwise directions (Figure 20.9).

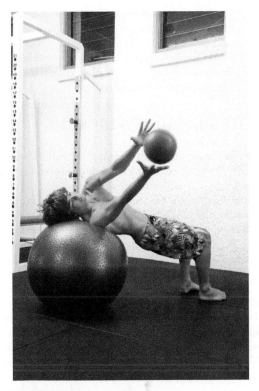

FIGURE 20-8.   Upper Russian twist.

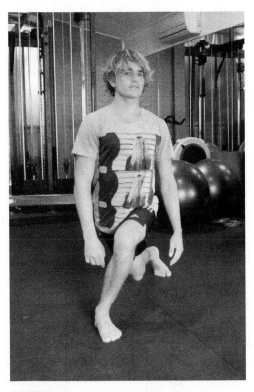

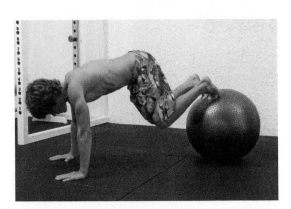

FIGURE 20-7.   Ball push to prone jack knife.

FIGURE 20-9.   Multidirectional clock lunges.

- Further progression: The surfer changes the center of the clock as they progress through the time sequences and adds unstable surfaces like Bosu/wobble board or sand as well as engages more high-speed ballistic medicine ball catch and throw sequences if functionally developed and able to perform.

ELITE SURFING DEVELOPMENT

Elite surfing requires the development and performance of progressive linked and complex ballistic maneuvers on high-speed, high-risk large waves. Training programs require a sound sensorimotor base and a high degree of functional flexibility and stability performed by physically, skeletally, and emotionally mature athletes. Elite surfing, however, is still "FUNdamentally" based on a lifestyle centered around freedom, adventure, and hydrotherapy where the emphasis is always on balance.

Explosive agility, power, and elite ABC are the goals of elite surfing advanced skills training and are added onto a skill base of strength and stability developed during the recreational stage. Breath-holding and breath enhancement training are also introduced at this time as are water-based heat drills and fatigue-based training, all periodized around competition requirements.

Swiss Ball Balance/Squats/Twists

- Initial: The surfer while being safely spotted learns to balance kneeling in a neutral spinal position on the correct pressure and sized Swiss ball, progressing to being unassisted and able to carry out sensorimotor rainbow and transverse plane rotation movements and catch passing patterns.
- Progression: The surfer learns to safely stand unassisted on the Swiss ball and proceeds to squatting routines, sensorimotor transverse plane rotation movements, and catching skills, progressing to ballistic medicine ball throwing routines (Figure 20.10).

TRX Pull-Up/Scapula Stabilizers

- Initial: The surfer lies in a supine spinal neutral plank position with shoulders at 90° and proceeds to sequentially activate scapular retraction and shoulder horizontal extension to an elbow 90° reverse push-up pattern while maintaining functional spinal neutral (Figure 20.11).
- Progression: The surfer maintains a more extended elbow position to perform a reverse fly pattern.

Cable Wood Chops

- Initial: The surfer holds the cable pulley handles at the starting position under load while maintaining a foundation stable standing posture. A functional

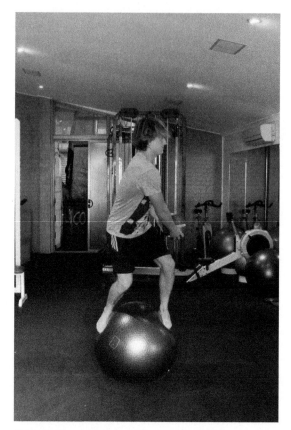

FIGURE 20-10. Swiss ball balance/squats/twists.

bracing pattern is engaged and the surfer smoothly rotates and steps into an open side lunge pattern while pulling the cable across the body to its final position under load (Figure 20.12) and returns to starting position and repeats. Cable pulley anchors can be set high or low to simulate multiple surfing

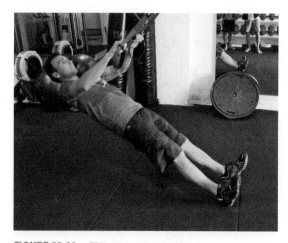

FIGURE 20-11. TRX pull-up/scapula stabilizers.

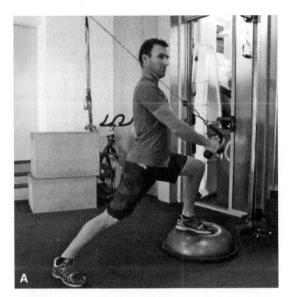

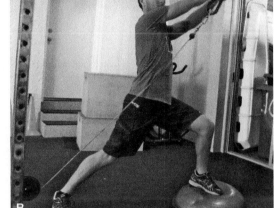

FIGURE 20-12.   (A, B) Cable wood chops.

maneuvers and weights set to allow 10 to 15 sets of functional repetitions.

- Progression: The surfer performs the above onto a Bosu, repeats at higher speed ballistic sequences, or engages in greater range of surfing functional movements toward end range.

TRX/Swiss Ball Scorpion Twist

- Initial: The surfer places hands shoulder width apart on the ground and lies with dorsum of feet in the

TRX straps in a braced neutral sagittal spine plank position and proceeds to bring one knee into an abducted and flexed position along the outside of the ipsilateral arm (Figure 20.13A) and repeats bilaterally. Alternatively, one leg can be anchored in the TRX straps allowing the unsupported knee to be flexed and rotated toward the opposite elbow while maintaining functional spinal neutral.

- Progression: These TRX patterns can be repeated on the Swiss ball progressing to unsupported hip extension and pelvic ipsilateral rotation while the

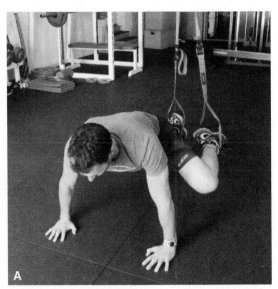

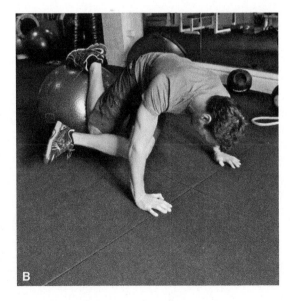

FIGURE 20-13.   (A, B) TRX/Swiss ball scorpion twist.

ball is drawn toward the chest with the supported leg (Figure 20.13B) and repeated. Alternatively, the unsupported hip is flexed and pelvis contralaterally rotated toward the chest and alternated bilaterally.

REFERENCES

1. Mendez-Villanueva A, Bishop D. Physiological aspects of surfboard riding performance. Sports Med 2005;35(1):55–70.
2. Treleaven J. Sensorimotor Disturbances in Neck Disorders Affecting Postural Stability, Head and Eye Movement Control. Neck Pain and Whiplash Research Unit, Division of Physiotherapy, University of Queensland; June 8, 2007.
3. Brown T, Prosser C. Professional Male and Female World Championship Tour Surfer Injury Incidence File Summary from over 1500 Unique Injury Presentations from Rip Curl Pro Bells Beach 1997 through Quiksilver Pro Fiji 2004. Association of Surfing Professionals Internal Injury Report, 2005.
4. Nathanson A, Bird S, Dao L, Tam-Sing K. Competitive surfing injuries, a retrospective study of surfing-related injuries among contest surfers. Am J Sports Med 2007;35:1.
5. Butel M, Carton J, Grainger R, McBride A, Prosser C, Uwland M. Professional Male and Female World Championship Tour Surfer Pre-participation Screen. Quiksilver Pro March 2004. Association of Surfing professionals Internal Injury Report, 2005.

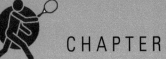

CHAPTER 21

Todd S. Ellenbecker, Mark Kovacs, and E. Paul Roetert

Tennis

INTRODUCTION

Tennis is a sport with unique, whole-body demands, played on four different surfaces that produce specific anatomical adaptations and injury profiles in its elite players. This chapter considers the injury patterns and biomechanical characteristics of tennis play and provides a tennis-specific training program template for both young developing players and more mature elite tennis players.

COMMON INJURY PATTERNS IN TENNIS

Tennis injuries have been reported throughout all regions of the body with more common areas being the shoulder, elbow, and knee (1). Most of the injuries in tennis can be defined as overuse injuries coming from the repetitive microtrauma inherent in the sport (1,2). Identifying the most commonly injured anatomical sites is important to target for both preventative and developmental training. Pluim and Staal published an extensive review paper summarizing epidemiological studies in tennis that report the lower extremity to be the most frequently injured region (39% to 65%), followed by the upper extremity (range 24% to 46%) and the head/trunk (8% to 22%) (1). These findings demonstrate the demands of tennis and highlight the importance of a complete conditioning program for repetitive players.

The most frequently injured parts of the lower body were the lower leg, ankle, and thigh, with ankle sprain and thigh muscle strain (hamstring, quadriceps, and adductors) as most frequent injuries. Upper extremity injuries were most frequently located in the elbow and shoulder regions, with tendon injuries of the shoulder and elbow (humeral epicondylitis) cited as most frequent.

BIOMECHANICS OF TENNIS

Shoulder

Overuse injuries in the shoulder typically involve rotator cuff and biceps tendon pathology (1,2), often secondary to not only the repetitive concentric and eccentric demands on the rotator cuff but also the underlying hypermobility and excessive laxity of the glenohumeral joint. Stability of the shoulder joint during tennis strokes requires a high level of muscular control. Ryu et al. reported high levels of normalized concentric and eccentric muscular activity using EMG (electromyography) for the rotator cuff and scapular stabilizers during virtually all strokes (3). For example, during the cocking phase of the tennis serve, muscular activity of the supraspinatus (53%), infraspinatus (41%), and serratus anterior (70%) functions to position the scapula and stabilize the glenohumeral joint, while during the follow-through phase eccentric activation of the rotator cuff (40%) and serratus anterior (53%) assists with further stabilization and deceleration of the shoulder (3). Due to the prevalence of over 75% forehands and serves used during points in modern tennis that inherently require powerful concentric internal shoulder rotation, there are consistent common findings of muscular imbalance between the posterior rotator cuff (external rotators) when compared to the internal rotators (3,4). Additionally, isokinetic testing (5) of the shoulder has repeatedly shown either equal or decreased dominant arm external rotation strength and 15% to 30% increases in dominant arm internal rotation strength compared with the nondominant arm in elite-level players. Greater dominant arm internal rotation strength and equal or decreased dominant arm external rotation strength create an external rotation/internal rotation muscle imbalance in elite players (5). This finding coupled with reports of scapular dysfunction and muscular weakness in the upper back and thorax among experts who routinely evaluate elite tennis players has led to the recommendation of the preventative exercises contained later in this chapter for both developing and elite-level players.

Range of motion loss in the shoulder in the direction of internal rotation has also been widely reported in junior and adult tennis players (6,7). Reduced internal rotation range of motion in the dominant arm greater than 20° compared with the nondominant arm has been termed glenohumeral internal rotation deficiency and advocates the use of specific stretches to increase internal rotation of the dominant shoulder in many players (8).

Elbow

Injuries to the elbow region in elite tennis players are primarily from repetitive overuse and center on the tendinous structures inserting at the medial and lateral humeral epicondyle (9). The reported injury rates for tennis elbow are quite high, with percentages ranging from 37% to 57% in elite and recreational players (1). These studies also show higher rates of incidence in elite players on the medial side of the elbow from overload on the serve and forehand strokes, compared with higher rates of lateral humeral epicondylitis in lower level recreational players from the overload on the backhand groundstroke (9,10).

Exercises recommended for prevention of elbow injury focus on increasing the strength and particularly the muscular endurance of the wrist and forearm musculature. In addition to the standard flexor and extensor wrist curls, use of a counterbalanced weight for forearm pronation and supination, and wrist radial and ulnar deviation is recommended (2,9,10). It is important to note that contrary to common beliefs among coaches, players, and even medical professionals, power generation does not come from the wrist and forearm in properly executed tennis strokes (11,12). Instead, the summation of forces from the entire body or kinetic chain produces the power that is transferred through the wrist, forearm, and ultimately to the racquet head to generate power (13). Overdependence on forearm musculature for power generation sustains the clinical hypothesis for the origin of elbow pathology due to nonoptimal contributions from other segments of the kinetic chain, poor overall stroke biomechanics, and inadequate fitness (13).

Lower Back

The motions required in tennis include repeated flexion, extension, lateral flexion, and rotation of the spine, a risk factor for low back pain (14). One of the motions that can particularly stress the spine in the elite player is the combined movements of extension, lateral flexion, and rotation that are inherent in the cocking or loading phase of the tennis serve. These combined repetitive motions have been shown to stress the lumbar spine and are believed to be a causative factor for spondylolysis (fracture of the pars interarticularis) and spondylolisthesis (pars fracture with graded anterior migration of the vertebral body) identified in many athletes participating in sports with repetitive extension-based movement requirements (15). Alyas et al.(15) studied the spine of 33 asymptomatic elite adolescent tennis players (mean age 17.3 ± 1.7 years) and reported 5 players (15.2%) with a normal magnetic resonance imaging examination and 28 (84.8%) with an abnormal examination. Nine players showed 10 pars lesions (3 complete fractures) and 23 patients showed signs of early facet arthropathy; therefore, tennis players are at risk from lumbar disc disease, sciatica, and facet syndromes secondary to excessive repetitive loading.

To combat the effects of this loading, preventative conditioning strategies for tennis players include extensive core stability training. Similar to research on the shoulder, isokinetic profiling studies of elite tennis players demonstrate characteristic muscle development likely induced from sport-specific demands. Roetert et al.(16) tested elite junior players and found the trunk extension/flexion ratio to be <100, indicating greater actual strength in the abdominals and trunk flexors compared with the back extensors. Research on normal populations (nonathletes and nontennis players) typically produces ratios >100 in the extension/flexion ratio whereby the low back extensor strength exceeds trunk flexor strength. Ellenbecker et al.(17) tested elite junior players and found symmetrical torso rotation strength using an isokinetic dynamometer, indicating that healthy uninjured players should have symmetrical strength ratio. Together, these studies suggest an important role for developing flexors, extensors, and rotational strength balance. Core stabilization exercises should load and stress the core musculature in all three planes (sagittal, frontal, and transverse).

Hip

Historically, injuries to the hip region were thought to focus on the powerful muscles that spanned not only the hip joint but also the knee joint (rectus femoris and hamstrings). An increased understanding of the evaluation and diagnosis of the hip has led to the identification of other forms of hip pathology in tennis due to the impact loading and multidirectional movement patterns coupled with abrupt stopping, starting, cutting, and twisting (18). Injuries to the hip including femoroacetabular impingement and labral tears can occur in elite tennis players (19). In addition to ensuring that proper flexibility exists around the hip and pelvic girdle, exercises for greater stabilization to the hip joint and core are recommended. Ellenbecker et al. (20) measured hip rotation range of motion and found no side-to-side differences in hip internal or external rotation range of motion in healthy uninjured elite tennis players. No additional present data are available on normal muscular strength and range of motion relationships in the hip and pelvis to guide strength and conditioning programming at this time.

ESSENTIAL BASE TRAINING EXERCISES FOR TENNIS PLAYERS

Elemental conditioning exercises are recommended for developing players to promote strength and balance with a primary focus on ensuring that the player has strength in the primary muscles. These exercises may be applicable for athletes in many sports; however, the tennis players' heavy emphasis on trunk rotation, and use of the lower body and trunk for power generation necessitate early development of strength in these important body regions. While it is beyond the scope of this chapter to show all of the base and tennis-specific exercises recommended for tennis players, several exercises will be highlighted with reference to other texts for further reading (21,22).

EXERCISE PROGRESSION IN THE PROGRESSIVE DEVELOPMENT OF A HIGH-PERFORMANCE PLAYER

From a developmental standpoint, exercise prescription is typically emphasized in the second and third phases of the developmental model. In tennis, one model of development can be considered for the purposes of this chapter and includes the three phases termed Introductory, Transition, and World Class/Elite.

Introductory Phase

In this phase, the emphasis is on the development of balance, coordination, throwing, and catching, and in essence, basic athletic skill development for tennis. Focus on activities from a tennis-specific movement pattern standpoint would be recommended such as lateral movement, recovery steps, balance during upper extremity, and trunk rotational movements as well as hopping, skipping, and multidirectional movements. Additionally, skills such as throwing assist with skill acquisition on the serve and are paired with catching as another form of basic athletic skill development. Players in this phase typically range between 6 and 11 years of age.

Transition and World Class/Elite Phases

Starting as early as 12 years of age, when on-court performance ranges from three to four times per week to nearly daily, the introduction of tennis-specific exercise outlined below are introduced for players to address sport-specific musculoskeletal muscle imbalances or adaptations as well as to improve strength, speed, power, and endurance. A balance between exercises for performance enhancement and injury prevention is followed as can be evidenced from the list of exercises focusing on posterior rotator cuff and scapular stabilization for the upper extremity and inclusion of core exercises. The progression to plyometric exercises in the world class and elite phase once a solid base has been achieved is highly recommended given the sport-specific nature of these types of exercises.

SPORT-SPECIFIC EXERCISES FOR TENNIS PLAYERS

The use of the exercises in a multiple set format in a periodized training model (21,22) is recommended. These exercises are broken down by body region for ease of understanding and presentation.

Shoulder/Scapula

The main focus of exercises for the shoulder and scapula involves the external rotators and scapular stabilizers. The imbalance mentioned in the earlier portion of this chapter develops from repetitive forehand and serving activity which utilize forceful shoulder internal rotation. The following exercises target the key stabilizing musculature of the shoulder and scapula using a low weight and multiple set training paradigm.

External Rotation with Retraction

In a standing position, grasp a piece of elastic resistance and externally rotate the shoulders by moving the hands apart about 4 to 6 inches (Figure 21.1). Once tension is developed in the band, the scapulae are maximally retracted for a count of 1 to 2 seconds. The player then returns to the starting position with a controlled eccentric response.

Step-Up with Thera-Band Loop Resistance

A loop of elastic resistance is used along with a 6 to 8 inch step (Figure 21.2). The athlete places the loop around the wrist and steps up onto the platform with one hand

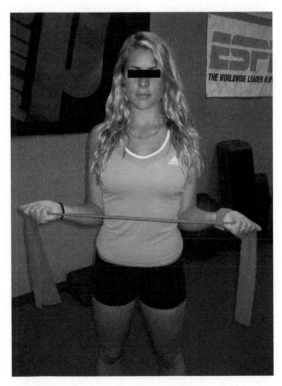

FIGURE 21-1. External rotation with retraction.

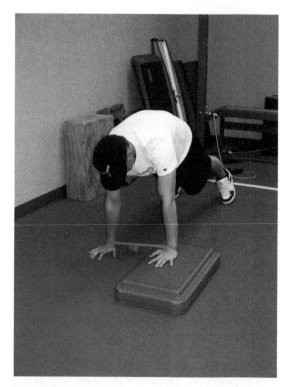

FIGURE 21-2.   Step-up with Thera-band loop resistance.

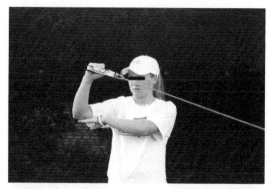

FIGURE 21-3.   90°/90° external rotation.

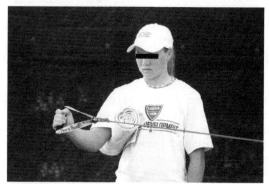

FIGURE 21-4.   Neutral external rotation.

followed by the second hand. An exaggerated protracted or "plus" position is held and the hands are one by one returned to the starting position. This exercise can be started off the knees initially and progressed to the full hands and toes position.

90°/90° External Rotation

In a standing position, secure a piece of elastic resistance to a fence or in a door (Figure 21.3). Start with the arm in 90° elevation in the scapular plane (30° forward from the coronal plane) and from a position of neutral rotation (forearm horizontal) externally rotate the shoulder until the forearm is nearly vertical. Slowly return to the starting position and repeat.

Neutral External Rotation

In a standing position, place a rolled up towel under the exercising arm (Figure 21.4). Secure elastic tubing in a door at nearly waist level. Begin with the hand nearly against the stomach (internal rotation). Keeping the elbow flexed 90°, externally rotate the shoulder gaining tension in the band until the hand is pointing direction straight ahead out in front of you. Slowly return to the starting position.

Prone Horizontal Abduction

Lie on a treatment table or counter top with arm hanging over the edge (see Figure 21.5A). Point the thumb outward

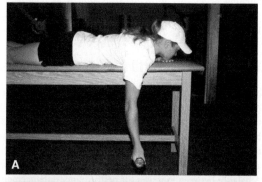

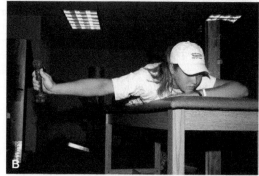

FIGURE 21-5.   Prone horizontal abduction. (A) Start position. (B) End position.

(externally rotate the extremity) and raise the arm out to the side until it is nearly horizontal (see Figure 21.5B). Keep the thumb pointed outward and elbow straight. Slowly return to the starting position.

Elbow

Ball Dribbling

Using a playground ball or basketball, repetitively and rapidly dribble the ball against a wall at eye level (shoulder is approximately 60° to 80° elevated) (Figure 21.6). This should be done for endurance and repeated maximally for sets of 30 seconds or more.

Medicine Ball Snaps

In a seated position and using a 1 kg medicine ball that bounces, snap the wrist downward into flexion catching the ball upon its return to the hand (Figure 21.7). Repeat for multiple sets of 15 to 20 repetitions. Note that it is important to isolate the movement such that only wrist flexion occurs and not elbow flexion extension as a substitution.

Tricep Extension in 90° Shoulder Elevation

This tennis-specific exercise involves resisted elbow extension with the shoulder in 90° elevation (shoulder level) (Figure 21.8). Using elastic resistance secured at shoulder level in a door or a fence, stand such that resistance occurs

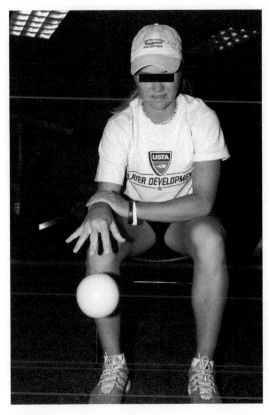

FIGURE 21-7.   Medicine ball snap.

as the elbow is extended or straightened against the resistance of the tubing. Slowly return to the starting position.

Trunk (Core)

Pointer (Bird-Dog) Exercise

This exercise emphasizes extensor muscle activation (Figure 21.9). The use of a tennis racquet can enhance

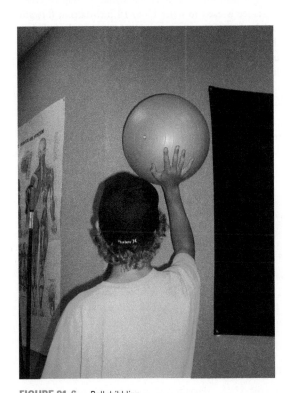

FIGURE 21-6.   Ball dribbling.

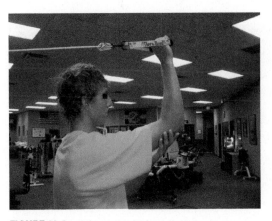

FIGURE 21-8.   Triceps extension.

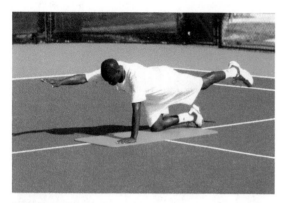

FIGURE 21-9. Pointer (bird-dog) exercise.

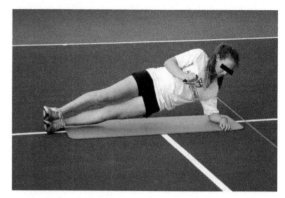

FIGURE 21-11. Side plank with unilateral row.

the control aspect of this exercise when placed in the low back of the player during the paired extremity movements.

Russian Twist

Use of a Swiss ball provides additional trunk activation while torso rotation occurs as pictured (Figure 21.10). A 4 to 6 lb medicine ball is initially used to provide additional resistance. Ensure that the pelvis remains elevated during the exercise as players often sag from a nicely extended initial position.

Side Plank with Unilateral Row

This plank variation combines important scapular stabilization with core stability training (Figure 21.11). A rowing motion is resisted with elastic resistance while a side or lateral plank exercise is executed.

Plyometric Sit-Up with Medicine Ball

This paired exercise allows for overload provided by the medicine ball to the player while lying across a Swiss ball (Figure 21.12).

Hip/Lower Body

Granny Toss Plyometrics

This explosive exercise involves using a medicine ball and using exaggerated leg drive to throw the ball upward with the entire lower extremity kinetic chain (Figure 21.13). The athlete tracks the ball and catches it after landing and repeats the exercise for multiple explosive repetitions and sets.

Thera-Band Kicks on Balance Platform

Using a platform and unilateral stance, a loop of elastic resistance is used to resist 12 to 18 inch lateral, forward, and backward repetitive movements to produce fatigue (Figure 21.14). Sets of 30 seconds of lateral, then forward, and finally backward movement are utilized to build hip and core strength and endurance.

Clam Shell/Reverse Clam Shell

Using a loop of elastic resistance, hip internal and external rotation are performed against resistance (Figure 21.15). The loop is applied at the level of the knees for external

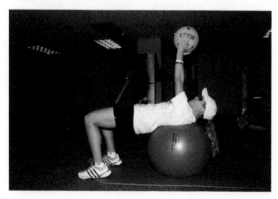

FIGURE 21-10. Russian twist.

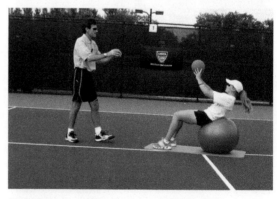

FIGURE 21-12. Plyometric sit-up with medicine ball.

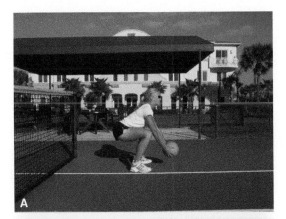

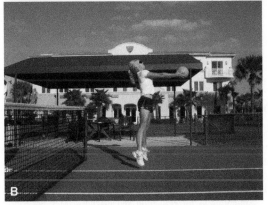

FIGURE 21-13. Granny toss plyometrics. (A) Start position. (B) Acceleration position.

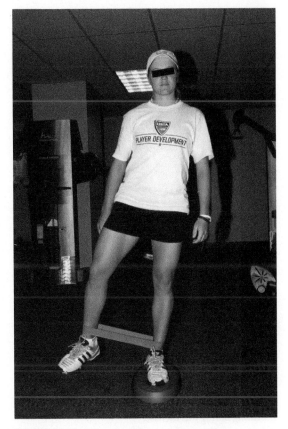

FIGURE 21-14. Thera-band kicks on balance platform.

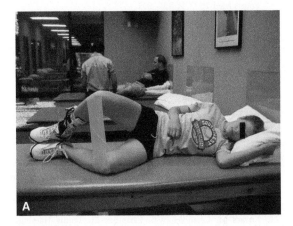

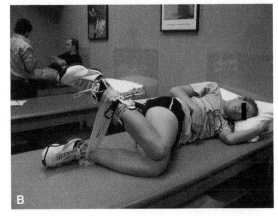

FIGURE 21-15. Clam shell/reverse clam shell. (A) External rotation. (B) Internal rotation.

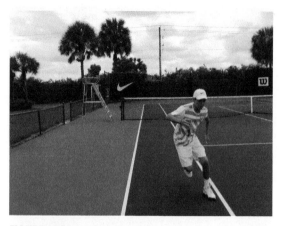

FIGURE 21-16. Alley hop.

rotation strengthening and around the ankles for hip internal rotation strengthening.

Alley Hops

A lateral lunging motion is used across the alley of the tennis court repetitively using a soft landing that promotes eccentric weight acceptance (Figure 21.16). Care is taken to maintain an upright body position with the upper body and keep the eyes forward as they would during tennis play instead of looking downward which can create slouched posturing during this exercise.

SUMMARY

The use of the exercises provided in this chapter can provide a valuable training stimulus to both developing and elite-level tennis players. The focus of these exercises is on both the injury patterns and tennis-specific demands reported in the sport science literature. Coupling these exercises with a complete conditioning and overall training program that includes optimal nutrition and hydration, as well as on-court tennis drills can assist players in achieving and maintaining their optimum potential.

REFERENCES

1. Pluim BM, Staal JB. Tennis injuries in Olympic sports. In: Caine D, Harmer P, Schiff M, eds. Encyclopedia of Sports Medicine. Hoboken, NJ: Wiley-Blackwell; 2009. ISBN 9781405173643.
2. Ellenbecker TS, Pluim B, Vivier S, Sniteman C. Common injuries in tennis players. Exercises to address muscular imbalances and reduce injury risk. Strength Cond 2009;31(4):50–58.
3. Ryu KN, McCormick J, Jobe FW, et al. An electromyographic analysis of shoulder function in tennis players. Am J Sports Med 1988;16:481–485.
4. Johnson CD, McHugh MP. Performance demands of professional male tennis players. Br J Sports Med 2006;40:696–699.
5. Ellenbecker TS, Roetert EP. Age specific isokinetic glenohumeral internal and external rotation strength in elite junior tennis players. J Sci Med Sport 2003;6(1):63–70.
6. Ellenbecker TS, Roetert EP, Piorkowski PA. Shoulder internal and external rotation range of motion of elite junior tennis players: a comparison of two protocols. J Orthop Sports Phys Ther 1993;17:65.
7. Ellenbecker TS, Roetert EP, Bailie DS, Davies GJ, Brown SW. Glenohumeral joint total rotation range of motion in elite tennis players and baseball pitchers. Med Sci Sports Exerc 2002;34(12):2052–2056.
8. Burkart SS, Morgan CD, Kibler WB. The disabled throwing shoulder: spectrum of pathology: part I. Arthroscopy 2003;19:404–420.
9. Nirschl RP, Ashman ES. Tennis elbow tendinosis (epicondylitis). Instr Course Lect 2004;53:587–598.
10. Nirschl RP, Sobel J. Conservative treatment of tennis elbow. Phys Sports Med 1981;9:43–54.
11. Elliott BC, Mester J, Kleinoder H, Yue Z. Loading and stroke production. In: Elliott BC, Reid M, Crespo M, eds. Biomechanics of Advanced Tennis. London: International Tennis Federation; 2003:93–108.
12. Segal DK. Tenis Sistema Biodinamico. Buenos Aires, Argentina: Tenis Club Argentino; 2002.
13. Kibler WB. Clinical biomechanics of the elbow in tennis. Implications for evaluation and diagnosis. Med Sci Sports Exerc 1994;26:1203–1206.
14. Hainline B. Low back injury. Clin Sports Med 1995;14(1):241–266.
15. Alyas F, Turner M, Connell D. MRI findings in the lumbar spines of asymptomatic adolescent elite tennis players. Br J Sports Med 2007;41:836–841.
16. Roetert EP, McCormick TJ, Brown SW, Ellenbecker TS. Relationship between isokinetic and functional trunk strength in elite junior tennis players. Isokinet Exerc Sci 1996;6:15–20.
17. Ellenbecker TS, Roetert EP, Bailie DS, Davies GJ, Brown SW. Glenohumeral joint total rotation range of motion in elite tennis players and baseball pitchers. Med Sci Sports Exerc 2002;34:2052–2056.
18. Kovacs M. Movement for tennis. The importance of lateral training. Strength Cond 2009;31(4):77–85.
19. Byrd JWT. Hip arthroscopy in athletes. Operative Tech Sports Med 2005;13(1):24–36.
20. Ellenbecker TS, Ellenbecker GA, Roetert EP, Silva RT, Keuter G, Sperling F. Descriptive profile of hip rotation range of motion in elite tennis players and professional baseball pitchers. Am J Sports Med 2007;35(8):1371–1376.
21. Kovacs M, Chandler WB, Chandler TJ. Tennis Training. Vista, CA: Racquet Tech Publishing; 2007.
22. Roetert EP, Ellenbecker TS. Complete Conditioning for Tennis. Champaign, IL: Human Kinetics; 1997.

CHAPTER 22

Kyle B. Kiesel and Phillip J. Plisky

Establishing Functional Baselines and Appropriate Training for Off-Season Conditioning and Injury Prevention

TESTING: WHY?

The goal is to keep athletes on the field performing at the highest level possible. But we need to take a step back and acknowledge something obvious: if athletes get hurt or play hurt, they cannot perform at their best. We need to think of testing for performance and injury prevention as two different sides of the same coin. Fortunately, with athletes we have multiple opportunities to improve performance and decrease injury risk. We strive for a continuum of injury prevention (Figure 22.1), and in this chapter we focus on the off-season.

As sports injury researchers, we know that we need to establish the extent of the problem, identify risk factors, implement preventative measures, and then reassess their effectiveness. This chapter takes the injury prevention research model and applies it to individual athletes. There are currently numerous prevention programs, but we have not seen a concomitant decrease in injury rates (1). Researchers are finding that while group prevention programs are effective, they do not reduce the risk of everyone and the risk reduction does not decrease each athlete's level to low risk (2).

SUCCESS IN INJURY PREVENTION: HOW ARE WE DOING?

The first reaction might be that we, as rehabilitation and strength and conditioning professionals, are doing all that we can for the athletes in our care and that injury is random and unpredictable. Further, we might think that once a player is sidelined with an injury, the course back to playing is certain and outcomes are good. However, research shows that may not be the case. A systematic review (48 studies evaluating 5,770 participants at a mean follow-up of 41.5 months) of anterior cruciate ligament (ACL) reconstruction outcomes found (3) that only 63% returned to preinjury level of participation and only 44% returned to competitive sport at final follow-up. Interestingly, approximately 90% achieved normal knee function based on traditional impairment measures such as strength. Further, 30% of these athletes will go on to tear the reconstructed or contralateral ACL (4,5). Clearly, as rehabilitation and strength and conditioning professionals, we are not as successful as we might have thought. We need to know how our athletes are doing at discharge, in the preseason, and in the off-season. This can be accomplished only through comprehensive, systematic testing.

INJURY RISK FACTORS IN SPORT

The modifiable intrinsic risk factors identified by prospective cohort studies include body mass index, dynamic balance, faulty movement patterns, and knee alignment with landing and training load (6–10). Previous injury is not frequently included in this list because it is considered nonmodifiable. Not surprisingly, previous injury is the most robust risk factor for future injury as identified by over 25 prospective cohort studies. Given the plethora of research demonstrating that modifiable motor control changes remain after injury, it would be prudent to include it in the list of modifiable risk factors. Since previous injury is the most robust risk factor for future injury, we need to understand and address it through the examination of the modifiable risk factors that remain after injury.

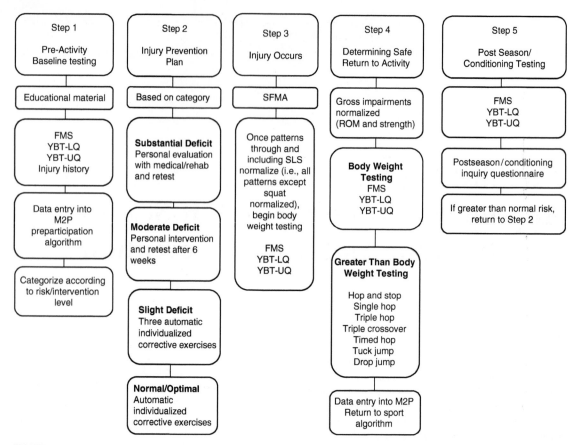

FIGURE 22-1. Systematic injury prevention for sports, military, and fitness. FMS, Functional Movement Screen™; M2P, Move2Perform; ROM, range of motion; SFMA, Selective Functional Movement Assessment; SLS, single-leg stance; YBT-UQ/LQ, Y Balance Test™ upper and lower quarter. (Copyright 2012 Balanced EBP, LLC. Reprinted with permission from Balanced EBP, LLC.)

MOTOR CONTROL IMPAIRMENTS REMAINING AFTER REHABILITATION

It should be disturbing to rehabilitation professionals that previous injury is such a strong risk factor for future injury in sports. There are a number of possible conclusions one can draw from this fact including inadequate rehabilitation, early return to sport, and poor compliance with recommended rehabilitation. Additionally, we have proposed the notion that motor control changes related to injury are often retained, despite our rehabilitation efforts, and ultimately contribute to subsequent injury (11).

When considering motor control changes as they relate to injury, the ankle and low back pain (LBP) literature provides substantial evidence that motor control changes exist after injury and help to support the need for proper motor control–oriented testing. For example, in individuals with chronic ankle instability, significant muscle activation latency differences were found in the gluteus medius muscle

when a simple inversion perturbation was applied (12). Another study demonstrated significantly delayed onset times for the ankle, hip, and hamstring muscles in subjects with a history of ankle sprain when compared with control subjects when performing a basic transition from double limb to single-limb stance (13). Yet another study reported a delay in onset of activation of the gluteus maximums in previously injured subjects, again when compared with controls (14). These data suggest that an altered motor control strategy persists following chronic ankle sprain and the deficits are identifiable during low-level, body weight tasks as simple as transitioning from bilateral to unilateral stance.

A series of well-designed and executed research studies on how LBP affects motor control have helped the understanding of true core muscle function and how this function changes after a painful episode. While studying various aspects of core muscle function in athletes (300+), Cholewicki et al. have shown that altered outer core muscle activation is present in athletes with a history of LBP who were pain-free at the time they were tested (15,16). This research has demonstrated that the central nervous system increases input into the muscles of the outer core and that outer core muscles tend to stay on longer during automatic reaction tasks in athletes with a history of LBP when compared with controls. This suggests that an alteration in the timing and coordination of outer core muscles exists in athletes with a history of LBP. This is not traditional muscle weakness; rather, it is another demonstration that motor control changes exist after injury. Although subtle, these motor control changes are thought to have consequences including increased compressive loads on the spine, increased metabolic cost, and breathing pattern changes (17–19), and ultimately they may contribute to impaired functional movement patterns such as lunging, reaching, balancing, or squatting.

A study demonstrating a functional representation of poor movement following LBP suggested again that altered movement patterns persist after the LBP has resolved. This research showed that athletes with a history of LBP, pain-free at the time of the study, demonstrated a slower time on a simple shuttle run as compared with matched controls without a history of LBP (20). This may, in part, be due to altered core muscle activation and subsequent attenuation of the functional movement required to change directions and bend down to touch the floor during a shuttle run and may, in part, be identifiable with functional movement-oriented testing.

It is important to recognize that all of these studies were performed on subjects who were pain-free and fully functional at the time they were tested. This helps us to understand that motor control changes occur following injury and not only at the site of injury, but rather muscles several joints away and on the contralateral side are affected. This demonstrates that a complete change in motor control has occurred. Taken as a whole, these studies provide evidence that profound changes occur and, as stated by one of the authors, support the need to "extend the assessment beyond the side and site of injury." We would suggest not only assessment beyond the side and site of injury, but a motor control–oriented assessment because traditional strength and range of motion testing may not be adequate to identify the motor control changes that are clearly present following injury.

FIELD-BASED OFF-SEASON TESTING

Since previous injury is the most commonly identified risk factor for future injury and modifiable risk factors remain after injury, we need easily implementable tests to perform in the off-season to identify the motor control changes that may have occurred from injury (known or unknown) during the season. Further, we complete this testing so we can identify what to remove from conditioning programs so as to

not compromise movement. Simultaneously, we can implement effective, individualized injury prevention education and training. This testing also provides a functional baseline as a checkpoint at the beginning of the season to ensure that athletes maintain functional patterns when they are not with us. This functional testing also serves an important role in the injury prevention continuum by providing a baseline for return to sport testing in the event of injury. This also ultimately helps the sports medicine team work together by ensuring that everyone is on the same page and using the same language to discuss the current status of all their athletes. Professional sports teams cite that this is one of the greatest benefits.

While we have described a number of research studies that utilize time-consuming tests that are not mass deployable, we also realize that this information can be overwhelming. Thus, we developed this comprehensive approach to off-season testing, utilizing the following guidelines. The tests selected should be

1. Evidence-based
2. Reliable
3. Predictive of injury
4. Valid (discriminate)
5. Modifiable
6. Practical

The tests that meet these criteria are the upper and lower quarter Y Balance Test™ (YBT-UQ and YBT-LQ, respectively) and the Functional Movement Screen™ (FMS). The YBT-LQ protocol has been shown to possess good inter- and intrarater reliability (21). The YBT-LQ protocol requires the athlete to maintain single-limb stance control while reaching with the free lower limb in the anterior, posteromedial, and posterolateral reach directions, followed by returning to the start position (Figure 22.2). It is designed to challenge the athlete's balance at her limit of stability. Overall performance score on the YBT is calculated by averaging the greatest normalized reach distance in each direction. Absolute differences between left and right lower limb reach distances are also examined to assess symmetry. High school basketball players and collegiate football players with asymmetry or scoring poorly compared with age, gender, and sport risk cut-point on the YBT-LQ were more likely to become injured (9,22). In addition, researchers have reported that poor performance on the YBT-LQ can identify individuals with an existing chronic lower extremity injury (ankle sprain, patellofemoral pain syndrome, or ACL tear) (23–29). That is to say, the YBT-LQ potentially identifies the motor control changes that remain after injury. Simply, the athlete must demonstrate symmetry (no greater than 4 cm difference in the anterior reach and 6 cm in the posterior reaches) and a composite score above the at-risk cut-point for the specific age, gender, and sport.

The YBT-UQ is a similar test for the upper extremity and trunk that challenges the athlete at the limit of stability

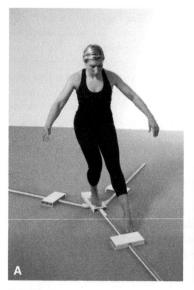
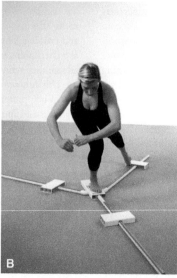
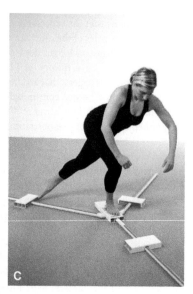

FIGURE 22-2.   Lower quarter Y Balance Test™ components. (A) Anterior reach. (B) Posteromedial reach. (C) Posterolateral reach.

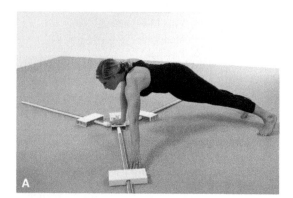
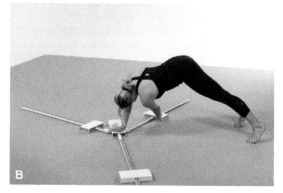
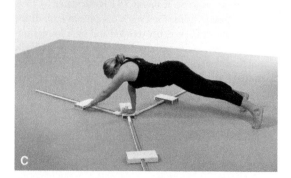

FIGURE 22-3.   Upper quarter Y Balance Test™ components. (A) Medial reach. (B) Inferolateral reach. (C) Superolateral reach.

while simultaneously requiring mobility of the entire upper limb and trunk. The YBT-UQ protocol requires the athlete to maintain a wide base push-up position with one arm while reaching with the free upper limb in the medial, inferolateral, and superolateral reach directions, followed by returning to the start position (Figure 22.3). The YBT-UQ has demonstrated excellent intra- and inter-rater reliability as well as discriminate and concurrent validity (30,31). The test has been suggested as a preparticipation as well as a return to sport test for athletes who heavily utilize overhead and rotational movement. One author concluded, "Similarity in performance bilaterally indicates that reach distances on this test using a non-injured UE (whether dominant or not) may serve as a reasonable baseline measure when comparing an injured and uninjured UE" (31) (UE signifies upper extremity).

Another test of movement competency is the FMS. The FMS ranks a series of seven fundamental movement patterns that require flexibility, mobility, and stability (Figure 22.4) (32,33). Three FMS clearing tests are also used to identify pain (Figure 22.5). The FMS has been

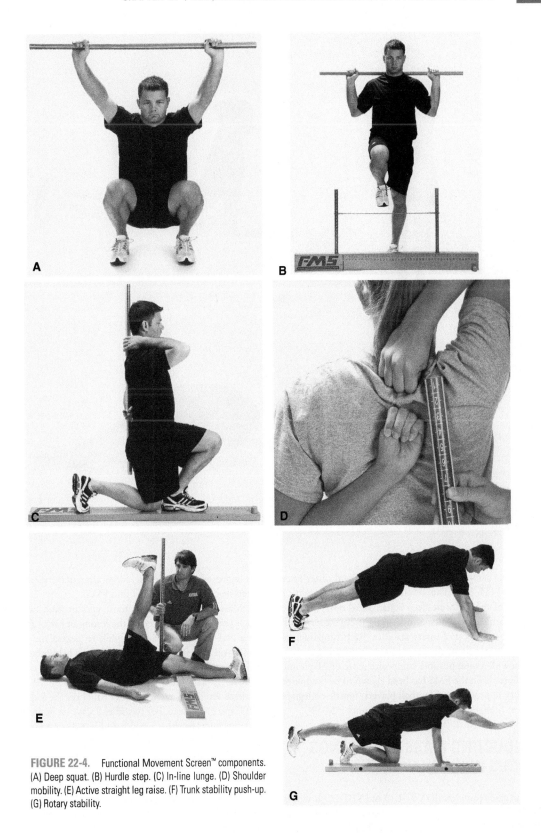

FIGURE 22-4. Functional Movement Screen™ components. (A) Deep squat. (B) Hurdle step. (C) In-line lunge. (D) Shoulder mobility. (E) Active straight leg raise. (F) Trunk stability push-up. (G) Rotary stability.

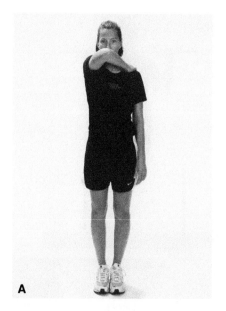

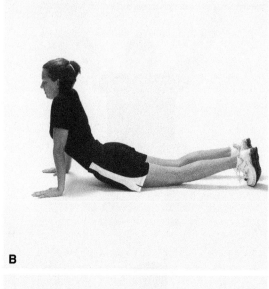

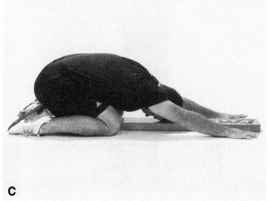

FIGURE 22-5. Functional Movement Screen™ (FMS) clearing tests. (A) Shoulder pain provocation test (used with shoulder mobility component of FMS). (B) Press-up extension test (used with trunk stability push-up component of FMS). (C) Posterior rocking test (used with rotary stability component of FMS).

shown to demonstrate excellent intra- and inter-rater reliability (34–38). The seven fundamental movement patterns of the FMS are deep squat, hurdle step, in-line lunge, shoulder mobility, active straight leg raise, trunk stability push-up, and rotary stability. Each fundamental movement is individually scored (0, 1, 2, 3) using scoring criteria with a total possible composite score of 21 points. A lower score on the FMS has been shown to be predictive of injury in professional football players, female collegiate athletes, firefighters, and military personnel (39–42).

CONDUCTING MASS SCREENINGS VERSUS INDIVIDUAL TESTING

You can easily complete the YBT-UQ and YBT-LQ as well as the FMS in 20 minutes per athlete. If you allow 30 minutes per athlete, you will have time to prescribe personalized corrective exercises to each individual. It is highly recommended

for improved consistency in scoring and intervention that all raters be certified in the YBT and FMS.

Mass screening requires more coordination and staff. Each year we are involved in the testing of over 1,000 athletes and it has taken quite a while to perfect the process, so we will describe our current system to help others avoid mistakes we have made. For example, we test 175 collegiate athletes in 2.5 hours and give approximately 100 of the athletes three corrective exercises based on the individual's YBT and FMS score. For the other 75, we set up individual appointments to either provide additional corrective strategies (e.g., isolated stretching or trigger point work) or complete a Selective Functional Movement Assessment (SFMA) from a trained healthcare provider to initiate treatment for pain identified.

As you read this, you may be thinking that you do not have the resources (time, staff, or money) to do all this screening and intervention. Most frequently, the programs that have successfully implemented systematic, comprehensive screening have limited staff and financial resources. One of the ways to manage this is to allocate the resources to those who need it. Current trends in evidence-based medicine are to individualize intervention programs by matching specific treatments to appropriate patients (43,44). Off-season testing and individualized programming requires a similar process, in which each athlete is categorized by a composite of individual risk factors. Sports medicine professionals can then more accurately direct appropriate treatments and allocate resources to those at increased risk for injury.

A study by Lehr et al. examined categorizing athletes into four groups according to resource allocation (based on risk). At the start of the season, 183 collegiate athletes across multiple sports (including soccer) were tested on YBT, FMS, and injury history. Their scores were then entered into the Move2Perform (Move2Perform, Evansville, IN) software that uses an evidence-based algorithm to classify the athlete into one of four risk categories. The algorithm calculates and weights the FMS composite score, individual FMS test scores, results of FMS clearing tests, presence of asymmetry on any of the five bilateral FMS movements, pain during testing, previous injury, YBT-LQ asymmetry, and YBT-LQ composite score below the risk threshold for the individual athlete (Table 22.1). The YBT-LQ composite score risk threshold is determined by the algorithm based on competition level (i.e., junior high, high school, college, and professional), sport, and gender of the athlete.

If the athlete was in the moderate or substantial risk category, they were 3.4 times (95% CI 2.0 to 6.0) more likely to get injured. Interestingly, no one in the normal category got injured. In a subsequent analysis, there were four noncontact ACL injuries: three were in the high-risk group and one in the slightly increased risk group.

Mass Screening Logistics

The key to screening large groups is preparation. Once you determine how many athletes you need to screen and which tests you are performing, you need to determine the staff and your equipment needs.

Choosing the Tests

Ideally, all athletes receive an FMS and a YBT-UQ and YBT-LQ. At a minimum, all athletes receive an FMS and a YBT-LQ. Only overhead athletes (e.g., swimmers, throwers, and volleyball players) additionally receive the YBT-UQ.

To make the screening as efficient as possible, the athletes should come in groups of about 20 and watch YBT instructional videos. These videos outline the instructions for performing the test. The athletes then go to "practice stations" with athletic tape affixed to the floor in the shape of the YBT. The athletes then practice six reach directions on each leg for the YBT-LQ and two practice trials on each arm for the YBT-UQ. We find that referring to this as a

| TABLE 22.1 | Sample Provider Risk Summary Report |

Lower Quarter Y Balance Test™

	Left	Right	Difference	Result
Anterior	65	62	3	Pass
Posteromedial	98	96	2	Optimal
Posterolateral	100	102	2	Optimal
Composite	92.3	91.2		Fail

Functional Movement Testing

Test		Raw Score	Final Score	Result
Deep squat		2	2	Pass
Hurdle step	L	2	2	Pass
	R	2		
In-line lunge	L	2	2	Pass
	R	2		
Shoulder mobility	L	2	2	Pass
	R	2		
Impingement clearing test	L	–		
	R	–		
Active straight leg raise	L	3	3	Optimal
	R	3		
Trunk stability push-up		2	2	Pass
Press-up clearing test		–		
Rotary stability	L	2	2	Pass
	R	2		
Posterior rocking clearing test		–		
Total			15	Pass

Injury risk: moderately increased.

Copyright 2009–2012 Move2perform, LLC. www.move2perform.com

"warm-up" improves athlete's compliance. You will want one person supervising the video and warm-up. This person also directs athletes to the open stations for testing. This is a great position for a coach or support personnel.

Great efficiency can be gained from using the station format for movement screening. Depending on the number of staff and athletes tested, the tests are broken up into stations. Each examiner performs two to three tests that are grouped by body position and complexity. Typically the following work well together, but any logical grouping works: FMS rotary stability/trunk stability push-up, in-line lunge/hurdle step, FMS shoulder mobility/upper limb length measurement/deep squat, and FMS active straight leg raise/lower limb measurement.

Analysis, Reporting, and Intervention

As with any measurement system, an in-depth understanding of the information gained from testing is required to reach the goals of the program. Analysis should be conducted on multiple levels including for the individual, group, as well as possibly player position. Each athlete should have an individual report of performance on the testing with specific action steps. Researchers have found that certain elements should be present to accomplish behavior change regarding risk reduction. These elements include providing information that is personalized, tailored, and at the appropriate reading level (45–47).

Also, researchers have found that in sports it is important to focus on the context of performance benefits rather than risk reduction benefits (50). For example, in the individual report, the athletes' performance on the test is compared to his specific peer group (e.g., male collegiate basketball players). In addition to individual reporting, an overall team report should demonstrate the number of athletes in each risk category and the number of athletes who tested positive for each of the main risk factors, such as movement asymmetry (Figure 22.6). An overall assessment of the data at this level will help the sports medicine professional in a number of ways, including

1) evidence-based understanding of current team risk
2) a sense of resources and time that will be required to decrease team injury risk
3) a team-level assessment to help determine if current group programming is detrimental to functional movement standards
4) an objective and easy-to-understand communication tool for all stakeholders, including management, coaches, players, and parents.

In addition to analysis of the data at the team level, some may find it beneficial to assess the data for each sports position. For example, in American football, it may be helpful to analyze how the linebackers perform compared with the defensive backs and so on (Table 22.2). Position-level assessment of team data will also help to gauge readiness and risk more precisely and identify potential program-level changes that may be required. For example, in baseball, much attention is given to the shoulder function of pitchers. This is a well-studied population and there are a number of group programs available to

prevent injuries. Interestingly, our experience in professional baseball is that in general the pitchers scored fairly well on the functional movement tests described, but when we analyzed other positions there were substantial deficits. On one team, nearly all middle infielders demonstrated a major asymmetry on the shoulder mobility test. This emphasized the importance of performing these basic functional tests on all players on a regular basis.

Analysis at the team level is insightful and can assist the sports medicine team in many ways. However, to correct motor control deficits identified in testing, an individualized and evidence-based program is required. The individual report and subsequent corrective program is the key to managing functional movement deficits, reducing injury risk and ultimately providing the greatest potential for performance enhancement. An in-depth look into the philosophy and details at the root of the individualized corrective strategy is beyond the scope of this chapter, but recognize that the basis is derived from the science of motor learning and motor control rather than traditional strength and conditioning.

A number of studies demonstrate that attributes of functional movement testing are modifiable. When an individual program is prescribed, based on the results of the FMS, improvements have been documented in professional football players as well as firefighters (11,48). A large number of studies have shown that performance on the YBT improves with training. These have been based on group programming, including plyometric training and balance training programs. While it may be tempting to just give group plyometric and balance programs, remember that approach is what got us in trouble in the first place. Group programs are for those who have demonstrated movement competence. That way, they are not wasting time trying to perform plyometrics correctly when, in fact, they have an ankle mobility issue that will not resolve without specific intervention. It is our opinion that those in high-level group programs, such as plyometrics, who do not have some level of movement competency, may actually be creating a motor control problem by reinforcing their dysfunction with high repetitions of faulty movement. We have described that as

Your Group's Overall Injury Risk

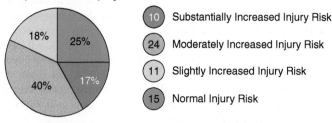

FIGURE 22-6.   Overall injury risk pie chart for active members of a football team using Move2Perform software, which synthesizes a variety of evidence-based factors to categorize each person's individual risk. Several published studies indicate that individuals who are in the substantially increased and moderately injury risk categories are three to six times more likely to get injured. (Copyright 2009–2012 Move2Perform, LLC. www.move2perform.com.)

TABLE 22.2 Report of Screening Tests to Determine Injury Risk for a Football Team

Lower Quarter Y Balance Test™

Direction	Left cm	Right cm	Difference Ave	# Asym	# Fail	# Pass	# Optimal
Anterior:	57.8	56.6	2.6	8	6	27	22
Posteromedial:	91.2	89.5	2.5	6	5	9	41
Posterolateral:	90.7	91.1	1.9	3	4	1	50
Composite:	89.9	89.1			13	30	12

Upper Quarter Y Balance Test™

Direction	Left cm	Right cm	Difference Ave	# Asym	# Fail	# Pass	# Optimal
Medial:	85	85.2	5.1	3	3	2	5
Inferolateral:	76.6	75.7	4.3	4	4	0	6
Superolateral:	58.2	54.4	6.7	4	4	0	6
Composite:	82.4	80.8			6	2	2

Functional Movement Testing

Test		Raw Score Ave	Final Score Ave	# Asym	# of 0's	# of 1's	# of 2's	# of 3's
Deep Squat:		1.7	1.7		0	11	32	0
Hurdle Step:	L	2	2	3	0	2	40	1
	R	2						
Inline Lunge:	L	2.1	2	3	0	2	37	4
	R	2.1						
Shoulder Mobility:	L	2	2	5	0	5	31	7
	R	2.2						
Impingement Clearing Test:	L	0						
	R	0						
Active Straight-Leg Raise:	L	2.5	2.5	2	0	2	19	22
	R	2.5						
Trunk Stability Pushup:		1.8	1.8		0	8	35	0
Press-Up Clearing Test:		0						
Rotary Stability:	L	1.9	1.8	6	1	7	34	1
	R	1.9						
Posterior Rocking Clearing Test:		0						
Total:			13.9	19	1	37	228	35

"adding strength and power to dysfunction" which yields a stronger or more powerfully dysfunctional athlete.

Individually prescribed programs, based on the results of functional movement testing, also include isolated trigger point work and stretching. This point is important as often an athlete will retain a muscle trigger point, possibly from a motor control response to a previous injury, that will otherwise go undetected and be reinforced and continue to contribute to dysfunctional patterns of movement. When such trigger points are addressed, the motor learning environment is enriched, contributing to movement restoration.

Individual corrective exercise prescription is time consuming and can be a substantial drain on team resources.

Technology can be helpful in this case. The sports medicine professional can consider the use of automated programming that has been proven to increase efficiency. Time saving gained from the utilization of the Move2Perform software was highlighted in a study by Teyhen et al. (49). This study demonstrated that automatically generated individual reports saved over 3 minutes per subject compared with manually generating reports. In addition, the researchers found a significant reduction in the time needed to prescribe an individual corrective program. For example, automatically prescribing three exercises-based FMS, YBT-LQ, and YBT-UQ score via the Move2Perform software saved 11.5 minutes/soldier relative to manual exercise prescription. From a practical implementation perspective, athletes who are at the lower risk/resource levels can be given evidence-based individual reports with three personalized exercises to incorporate into the warm-up with little time cost to the tester.

Proper analysis and use of the information gained from functional movement testing can be utilized in a number of ways to improve the readiness and reduce risk for any team. The team report will allow for communication while the team and position analysis will help to successfully modify the group program to avoid the perpetuation of dysfunctional patterns. Ultimately, the individual report provides each athlete with a functional movement profile and risk level allowing for an individualized approach to injury prevention and performance enhancement. This sets the stage for appropriate retesting postinjury if needed, and across the continuum of a strength and conditioning year.

SUMMARY

To address the high prevalence of injury in sport as well as the suboptimal outcomes after injury, we need to implement a comprehensive system of testing. This should include testing prior to start of season, testing as part of return to sport protocol postinjury, testing at end of season, and testing as needed at the start of each major strength cycle. Integrating intermittent testing with individually tailored programs based on the potential for repeated injury dramatically improves the performance of individual athletes and, therefore, the team's success.

Practical Example of Comprehensive, Systematic Off-Season Testing

A college conducts a systematic, comprehensive off-season testing program of 250 athletes from multiple sports. From the Move2Perform software it is determined that 37 athletes are in the high-intervention (high-risk) group, 55 athletes are in the moderate-intervention (moderate-risk) group, 118 athletes are in the slight-intervention (slight-risk) group, 40 athletes are in the normal-intervention (normal-risk) group. The athletes in the high-risk group are seen by the rehabilitation staff since they have pain or injury and are evaluated and treated with the SFMA until the top tier patterns of the SFMA normalize. They are then retested with the FMS, YBT-LQ, and YBT-UQ. The moderate group is seen individually by a member of the rehabilitation or strength and conditioning staff and given corrective exercises, manual therapy techniques as needed, and partner stretching. The moderate group is retested after 6 weeks of corrective activities to ensure they have moved to the lower risk categories. The slight and normal groups are

given three corrective exercises to incorporate into the team warm-up. From the group reporting, it is noted that most of the football linemen have asymmetrical shoulder mobility pattern and so in the linemen's program, additional shoulder mobility corrective exercises are added. Most importantly, strength-related pressing may be modified in the lineman's strength and conditioning program since it is likely contributing to or at least exacerbating the asymmetrical patterns.

REFERENCES

1. Bahr R, Krosshaug T. Understanding injury mechanisms: a key component of preventing injuries in sport. Br J Sports Med 2005;39(6):324–329.
2. Myer GD, Ford KR, Brent JL, Hewett TE. Differential neuromuscular training effects on ACL injury risk factors in "high-risk" versus "low-risk" athletes. BMC Musculoskelet Disord 2007;8:39.
3. Ardern CL, Taylor NF, Feller JA, Webster KE. Return-to-sport outcomes at 2 to 7 years after anterior cruciate ligament reconstruction surgery. Am J Sports Med 2012;40(1):41–48.
4. Paterno MV, Rauh MJ, Schmitt LC, Ford KR, Hewett TE. Incidence of contralateral and ipsilateral anterior cruciate ligament (ACL) injury after primary ACL reconstruction and return to sport. Clin J Sport Med 2012;22(2):116–121.
5. Ververidis A, Verettas D, Kazakos K, Xarchas K, Drosos G, Psillakis I. Anterior cruciate ligament reconstruction: outcome using a patellar tendon bone (PTB) autograft (one bone block technique). Arch Orthop Trauma Surg 2009;129(3):323–331.
6. Dahle LK, Mueller MJ, Delitto A, Diamond JE. Visual assessment of foot type and relationship of foot type to lower extremity injury. J Orthop Sports Phys Ther 1991;14(2):70–74.
7. Gomez JE, Ross SK, Calmbach WL, Kimmel RB, Schmidt DR, Dhanda R. Body fatness and increased injury rates in high school football linemen. Clin J Sport Med 1998;8(2):115–120.
8. Krivickas LS, Feinberg JH. Lower extremity injuries in college athletes: relation between ligamentous laxity and lower extremity muscle tightness. Arch Phys Med Rehabil 1996;77(11):1139–1143.
9. Plisky PJ, Rauh MJ, Kaminski TW, Underwood FB. Star Excursion Balance Test as a predictor of lower extremity injury in high school basketball players. J Orthop Sports Phys Ther 2006;36(12):911–919.
10. Turbeville SD, Cowan LD, Owen WL, Asal NR, Anderson MA. Risk factors for injury in high school football players. Am J Sports Med 2003;31(6):974–980.
11. Kiesel K, Plisky P, Butler R. Functional movement test scores improve following a standardized off-season intervention program in professional football players. Scand J Med Sci Sports 2011;21(2):287–292.
12. Beckman SM, Buchanan TS. Ankle inversion injury and hypermobility: effect on hip and ankle muscle electromyography

onset latency. Arch Phys Med Rehabil 1995;76(12): 1138–1143.

13. Van Deun S, Staes FF, Stappaerts KH, Janssens L, Levin O, Peers KK. Relationship of chronic ankle instability to muscle activation patterns during the transition from double-leg to single-leg stance. Am J Sports Med 2007;35(2):274–281.

14. Bullock-Saxton JE, Janda V, Bullock MI. The influence of ankle sprain injury on muscle activation during hip extension. Int J Sports Med 1994;15(6):330–334.

15. Cholewicki J, Greene HS, Polzhofer GK, Galloway MT, Shah RA, Radebold A. Neuromuscular function in athletes following recovery from a recent acute low back injury. J Orthop Sports Phys Ther 2002;32(11):568–575.

16. Cholewicki J, Silfies SP, Shah RA, et al. Delayed trunk muscle reflex responses increase the risk of low back injuries. Spine 2005;30(23):2614–2620.

17. Kolar P, Sulc J, Kyncl M, et al. Postural function of the diaphragm in persons with and without chronic low back pain. J Orthop Sports Phys Ther 2012;42(4):352–62.

18. McLaughlin L, Goldsmith CH, Coleman K. Breathing evaluation and retraining as an adjunct to manual therapy. Man Ther 2011;16(1):51–52.

19. Whittaker JL. Ultrasound imaging of the lateral abdominal wall muscles in individuals with lumbopelvic pain and signs of concurrent hypocapnia. Man Ther 2008;13(5): 404–410.

20. Nadler SF, Malanga GA, Feinberg JH, Rubanni M, Moley P, Foye P. Functional performance deficits in athletes with previous lower extremity injury. Clin J Sport Med 2002;12(2):73–78.

21. Plisky PJ, Gorman PP, Butler RJ, Kiesel KB, Underwood FB, Elkins B. The reliability of an instrumented device for measuring components of the Star Excursion Balance Test. N Am J Sports Phys Ther 2009;4(2):92–99.

22. Lehr M, Plisky P, Bulter R, Kiesel K. Field expedient screening and an injury risk algorithm categories as predictors of non-contact lower extremity injury in collegiate athletes. Br J Sports Med 2013;23(4):e225–232 .

23. Akbari M, Karimi H, Farahini H, Faghihzadeh S. Balance problems after unilateral lateral ankle sprains. J Rehabil Res Dev 2006;43(7):819–824.

24. Aminaka N, Gribble PA. Patellar taping, patellofemoral pain syndrome, lower extremity kinematics, and dynamic postural control. J Athl Train 2008;43(1):21–28.

25. Hale SA, Hertel J, Olmsted-Kramer LC. The effect of a 4-week comprehensive rehabilitation program on postural control and lower extremity function in individuals with chronic ankle instability. J Orthop Sports Phys Ther 2007;37(6):303–311.

26. Herrington L, Hatcher J, Hatcher A, McNicholas M. A comparison of Star Excursion Balance Test reach distances between ACL deficient patients and asymptomatic controls. Knee 2009;16(2):149–152.

27. Hertel J, Braham RA, Hale SA, Olmsted-Kramer LC. Simplifying the Star Excursion Balance Test: analyses of subjects with and without chronic ankle instability. J Orthop Sports Phys Ther 2006;36(3):131–137.

28. Hubbard TJ, Kramer LC, Denegar CR, Hertel J. Contributing factors to chronic ankle instability. Foot Ankle Int 2007;28(3):343–354.

29. Olmsted LC, Carcia CR, Hertel J, Shultz SJ. Efficacy of the Star Excursion Balance Tests in detecting reach deficits in subjects with chronic ankle instability. J Athl Train 2002;37(4):501–506.

30. Gorman PP, Butler RJ, Plisky PJ, Kiesel KB. Upper Quarter Y Balance Test™: reliability and performance comparison between gender in active adults. J Strength Cond Res 2012;26(11):3043–3048.

31. Westrick R, Miller J, Carow S, Gerber JP. Exploration of the Y-balance test for assessment of upper quarter closed kinetic chain performance. Int J Sports Phys Ther 2012;7(2): 139–147.

32. Cook E. Movement. Aptos, CA: On Target Publishing; 2010.

33. Cook G, Burton L, Hoogenboom B. Pre-participation screening: the use of fundamental movements as an assessment of function—part 2. N Am J Sports Phys Ther 2006;1(3): 132–139.

34. Butler RJ, Plisky PJ. Reliability of the functional movement screen™ using a 100-point grading scale. Athl Train Sports Health Care 2012;4(3):103–109.

35. Frohm A, Heijne A, Kowalski J, Svensson P, Myklebust G. A nine-test screening battery for athletes: a reliability study. Scand J Med Sci Sports 2012;22(3):306–15.

36. Minick KI, Kiesel KB, Burton L, Taylor A, Plisky P, Butler RJ. Interrater reliability of the functional movement screen™. J Strength Cond Res 2010;24(2):479–486.

37. Schneiders AG, Davidsson A, Horman E, Sullivan SJ. Functional movement screen™ normative values in a young, active population. Int J Sports Phys Ther 2011;6(2):75–82.

38. Teyhen DS, Shaffer SW, Lorenson CL, et al. The functional movement screen™: a reliability study. J Orthop Sports Phys Ther 2012;42(6):530–540.

39. Butler RJ, Contreras M, Burton L, Plisky PJ, Kiesel KB. Modifiable risk factors predict injuries in firefighter during training academies. Work 2013;46(1):11–7.

40. Chorba RS, Chorba DJ, Bouillon LE, Overmyer CA, Landis JA. Use of a functional movement screening tool to determine injury risk in female collegiate athletes. N Am J Sports Phys Ther 2010;5(2):47–54.

41. Kiesel K, Plisky PJ, Voight ML. Can serious injury in professional football be predicted by a preseason functional movement screen™? N Am J Sports Phys Ther 2007;2(3): 147–158.

42. O'Connor FG, Deuster PA, Davis J, Pappas CG, Knapik JJ. Functional movement screening: predicting injuries in officer candidates. Med Sci Sports Exerc 2011;43(12):2224–30.

43. Brennan GP, Fritz JM, Hunter SJ, Thackeray A, Delitto A, Erhard RE. Identifying subgroups of patients with acute/subacute "nonspecific" low back pain: results of a randomized clinical trial. Spine (Phila Pa 1976) 2006;31(6): 623–631.

44. Childs JD, Fritz JM, Flynn TW, et al. A clinical prediction rule to identify patients with low back pain most likely to benefit from spinal manipulation: a validation study. Ann Intern Med 2004;141(12):920–928.

45. Guillen S, Sanna A, Ngo J, Meneu T, del Hoyo E, Demeester M. New technologies for promoting a healthy diet and active living. Nutr Rev 2009;67(Suppl 1):S107–S110.

46. Hovell MF, Mulvihill MM, Buono MJ, et al. Culturally tailored aerobic exercise intervention for low-income Latinas. Am J Health Promot 2008;22(3):155–163.

47. Kreuter MW, Strecher VJ. Changing inaccurate perceptions of health risk: results from a randomized trial. Health Psychol 1995;14(1):56–63.

48. Peate WF, Bates G, Lunda K, Francis S, Bellamy K. Core strength: a new model for injury prediction and prevention. J Occup Med Toxicol 2007;2:3.

49. Teyhen DS, Shaffer SW, Umlauf JA, et al. Automation to improve efficiency of field expedient injury prediction screening. J Strength Cond Res 2012;26(Suppl 2): S61–S72.

50. Cite Finch et al Finch C, White P, Twomey D, Ullah S. Implementing an exercise-training programme to prevent lower-limb injuries. Br J Sports Med. 2011;45(10): 791-796.

Running in Sport

INTRODUCTION

"When can I start running?" This is a common question clinicians hear in the office all the time. "My doctor said I could start running at 8 weeks after my injury." This is another common phrase rehabilitation specialists will hear. As if something miraculous were to happen on a physiological level between 7 weeks and 6 days, and 8 weeks. We are well aware that human physiology simply does not work that way. We know the body needs time to adapt to stress and we need to gradually load tissue in order to have it adapt to the load placed on it (1). If we allow the principles of supercompensation to work, our body will respond with stronger, more resistant tissue. If we do not follow these principles, the tissues we are stressing will sustain microtrauma, which will gradually become pain and injury. No matter what tissue in the body is trying to heal (bone, muscle, tendon, and ligament), these basic physiological overloading principles apply (1). We must gradually and precisely introduce movement patterns, at various loads and speeds, in order to prepare the body for what it needs to do. In this chapter, we will focus on return to running. How do we take a patient who has just undergone some sort of ankle, knee, hip, low back, or shoulder injury, and gradually introduce linear movement at various speeds? How do we return someone who is lying on the table, just attaining full range of motion at an injured joint, to this complex movement pattern? In order to do this, we need to understand the components of linear movement, the components of transitional movements, the requirements of each joint during different phases of linear movement, and then select appropriate exercises using the contractile continuum to reinforce the requirements of these phases.

EPIDEMIOLOGY OF RUNNING INJURIES IN SPORT

Injuries associated with high-speed, high-velocity movements are prevalent in the literature (2–11). In 2004, Weist et al. found different plantar pressures in the foot during soccer-specific movements (run to cutting, run to sprinting, and run to shooting) that may be correlated with certain overuse injuries and stress fractures of the lower extremity (2).

Several studies have shown the increase in hamstring eccentric loads during sprinting movements, leading to overstress of the hamstring tissue, causing a strain (3–5). Sugiura et al. (6) found an association between hamstring injuries and decreased concentric hip extensor strength and eccentric hamstring strength. Still others have found ankle sprains can have a proprioceptive and strength deficit–causing relationship to the gluteus medius, thus decreasing frontal plane stability of the pelvis during gait, potentially leading to a multitude of lower extremity injuries (7,8). Given the amount of varying intensity and speed of movement during sport, and the chaotic nature of sport movement, virtually any injury is possible. From fractures anywhere in the lower extremity, to strained or torn tendons, to ruptured ligaments at the foot, ankle, or knee, the type of injury sustained is the result of many intrinsic and extrinsic factors. The type of shoes, surface of training or competition, weather, and movement pattern can all play a role in the type of injury that can be sustained. Although we have seen asymmetries of movement (9) and torsion (10,11) to have a strong correlation to lower extremity injuries, there is much research that still needs to be done in this area to understand the cause and potential reduction of these injuries.

BIOMECHANICS OF RUNNING

Linear movement consists of acceleration (sprinting), absolute speed (distance running greater than 30 to 40 yards in the same direction), and deceleration. Posturing for these three variants of linear movement is vastly different and requires different demands (12,13).

Acceleration

In acceleration, the athlete is in a total body lean, not flexed at the hip. There is a significant amount of arm action using the shoulder as the pivot point. The ankle is dorsiflexed and utilized as an active force transducer. Hip separation is ideally large, allowing the femur to be parallel to the ground. The more hip separation there is, the more energy can be driven into the ground. This allows for an equal and opposite reaction to propel the body forward (Figure 23.1). Let us break down these components more specifically.

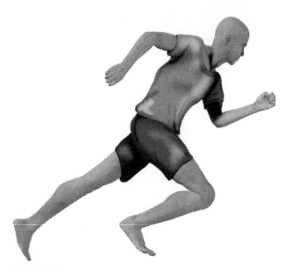

FIGURE 23-1. Acceleration posture.

Total Body Lean

The ear, shoulders, hip, and ankle are in a straight line, with no breaking point at the low back. The spine should be in a neutral posture, with the head being a natural extension of the spine. This requires a significant amount of abdominal, low back, pelvic floor, hip, and shoulder musculature working to maintain a stable posture from which the legs can create power. If we do not have enough stability in the sagittal or frontal planes, we will break down our stable base, creating an energy leak. These energy leaks cannot be made up. Once the energy is lost, we cannot recreate it. We will simply have less power going into the ground, which means less ground reaction force to propel us forward in a powerful manner. This will decrease our movement efficiency and productivity. Also, the torso is meant to be in a stable position, with the arms and legs moving on it to create movement. The back cannot be moving in a compensatory fashion to make up for something the hips or shoulders cannot do. This extraneous movement at the low back will not only cause the energy leaks described above, but also place strain on the musculature, joints, ligaments, and disks, causing potential back pain in our athletes.

Arm Action

The pivot point for the upper extremity during running is the shoulder, not the elbow. The shoulder has a direct connection to the hip through the latissimus dorsi via the lumbodorsal fascia. This reciprocal movement between opposite arms and legs creates a stretch–shorten cycle, allowing us to use elastic energy and the principles of plyometrics during our running movement. When our elbows open up and become the focus of upper extremity movement, we lose this cross-patterning between shoulder and opposite hip, we lose the ability to utilize

the stretch–shorten cycle for energy, and our movement becomes much more concentric. This is generally fatiguing and can lead to global fatigue of the entire system, potentially leading our body to overall injury as we get tired. A phrase sometimes heard during coaching is "Hips to Lips," meaning a runner's shoulder should move so their thumb moves all the way from their hips during shoulder extension, to lips during shoulder flexion. A caution if using this phrase—a runner can sometimes interpret that too literally, by taking their hands directly to their lips, across mid-line. We want to avoid cross midline motion. If the arms move across mid-line during running, an unnecessary torsion is created in the trunk, wasting energy, and ultimately slowing the body down.

Leg Action

In an acceleration position, the legs move up and down in a very piston-like manner. If this is not happening, and the lower leg "casts out" in front of the leaning body, the athlete will land with the heel in front of the body, causing the leg to absorb the force of the body, slowing it down. The athlete must then reaccelerate by pulling the body forward. This initial slowing of the body, coupled with the reacceleration, places a lot of stress at the distal hamstring. Athletes who are constantly dealing with distal hamstring strains may have some faulty mechanics, causing the hamstring to become overloaded and painful.

Ankle Dorsiflexion

The ankle, including the subtalar joint and talocrural joint, needs to be in a congruent position for optimal force transfer. We know a stiff rod will transfer force better than a wet stick that has "give," or bend, to it. If something has "give" to it, we again see the energy leaks described above, with a decrease in the ability for the body to get back the maximum return on investment that it put into the ground. Having our ankle in a dorsiflexed position, rather than a plantarflexed position, allows us to use this principle and transfer force from the lower extremity to the ground and vice versa. Biomechanically, the ankles will plantarflex during the push-off phase. However, we do not train this consciously. We train the athlete to maintain ankle dorsiflexion, allowing whatever amount of plantarflexion they naturally achieve to occur. If the ankle remains and is focused on being in a plantarflexed position, and the athlete hits the ground with the tip of his toes first, energy is lost as the heel comes to the ground, and the body then needs to try and reproduce force as it pushes off the ground. This can add tenths of seconds onto someone's time, which can have a detrimental effect on their performance. Also, landing in a plantarflexed position places our ankle joint at risk for increased incidence of ankle sprains, which can involve both the anterior talofibular and calcaneofibular ligaments. Therefore, we teach "pull your foot up to your shin" and allow the athlete to focus on quick recovery into ankle dorsiflexion.

Hip Separation

Every action has an equal and opposite reaction. If we lift our foot off the ground only a few inches, we only have so much ground reaction force returning to our body to move us. So we want enough hip separation that we will utilize the principles of physics in the most efficient manner possible, giving us the biggest return on our investment on the utilization of ground reaction forces. But we do not want so much hip separation that our posturing is compromised, and we lose our total body lean, break at our low back, and cause low back pain.

Absolute Speed

In absolute speed, the body is at a top end speed and gliding efficiently across the ground. This occurs after about 10 yards of sprinting, depending how strong the athlete is. If an athlete has a very strong core, they may be able to stay in acceleration speed mechanics for up to 15 yards. If they are weaker, they may pop up into absolute speed mechanics around 5 yards. For the purpose of this discussion, we will say absolute speed mechanics begin around 10 yards of sprinting. The principles of hip separation, ankle dorsiflexion, and arm action remain the same in absolute speed as in acceleration. The biggest differences in absolute speed come in during posturing and leg action.

Upright Posture

The body is no longer in a total body lean, but in an upright posture (Figure 23.2). Ears, shoulders, hips, and ankles are still in a line, just now underneath each other with the head remaining a natural extension of the spine. If the athlete is unable to maintain this upright posture, he or she will be slightly flexed at the trunk and the head will be jutted forward. This forward head posture can increase stress put on the upper trapezius and neck, causing tension at the upper back and headaches, and it can even change our breathing pattern. When our head is in this position, and our body is not upright, we will have a difficult time utilizing our diaphragm, pelvic floor, abdominals, and intercostals to breathe. Instead, our accessory muscles become overactive, less oxygen gets into our lungs, and we reach our anaerobic threshold faster than maybe we normally would. This will be difficult to maintain for a long period of time as a primary energy resource and can be tiring, again causing global fatigue issues.

Leg Action

Leg action during absolute speed is more cyclical, rather than piston-like. Yet similar to the acceleration leg action, if the lower leg is casted out in front of the body, the leg will absorb excessive force of the body moving forward as the leg is stopping the body, causing a slowing down of the body and a reacceleration action to move forward. Again,

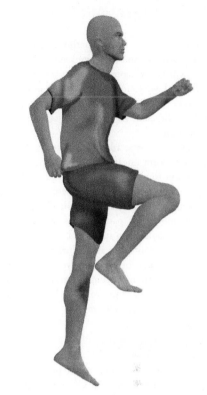

FIGURE 23-2.   Absolute speed posture.

we see an increase in hamstring strain as the body is trying to adapt to this inefficient movement pattern.

Deceleration

Deceleration is a transitional movement where the athlete attempts to eccentrically control momentum in order to slow or stop the body with the potential for reinitiating movement in a different direction (see Chapter 9). In sport, an athlete will often decelerate in order to reaccelerate in the same direction, accelerate into a different direction (so they may cut to the left, right, backward, or jump into the air), or to stop body movement altogether. The goal of deceleration is to control eccentric forces properly to avoid injury and prepare the body for the next possible movement pattern. There is no one pattern that someone uses to decelerate. Deceleration is dependent on the next movement pattern that is going to be performed. Deceleration will prepare the body to get into an optimal position to initiate the next motor program. Therefore, when teaching deceleration, one must know what pattern will be taught next. This will influence body position, posture, and the height of the athletes' center of gravity. We must consider the stretch–shorten cycle (plyometrics) postural alignment; the body orientation relative to the ground; foot to ground contact; and strength of the torso, pelvis, and lower extremities.

MULTIDIRECTIONAL MOVEMENT

Unless an athlete is a sprinter or marathoner, most athletics require some combination of acceleration with multidirectional movement (see Chapter 9). Very rarely will an athlete sprint forward, without having to change direction and accelerate again. Understanding multidirectional movement will help the clinician prepare the athlete for these movement patterns.

The overall key to true athletic movement is not only being able to perform linear and multidirectional movement patterns but to be able to transition from any movement pattern into any other movement pattern. This chapter does not focus on jumping or landing, but these are important movement patterns that also need to be considered. As rehabilitation specialists, we need to break down and introduce different individual movement patterns to an athlete, and then progressively and systematically combine them into more complex movement patterns to prepare the athlete for return to sport, bridging the gap between rehabilitation and performance.

Achieving Athletic Base

Athletic base is the most fundamental posture for multidirectional movement (Figure 23.3). An athlete needs

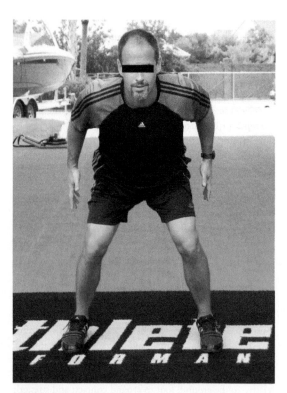

FIGURE 23-3. Athletic base.

to be able to achieve a wide stance in order to anticipate movement in any direction. Feet need to be wider than the knees, and knees wider than the hips. Keep in mind—this wide base does not mean femoral internal rotation with no hip control. Athletic base is very much an active posture with hips and torso activated, prepared to move the body in any direction. This requires appropriate amounts of hip flexion, knee flexion, and ankle dorsiflexion to maintain such a posture, along with proper stability and strength in each segment to support the position. Hence, "isolative" mobility, stability, and strength are required at the trunk, hips, knees, and ankles to be able to achieve such a posture and therefore build upon it with the following movements.

Shuffle

An athlete needs to be able to maintain this athletic base while pushing himself or herself to the left or the right. Focusing on the pushing part of the movement using the outside leg will allow the athlete to use the big gluteal muscles for power production into hip extension and external rotation. When using the front leg to pull themselves forward, the athlete will use the smaller, less powerful hip adductors and hamstrings, potentially creating an opportunity for injury (think of your chronically strained "high" hamstring or groin patients). Emphasizing the push portion of this movement pattern allows improved efficiency in the movement and potentially more power production.

Change of Direction

This movement pattern allows the athlete who is shuffling to the left to change direction and begin shuffling to the right. Although technically it is simply a weight shift change and directional change, it can be very challenging for the athlete who is rehabilitating a leg injury, who is hesitant to place stress and load on one lower extremity. The ability to load and push of both legs is a must for any athletic event.

Crossover

The crossover maneuver (Figure 23.4) allows the athlete who is in an athletic base position, moving laterally in one direction, to cross the back leg over the front, going from a lateral position to an acceleration position. This drill is used as a transitional movement from lateral to linear movement and is challenging for the rehabilitating athlete. This move should be introduced at the later stages of rehabilitation, when beginning to combine already established linear and multidirectional movement patterns.

Drop Step

Like the crossover, the drop step (Figure 23.5) is a transitional movement used when an athlete is facing one

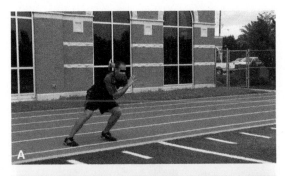

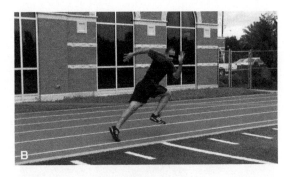

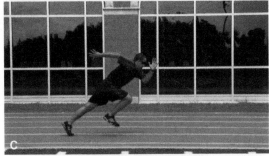

FIGURE 23-4. (A–C) Crossover.

direction and needs to turn around at an angle greater than 90° from where they are facing. This move can be transitioned from any movement pattern and can lead into acceleration movements.

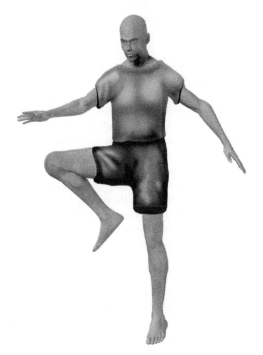

FIGURE 23-5. Drop step.

TRAINING STAGES

Youth

In the Balyi model, youth "FUNdamentals" are aimed at promoting general athletic development, posture, balance, and coordination.

Acceleration Exercises

Total body lean requires a significant amount of trunk stability. The stronger someone is in his or her trunk, the more total body lean, or aerodynamic, they can be. There are thousands of exercises to improve someone's core stability. Some are better than others. Consider the pillar bridge (Figure 23.6). The pillar bridge is a commonly prescribed exercise in rehabilitation and performance. How can the pillar bridge become more specific to acceleration? Place the athlete up against gravity, on the wall, with good hip separation and ankle dorsiflexion (Figure 23.7). This position requires proper ankle and hip mobility on the top leg and proper frontal plane stability of the down leg. Hold this posture for each side up to 30 seconds. These are tangible, objective observations that the health-care professional can address in an attempt to return the athlete to a specific athletic movement. If the athlete lacks ankle dorsiflexion, hip

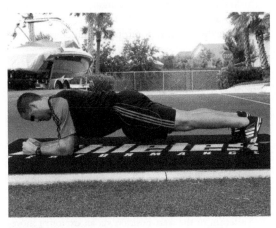

FIGURE 23-6. Pillar bridge.

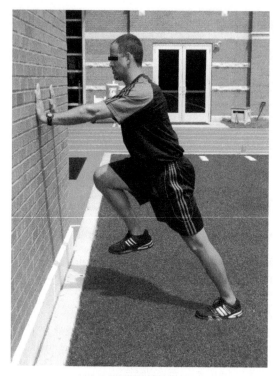

FIGURE 23-7.   Wall acceleration posture.

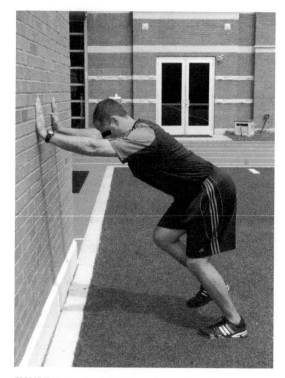

FIGURE 23-8.   Load and lift.

flexion mobility, or any other component required of the position of acceleration, the athlete will be unsuccessful at returning to this movement pattern. The clinician must provide each joint with the proper fundamental mobility, stability, and strength that is necessary in order to be used in the larger, more integrated system.

After acceleration wall posture stability is achieved, progress the athlete to the following:

Wall Marching

- Begin in wall posture as in Figure 23.7.
- Maintain arm and trunk position; nothing above the hips moves.
- Place the foot that is in triple flexion down into the ground.
- Once the foot makes contact with the ground, lift the opposite foot up into triple flexion.
- Repeat, simply exchanging leg positions from triple flexion to triple extension, not allowing the total body lean to be lost.

Load and Lift

- Place yourself into a position as in Figure 23.7.
- Load back into your hips, avoiding dropping down into your knees. Movement should be back, so your hips feel as if they are loaded (Figure 23.8).
- Return to the start position via an explosive movement from your hips, taking care not to run your face

into the wall; use your arms to support you as you explode up and into the wall (see Figure 23.7).
- Progress this exercise from two legs (not pictured) to one-leg support as shown.

Wall Up/Downs

- Begin in the wall posture position, as in Figure 23.7.
- Explosively drive your leg into the ground just slightly ahead of the down leg, trying to maintain ankle dorsiflexion. After performing on one leg, switch and perform on the other leg.
- Allow the leg to return to the original position. This should be done in the similar action as dribbling a basketball. You do not think about the basketball coming from the floor to your hands; you simply drive the basketball into the ground and know it will return to your hand. Use this same concept as you drive your leg into the ground, allowing it to return to the original position.

Absolute Speed Exercises

Absolute speed requires a totally different posture and leg action from acceleration. Maximizing trunk stability is the key, so the shoulders and hips have the ability to create force to propel us forward. Any extraneous movement at the trunk will cause compensatory movement patterns, decreased movement efficiency, and poor performance, and

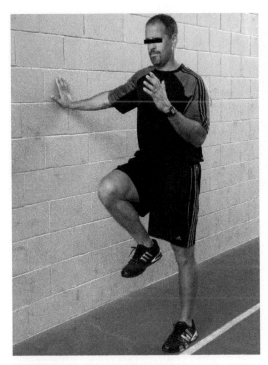

FIGURE 23-9. Wall absolute speed posture.

it potentially increases the risk of injury, specifically to the hamstrings and low back.

Wall Absolute Speed Posture (Figure 23.9)

- Maintain an upright posture with the inside leg triple flexed as pictured.

Wall Absolute Speed Posture Cycle

- Begin in the posture as shown in Figure 23.9.
- Place the foot about a half foot in front of the down leg, pressure on the forefoot.
- Pull the foot through until the hip is in extension.
- Keep the leg tight and quickly return to the starting position and hold.
- Repeat this exercise five to ten times slowly.

Deceleration Exercises

Deceleration is eccentric control of the body, using the stretch–shorten cycle to absorb force and control body movements, preparing the body for the upcoming movement pattern. Recognition of lower extremity muscles being worked, building general lower body eccentric strength and pillar strength, and developing both feed-forward and feedback mechanisms for motor control are crucial to introducing deceleration at this stage.

Red Light/Green Light Games

- We all have played the games when we were young. Repeat these same games with your younger athletes.

- Have an athlete run in any direction and yell "red light" for them to stop on a dime wherever they are.
- Make them hold this position until you yell "green light," at which time they can begin running in any direction again.

Star Drill

- Place the athlete at the center of a six-point "star."
- Place cones or markers at the end of a predetermined distance to delineate the six directions.
- Point an athlete in any direction and have him/her accelerate from the starting position, stopping at the designated end position.
- Return to the center point and repeat.

Recreational/High School

In the Balyi model, emphasis is on technique of the movement during the high school or recreational level.

Acceleration Exercises

Wall Singles/Triple Exchanges

- Begin at the starting posture shown in Figure 23.7.
- Essentially, combine the previously mentioned march and up/down exercises.
- Maintain stability on one leg, drive the leg that is up into triple flexion into the ground, creating the "basketball effect" previously described to drive the *opposite* leg up into the triple flexion position.
- Repeat this exercise in sets of one until fatigue, or breakdown of technique, is noted.

Get-Ups

- Start on the ground, laying on your stomach, with your hands at your shoulders and toes pulled under you as if you were about to do a push-up.
- On the coach's word, get up off the ground using your arms and legs and drive forward into a sprint.
- You will be in an acceleration-type posture.

Sitting Arm Action (Figure 23.10)

- Sit up tall on the ground with your legs extended out in front of you.
- Bend your elbows to a 90° angle.
- Begin driving your elbows backward, gradually increasing the speed until you are moving so fast you are bouncing slightly off the ground.

Partner Marches

- Begin in a total body lean, having your partner stand in front of you and hold your shoulders, a big game of trust. Be comfortable in this position before moving on.
- Maintain your acceleration posture, and begin to march forward into your partner as they move backward, supporting your shoulders.

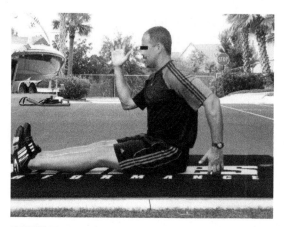

FIGURE 23-10. Sitting arm action.

- Be sure to maximize your arm action and hip separation.
- Your partner is there to allow you to maintain a total body lean.

Absolute Exercises

Wall Singles

- Repeat the fundamental exercise, with an increase in speed. It is the same movement.
- Progress this exercise by increasing the speed, performing 5 sets of 1, instead of a slow set of 5 as in the fundamental stage.

Wall Triples

- Repeat the above "singles" exercise. However, instead of one rep, perform three quick cycles and end in the top starting/ending position.

Pillar Marching

- Move away from the wall and allow yourself 10 to 15 yards of movement.
- Maintain the upright posture, the quick downward movement of the leg, the triple flexion action of the lower extremity, and the arm action.
- Move forward without any support from the wall (Figure 23.11).

Pillar Skipping

- Repeat the above marching exercise in a quick fashion, allowing two hits per foot contact.
- The difference between the march and skip is that during the march, there is always foot contact. During the skip, there is a point in time where both feet are off the ground.
- The general movement of the march and skip remains the same.

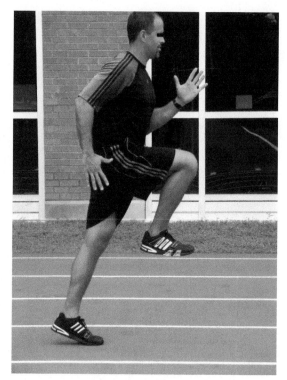

FIGURE 23-11. Linear pillar marching.

Deceleration Exercises

Mirror Drill/Wave Drill

- The athlete will begin running forward toward you.
- You will point to what direction (left, right, forward) the athlete is to proceed to.
- The athlete will need to react to whatever direction you tell him or her to go.

"Stop on a Dime"

- Allow the athlete to run forward, aiming for a marker that you have laid down.
- Ask the athlete to run as fast as he or she can to that marker and "stop on a dime" when they reach the marker.

Elite/Professional

In the Balyi model, emphasis at this stage is development of power and speed within the movement pattern. I would also suggest a continued emphasis on the quality of movement patterns. At the elite level, athletes have likely sustained an injury at some point along the way. Injury can cause pain, and pain will cause altered movement patterns. Synergistic dominant patterns can be prevalent during movement at this stage, often requiring a return to fundamental movement patterns and tasks.

Acceleration Exercises

Wall Exchanges for Time

* Repeat the above-stated exercises for time (under 6 seconds), instead of for repetitions.

Sled (Figure 23.12)

* Attach a sled with shoulder harness to the athlete.
* The sled should be behind the athlete and contain enough weight to allow the athlete to maintain a total body lean forward and drive into the ground as he moves forward in an acceleration-type movement.

Overspeed

* Utilize bungees to create an overspeed moment with the athlete, requiring the athlete to control the additional speed the bungee is creating.

Absolute Exercises

Single-Leg Walks

* Perform the pillar marching exercise described above, but keep one leg "a dead leg."
* This "dead leg" will allow you to focus on the moving leg, creating large hip separation, and clawing into the ground.
* The "dead leg" simply goes along for the ride and does not actively flex.
* Repeat on both sides.

Single-Leg Runs

* Maintain the above-stated position and turn the walk into a run.
* This will require a significant amount of coordination.

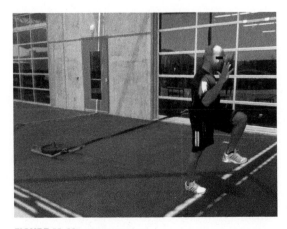

FIGURE 23-12. Sled marching.

Deceleration Exercises

5-10-5

* You can do this on a football field. Have the athlete run 5 yards and touch the line, then run 10 yards and touch the line, and finally accelerate back through 5 yards.
* Repeat for time.

General Eccentric Strengthening

* Maximizing general eccentric leg strength in the weight room as well as during all movement patterns will help maintain and improve all deceleration movements. We will leave the exercise selection to the imagination of the clinician.

Continue with the Mirror Drill/Wave Drill

* The athlete will begin running forward toward you.
* You will point to what direction (left, right, forward) the athlete is to proceed to.
* The athlete will need to react to whatever direction you tell him or her to go.

FINAL THOUGHTS

In order to return an athlete to any movement, we must fully understand the pattern and its component parts. Returning someone to running is a complex task, one that requires the knowledge of not only running but also the demands of the sport and the athlete's particular position. Once you understand the movement pattern and the athletes' sport/position demands, a comprehensive program can be developed to return or enhance this movement. When this happens, the physician, the rehabilitation specialist, the performance coach, and the skill coach can all work together to bridge the gap between rehabilitation and performance, allowing an athlete to return to his or her sport and be better than before the injury.

REFERENCES

1. Bompa T, Haff G. Basis for training. In: Periodization: Theory and Methodology. 5th ed. Champaign, IL: Human Kinetics; 2009:1–30.
2. Weist R, Eils E, Rosenbaum D. The influence of muscle fatigue on electromyogram and plantar pressure patterns as an explanation for the incidence of metatarsal stress fractures. Am J Sports Med 2004;32(8):1893–1898.
3. Schache AG, Kim HJ, Morgan DL, et al. Hamstring muscle forces prior to and immediately following an acute sprinting-related muscle strain injury. Gait Posture 2010; 32(1):136–40.
4. Heiderscheit BC, Hoerth DM, Chumanov ES, et al. Identifying the time of occurrence of a hamstring strain injury

during treadmill running: a case study. Clin Biomech 2005;20(10):1072–1078.

5. Chumanov ES, Heiderscheit BC, Thelen DG. The effect of speed and influence of individual muscles on hamstring mechanics during the swing phase of sprinting. J Biomech 2007;40(16):3555–3562.

6. Sugiura Y, Saito T, Sakuraba K, et al. Strength deficits identified with concentric action of the hip extensors and eccentric action of the hamstrings predispose to hamstring injury in elite sprinters. J Orthop Sports Phys Ther 2008;38(8):457–464.

7. Friel K, McLean N, Myers C, et al. Ipsilateral hip abductor weakness after inversion ankle sprain. J Athl Train 2006;41(1):74–78.

8. Bullock-Saxton J. Local sensation changes and altered hip muscle function following severe ankle sprain. Phys Ther 1994; 74:17–31.

9. Knapik JJ, Jones BH, Bauman CL, et al. Strength, flexibility and athletic injuries. Sports Med 1992;14(5):277–288.

10. Boden BP, Dean GS, Feagin JA, Garett WE. Mechanisms of ACL injury. Orthopedics 2000;23:573–578.

11. Howse C. Wrist injuries in sport. Sports Med 1994;7(13): 163–175.

12. Verstegen M. Core Performance. Emmaus, PA: Rodale; 2004.

13. Seagrave L, Mouchbahani R, O'Donnell K. Neuro-Biomechanics of Maximum Velocity Sprinting. IAAF NSA; 12009.

The Dead Lift

Many traditional free weight training choices have earnestly stood the test of time over years and years of resistance training for rehabilitation and athletic enhancement. While there is solace in "what is old becomes new again" with these lifts, many clinicians and individuals still do not embrace free weight compound lifts in their programming (1). Rejection of these functional training choices may be the relative simplicity to using supported environments or the requirement for some teaching and learning of the lift prior to executing it with progression (2).

One such lift that fits the above scenario is the dead lift (DL). The very name of the lift often strikes concern or rejection by the inclusion of the word "dead" in the name. There is lore that the term was coined as early as 200 BC when young Romans returned to the battlefield trenches to "lift the dead" onto carts and return them to their townships for a proper burial. Lifting a limp mass such as the above requires ideal body control, technique, and limit strength (3–5). When applying these qualities to a weight training implement such as a barbell, dumbbell, kettlebell, or really any resistance or load, we have a premiere choice for patterning and strength gains (5–7).

Perhaps the DL is one of the best functional choices we have, given its wide-reaching targets of adaptation for the body and variations of the lift that can accommodate the desires of variety and the uncommon variables of body control and somatotype. Some of the regional targets of the DL are the posterior chain, hip mobility and stability, lumbar spine stability, and scapular stability. Depending on the implement or how far off the floor you pull from can accommodate a great training effect for folks that are working concurrently on physical limitations or a longer torso and neck.

The common denominator of all forms of the DL is the vertical tibia. Variations that we do not explore in this chapter are the "good morning," kettlebell swing, and hip-dominant "powerlifting" box squat. None of these techniques involves lifting a "dead" object from the ground, but they do employ the vertical tibia as described in the drills below. We choose the true DL patterns as most lifts incur an eccentric phase prior to a concentric phase. While many drills enjoy a "presetting" integrity with eccentric before concentric, the nature of the DL is potentially best suited to pulling from a still position. Overcoming Newton's first law that an object at rest tends to stay at rest reminds the client to establish excellent integrity statically before engaging the load in a dynamic fashion.

By definition, you are able to perform a DL with quite dominant mobility restrictions through the trunk and hips (8). The range of the lift may not be very far, but the movement can technically be executed. Certainly, the efficiency of this choice could be questioned. The challenge is the urge to exceed a small range and run into compensatory relative flexibility through the spine or scapulae.

In terms of a loss of spinal flexion in a multisegmental flexion test, the inability to flex the spine may yield poor proprioception as the mechanoreceptors of the spine are not stimulated without the spine able to explore that range. Certainly, this exploration should not be at all regular, repetitive, or loaded, but it should be capable prior to engaging a loaded DL pattern (3,4,9–11).

The techniques reviewed in this chapter are the toe touch, dowel DL, conventional DL, one-leg DL, sumo DL, and trap bar DL. The trap bar DL does not employ a vertical tibia, but given its pulling from a dead stop, it will be reviewed. Repetitions are typically performed as multiple sets of 1 with a regrip or reset between each repetition.

The toe touch as described by the standards set in the Selective Functional Movement Assessment (http://www.functionalmovement.com) requires (1) the finger tips touching the toes, (2) a posterior weight shift of the hips, (3) a rounding of the lumbar spine, (4) no lateral sway, and (5) appropriate respiration stereotype at the bottom of the movement (Figure 24.1). Keen judgment is required to determine whether excursion is excessive or if progression is warranted despite failing this movement screen. Pain and/or dysfunction should be assessed and trained appropriately.

The dowel DL is the first step in challenging the neutral spine during the hip hinge.

1. Use a small polyvinyl chloride pipe or very light short bar or dowel aligned along the spine, holding it in place with one arm flexed and laterally rotated and the other arm extended and medially rotated. The hand holds should fit into the natural lordoses of the cervical and lumbar spines (see Figure 24.2A, B).
2. Maintaining constant contact with the dowel with the posterior cranium, the thoracic spine, and the superior sacrum, drive the hips backward, maintaining a 20° knee bend (see Figure 24.2C).

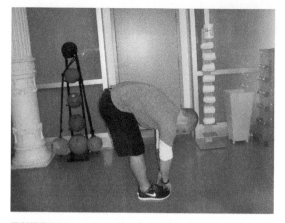

FIGURE 24-1. Toe touch in sagittal plane.

3. This technique can also be employed with a single-leg technique. The hinging lower extremity should correlate to the same side upper extremity in medial rotation and extension (see Figure 24.2D).

The conventional DL is typically performed with a straight bar, which is demonstrated (12) in Figure 24.3A–D.

1. Setup begins with feet at a width where you feel like you can jump the highest, and the bar hovered over the middle of the foot.
2. Squat down to grip the bar just outside the shoulder width. The shins will be angled as it touches the bar. A large diaphragmatic breath should occur before the lift and held through the lockout. The bar is on the ground or elevated as described below in a "rack pull."
3. With neck packed (retruded) if necessary and gripping as strongly as possible, the bar's path begins moving into the shins by sitting backward into the hip hinge.
4. As the bar ascends, the tibia becomes vertical, and the pull continues with a measure of pushing down into the floor.
5. Neither feet nor knees should demonstrate valgus collapse. The shoulders should not shrug. Neither the thoracic nor lumbar spines should flex.
6. A high DL or "rack pull" should start with vertical tibia.

I would consider the options where you tap the wall to encourage hip hinge patterning. These are no-load or reactive loads meant to provide the right proprioception to achieve an efficient hip hinge. I would look to clear the toe

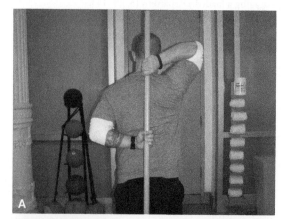

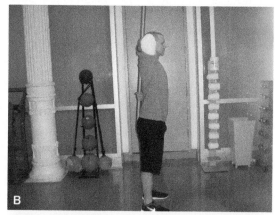

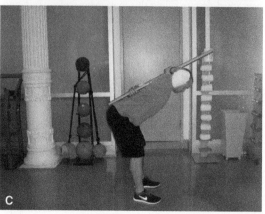

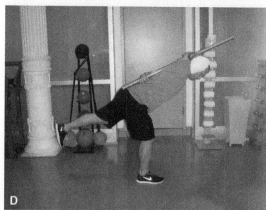

FIGURE 24-2. Dowel dead lift. (A) Setup, rear view. (B) Start, sagittal plane. (C) Finish, one-leg, sagittal plane. (D) Finish, two-leg, sagittal plane.

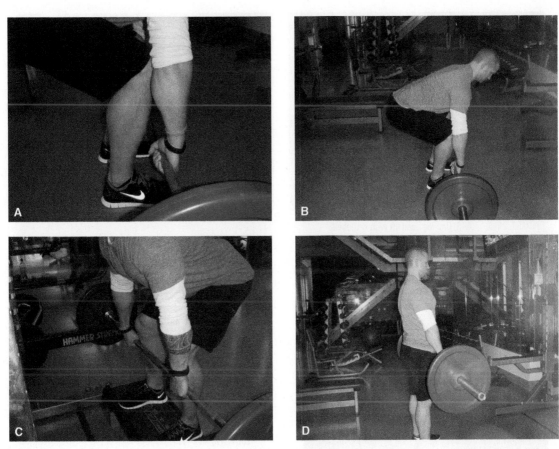

FIGURE 24-3. High dead lift or rack pull. (A) Setup demonstrating daylight between bar and shin. (B) Setup off floor. (C) Pull to vertical tibia. (D) Lockout.

touch and dowel DL or use the reactive patterns to pattern the hip hinge if the toe touch was capable but the stability in the hip hinge was not (3–5,13).

The hamstring lengthening is a by-product of a well-executed hip hinge or any kind of DL. I would coach caution in aggressively using an anterior tilt so as not to foster form closure at L5-S1. Otherwise, these options are solid. I especially like the bottom-up approach as that is the natural neurodevelopmental pattern of squatting down and dead lifting up (4,5,14,15).

The sumo DL is also typically performed with the straight bar (12,16).

1. The setup is with feet considerably wider than shoulders and toes pointed out. The bar will be up against the shins during setup. There is no daylight between the bar and shins (Figure 24.4).
2. The bar path begins with pulling into the shins and pushing backward.
3. When the bar leaves the floor, immediately push through the heels to finish the return from the hip hinge.

The one-leg DL can be performed with a bar, individual load in each hand, or individual load in one hand. It is not typical for someone to be able to address a load off the floor

with this one-leg technique. The one-leg DL with a reach with ball is another reactive exercise to pattern the movement (Figure 24.5A–B).

1. Perform the one-leg hip hinge to address the load. The load should be set up to allow for 20° of knee flexion. Grip as hard as you can to set the shoulder(s).

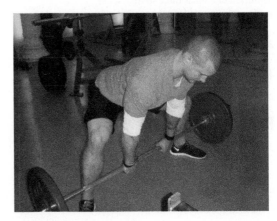

FIGURE 24-4. Sumo dead lift.

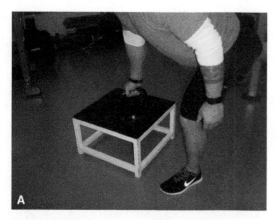 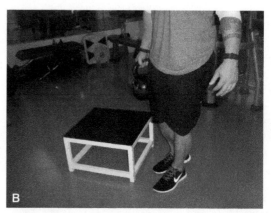

FIGURE 24-5. (A–B) One-leg dead lift with kettlebell.

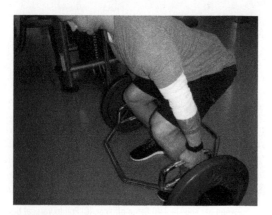

FIGURE 24-6. Trap bar dead lift.

2. Push through the heel and ball of first toe to return to standing position.
3. Return the load to the starting point with the one-leg hip hinge pattern.

The trap bar (hex bar) DL can be performed with a vertical or angled tibia, but it is typically and more naturally performed with the angled tibia position. This meets the definition of a squat more so than a DL.

1. Setup begins with feet at a width where you feel like you can jump the highest, centered inside the bar.
2. Grip the bar as hard as you can to set the shoulders (Figure 24.6).
3. Pack the neck back and push into the heels and big toe in a jumping fashion to pull the bar to lockout.

REFERENCES

1. McGill SM. Low back exercises: evidence for improving exercise regimens. Phys Ther 1998;78(7):754–765.
2. Dylla J, Forrest JL. Fit to sit—strategies to maximize function and minimize occupational pain. J Mich Dent Assoc 2008;90(5):38–45.
3. McGill SM, Karpowicz A. Exercises for spine stabilization: motion/motor patterns, stability progressions, and clinical technique. Arch Phys Med Rehabil 2009;90(1):118–126.
4. McGill SM. Low back stability: from formal description to issues for performance and rehabilitation. Exerc Sport Sci Rev 2001;29(1):26–31.
5. McGill SM. Distribution of tissue loads in the low back during a variety of daily and rehabilitation tasks. J Rehabil Res Dev 1997;34(4):448–458.
6. Kibler WB. Closed kinetic chain rehabilitation for sports injuries. Phys Med Rehabil Clin N Am 2000;11(2):369–384.
7. Kibler WB, Livingston B. Closed-chain rehabilitation for upper and lower extremities. J Am Acad Orthop Surg 2001;9(6):412–421.
8. Scannell JP, McGill SM. Lumbar posture—should it, and can it, be modified? A study of passive tissue stiffness and lumbar position during activities of daily living. Phys Ther 2003;83(10):907–917.
9. Wallden M. The neutral spine principle. J Bodywork Movement Ther 2009;13(4):350–361. Epub 2009 Aug 26.
10. Keller TS, Colloca CJ, Harrison DE, Harrison DD, Janik TJ. Influence of spine morphology on intervertebral disc loads and stresses in asymptomatic adults: implications for the ideal spine. Spine J 2005;5(3):297–309.
11. Kavcic N, Grenier S, McGill SM. Determining the stabilizing role of individual torso muscles during rehabilitation exercises. Spine (Phila Pa 1976) 2004;29(11):1254–1265.
12. Escamilla RF, Francisco AC, Kayes AV, Speer KP, Moorman CT 3rd. An electromyographic analysis of sumo and conventional style deadlifts. Med Sci Sports Exerc 2002;34(4):682–688.
13. Smith J. Moving beyond the neutral spine: stabilizing the dancer with lumbar extension dysfunction. J Dance Med Sci 2009;13(3):73–82.
14. Bliss LS, Teeple P. Core stability: the centerpiece of any training program. Curr Sports Med Rep 2005;4(3):179–183.
15. Cholewicki J, Panjabi MM, Khachatryan A. Stabilizing function of trunk flexor-extensor muscles around a neutral spine posture. Spine (Phila Pa 1976) 1997;22(19):2207–2212.
16. Escamilla RF, Francisco AC, Fleisig GS, et al. A three-dimensional biomechanical analysis of sumo and conventional style deadlifts. Med Sci Sports Exerc 2000;32(7):1265–1275.

25

Eric Cressey

Off-Season Considerations for Baseball

Adequate preparation for baseball at the collegiate and professional levels mandates that strength and conditioning specialists and coaches appreciate a number of different qualities about the biomechanics of the sport. However, important considerations do not just end here; one must also appreciate the nature of the competitive season's structure; the energy systems demands of baseball; and the individual differences among position players, catchers, and pitchers.

One thing I mention to all my baseball players is that it is important to realize throwing a baseball can hardly be considered a natural act. In fact, the velocities one encounters during overhead throwing of the baseball are actually the fastest encountered in sports. During acceleration, the humerus can internally rotate at velocities faster than 7,000°/s (1), while the elbow may extend at greater than 2,300°/s (2). This act of acceleration imposes tremendous stresses on osseous, musculotendinous, ligamentous, and labral structures at the elbow and shoulder girdle. These stresses are magnified when throwing off the mound as compared with flat-ground throwing.

Equally important, though, are the chronic adaptations that occur in response to the eccentric stress imposed during deceleration of this motion. Research from Reinold et al. demonstrated that pitchers lose both shoulder internal rotation and elbow extension over the course of a competitive season, but that this loss can be prevented with appropriate stretching (3). Previous research has demonstrated that a glenohumeral internal rotation deficit greater than 20° markedly increases one's risk of shoulder pain (4), and we have also seen it as a fundamental flaw in many of those who present with elbow pain.

That said, in light of research from Wilk et al. (5) our approach typically focuses on normalizing total motion, which should be the same on the dominant and nondominant sides, even if the specific arc of each range of motion is not the same. Overhead throwing athletes may present with markedly more external rotation and less internal rotation in the dominant shoulder compared with the nondominant shoulder, but if total motion is the same on both sides, this asymmetry may be normal. An example of this may

be (measured in supine, at 90° abduction with the scapula stabilized):

- Dominant shoulder internal rotation: 50°
- Dominant shoulder external rotation: 130°
- Dominant shoulder total motion: 180°
- Nondominant shoulder external rotation: 115°
- Nondominant shoulder internal rotation: 65°
- Nondominant shoulder total motion: 180°

While there is a 15° internal rotation deficit, total motion is symmetrical, which would indicate that the differences are likely due to osseous adaptations (retroversion) acquired before skeletal maturity. This asymmetry is likely completely normal and acceptable. However, when this total motion is asymmetrical, one should look to flexibility deficits in the soft tissues, particularly the posterior rotator cuff.

Anecdotally, the same aforementioned responses to eccentric stress can be observed in lower body flexibility measurements of pitchers; we have noted marked losses in lead-leg knee flexion and hip internal rotation in just about every pitcher we have seen who has not been involved in adequate flexibility programs. Additionally, research has demonstrated that 49% of athletes with arthroscopically diagnosed superior labrum anterior posterior lesions present with contralateral hip range of motion or abduction strength deficit (6). It is important to recognize that these same deficits may also be observed in healthy pitchers and could be a nonsignificant finding, so further research is warranted, but we can work to address the issues in the interim.

Many pitchers acquire a low dominant shoulder in conjunction with shortness of the pectoralis minor and weakness of the muscles—particularly lower trapezius and serratus anterior—that are responsible for upwardly rotating the scapula. Flexibility and resistance training exercises should take this problem into account, although subtle asymmetries may (again) be completely normal (7).

The demands of hitting, while not as extreme as those of pitching, certainly must be appreciated in a good training plan. During hitting, the rotational position of the lead leg changes substantially from foot off to ball contact.

After hitting a maximal external rotation of 28° during the foot off "coiling" that takes place, the hips go through some violent internal rotation as the front leg gets stiff to serve as a "block" over which dramatic rotational velocities are applied. In professional hitters, this velocity averaged 714°/s at the hips—and was accompanied by a stride length averaged 85 cm—or roughly 380% of hip width. In other words, hitting requires a tremendous amount of both hip power and mobility. To make matters more complex, hitters encounter maximum shoulder and arm segment rotational velocities of 937°/s and 1,160°/s, respectively. All of this happens within a matter of just 0.57 seconds (8)!

Previous research from Shaffer et al. has demonstrated that during the hitting motion, the electromyography (EMG) of the erector spinae and oblique muscles is not significantly different between sides (9). In other words, these muscles act as isometric stabilizers of the spine to effectively transfer force from the lower body to the upper extremity, where it is carried to the bat; you want to move at your hips and thoracic spine, not your lumbar spine—or else you will be at a greater risk for back pain. This recruitment strategy must be taken into account in an effective core stability program; good exercises should focus on creating lumbar stability through isometric and eccentric muscle actions, not those (crunches, sit-ups, lumbar rotation drills) that create motion.

While pitching and hitting are different actions, they do share one thing in common: in both motions, the hip segment begins counterclockwise (forward) movement before the shoulder segment (which is still in the cocking/coiling phase). This creates the "whip" that increases muscular power via the stretch-shortening cycle—and it demands precise integration of muscles all the way from the feet up to the hands. Along this kinetic chain, we have found that the most crucial considerations are

- Ankle mobility (particularly dorsiflexion range of motion)
- Hip mobility (particularly in internal rotation and extension)
- Core stability (both in resisting extension and resisting rotation)
- Thoracic spine mobility (particularly in extension and rotation)
- Scapular stability (particularly of the lower trapezius and serratus anterior)
- Glenohumeral mobility (symmetrical total motion) and dynamic stability (adequate rotator cuff function)
- Lower body strength/power (particularly of the hip and knee extensors)

When one of these factors is insufficient, the rest are negatively affected. For instance, a lack of hip mobility can cause an individual to rotate excessively at the lumbar spine or knee. Poor thoracic spine mobility negatively affects scapular stability, so a pitcher may sacrifice glenohumeral motion to move the less-stiff segment: the scapula.

Biomechanics and asymmetries aside, the nature of the competitive season in baseball must be taken into account. At the professional level, in consideration of spring training, the regular season, and postseason play, a baseball player may participate in over 200 games between February and the beginning of November. As a college player, this number may be over 120, in consideration of fall scrimmages, the spring competitive season, and then the summer calendar. And, some high school athletes may approach 100 games per year on top of camps and showcases. In fact, showcase participation is associated with an increased incidence of arm injuries in adolescent baseball players (9)—and it may be due to the poor timing of many of these events (fall/winter).

With all this participation in game play, one realizes that it is a short off-season, and the fact that games occur just about every day at the highest level cannot be overlooked. As a result, it can be challenging to improve/maintain strength, power, flexibility, tissue quality, immunity, endocrine function, and body composition for a large portion of the year. As a result, the off-season period is absolutely crucial for those looking to improve performance and stay healthy.

The nature of the game itself also poses a threat on the injury front. Rarely will a player have to run longer than 30 to 60 yards at a time, and the acts of throwing and hitting are about as far to the left of the anaerobic–aerobic continuum as one can get. While this makes energy systems considerations quite simple (train with short bursts of activity, not aerobic exercise), the stop-and-go nature of the sport can increase the likelihood of acute injuries (e.g., hamstrings, hip flexor, and adductor strains). Maintaining adequate flexibility and muscular recruitment patterns works hand-in-hand with "staying warm" throughout the game to keep athletes healthy.

One could write an entire book on how to train pitchers, position players, and catchers differently. However, for the sake of brevity, it is safe to say that they are largely similar in the way that their training must be approached. While I outline specific contraindicated exercises for baseball players, the main changes across positions I make are as follows:

- a larger focus on arm care exercise in pitchers and catchers (although it is still important with position players)
- fewer (or no) squats in training for catchers
- less upper body and medicine ball training volume for pitchers during points of the year when they are throwing off the mound

Unfortunately, based on reports of injury rates in players at all levels, the status quo from an injury prevention standpoint is wholly inadequate. Elbow and shoulder injuries—particularly among youth pitchers—have increased exponentially in the past decade alone (10). For example, a 2003 review reported that more than 57% of pitchers suffer some sort of shoulder injury during a playing season (11), and that does not even take into account issues at any other joints.

ASSESSMENTS FOR ALL BASEBALL PLAYERS

With these injuries in mind, let us start breaking away from the status quo and take a look at just a few assessments I use with all my baseball players. This list is certainly far from exhaustive, but it is a good start. In addition to flexibility assessment, I also test vertical jump and take front, side, and back pictures to assess posture and body composition with each of my baseball athletes.

Shoulder Motion: Internal, External, and Total

When assessing glenohumeral range of motion, it is important to stabilize the scapula (particularly with the internal

rotation measurement) (Figure 25.1). The humerus can be elevated slightly to the scapular plane, and the examiner should be sure to avoid pressing down on the humeral head. Our goal is a symmetrical total motion (internal rotation + external rotation = total motion). Most baseball players will present with an internal rotation deficit on their throwing shoulder; this deficit may be completely normal and should be considered alongside total motion to determine the appropriate course of action.

Supine Shoulder Flexion

The hips and knees should be flexed with the lower back flat on the table (Figure 25.2). In an acceptable test, the upper arms should rest on the table.

Hip Rotation: Internal and External (90°)

When assessing hip rotation, it is important to not allow the pelvis to hike (Figure 25.3). The goal for both tests is greater than 40° of rotation.

Push-Up

The push-up test is a basic fitness test used to assess upper body fitness and to monitor progress during strength and fitness training (Figure 25.4).

Overhead Squat

This test should be performed with the shoes off (Figure 25.5). The overhead squat can quickly assess a wide variety of shortcomings: thoracic spine mobility, upper extremity mobility, core stability, hip mobility, and ankle mobility.

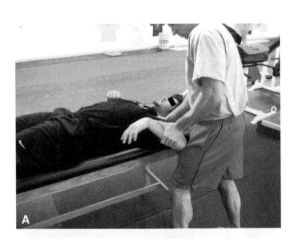

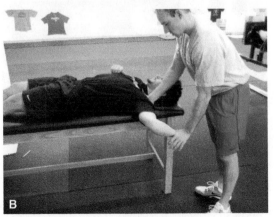

FIGURE 25-1. Shoulder motion: internal (A) and external (B).

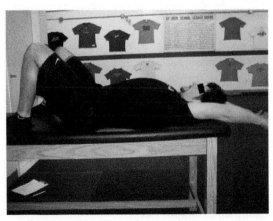

FIGURE 25-2. Supine shoulder flexion.

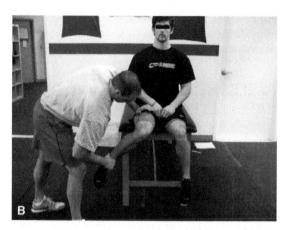

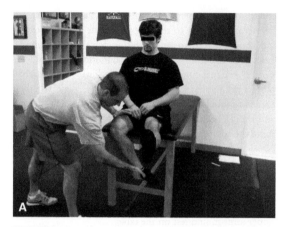

FIGURE 25-3.   (A and B) Hip rotation: internal and external (90°).

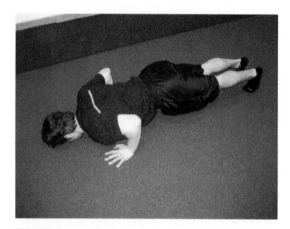

FIGURE 25-4.   Push-up.

Overhead Lunge Walk

The overhead lunge walk assesses many of the same issues as the overhead squat, but it also gives information on how well an athlete stabilizes in single-leg stance (Figure 25.6). We pay close attention to not only balancing proficiency but also stride length and upper extremity function.

EXERCISES IN KEY TRAINING CATEGORIES

With those assessments in mind, let us look at a few quick examples of exercises in each of the key training focus categories I outlined earlier. For the sake of brevity, the focus in the pages that follow will be primarily static and dynamic flexibility, medicine ball training, and resistance training—but one should not overlook the role of both linear and

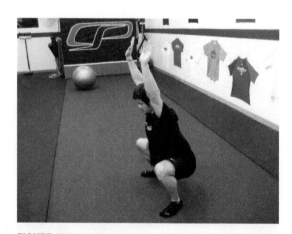

FIGURE 25-5.   Overhead squat.

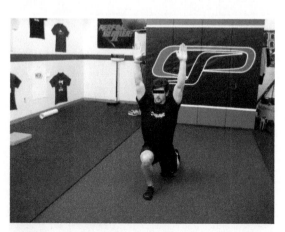

FIGURE 25-6.   Overhead lunge walk.

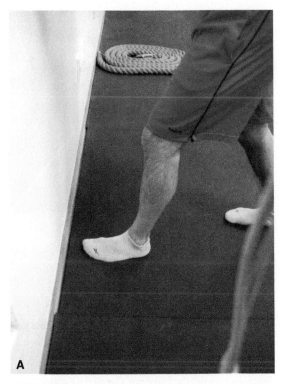
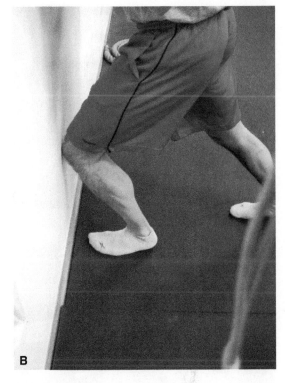

A **B**

FIGURE 25-7. (A and B) Wall ankle mobilization.

lateral movement training in preparing the baseball player for the competitive season.

Ankle Mobility: Wall Ankle Mobilization

Work the front foot as far away from the wall as possible without allowing the heel to come off the ground (Figure 25.7). Do not allow the foot to externally rotate, and do not let the knee cave in. The athlete should aim the knee directly over the middle toe as he or she rocks forward. The stretch should be felt in the Achilles tendons/calves.

Hip Mobility

Alternating Lateral Lunge Walk (Figure 25.8)

Be sure to keep the chest out. Do not allow the leading foot to externally rotate or the lower back to round. The stretch should be felt along the inner thigh.

Wall Hip Flexor Mobilization (Figure 25.9)

Do not lean forward at the trunk. Push the chest out. The stretch should be felt along the front of the hip and all along the quadriceps.

Lying Knee-to-Knee Stretch (Figure 25.10)

Keep the feet flat on the floor. The stretch should be felt along the outside of the hamstrings and/or glutes.

One-Leg Supine Bridge (Figure 25.11)

Make sure that the movement comes at the hips, not at the lower back. Push through the heels and squeeze the support-leg glutes at the top of the movement.

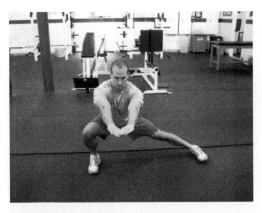

FIGURE 25-8. Alternating lateral lunge walk.

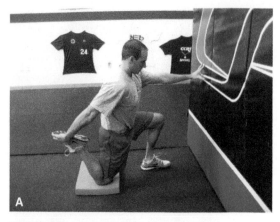
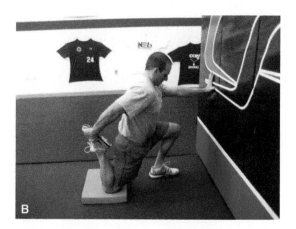

FIGURE 25-9.   (A and B) Wall hip flexor mobilization.

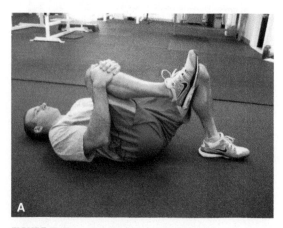

FIGURE 25-10.   Lying knee-to-knee stretch.

Core Stability

Rotational Medicine Ball Shot Put (Figure 25.12)

Be sure to brace the core tightly. Make sure that all the rotation comes from the hips and thoracic spine.

Recoiled Rollover Stomps to Floor (Figure 25.13)

Brace the core tightly. Make sure that all the rotation comes from the thoracic spine.

Split-Stance Cable Lift (Figure 25.14)

Brace the core tightly. Do not allow the pull of the cable to provide your rotation.

Stability Ball Rollout (Figure 25.15)

Brace the core tightly, and activate the glutes to prevent lumbar extension. The movement should be initiated with the hips, and the athlete should descend until the nose gently touches the ball.

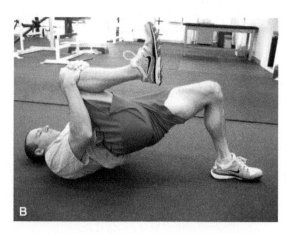

FIGURE 25-11.   (A and B) One-leg supine bridge.

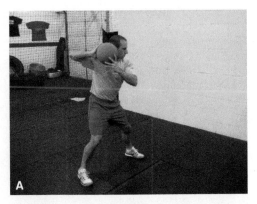
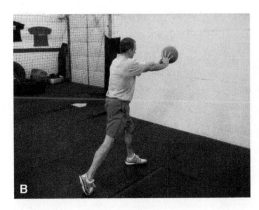

FIGURE 25-12.   (A and B) Rotational medicine ball shot put.

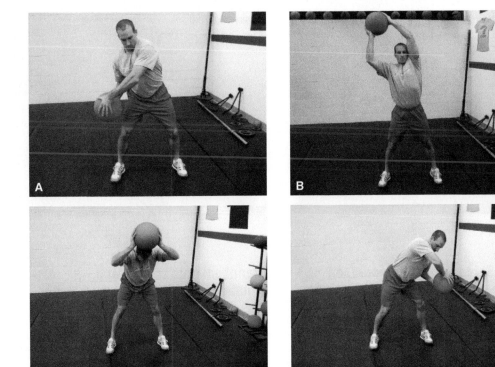

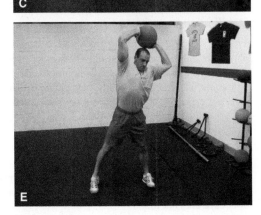
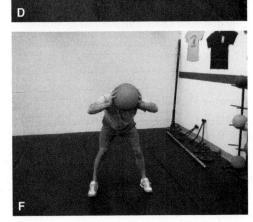

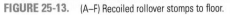

FIGURE 25-13.   (A–F) Recoiled rollover stomps to floor.

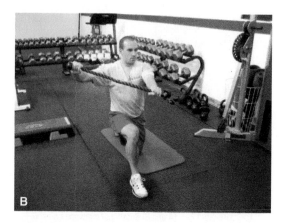
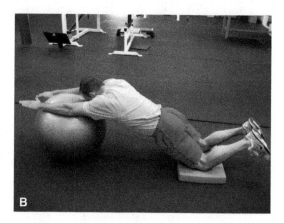

FIGURE 25-14.   (A and B) Split-stance cable lift.

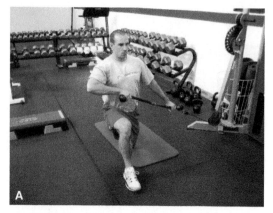
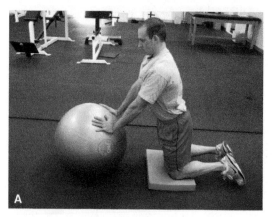

FIGURE 25-15.   (A and B) Stability ball rollout.

Thoracic Spine Mobility: Quadruped Extension–Rotation

Brace the core tightly to ensure that all the rotation comes from the thoracic spine (Figure 25.16).

Scapular Stability/Upper Body Strength

Standing One-Arm Cable Rows (Figure 25.17)

The shoulder blade should be pulled down *and* back to prevent it from rolling forward into anterior tilt at the end of the rowing motion.

Feet-Elevated Push-Up (Figure 25.18)

Make sure that the chest reaches the floor before the chin to prevent forward head posture. Also, brace the core and activate the glutes to prevent the hips from sagging.

Neutral Grip Pull-Up (Figure 25.19)

The chin should remain tucked. The chest should reach the bar at the top.

Glenohumeral Mobility and Dynamic Stability

Side-Lying External Rotation (Figure 25.20)

Place a towel or half foam roller between the upper arm and the torso. A weight plate, dumbbell, or partner-provided resistance can be used. The arm is abducted 30°.

Three-Position Split-Stance Rhythmic Stabilization (Figure 25.21)

A partner should apply gentle perturbations to dynamic stability as the athlete braces the core tightly, retracts the scapula, and attempts to stabilize the shoulder against the destabilizing torques. The movement can be made more challenging by having the athlete close his eyes during the drill.

Lower Body Strength/Power

Front Squat (Figure 25.22)

We prefer the cross-face grip set-up with baseball players to protect the hands, wrists, and forearms. Make sure that the lower back does not round.

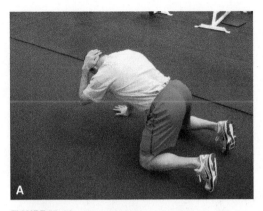
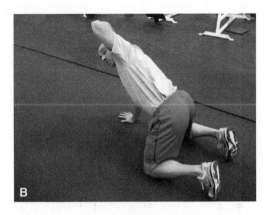

FIGURE 25-16.   (A and B) Quadruped extension–rotation.

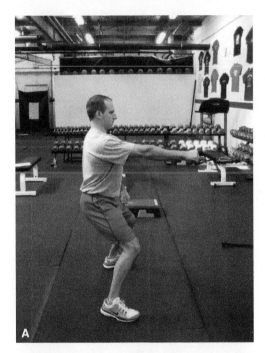
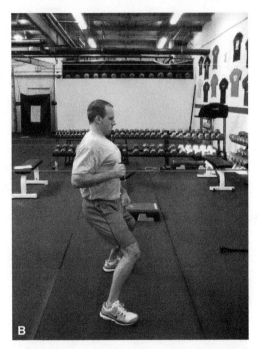

FIGURE 25-17.   (A and B) Standing one-arm cable rows.

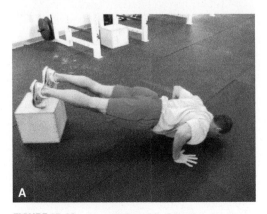
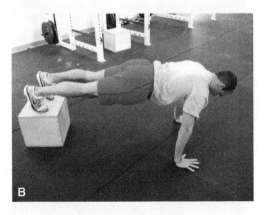

FIGURE 25-18.   (A and B) Feet-elevated push-up.

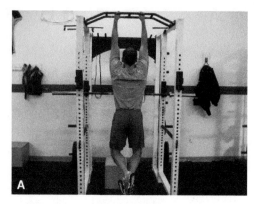

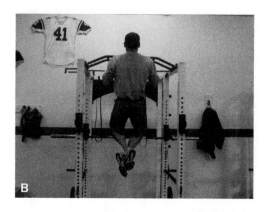

FIGURE 25-19.   (A and B) Neutral grip pull-up.

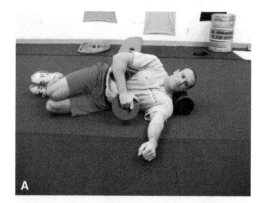

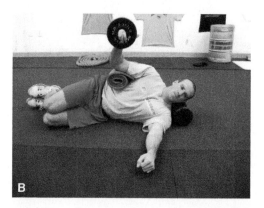

FIGURE 25-20.   (A and B) Side-lying external rotation.

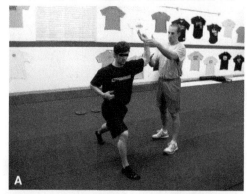

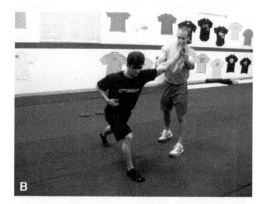

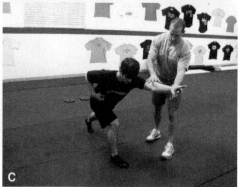

FIGURE 25-21.   (A–C) Three-position split-stance rhythmic stabilization.

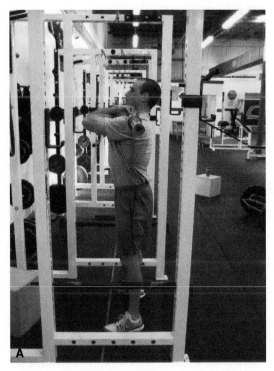

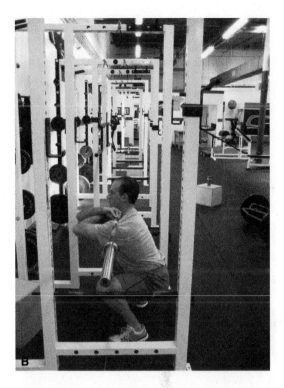

FIGURE 25-22. (A and B) Front squat.

Trap Bar Deadlift (Figure 25.23)

The athlete should push through the heels, and the knees, hips, and shoulders should all rise together. The glutes should be activated at the top of the movement to prevent excessive lumbar extension. The lower back should never round.

Dumbbell Reverse Lunge from Deficit (Figure 25.24)

Make sure that the torso does not tilt forward; the chest should be held up and out.

A Note on Overhead Pressing for Baseball Players

While some may disagree, it is my opinion that overhead pressing in baseball players is not worth the risk it imposes with this specific population. My rationale for this contra-indication includes:

1. The high incidence of players with asymptomatic rotator cuff tears (12) and labral defects (13); these two adaptations lead to impaired muscular and structural stability.

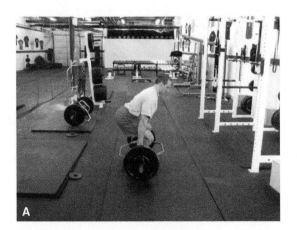

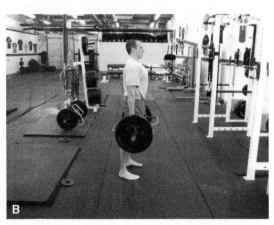

FIGURE 25-23. (A and B) Trap bar deadlift.

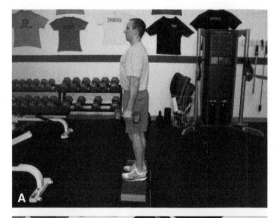

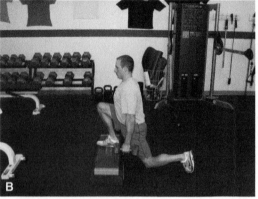

FIGURE 25-24. (A and B) Dumbbell reverse lunge from deficit.

2. The aforementioned limited scapular upward rotation demonstrated in pitchers (7); this adaptation may negatively influence scapular stability in the overhead position, particularly since overhead pressing typically mandates more shoulder elevation than overhead throwing.
3. The inherent differences between overhead pressing (an approximation stress on the glenohumeral joint) and the throwing motion (a traction stress); approximation stress is typically more stressful on the glenohumeral joint.
4. The nonneutral position of the humerus (with respect to population "norms") that results from humeral retroversion and an acquired internal rotation deficit.
5. The high incidence of congenital laxity in both pitchers and position players at the professional level. Bigliani et al. reported that 89% of pitchers and 47% of position players had positive sulcus signs in their throwing shoulder, and 89% and 100% of them, respectively, also had that laxity in their nonthrowing shoulder (14).

CONCLUSIONS

Baseball players—and certainly pitchers, more specifically—are a population with a wide array of unique functional demands. Appropriate training should take into consideration not only these demands but also the structure of the competitive season and the individual differences among position players, catchers, and pitchers.

REFERENCES

1. Dillman CJ, Fleisig GS, Andrews JR. Biomechanics of pitching with emphasis upon shoulder kinematics. J Orthop Sports Phys Ther 1993;18(2):402–408.
2. Escamilla RF, Barrentine SW, Fleisig GS, et al. Pitching biomechanics as a pitcher approaches muscular fatigue during a simulated baseball game. Am J Sports Med 2007;35(1):23–33.
3. Reinold MM, Wilk KE, Macrina LC, et al. Changes in shoulder and elbow passive range of motion after pitching in professional baseball players. Am J Sports Med 2008;36(3):523–527.
4. Myers JB, Laudner KG, Pasquale MR, Bradley JP, Lephart SM. Glenohumeral range of motion deficits and posterior shoulder tightness in throwers with pathologic internal impingement. Am J Sports Med 2006;34(3):385–391.
5. Wilk KE, Meister K, Andrews JR. Current concepts in the rehabilitation of the overhead throwing athlete. Am J Sports Med 2002;30:136–151.
6. Kibler WB, Press J, Sciascia A. The role of core stability in athletic function. Sports Med 2006;36(3):189–198.
7. Oyama S, Myers JB, Wassinger CA, Daniel Ricci R, Lephart SM. Asymmetric resting scapular posture in healthy overhead athletes. J Athl Train 2008;43(6):565–570.
8. Welch CM, Banks SA, Cook FF, Draovitch P. Hitting a baseball: a biomechanical description. J Orthop Sports Phys Ther 1995;22(5):193–201.
9. Shaffer B, Jobe FW, Pink M, Perry J. Baseball batting. An electromyographic study. Clin Orthop Relat Res 1993;292:285–293.
10. Olsen SJ 2nd, Fleisig GS, Dun S, Loftice J, Andrews JR. Risk factors for shoulder and elbow injuries in adolescent baseball pitchers. Am J Sports Med 2006;34(6):905–912.
11. Ouellette H, Labis J, Bredella M, Palmer WE, Sheah K, Torriani M. Spectrum of shoulder injuries in the baseball pitcher. Skeletal Radiol 2008;37(6):491–498. Review.
12. Connor PM, Banks DM, Tyson AB, Coumas JS, D'Alessandro DF. Magnetic resonance imaging of the asymptomatic shoulder of overhead athletes: a 5-year follow-up study. Am J Sports Med 2003;31(5):724–727.
13. Miniaci A, Mascia AT, Salonen DC, Becker EJ. Magnetic resonance imaging of the shoulder in asymptomatic professional baseball pitchers. Am J Sports Med 2002;30(1):66–73.
14. Bigliani LU, Codd TP, Connor PM, Levine WN, Littlefield MA, Hershon SJ. Shoulder motion and laxity in the professional baseball player. Am J Sports Med 1997;25(5):609–613.

Off-Season Considerations for Basketball

Basketball is one of the world's most popular sports and can be played nearly year-round with only a hoop and a basketball. Any interested athlete may work on specific basketball skills, playing each and every day. While this may not be the best method to improve upon overall game preparation, this effort is what the majority of basketball coaches and the basketball culture in general espouse. To this end, basketball athletes prefer playing and show little interest in the physical preparation required to actually increase skill. In contrast, football and ice hockey athletes typically enjoy physical preparation to improve their performance. The fact that basketball can be played year-round makes it difficult for many to devote the necessary time to improve strength and other physical measures. With such an incredible amount of emphasis placed on skill development by coaches, the average athlete has a limited amount of time and resources. Hence, basketball strength coaches are faced with a cumbersome task when designing a comprehensive program.

DEMANDS OF THE SPORT

Basketball involves a variety of movement skills including running, jumping, jogging, walking, hopping, shuffling, crossing over, backpedaling, skipping, bounding, and balancing in all three planes of movement. All players on the court perform similar movements (e.g., rebounding, guarding, shooting, and boxing out) as play transitions from offense to defense. These movements occur at varying intensities, lengths, and distances over the course of any given game.

Basketball is an intermittent sport (continuous with brief stoppages in play) with the intensity typically based upon the coach's preference (up-tempo, pressing vs. slow deliberate half-court style). In a study of an Australian National League game, close to 1,000 changes in movement were reported during a 48-minute game (1). This equated to a change in movement every 2 seconds. Interestingly enough, shuffling movements were seen in 34.6% of the activity patterns of a game, while running at intensities ranging from a jog to a sprint were observed in 31.2% of all movements (1). Many think that jumping is a large part of basketball. However, jumps only compromised

4.6% of all movements and 15% of actual playing time when high-intensity shuffles and jumps were considered together. Additionally, movements characterized as high intensity were recorded once every 21 seconds of play in this study. Standing or walking was observed during 29.6% of playing time (1).

The results of this well-known study suggest that movements occurring during a basketball game are performed at an intensity that is primarily aerobic in nature, which is in contrast to other reports that suggest successful basketball performance is dependent upon anaerobic performance (2). These contrasting results are likely related to the different styles of play between different levels of basketball as mentioned previously. Monitoring heart rate measures during actual play and other activities is excellent when determining the intensities at which athletes are working. As noted in the previous study, 75% of the actual play occurred at a heart rate that was 85% of the athlete's peak heart rate, while 15% of the contest heart rate exceeded 95% of peak heart rate (1).

Lactate along with hydrogen ions are by-products of anaerobic metabolism and thus can affect pH levels via metabolic acidosis which impairs muscular contractions. Lactate concentrations during a basketball game are likely influenced by the intensity at which the game is played and can vary considerably from game to game. Significant correlations exist between lactate concentration and both the time spent in high-intensity activity and the mean percentage of peak heart rate (1). It appears that the aerobic component to successful basketball performance is more important in the recovery processes (e.g., lactate clearance, cardio-deceleration patterns) than in providing a direct performance benefit (2). Interestingly enough, a high aerobic capacity has been reported to have a negative relationship with playing time in elite male college basketball players (3)—meaning that those with a higher VO_2 max tend to also be less powerful and slower. In contrast, maximal aerobic capacity in female basketball players clearly discriminates between higher and lesser skilled players (4).

Actual on-court success, however, appears to be more dependent upon an athlete's anaerobic power and endurance (2). Although only 15% of the playing time in a basketball game has been described as high intensity (1), it is clear that these actions weigh most heavily on the outcome of a contest. The quick change of direction and explosive power needed to free oneself for an open shot or defend an opponent, jump for a rebound, or the speed needed to reach a loose ball are all examples of activities that fall under this category and have also been demonstrated to be strong predictors of playing time in male college basketball players (3).

BASKETBALL ASSESSMENT AND INJURIES

Basketball, like many sports, is deeply entrenched in both "tradition" and the mindset of "the way we have always done things." This is evident in almost all collegiate and professional sports medicine and strength and conditioning areas when considering basketball athletes during both injury or preinjury *evaluation* screening and *performance* testing. Unfortunately, as is the case with so many other sports, evaluation and performance testing often neither reflect the actual demands of the sport as outlined above nor contribute to or predict actual on-court performance measures (e.g., points scored, rebounding).

As an example, for many years the National Hockey League's combine draft has been scrutinized for evaluating draft picks by running them through a number of tests only to have those tests demonstrate a poor or negative correlation to actual on-ice performance measures (e.g., goals scored, minutes played)(5). Most recently, the individuals responsible for the National Basketball Association (NBA) draft combine have considered changing or adding additional tests in the hopes of addressing this problem. The on-court tests currently utilized in the NBA combine—the 3/4 court sprint time (similar to the 40-yard dash in football), the lane agility test (instituted only because of dimensions clearly painted on all courts), along with the vertical jump test show little, if any, correlation to actual on-court success.

THE NEED FOR ASSESSMENT

Why assess? With all things being equal, the athlete who has the least number of injuries throughout a playing career—high school, college, and professional—should be able to make significant strides forward by virtue of simply having more opportunities to both practice and play. Therefore, an evaluation process that is able to identify causative injury factors, in addition to a comprehensive strength program which not only addresses these concerns but increases actual on-court performance, is paramount if the basketball athlete is hoping to play and compete at elite levels.

On evaluation, gross movement patterns such as the overhead squat, multisegmental flexion (toe touch) (Figure 26.1), and multisegmental extension (backward bend) (Figure 26.2) give the clinician or strength coach opportunities to evaluate

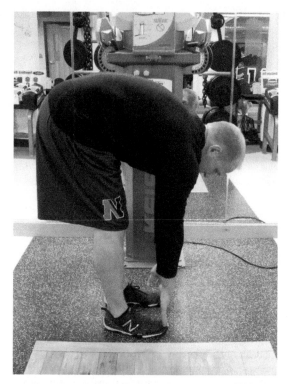

FIGURE 26-1   Multisegmental flexion.

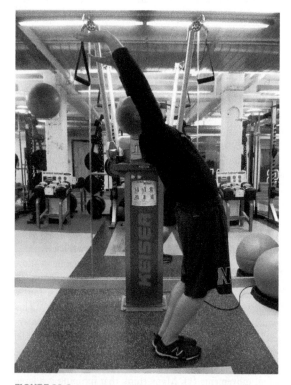

FIGURE 26-2.   Multisegmental extension.

limitations within whole-body movements that may either limit performance or potentially result in pain or disability down the road. Once major flaws are identified, these limitations should of course be followed up by a more specific joint or tissue evaluation and treatment by a skilled clinician. Since basketball athletes are placed within the aforementioned positions repeatedly during the course of a game, such as during the course of establishing an advantageous post position or while defending a ball handler, it behooves us to provide each athlete with the mobility and stability required to do these movements efficiently and successfully.

Since ankle sprain ranks first in both games and practices for most common injuries (6), it makes sense to evaluate limitations within this specific joint, particularly discrepancy between left and right ankle range of motion and strength. In addition, evaluating how the ankle and its limitations contribute to more global affects including aches and pains up the kinetic chain such as anterior knee and low back pain is of upmost importance. By evaluating the aforementioned overhead squat pattern as well as the star excursion balance test, evaluators can easily identify these differences as well as identify increased risk of future injury (7).

Continuing with the lower extremity assessment, equality and discrepancy between left and right power output and landing ability can be easily evaluated and recorded during a single leg hop test. During this test athletes keep both hands on hips, jump off of one foot, and land on the same foot while maintaining balance upon landing for a 2-second count. A red flag is placed beside any left to right discrepancy greater than 15%, and the athlete is directed to more comprehensive follow-up assessment and care. In addition to identifying those athletes with large asymmetries, prescreening evaluations provide excellent return to play criteria.

After ankle and knee pathology, low back pain ranks fourth in injury occurrence in collegiate men's basketball practices (behind ankle, knee, and pelvis/hip) in time lost due to injury (6) among basketball athletes. Although identifying individual causes of low back pain is certainly not the focus of this chapter, it is worth noting here that many basketball athletes lack the required strength to provide appropriate stabilization about the lumbar spine and that, as with most individuals, those suffering from a previous episode of low back pain predict future episodes of low back pain as indicated in the literature (8). Not only do appropriate levels of strength provide a protective effect against low back pain, its importance cannot be overstated with regard to measures of performance success on the basketball court (9). The ability to stiffen the torso and pelvis to allow frontal plane loading is enabled with lateral torso strength (10). This stability requirement is why carrying enhances frontal plane strength needed for single-leg takeoff jumps.

To ensure appropriate levels of lumbar strength and endurance, a simple side plank test for time can be instituted to evaluate the endurance of the lateral core musculature both in relation to the opposite side and also in comparison with the back extensor strength/endurance, which can be measured and recorded using the Biering-Sorensen test. Side plank times should be within ±5% of each other and measure at 75% of the back extensor strength to ensure appropriate symmetry and protection against future injury (11,12). In hockey, research demonstrates that holding the side bridge longer than 70 seconds reduces the risk of abdominal wall injury (12). Inappropriate ratios between the left and right side plank times and back extension time may indicate poor overall symmetry of torso function and should raise a red flag in both injury and performance areas and again be referred out for further evaluation and treatment (12). The inability to hold the torso upright in a controlled manner (extensor strength) precipitates itself into a poor defensive posture that decreases performance. Jump performance is also enhanced with a stiffer torso.

Performance measurements should also be taken into account when looking at developing an appropriate athletic development program. Strength tests such as squats, deadlifts, bench press, push-ups, and pull-ups are common exercises used to measure an athlete's ability to produce force, but their power (or how quickly they can produce force) must be measured as well. Two different vertical jump tests can give you an idea on which direction to take an athlete, the vertical jump with countermovement and the vertical jump with approach. The vertical jump with countermovement is reliant on strength as the athlete has to propel the body from a dead stop and this requires greater levels of muscular force. The vertical jump with approach is reliant on elastic energy as the steps prior to the jump build up kinetic energy that is stored within the tendon and can be used in the subsequent contraction. If there is greater than a 4-inch difference between the two, the focus should be on developing strength (they are more elastic). If there is less than a 4-inch difference, the athlete can spend more time devoted to developing power (strength–speed, speed–strength methods). Understanding this idea can provide a clear direction on how to develop an appropriate program.

TRAINING CONSIDERATIONS

Knowing the specific demands of the sport along with the most common injuries now provides us a map for training basketball athletes more successfully. As mentioned earlier, basketball athletes play year-round, which often makes it difficult to dedicate the time needed for comprehensive physical preparation. Playing and running up and down the court reduces "resources" from the body that can be used toward developing speed, strength, and power. And these physical attributes often determine which athletes are able to make plays. Just as movement restrictions may cause potential injuries, physical limitations most certainly affect performance. The goal of a well-designed strength and conditioning program then is to minimize these weaknesses and improve the specific qualities needed to be successful while on the court.

The qualities needed to be successful on the court are
a. Mobility/stability
b. Strength
c. Speed
d. Power
e. Fitness (basketball-specific power endurance)

The following are the major questions to address:

- Can the athlete get into position correctly? (mobility)
- Can the athlete hold position correctly? (stability)
- Can the athlete move in and out of position? (strength)
- Can the athlete move in and out of position with speed? (speed/power)
- Can the athlete move in and out of position with speed continuously? (power endurance)

Mobility is the quality of moving freely while stability describes the ability to control that movement. Each joint throughout the body has an inherent degree of either more mobility or stability and this helps to guide decision-making regarding proper and safe training methods (see Chapter 25, which describes this relationship in more detail).

Strength is the ability to exert force. Strength development is fundamental for basketball athletes because it serves as the foundation for all other qualities (e.g., speed, strength endurance, power, and agility). Improved strength allows all other movements to be performed at a lower energy cost because an athlete can now work at a lower percentage of exertion to perform the same tasks, which prior required increased strength levels. This improvement in strength clearly improves movement economy by increasing total capacity, which yields extra energy that can be used for other facets of the game.

Strength is a motor skill and must be done year-round to improve. Coaches that only have their athletes strength train in the off-season are doing them a disservice, with many players losing the gains they had made during the season. If a player wanted to improve their shooting ability, would they practice shooting for one month and then stop the next, expecting to be a better shooter? Of course not, so why would one expect to have their strength maintained when training is ceased during certain parts of the year?

Many coaches believe that speed and power development are far more important than simply strength training; however, both attributes are heavily influenced through strength training. Speed is the ability to reach a high velocity of movement, while power is the ability to produce a large amount of force in a short period of time. Power has components of force and speed. It is important to understand that both speed and power require force and force development to enhance each of their qualities. Training for power or speed does not improve the ability to produce

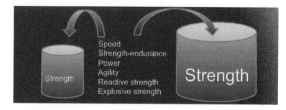

FIGURE 26-3. Strength diagram—analogy of strength to other attributes as cup volume is to contents.

maximal force, but training for strength (force) can enhance speed and power because ultimately the force component of their equations is improved.

Cressey uses a cup as an analogy that describes the importance of strength development and its relationship to other physical qualities (Figure 26.3). Strength is like the size of a glass, and all other aspects of performance are like fluid that is bound by the dimensions within the glass. The size of the glass must increase in order for improvement in speed, power, and other similar attributes past a training plateau. For example, speed and agility are both reported to be a consistent predictor of playing time in National Collegiate Athletic Association (NCAA) Division I male basketball athletes (2), and developing a foundation of strength is essential to improve these qualities.

Think of speed and strength as a continuum (Figure 26.4). As one gets closer to the left side, one will display a high degree of speed, with strength being a secondary factor. On the right side of the continuum, speed will not be as prevalent as strength. What does this mean when training the basketball athlete? If everything basketball athletes do are things on the left side of the continuum, their potential for improvement will not be as great as if they included tasks from the right side of the continuum. As mentioned previously, the majority of basketball athletes get plenty of work on the left side by simply playing, and very little on the right or middle sections.

MAJOR LIFTS

The central nervous system (CNS) controls the entire body by recruiting specific motor units to produce various movements. All athletes walk, lunge, squat, run, push, pull, rotate, and bend, and these movements should form the foundation for functional training in order to enhance the full potential of the CNS. Thinking in movements not only makes sense but also creates a large, accessible exercise menu.

BODY BREAKDOWN

When establishing an exercise menu, it is important to first lay out how the movements will be broken up; doing so ensures that there will be a balance between all muscle

Speed–strength continuum			
ABSOLUTE SPEED	**SPEED–STRENGTH**	**STRENGTH–SPEED**	**ABSOLUTE STRENGTH**
Vertical jumps/Basketball	*Weight vest jumpss (10% body weight)*	*Jump squats (30–40% of squat max*)*	*1 repetition maximum*

*Wilson, GJ, Newton, RU., Murphy, AJ., Humphries, BJ. The optimal training load for the development of dynamic athletic performance. *Medicine and Science in Sport and Exercise* 1993;25:1279–1286.

FIGURE 26-4. Speed–strength continuum. On the far left is absolute speed. On the right is absolute strength. In between is the interplay of the two and how they affect power.

groups and movements. The setback encountered with training muscles and not movements is that certain muscles (agonists) will get more work than their counterparts (antagonists). An example of this occurs when trainees work the "chest" and "back" together. Most people will train pressing movements, such as bench and incline, for their chest, and will perform pulling movements, such as "lat" pull-down and pull-ups for the back. The problem is that vertical pulling movements such as "lat" pull-downs and pull-ups internally rotate the humerus; this internal rotation also occurs in most pressing movements, and thus, the combined effect may actually exasperate a previous injury or precipitate itself as a future problem. Movements should be paired to create balance and minimize kinetic chain dysfunction. There are three types of movements:

- Total body movements
- Lower body movements
- Upper body movements

Table 26.1 shows how these movements are subdivided.

Create a basic menu of exercises that you commonly perform for each category. See Table 26.2 for a simplified example.

Explosive movements are not likely the weak link due to the plyometric nature of the sport and the volume that is conducted throughout the year, so they will not be mentioned in this discussion; rather, strength will be the area of focus as the majority of basketball athletes can impact their development the most by improving force capacity. This focus is particularly true with both single-leg and posterior chain strength development as they play a large role in reducing a number of injuries.

Single-leg strength is frequently overlooked in strength programs, but it is essential to the improvement of speed, development of balance, and prevention of injury. The majority of strength programs focus on conventional double-leg exercises such as squats, which are very beneficial and serve a purpose in improving general strength; however, single-leg strength helps to bridge the gap from training to sport as the majority of sport skills are performed on one leg. In addition, single-leg exercises, such as the single-leg squat, recruit the pelvic stabilizers, which are not called upon in the same way during double-leg stance exercises. For example, during single-leg exercises the gluteus medius

TABLE 26.1	**How Body Movements Are Subdivided**

Total Body Movements

Explosive movements (goal is a high rate of force development/power)
    Olympic (snatch)
    Jumps and throws (jump squats/medicine ball scoop throw)
Combination movements (combine two movements together)
    Upper–lower (squat to press)
    Upper–upper (upright row to press)

Lower Body Movements

Squat movements (knee/quad dominant)
    Two leg (Squat)
    One leg (lunge)—supported vs. unsupported
Bend movements (hip/glute/hamstring dominant)
    Straight leg (straight leg deadlift)
    Bent leg (glute hamstring)

Upper Body Movements

Pushing movements (moving a load away from body)
    Horizontal (bench press)
    Vertical (shoulder press)
Pulling movements (moving a load closer to body)
    Horizontal (bent over row)
    Vertical (pull-up)

is forced to operate as a stabilizer, which is critical in reducing the chance of injury.

Single-leg strength can be broken down into supported and unsupported movements. Supported single-leg exercises involve both legs on the ground with the majority of the work performed by only one leg, while single-leg unsupported exercises have the uninvolved leg in the air. Both classifications need to be trained as the demand on the pelvic musculature is quite different. Single-leg supported work allows the pelvis to be relatively fixed as the other leg helps to provide stability. Single-leg unsupported work challenges the pelvic and foot stabilizers to a greater degree as stability must be attained at the proper joints for successful movement. Both challenges are important and must be included into basketball strength training

TABLE 26.2	Body Exercises: Basic Menu		
Explosive—Olympic	**Explosive—Jumps and Throws**	**Combo—Up/Low**	**Combo—Up/Up**
Total Body Exercises			
Snatch	Jump squats	Squat to press	Up row to press
Clean	Medicine ball chest pass throw	Lunge to up row	Bent row to curl
Lower Body Exercises			
Squat—Two Leg	**Squat—One Leg (Supported)**	**Squat—One Leg (Unsupported)**	**Bend—Straight leg**	**Bend—Bent Leg**
Back squat	Split squat	One-leg squat	One-leg deadlift	Deadlift
Front squat	Lateral squat	One-leg cross-behind squat	Straight leg hip lift	Glute ham raise
Upper Body Exercises **Push—Horizontal**	**Push—Vertical**	**Pull—Horizontal**	**Pull—Vertical**
Bench press	Military press	Bent over row	Chin-up
Push-up	Dumbbell shoulder press	Inverted row	Pull-up

programs to address athletes with longer levers that render a mechanical disadvantage to hip stabilizers. The emphasis for single-leg work is not only to enhance large force-producing muscles but also the smaller muscles that help control movement occurring at the femur, knee joint, and even the ankle and foot. Figures 26.5 to 26.10 illustrate several single-leg exercises.

The posterior chain is primarily made up of the gluteal complex, hamstrings, and erectors. Strength in these muscles is necessary for both maximum force production and control of these large forces at the femur and knee. The gluteal complex concentric function is hip extension and hip external rotation; therefore, their eccentric function is to control hip flexion and hip internal rotation, which occurs during deceleration at landing each time the foot hits the ground. If the glutes do not adequately

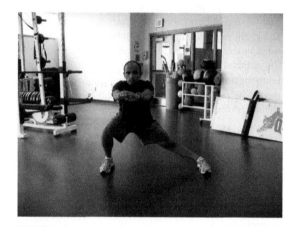

FIGURE 26-6. Lateral squat.

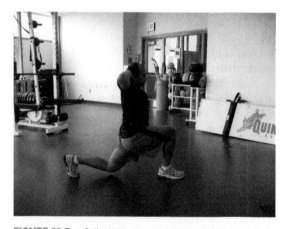

FIGURE 26-5. Split squat.

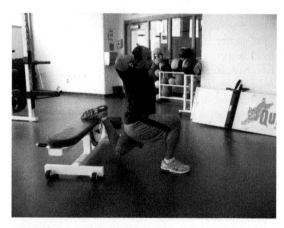

FIGURE 26-7. One-leg bench squat.

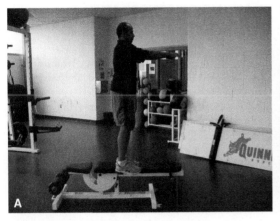

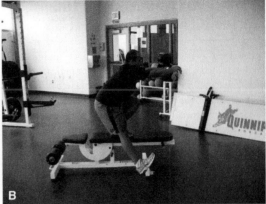

FIGURE 26-8.   (A and B) One-leg squat on bench.

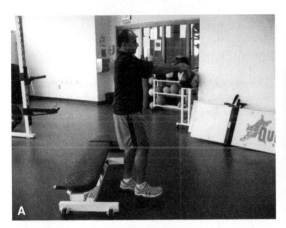

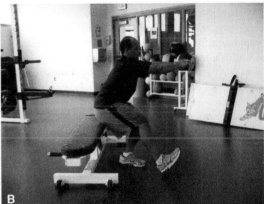

FIGURE 26-9.   (A and B) One-leg squat to bench.

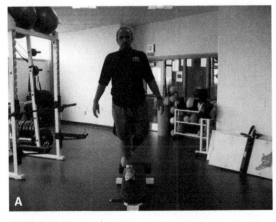

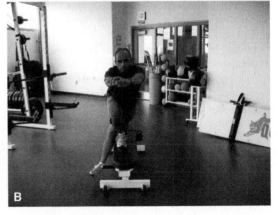

FIGURE 26-10.   (A and B) One-leg cross-behind squat on bench.

control these forces, the knee will experience excessive stress that can lead to injuries. Examples of exercises that target the posterior chain are deadlifts and their variations (rack pulls, sumo deadlifts, trap bar deadlifts, single-leg deadlifts), bridges and their variations (glute bridge, shoulder-elevated glute bridge, hip lifts), and a combination of the two (glute ham raise, ball leg curl) (see Chapter 29 for further information).

TRAINING FOR SUCCESS ON THE COURT—WHAT REALLY MATTERS

As mentioned previously, very few, if any, traditional strength testing measures actually relate to, or indicate, performance success within the context of a basketball game, and since many of the traditional strength training programs are geared toward producing the greatest end score on these tests, it may be reasonable to assume that many of our strength and conditioning practices are simply off the mark when it comes to quantifiably improving on-court statistics. While it is difficult to assign a level of importance for exercises that benefit "hustle plays," it is quite easy to evaluate preseason strength and performance measures and compare them with postseason statistics such as points scored, rebounds, block shots, assists, minutes played, and games lost due to injury.

With regard to points scored, the ability to express spine stiffness correlates strongly, as does the lane agility test in college male athletes utilizing collegiate lane dimensions. And while the relentless pursuit of vertical jumping ability does not prove advantageous when compared with both rebounding and shots blocked, long jump ability correlates favorably when examining preseason strength and performance measures against end-of-year statistical success (9).

Even though most fans of basketball and certainly the athletes who participate within the sport itself enjoy action above the rim, the amount of time dedicated to this movement during actual game play is minute compared with other movements previously mentioned. Movements requiring athletes to quickly take up space and/or "take an opponent off the dribble" happen much more frequently and thus should be addressed more so during dedicated training time. These maneuvers or movements require athletes to express a superstiffness within their trunk and core followed by relaxation, followed again by superstiffness on the contralateral side. This athletic phenomenon has been measured and demonstrated in elite mixed martial arts athletes in whom an extreme stiffening takes place within the core as the athlete prepares to kick followed by relaxation as the leg travels through the air, followed again by extreme stiffening just prior to impact, essentially turning the fighters' leg and body into stone just prior to contact with their opponent. The ability to create "impulses" allows the fighter to strike their opponent not just with their foot but with their entire mass, and this process is ubiquitous throughout many sports (13).

The "stiffening–relaxation–stiffening" cycle takes place in elite basketball athletes as they create "impulses" that allow them to change direction quickly during a crossover dribble, creating scoring opportunities. The same cycle occurs during defense against elite ball handlers. Those basketball athletes with superior core stiffening and relaxation abilities are able to respond and change direction much more quickly, staying in front of their opponent on the defensive end.

TRAINING STIFFNESS IN THE BASKETBALL ATHLETES

It is clear then that specific core training is required in the programming of the basketball athlete to improve on-court performance measures. Examples include:
1. Chops (Figure 26.11) and lifts (Figure 26.12)
2. Rotational planks (Figure 26.13). Transition from a traditional side plank to a front plank and return, maintaining low back and pelvis alignment. Hold each position for 5 seconds
3. Antirotation presses (Figure 26.14)
4. Asymmetrical carries (farmer walk) (Figure 26.15)
5. Asymmetrical reverse lunges (Figure 26.16)

PROGRAMMING THROUGHOUT THE YEAR

Postseason

The postseason occurs directly as the season ends, typically lasting 3 to 6 weeks, depending upon season length for the competitive age group and injuries that occurred during the season.

Postseason goals include:
1. Restore range of motion that was lost during the season.
2. Build work capacity for the off-season so higher volumes of training can be handled.
3. Reinforce technique in the major primary lifts.
4. Provide rehabilitation to those athletes suffering injuries during the season.
5. Build connective tissue strength through higher eccentrics, isometrics, and longer duration movements.
6. Teach proper position of movement skills.
7. Establish sound team mentality.
8. Establish individual goals for physical improvement.
9. Build a flexibility reserve.
10. Teach movements/exercises that will be performed during the off-season.

It is important to address these areas of training before we begin developing maximum strength, speed, power, and special conditioning. This will ensure a proper foundation before engaging in higher volumes, higher loads, and higher speeds of training. A good recipe must always start with a checklist of the ingredients.

Off-Season

The off-season can last anywhere from 10 to 18 weeks again depending on the length of the season. This window of time provides the best opportunity for physical improvement in preparation for the rigors of the preseason period. The off-season consists of two phases: the early off-season and the late off-season.

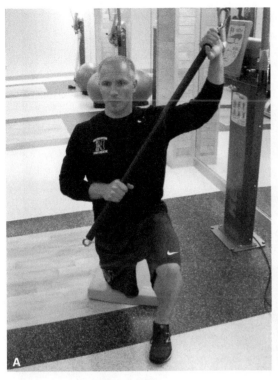
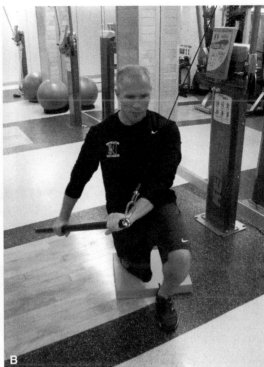

FIGURE 26-11. Chop. (A) Start. (B) End.

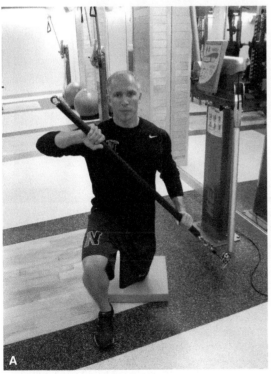
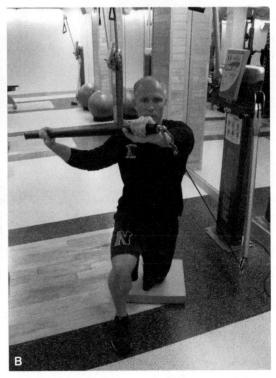

FIGURE 26-12. Lift. (A) Start. (B) End.

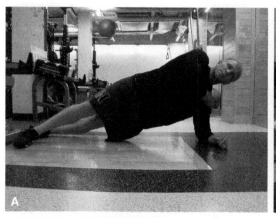

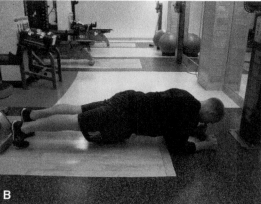

FIGURE 26-13. Rotational planks. (A) Side bridge. (B) Front bridge.

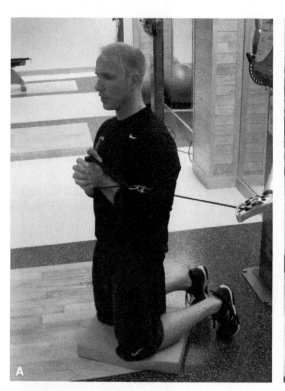

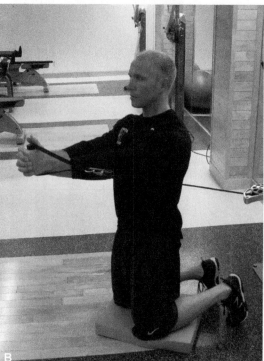

FIGURE 26-14. Antirotational press. (A) Start. (B) End.

The early off-season is much more general and has the following goals:

1. Develop hypertrophy (if needed)
2. Develop maximal strength (focusing on compound, multijoint movements)
3. Develop aerobic base through continuous aerobic work and aerobic intervals
4. Emphasize and teach proper landing mechanics for future plyometric work
5. Teach linear and lateral speed mechanics

As the off-season progresses the exercises and movements become more specific and include:

1. Developing strength but with emphasis on speed/velocity
2. Transition to rate of force development work/power
3. Transition to anaerobic power and anaerobic capacity intervals
4. Transition to true plyometrics emphasizing short response time
5. Transition to specific linear and lateral speed drills emphasizing acceleration coupled with deceleration

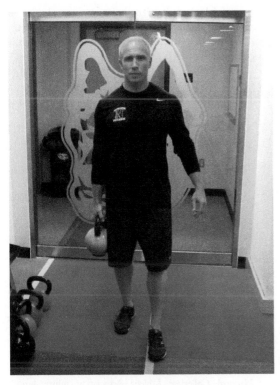

FIGURE 26-15. Asymmetrical carry: farmer walk.

Preseason

The preseason employs practice and games nearly every day. The preseason is the last chance to prepare for the season and requires the qualities that are developed in the off-season because practice time should not be wasted upon developing fitness. Practice time should be geared toward developing skills and strategies.

The goals of training in the preseason include:

1. Continue emphasizing speed of contraction and power development.
2. Transition to sport-specific conditioning using distances, time intervals, and movement patterns used during play (shuffling, backpedaling, sprinting, crossovers, jumping, etc.) while prioritizing anaerobic capacity.
3. Transition plyometric work to multiplanar jump and leg circuits to simulate stresses encountered during the season.
4. Linear and lateral speed development should be open loop drills where change of direction is reactionary versus programmed.

In-Season

In-season training may be the most confusing, challenging, and misunderstood component of the year-long training cycle because in-season training might be one of the most

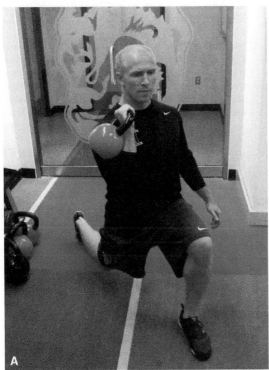

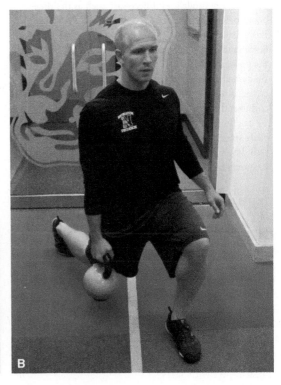

A

B

FIGURE 26-16. (A and B) Asymmetrical reverse lunge.

important times of the year to train. Sure, the off-season and preseason are important, but the current goal should aim toward maintaining physical peak through the end of the regular season and postseason tournaments.

"DO THE OPPOSITE OF THE SPORT"

Huh? What does this mean? Trainers should be doing things specific to make athletes better at their sport, right? We strongly disagree.

In an effort to avoid overuse-type injuries, in-season practice characteristics include:
1. High volume of activity
2. Low loads being used—typically just body weight
3. Low amplitude of movement—never experience full joint range of motion during most sporting activities.

And in-season training characteristics include:
1. Use low volume of in-season strength training. Two days a week has demonstrated that strength can be maintained or improved (14).
2. Use high load to stimulate maximum motor unit activation for strength maintenance or gains.
3. Use high amplitude of movements to restore and enhance joint mobility.

Additional guidelines to help direct basketball programming and progressions during a basketball season include:
1. Basketball athletes experience heavy impact (running, jumping), so limit extra runs and jumps. Choose other conditioning modalities if necessary such as the slide board or swimming pool.
2. Basketball athletes typically demonstrate anterior chain dominance. An emphasis should be placed on training the posterior chain.
3. Basketball athletes have tendencies to lose mobility in typical areas (i.e., ankles, hips). Address these issues consistently and aggressively.
4. Be careful to avoid losing conditioning levels, especially since coaches prefer to do half-court work or skill development versus up-tempo full-court drills or scrimmaging.

CONCLUSIONS

Basketball athletes have been historically and unfairly painted as long-levered athletes incapable of strength training. A quick look at any elite basketball athlete today will validate strength training as an integral part of all basketball performance training and a necessity for achieving elite success. Caution should, however, be given to those attempting to increase absolute strength within this group as this population is faced with a unique set of injury trends, body types, and sport demands requiring special attention to programming detail and exercise selection.

A successful basketball strength program can be implemented that not only addresses common injuries for injury prevention but also increases attributes directly related to on-court success.

REFERENCES

1. McInnes SE, Carlson JS, Jones CJ, McKenna MJ. The physiological load imposed on basketball players during competition. J Sport Sci 1995;13:387–397.
2. Hoffman JR, Maresh CM. Physiology of basketball. In: Garrett WE, Kirkendall DT, eds. Exercise and Sport Science. Philadelphia, PA: Lippincott Williams & Wilkins; 2000: 733–744.
3. Hoffman JR, Tennenbaum G, Maresh CM, Kraemer WJ. Relationship between athletic performance tests and playing time in elite college basketball players. J Strength Cond Res 1996;10:67–71.
4. Riezebos ML, Paterson DH, Hall CR, Yuhasz MS. Relationship of selected variables to performance in women's basketball. Can J Appl Sport Sci 1983;8:34–40.
5. Vescovi JD, Murray TM, Fiala KA, VanHeest JL. Off-ice performance and draft status of elite ice hockey players. Int J Sports Physiol Performance 2006;1:207–221.
6. Dick R, Hertel J, Agel J, Grossma J, Marshall SW. Descriptive epidemiology of collegiate men's basketball injuries: National Collegiate Athletic Association injury surveillance system, 1988–1989 through 2003–2004. J Athl Train 2007;42(2):194–201.
7. Plisky P, Rauh M, Kaminski T, Underwood F. Star excursion balance test as a predictor of lower extremity injury in high school basketball players. J Orthop Sports Phys Ther 2006;36(12):911–919.
8. McGill SM, Grenier S, Bluhm M, Preuss R, Brown S, Russell C. Previous history of LBP with work loss is related to lingering effects in biomechanical physiological, personal, and psychosocial characteristics. Ergonomics 2003;46(7):731–746.
9. McGill SM, Anderson J, Horne AD. Predicting performance and injury resilience from movement quality and fitness scores in a basketball player population. J Strength Cond Res 2012;26(7):1731–1739.
10. McGill SM, McDermott A, Fenwick C. Comparison of different strongman events: trunk muscle activation and lumbar spine motion, load and stiffness. J Strength Cond Res 2008;23(4):1148–1161.
11. McGill SM. Ultimate Back Fitness and Performance. 4th ed. Waterloo, Canada: Backfitpro Inc.; 2009.
12. McGill SM. Low Back Disorders: Evidence Based Prevention and Rehabilitation. 2nd ed. Champaign, IL: Human Kinetics Publishers; 2007.
13. McGill SM, Chaimber JD, Frost DM, Fenwick CM. Evidence of a double peak in muscle activation to enhance strike speed and force: an example with elite mixed martial arts fighters. J Strength Cond Res 2010;24(2):348–357.
14. Hoffman JR, Fry AC, Howard R, Maresh CM, Kraemer WJ. Strength, speed and endurance changes during the course of a division 1 basketball season. J Appl Sport Sci Res 1991;5:144–149.

Off-Season Considerations for Hockey

GENERAL OVERVIEW

The key to training an ice hockey player, and really the key to training any athlete, is realizing that although there are unique areas that need special attention, the true key lies in identifying and training the basics. One of the major problems in training ice hockey players and in training many modern-day athletes is actually the perceived need for sport-specific training.

In the simplest analysis, an ice hockey player is a sprinter, a sprinter who moves faster than any other team sport athlete. Estimates of top speed in skating have run as high as 30 miles/h. Imagine the collisions produced by two masses, each moving at full speed, or one mass striking a relatively immovable object such as the boards of the rink at these rates. Strength, particularly in the often neglected upper body, becomes critical to protect joints at this velocity.

Additionally, to develop the speed necessary to play ice hockey, the development of lower body strength is vital. The ice hockey player must also train like a track sprinter to develop the speed and power that has become such a critical part of the game. The only way to do this is to employ the same multijoint lifts and jumps that comprise the majority of the program in any sprint-dominant sport.

There exists a culture of misinformation that is often perpetuated, even at the highest levels, and this is a fundamental problem in training ice hockey players. Years ago, the simplistic perception was that hockey players were poorly conditioned based on low VO_2 values. This led to a long period of training that emphasized the development of aerobic capacity for hockey players, particularly at the professional level. This push to develop aerobic capacity was spearheaded by exercise scientists with limited experience in team sports and with a bias toward aerobic metabolism. In fact, it is quite natural for sprinters to have relatively low levels of oxygen consumption (1). In my experience it is not uncommon for a well-trained hockey player to have a VO_2 value in the high 40s to mid-50s. Values higher than this probably indicate a lower percentage of fast twitch muscle fibers and would present a less-than-desirable adaptation. Training to raise values beyond the low 50s is a poor use of time and could result in reduced speed and power.

Many coaches and strength and conditioning coaches lose sight of these big picture goals of size and strength in their ice hockey players, and instead focus on the small areas specific to hockey. As an example, in the 1980s, I forbade my players from doing wrist curls, which some consider important in stick handling. My feeling was if the players did not develop the important muscles of the lower body, the smaller muscles of the arms would not be highly relevant. I continue to practice that philosophy today.

There are unique characteristics in ice hockey that should be addressed if time allows. However, the primary emphasis should be on developing lower body strength and power, and on building the proper energy systems. Once these areas are addressed, then, and only then, should coaches and players begin to look at specifics.

Important as the foundation of all my program designs is the concept of joint-by-joint training, developed during a conversation with physical therapist Gray Cook. Gray's analysis of the body is a straightforward one: In his mind, the body is just a stack of joints. Each joint or series of joints has a specific function and is prone to predictable levels of dysfunctions. As a result, each has particular training needs.

Table 27.1 looks at the body on a joint-by-joint basis from the bottom-up, illustrating that joints alternate between mobility and stability. The ankle needs increased mobility, and the knee needs increased stability. Moving up the body, it becomes apparent the hip needs mobility. And so the process goes up the chain—a basic, alternating series of joint purpose.

Loss of function in the joint below seems to affect the joint or joints above. In other words, if the hips cannot move, the lumbar spine will. The problem is that the hips are designed for mobility and the lumbar spine for stability. Of course, this is a surface view; the hips need both mobility and stability, and certainly they need power.

Also, it should be noted that when the intended mobile joint becomes immobile, the stable joint is forced to move as a compensation, becoming less stable and subsequently painful.

The process is simple.

- Losing ankle mobility → knee pain
- Losing hip mobility → low back pain
- Losing thoracic mobility → neck and shoulder pain or low back pain

TABLE 27.1	Joints and Their Primary Needs
Ankle—Mobility (sagittal)	
Knee—Stability	
Hip—Mobility (multiplanar)	
Lumbar spine—Stability	
Thoracic spine—Mobility	
Scapula—Stability	
Glenohumeral—Mobility	

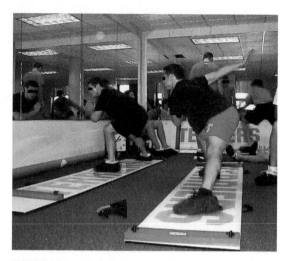

FIGURE 27-1. Slideboard—lateral slides.

When looking at the body on a joint-by-joint basis beginning with the ankle, this makes sense. Once this is understood, it is possible to build this philosophy into your programming, and your athletes will be less susceptible to injury.

OFF-SEASON TRAINING

From a specificity standpoint, it is important for ice hockey players to run in the off-season. Please note I am not advocating jogging. By running, I mean a well-planned program of interval training. Interval training means simply alternating periods of work and rest to develop conditioning. Think of interval training as the opposite of steady-state aerobic training. Although this may seem counterintuitive, interval running in the off-season actually makes sense. In ice hockey, the hips are flexed the majority of the time. This results in adaptive shortening of the hip flexors, and in many cases of the abdominals and pectorals. Running allows the body to readapt to upright posture and may prevent the long-term deterioration of the hips and back.

Contrast the concept of off-season running to the common practice of stationary cycling advocated by many professional team coaches. On the stationary bike, the player assumes the same posture used during the entire season. This, in my opinion, drastically accelerates the deterioration of the hips and core and may be strongly related to the increasing incidence of hip and abdominal injuries in hockey players. In addition, the hip flexors are severely neglected on the bike because the recovery of the hip is passively accomplished by the rotation of the pedals. This is a benefit in-season as a player can do energy system work without overstressing the often-injured groin area, but is a detriment in the off-season.

We deliberately use running as an injury prevention tool. This is not popular with hockey players but must be implemented if the players are healthy. Many players complain of the inability to run due to various orthopedic issues; however, what they most often mean is they cannot jog. Running is usually not an issue.

In addition to a program of interval sprinting, it is recommended that hockey players also use the slideboard (Figure 27.1) in the off-season. Although the slideboard mimics the skating position, it also stresses the hip abductors and adductors. The slideboard generates both concentric and eccentric stress on the hip flexors and adductors in the pattern of flexion and adduction so critical to groin health.

BUILDING THE BASE—INVERTING THE PYRAMID FOR TEAM SPORT CONDITIONING

The conventional model of interval training espouses the development of conditioning in a pyramidal concept. Experts in the fields of training and coaching have continually advocated the concept that the peak could only be as high as the base allowed. The base in theory was the development of a level of aerobic capacity onto which a series of anaerobic blocks could be placed. This was a mechanical or architectural model based on a mechanical system that probably does not apply to exercise. Interestingly enough, coaches have rejected this model as unworkable, yet physiologists continue to spread what I call "the myth of the aerobic base."

In all of my programming and writings since the early 1980s, I have indicated that the concept of the aerobic base was flawed and counterproductive. Numerous studies have proven exactly this over the past 10 years, yet we still have exercise scientists advocating a period of general aerobic training. The most notable recent studies are the Tabata study and Gibala's work at McMaster University (2,3) (see Table 27.2).

TESTING FOR ICE HOCKEY

The most important aspect of preseason testing for ice hockey is that tests must reinforce the desired training concepts. The specific adaptation to imposed demands (SAID) principle

TABLE 27.2	Work Capacity Model for Energy System Development		
Week	Number of Reps	Intervals	Total Time (Min)
1	3	30 s, 30 s, 30 s	1:30
2	4	30 s, 30 s, 30 s, 30 s	2:00
3	5	30 s, 30 s, 30 s, 30 s, 30 s	2:30
4	6	30 s, 30 s, 30 s, 30 s, 30 s, 30 s	3:00

shows clearly that the body adapts to imposed or implied demands. It makes no sense to ask an athlete to interval train and then administer a steady-state test, in the same way we should not ask an athlete to strength train and then administer an endurance test. If we want athletes to interval train, we should use an interval test. If we want athletes to strength train, we administer a strength test. Athletes will train for the tests rather than follow the program. They know they are not being evaluated on program compliance, but rather on results. The key is to make program compliance produce the desired results. If testing is performed, strict attention must be paid to form and technique. Do not allow athletes to cheat, as this creates another layer of problems.

If we are going to perform off-ice testing, there are a few key areas of concern. Although I am a huge believer in lower body strength, I think coaches need to be careful in testing lower body strength due to an element of danger. Although I consider lower body strength the number one goal for an ice hockey player, I urge caution in testing. Instead, focus lower body testing on the vertical jump and the 10-yard dash.

The only way to improve these quantities is to follow a well-designed lower body strength program. Increases in vertical jump and improvements in speed will indirectly test the compliance in lower body training. It is also important to track body weight and body fat percentage. Young players who are gaining muscle mass may not improve in speed and power; however, if a player gains lean body mass and maintains vertical jump and speed, the net result is a gain in power as more mass is being moved at the same speed. This will not be as great a problem for older veteran players, as they will not tend to have large changes in lean body mass from year to year. In fact, when testing older players, it is important to note that power is not decreasing. It is very common for older players to focus on aerobic fitness and see decreases in speed. In order to not "lose a step," the older player must work diligently to increase or at least maintain speed and power.

Vertical Jump

This is the standard standing two-foot jump. Coaches can use a Vertec or the new jump pads such as the Just Jump.

It is important to accurately measure reach on the Vertec and to monitor technique on the Just Jump. The Just Jump measures time in the air and converts time to distance. This can be influenced by jumping from the back of the mat and landing on the front, or by an exaggerated landing on the heels. The key to any of the jump mat systems is that the jump appears "normal." The idea of *normal* is one you will understand after observing athletes jump—there are no standards and no published norms for this.

10-Yard Dash

I strongly prefer electronic timers for 10-yard-dash timing, since an electronic timer eliminates the margin of error. Electronic timers yield slower times, but the times are far more reliable. Off-ice speed has been shown in numerous studies to correlate to on-ice speed. Hockey speed expert Jack Blatherwick has been preaching this since the early 1980s (4).

300-Yard Shuttle Run (or Goal Line to Blue Line [×7])

Conditioning testing should be interval in nature and should test performance. Do not test physiology and assume physiology predicts fitness—performance predicts fitness. The 300-yard shuttle run is an excellent, valid, and reliable test that will accurately measure fitness in a competitive environment. The athlete with the lowest average time is in the best shape … simple.

To perform the 300-yard shuttle test, athletes run 12 × 25 yards, rest 5 minutes, and repeat—the score is the average of the two times. We also make note of the differential between the first and the second time. This is important, as a fast athlete may be able to obtain a passing score, but have a large differential between the two times. My guideline is to consider differentials greater than 5 seconds a failed test.

The Goal Line to Blue Line (×7) test is almost identical to the 300-yard shuttle. We developed this test to mimic what we did off-ice, and the correlation has been perfect. We administer this test in week 3 of our preseason to allow some adaptation to skating. Professional teams could do this early in training camp, since players are expected to begin skating well in advance of camp. For this test, we have the players begin on the blue line and skate to the goal line and back seven times. As in the 300-yard shuttle run, the rest is 5 minutes. Some coaches have argued this rest is too long, but for comparative purposes we keep the rest consistent.

Upper Body Pushing

Many coaches prefer push-ups for upper body strength, but push-ups actually test upper body endurance. As stated above, if you want athletes to develop strength for injury prevention, a test of strength must be administered. For this reason we use some version of the bench press. When I am familiar with an athlete, I use a one-repetition (one-rep) maximum (max). With other athletes such as draft choices or athletes involved in trades, we will use a rep max test. My current choice is to ask the athlete to select a load perceived to be a five-rep max and go to failure. Maximums can easily be estimated from this data.

To test a one-rep max, it is necessary to have an accurate estimate of the athlete's strength. Therefore, do not perform one-rep max tests with athletes you do not coach on a regular basis. To perform a one-rep max, the athlete does two or three warm-up sets with increasing loads. After the initial warm-up set of 5 to 10 reps, the athlete performs single reps. The first attempt in a one-rep max test should be done at a weight of which both the athlete and coach are confident. The key is for the bar to descend under control, touch the chest with no bounce, and be pressed back to the starting position. This attempt then determines the load for the next attempt.

At this point, the science of strength and conditioning becomes the art of strength and conditioning. Deciding what the next attempt will be takes an experienced eye. This is the reason I do not recommend that inexperienced coaches undertake one-rep max testing. Instead, a rep max test can be performed. For a rep max test, use a load the athlete is confident of five successful reps. Again, the weight must be raised and lowered under control. No bouncing of the bar is allowed, and the hips must stay in contact with the bench. In addition, the elbows must extend at the end of every rep. It is critical that testing be done strictly if the testing is to have any validity.

Upper Body Pulling

For upper body pulling, a pull-up test is simple to administer (Figure 27.2). Although this test tends to also test endurance, in stronger athletes we generally use a rep max test. It is critical that the test is strictly administered and that no cheating is allowed.

Body Fat Percentage

Testing body fat is relatively simple, although two things are important to note. First, reliability is always an issue. In an ideal situation, the same person should function as the tester for all athletes. Second, do not use age adjustments for athletes. Athletes, particularly those in the professional ranks, do not age normally. Body fat calculation formulas assume we get fatter as we get older. As a result, the formula calculates additional body fat with age. Many professional athletes have much "younger" bodies. When an athlete moves to another age category, the same skinfolds yield a higher body fat percentage using the automated calculations. I test all my athletes as 18- to 25-year-olds regardless of age.

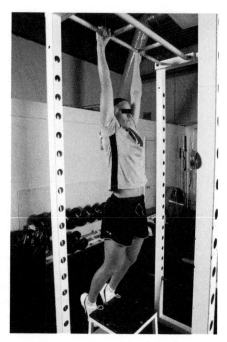

FIGURE 27-2. Pull-up.

To test body fat, we use a Cramer Skyndex. The Skyndex is an electronic caliper that takes a three-site measurement and immediately calculates a body fat percentage. This device has proven to be both valid and reliable provided it is calibrated as described in the manual.

SPORT-SPECIFIC EXERCISES FOR ICE HOCKEY

We use sport-specific exercises for ice hockey, but these exercises are actually multijoint lower body exercises designed to positively impact the skating muscles while minimizing lower back loads. These specific exercises can be used year-round. As a general rule of thumb, three sets of 5 to 10 reps are used. Lower body training is generally done twice per week on a year-round basis. In-season training would result in a decrease in the number of sets as athletes try to decrease volume. The beauty of these exercises is they incorporate all levels of hockey. Adolescent players might begin these exercises with bodyweight, while older players might use significant external loads.

Rear-Foot-Elevated Split Squats (Figure 27.3)

These are the base lower body strength exercise we currently use for our players. Commonly and incorrectly referred to as Bulgarian lunges, it is important to note that the exercise did not originate in the Eastern block and is not a lunge. The rear-foot-elevated split squat develops the unilateral

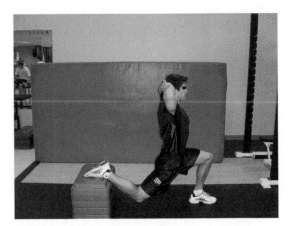

FIGURE 27-3. Rear-foot-elevated split squat.

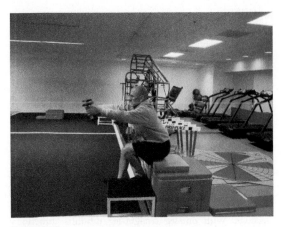

FIGURE 27-5. Single-leg two-box squat.

strength so necessary in skating, while also allowing the use of heavy loads. The ideal way to load is with a bar in the back squat position, but we have also used dumbbells and kettlebells.

One-Leg Squats

Like the rear-foot-elevated split squat, a true one-leg squat is also a key exercise we use to develop lower body strength. The one-leg squat is a more advanced exercise and develops the strength of the hips in three planes. The ideal situation is to use a combination of rear-foot-elevated split squats and one-leg squats. Although we load both exercises as heavy as possible, the additional stability of the rear-foot-elevated split squats allows significantly higher loads. Our strongest athletes will routinely use over 225 lb in a rear-foot-elevated split, but will rarely use over a hundred pounds in a one-leg squat.

In the one-leg squat, unlike the pistol, which is done off the floor, these are normally done off a standard exercise bench or an 18" Plyo Box (Figure 27.4). To control descent we have actually taken to using a combination of two Plyo

Boxes and a cone (Figure 27.5). The cone encourages the athlete to descend under control. Another version is the single-leg box squat (Figure 27.6). This can be done to a 12" Plyo Box placed on the floor. For most athletes an Airex pad is placed on the box to get a depth of 14.5 inch. Load is most often obtained through a combination of a weight vest and dumbbells.

POSTERIOR-CHAIN TRAINING

The glutes and hamstrings, and in fact the long adductors, are often referred to as the posterior chain and are worked

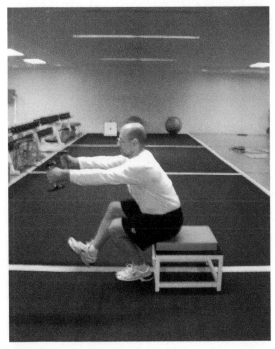

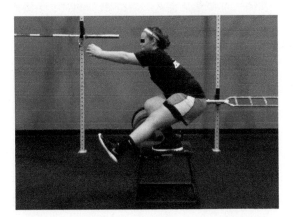

FIGURE 27-4. Single-leg squat off box.

FIGURE 27-6. Single-leg box squat.

with exercises that prioritize the motion of the hip over the knee. These exercises can also be referred to as hip-dominant exercises. This is in contrast to the previously illustrated one-leg squat variations most frequently referred to as anterior-chain or knee-dominant exercises.

Knee-dominant or anterior-chain exercises all bear a strong resemblance to squats. However, there are four critical areas of posterior-chain training.

Hip-Hinge Exercises

Straight-leg deadlifts (Figure 27.7) and another poorly named exercise, the Romanian deadlift, are examples of hip-hinge exercises. My preference is for the single-leg versions. With one-leg straight-leg deadlifts, functional capability of the hips is enhanced while lumbar loads are minimized.

Bridge Variations

Bridge variations include double-leg (Figure 27.8) and single-leg (Figure 27.9) versions, which progress into slide-board leg curl exercises. Bridge exercises allow a functional, closed-chain leg curl. The glute is used initially to extend the hip and later is used as a stabilizer while the hamstrings

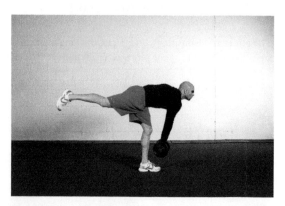

FIGURE 27-7. Single-leg deadlift.

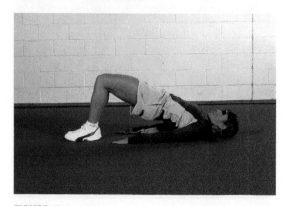

FIGURE 27-8. Bridge.

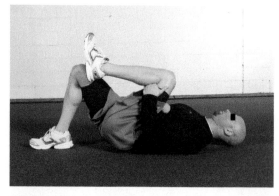

FIGURE 27-9. Single-leg bridge.

flex and extend the knee. These are excellent exercises to train the hamstrings.

Hip Lifts

The hip lift (Figure 27.10) takes the bridge variation to a higher level and is actually the best way to train the glutes. I call the shoulder-elevated hip lifts "the best exercise we never do." These can be done off any surface approximately tibial height, usually an 18" Plyo Box or a standard exercise bench is used.

Lower Pulls

The fourth category is best described as lower pulls. Both walking lunges and slideboard lunges (Figure 27.11) fall in the lower pull category. Many people consider these knee-dominant exercises; however, I disagree. The best way to describe these exercises is by the comparison of horses and zebras. By appearance, we would assume the animals are related, but they are not. The same applies to lower pulls and knee-dominant exercises. Although they look similar, the effect is far different. Lower pull exercises, like hip

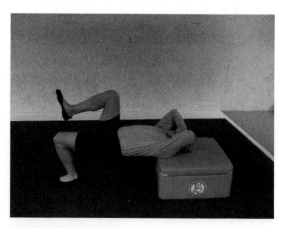

FIGURE 27-10. Shoulder-elevated hip lift.

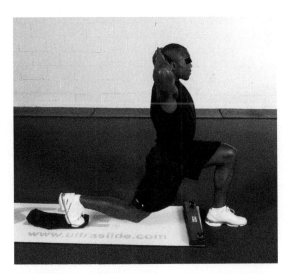

FIGURE 27-11. Slideboard lunge.

hinges and hip lifts, affect the glutes and hamstrings to a greater degree than the quadriceps.

CONCLUSIONS

The process of developing ice hockey players is complicated by the need to develop strength, speed, power, and conditioning. To train ice hockey players, all quantities must be trained and treated relatively equal. Too much work in one area can result in decreases in others or in injuries. In order to develop an effective program, it is important to analyze the demands of the game and not be a slave to conventional wisdom. When I began training hockey players over 20 years ago, the sport was dominated by stereotypes. Weight training was frowned upon and aerobic training was viewed as the key to improvement. By examining the training of speed and power athletes and applying the same concepts, we were able to change the paradigm of hockey training and develop programs that improve performance and prevent injury. In the process, we were able to develop some of the world's fastest skaters.

Remember, the ice hockey player is a sprinter who is going to experience high-speed collisions. Preparation must match the demands of the sport: hockey demands strength and power.

REFERENCES

1. Francis C. Training for Speed. Faccioni Speed and Conditioning Consultant; 1997.
2. Gibala, M. Short term sprint interval versus traditional endurance training: similar initial adaptations in human skeletal muscle and exercise performance. J Physiol 2006:575(3).
3. Tabata I, Nishimura K, Kouzaki M, et al. Effects of Moderate-Intensity Endurance and High-Intensity Intermittent Training on Anaerobic Capacity and VO_{2max}. Department of Physiology and Biomechanics, National Institute of Fitness and Sports, Kagoshima Prefecture, Japan.
4. Blatherwick J. Overspeed Skill Training for Hockey. 2nd ed. USA Hockey; 1994.

Training Strategies for Developing Explosive Power in Mixed Martial Arts and Other Sports

For a mixed martial arts (MMA) athlete, or any explosive power athlete, the ability to quickly induce and sustain high levels of muscular force is paramount. No MMA athlete ever knocked out his/her opponent by throwing a slap to the cheek; and no athlete benefits by fatiguing too early.

The sport of MMA requires a myriad of contractions, from high-velocity low-load movements (e.g., punch, kick) to low-velocity high-load movements (e.g., grappling), and everything in between. Each type of movement is enhanced when an athlete improves the rate of force development (RFD), a measure of how quickly peak levels of force are achieved. Indeed, an explosive athlete benefits by reaching peak levels of force in less than 0.3 seconds (1).

Since MMA is a relatively new sport, many trainers and coaches have borrowed strength training techniques from other realms such as boxing, power lifting, and bodybuilding. However, a boxer only needs to stand and exchange punches without worrying about a takedown, hip throw, or a lightning fast kick to the head. A power lifter must be able to quickly produce huge amounts of force, but only for a few seconds, and this force does not have to be reproduced seconds later like it does in a fight. A bodybuilder needs bigger, stronger muscles without regard for the explosive movements necessary in MMA.

Therefore, the strength and conditioning demands of MMA go far beyond those sports. Indeed, a unique, multi-faceted approach is required to optimally develop the kind of power and physical prowess that a fighter needs. The MMA fighter benefits from being conditioned to quickly reach peak levels of force, and sustain power output at the highest level possible for the duration of the event.

Numerous mechanical and morphological elements contribute to maximal power (2). However, this chapter focuses mainly on the neural factors that influence it.

HOW FORCE IS DEVELOPED

The human body relies on an elegant, orderly system to develop muscular force by recruiting and increasing the firing rates of its motor neurons. This fixed process is based on the physiological properties of the spinal motor neurons that sit in the anterior horn of the spinal cord. Motor neurons that are smallest in diameter are most easily excitable due to their electrical properties, so they require the lowest level of synaptic input to fire. As the synaptic drive to the motor neuron pool increases, larger motor neurons reach threshold and fire. This is known as the size principle (3) (Figure 28.1).

Each motor neuron is connected to a group of muscle fibers that can range from a few fibers to a thousand or more (4). When a motor neuron reaches threshold, a signal travels down its axon and initiates a cascade of events that result in muscle contraction. The combination of a motor neuron and all the fibers it innervates is a motor unit (Figure 28.2). To quickly induce peak levels of force and enhance RFD, it is necessary to recruit the largest number of motor units possible.

Since there are three primary skeletal muscle fiber types in humans (type I, type IIa, type IIb), there are three primary types of motor units (5). As the synaptic drive to the anterior horn increases, motor units are recruited in a fixed order from smallest/weakest to largest/strongest:

- Slow (S) motor units: These are the smallest motor units since they contain a small bundle (e.g., 10 muscle fibers) of type I slow-twitch, endurance muscle fibers. The S motor unit contains a skinny motor neuron and it produces modest increases in force when activated. The S motor units can sustain their activity for hours.
- Fast, fatigue-resistant (FFR) motor units: A FFR motor unit contains a medium-sized motor neuron that is connected to a medium bundle (e.g., 100 muscle fibers) of moderately strong type IIa fast-twitch muscle fibers. The FFR motor units produce more force than S motor units because they contain a larger bundle of stronger muscle fibers. FFR motor units have moderate endurance capabilities and can fire for minutes before fatigue sets in.

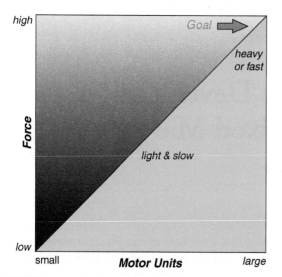

FIGURE 28-1. Size principle.

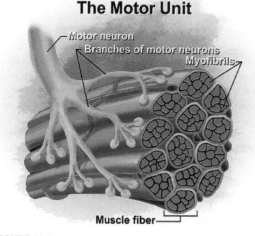

FIGURE 28-2. The motor unit.

- Fast-fatigable (FF) motor units: The FF motor units produce the most force because they contain a large bundle (e.g., 1,000 muscle fibers per bundle) of strong, type IIb fast-twitch muscle fibers. However, they can only sustain contractions for less than a minute due to their very low endurance characteristics. The largest, strongest FF motor units have the lowest endurance capacity of all motor units. They stop firing within 10 seconds due to the energy limitations of the ATP-PC system that supplies the type IIb fibers.

The S motor units are activated first and as they fire faster, FFR motor units are recruited. After FFR motor units fire faster, FF motor units are activated (5). An important element that is often overlooked is FF motor units are recruited last as determined by Henneman's size principle, but they are first to drop out due to their low endurance capabilities.

It should be noted here that in 2006 research by Wakeling et al. (6) conflictingly demonstrated out-of-sequence selective recruitment of high-threshold motor units in the medial gastrocnemius during ballistic contractions. However, the current overreaching view in the scientific community is that the size principle is preserved in all types of contractions. In a review of power training methods by Cormie et al. (2) the authors stated, "While preferential recruitment of type II fibres remains a possibility, the current evidence for it occurring in response to exercise in humans is not convincing."

Motor neurons within a motor unit receive synaptic input from many different sources. The simplest explanation of a voluntary contraction starts with the cerebellum, association cortex, and basal ganglia which feed information via the upper motor neurons directly to the spinal motor neurons. However, these upper motor neurons can also communicate with motor programs and reflexes within the spinal cord that, in turn, relay information to the motor neurons.

The key point in mentioning the complexity of neural communication is that any activity that enhances the higher brain centers, descending pathways, and/or built-in neural patterns could enhance motor neuron activity and potentially increase force production. For example, Yue and Cole (7) demonstrated that it is possible to improve a muscle's force-producing capabilities by having subjects simply imagine they are performing muscle contractions.

Training Tip

Fighters must be able to produce high levels of force while striking and grappling, and the most forceful contractions occur when the largest motor units are recruited. Since the largest motor units (FF) consist of motor neurons that require the highest synaptic input to reach threshold, these motor units are often referred to as "high-threshold motor units" (8). And given that the FF motor units produce the most force, and contract fastest, they could just as easily be referred to as "high-force" or "high-acceleration" motor units. In other words, only movements that produce high levels of force or acceleration will recruit the FF motor units that are responsible for the most powerful muscle contractions.

WHY SHOULD FIGHTERS LIFT HEAVY?

A commonly held belief in martial arts, and other sports that demand fast movements, is that heavy resistance training will make an athlete slower. This assumption often stems from three factors.

First, training with near-maximal loads forces the muscles to contract much slower than many movements that the sport demands. However, Behm and Sale (9) demonstrated that the intended velocity, rather than the actual movement velocity, determines the velocity-specific training response. Sixteen subjects applied maximum force to resistance that resulted in an isometric (zero-velocity) or dynamic (high-velocity) contraction. The zero-velocity contractions improved the subject's ability to produce high-velocity strength just as well as the high-velocity contractions did. Importantly, in other studies where no improvement in high-velocity strength was demonstrated with isometric training, no emphasis was put on attempting to move as rapidly as possible (10,11). Even though subsequent research with Dinn and Behm (12) suggests that high-velocity training is more effective than isometric training for increasing punching velocity, the benefits of maximal strength training to improve power should be appreciated.

The second assumption is that training with heavy loads will diminish an athlete's endurance. Using 17 well-trained male and female runners, Storen et al. (13) demonstrated that four sets of four repetitions (reps) of the half-squat three times per week for 8 weeks at the subjects' individual four-rep maximum (RM) improved running economy by 5% and increased time to exhaustion at maximal aerobic speed by 21.3%. Other studies (14,15) have demonstrated an increase in running economy with heavy-load training.

> **Training Tip**
>
> Therefore, there is solid evidence to support the notion that strength training can improve an athlete's aerobic capacity by lowering perceived rate of exertion and increasing time to exhaustion.

Third, any additional muscle mass may make an athlete move slower due to heavier body weight. It is well accepted that strength training does not necessarily lead to significant amounts of hypertrophy. Appreciable levels of muscle growth require additional nutritional support from increased calories, and higher volume training protocols produce more hypertrophy than lower protocols do (16). Therefore, by controlling calories and training volume, an athlete can become stronger without adding significant muscle mass. Nevertheless, since cross-sectional area is positively correlated with maximal power, even small additions of muscle mass that minimally increase an athlete's body weight can improve performance (17,18). Training with maximal loads coincides with high levels of synaptic input to the motor neuron pool that recruits the high-threshold motor units that produce the most force.

An often underappreciated benefit of training with heavy loads is the positive effect it has on increasing bone mineral density (19). Using 12 college-age men, Almstedt et al. demonstrated a 2.7% to 7.7% increase in bone mineral density after 24 weeks of resistance training (20). The benefits of a stronger skeletal structure cannot be overstated for any combat athlete.

POTENTIAL PROBLEMS WITH TYPICAL RESISTANCE TRAINING PARAMETERS

Building maximal power requires exercises that produce the highest levels of muscular force. When training for strength or hypertrophy, it is common for athletes to perform three or four sets of 10 to 12 reps to failure with a purposely slow-lifting tempo. There are two shortcomings with this bodybuilding-style approach when considering the science of motor unit recruitment.

First, a purposely slow-lifting tempo at the beginning of a set with submaximal load will not recruit high-threshold motor units. In order to recruit the high-threshold motor units, high levels of muscular force must be produced. By purposely slowing down the concentric phase of muscle contraction, acceleration and force are not at their peak. Therefore, the largest motor units remain inactive because force is less than maximal.

Second, as an athlete approaches failure the ability to accelerate the lift is diminished. This fatigue restricts an athlete's ability to recruit the high-threshold motor units that only come into play with high-force contractions. Research demonstrates that a loss of velocity is an accurate indicator of neuromuscular fatigue (21). High levels of force require high levels of acceleration when training with submaximal loads. By the time an athlete reaches rep 12, neuromuscular fatigue blocks his ability to recruit the largest motor units. Rather, if high-threshold motor units came into play toward the end of a set, velocity of the lift would increase.

MAXIMAL STRENGTH TRAINING FOR POWER ATHLETES

An athlete cannot develop high levels of power unless he or she is strong. Developing maximal strength in the hips and core enhances force transfer throughout the body by minimizing "energy leaks," a term popularized by Stuart McGill (22). Therefore, it is important to develop maximal strength before implementing explosive strength training protocols.

> **Training Tip**
>
> It is common practice for coaches to have athletes rest for 3 minutes or more between sets of heavy resistance exercises. Long rest periods are typical in sports like powerlifting or sprinting where endurance is not important. However, an MMA athlete can benefit by building cardiovascular capacity while training for maximal strength.

Alcaraz et al. (23) had subjects train with a 6 RM load to compare the strength and cardiovascular responses between straight sets with 3-minute rest periods and circuit training with 35 seconds rest between each exercise. In either case, the subjects rested 3 minutes before repeating an exercise; however, the circuit training group performed exercises for other muscle groups (active rest) during those 3 minutes. The research demonstrated similar strength gains between the two protocols while the cardiovascular demand was substantially greater with the heavy resistance circuit. This combined enhancement of strength and cardiovascular endurance is essential to an MMA athlete.

DETERMINING INITIAL MAXIMAL STRENGTH LEVELS

When determining an athlete's initial strength levels, great care should be taken to not push the athlete beyond his physical capabilities. Before performing any maximum attempt, three warm-up sets of three reps (3 × 3) with progressively heavier loads are recommended. The first set should be with a load the athlete rates as moderate, or a 4 to 5 rate of perceived exertion (RPE) with the Borg CR10 scale. The second set should be rated 6 to 7. The third should be 7 to 8. If an athlete feels he needs an additional warm-up set, he should do it.

Strength exercises to test include the following:

- Deadlift with unmixed, snatch grip (Figure 28.3): 1 RM.
- Bulgarian split squat (Figure 28.4): 3 RM for each leg. For safety reasons, it is recommended to hold a dumbbell in each hand with the arms hanging down at sides.
- Dumbbell push press (Figure 28.5): 3 RM. This can also be performed with a barbell.
- Pull-up with neutral grip: 3 RM. If the athlete can perform more than three reps, load should be added using a chin/dip belt or weighted vest, or a dumbbell can be held between the feet.
- Dip: 3 RM. If the athlete can perform more than three reps, load should be added using a chin/dip belt or a weighted vest, or a dumbbell can be held between the feet.
- Abdominal (Ab)-wheel rollout (Figure 28.6): should first be performed with the knees down. If the athlete can complete 10 full reps, the version with the knees up can be tested to determine whether the athlete can perform one rep.
- Pallof press: 10-second hold with the maximum load for each side.

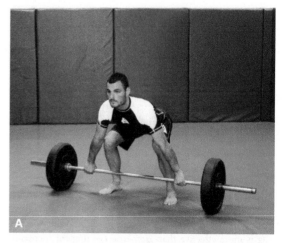

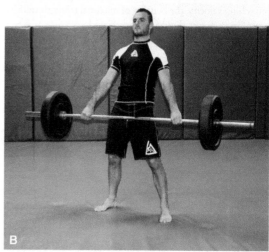

FIGURE 28-3.   (A, B) Deadlift.

> **Training Tip**
>
> The following maximal strength goals are for lean male athletes (<15% body fat) who weigh less than 200 lb. For athletes over 200 lb, the maximal strength loading goals can be decreased by approximately 10%.
>
> - Deadlift with unmixed, snatch grip: one rep with a load equal to double body weight.
> - Bulgarian split squat: three reps with a load equal to body weight.
> - Push press: three reps with a load equal to body weight.
> - Pull-up with neutral grip: three reps with an additional 25% of body weight.
> - Dip: three reps with an additional 25% of body weight.
> - Ab-wheel rollout (legs straight, knees off the ground): one full rep.
> - Pallof press (or cable core press): 10-second hold with 50% of body weight for each side.

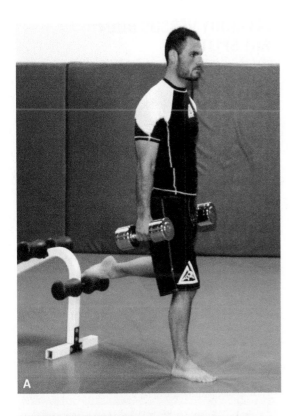

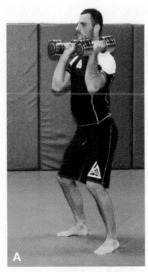

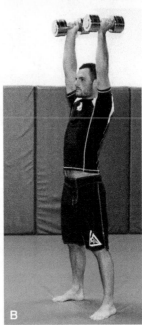

FIGURE 28-5. (A, B) Dumbbell push press.

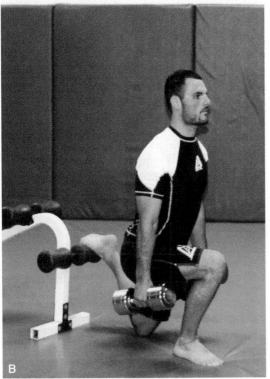

FIGURE 28-4. (A, B) Bulgarian split squat.

MICROCYCLE MAXIMAL STRENGTH TRAINING GUIDELINES FOR MIXED MARTIAL ARTS ATHLETES

- Frequency: Two sessions per week, evenly spaced (e.g., Monday/Thursday or Tuesday/Friday) for any exercise that falls short of the aforementioned maximal strength goals. If an athlete can achieve the maximal strength goal for an exercise, the exercise needs to be trained for maximal strength only once per week.

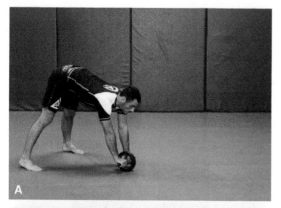

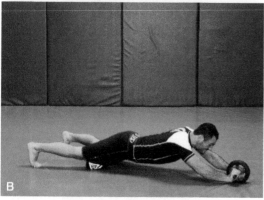

FIGURE 28-6. (A, B) Abdominal-wheel rollout.

- Work sets: Three. Before any exercise, an athlete can warm up by performing three sets of two reps with loads that progress from light to moderately heavy.
- Exercise sequence: To minimize a carryover of fatigue between exercises, it is recommended to perform the circuit in the following sequence, with 30 seconds of rest between exercises: 1, deadlift for 3 reps; 2, dip for 3 reps; 3, pull-up for 3 reps; 4, Pallof press for 10-second hold, each side; 5, Bulgarian split squat for 3 reps, each leg; 6, push press for 3 reps; 7, Ab-wheel rollout for 3 reps. Do three rounds total. (Or the workout can be split into two mini-circuits.)

This entire workout should be performed once per week when the athlete is least fatigued (earlier in the week typically works best). The second maximal strength workout (3 days later) consists only of the exercises that fall short of the maximal strength goals mentioned earlier.

> **Training Tip**
>
> The further an athlete is from his genetic strength limit, the greater the benefit that maximal strength training will provide. Since many MMA athletes train, or have trained, with low-load endurance protocols, training with heavy-load/low-velocity movements will not only increase maximal strength but also increase power (24).

FULL-BODY VERSUS BODY PART SPLITS

The aforementioned maximal strength training exercises can be performed throughout the week with an upper/lower body split.

- Monday and Thursday (upper body): 1, pull-up; 2, push press; 3, Pallof press; 4, dip
- Tuesday and Friday (lower body): 1 deadlift; 2, Bulgarian split squat; 3, Ab-wheel rollout

> **Training Tip**
>
> Some strength coaches favor a body part split; however, this approach can have limitations. The first limitation of an upper/lower split is that it requires four training sessions per week to train the entire body instead of two. Given an athlete's time constraints to practice wrestling, striking, jiu-jitsu, and so on, fewer strength workouts are often more conducive to the weekly training schedule. Second, a body part split workout takes less time to complete than a full-body workout. The benefit of a full-body strength workout is that the athlete must sustain his performance across a wider range of exercises for more time. This could carry over more effectively to the physical demands of a long fight.

MAXIMAL STRENGTH DELOADING PROTOCOL

Strength gains do not occur in a steady, linear fashion. Factors such as stress, nutrition, and sleep habits can influence an athlete's performance. The goal of maximal strength training is to steadily increase the load an athlete can lift until he reaches the maximal strength goals mentioned earlier. However, it is important to note how an athlete is feeling in any given training session.

> **Training Tip**
>
> An important, but often under-recognized role of the coach or trainer is to assess an athlete's readiness. This may be subjective or could be identified quantitatively via such methods as RPE with warm-up sets, grip strength, vertical leap, or omega wave assessment.
>
> When an athlete shows signs of fatigue, he should not be pushed to improve his maximal strength performance that day. Instead, the trainer should decrease the load of the athlete's work sets by approximately 30% for that session. A deload allows an athlete to recover, and possibly supercompensate, from the loading stress in previous training sessions.
>
> Elite, strong, motivated athletes with years of strength training experience are closer to their genetic strength

limit. It is likely that each maximal strength workout for an advanced strength athlete is more stressful than it is for a novice lifter who is far from his genetic strength limit. Therefore, an advanced athlete might benefit from more frequent periods of deloading.

It is common for elite coaches to plan deloading workouts into an athlete's training schedule. As a gross generalization, one or two consecutive deloading workouts performed every 4 weeks is a good starting point.

There are two ways to incorporate deloading workouts into a maximal strength training cycle. The first method is to continue adding load to an athlete's lifts each week until his strength gains plateau. At that point, one or two workouts with 30% less load is performed. After one or two lighter workouts, the athlete will revert to the previous predeload numbers and the load progression will continue. The second method is to plan periods of deloading into an athlete's training. An advanced strength athlete might perform two consecutive deloading workouts every fourth week, while a novice strength athlete might plan the deloading workouts every sixth week.

Another crucial factor to consider with respect to an athlete facing fatigue or a training plateau is the need for recovery. Besides deloading workouts such an athlete likely requires the following:

- A functional movement assessment to identify potential sources of "energy leaks" (see Chapters 5, 6, and 22)
- Recovery care such as soft tissue manipulation, cryobaths, and so on
- Corrective exercise strategies to stabilize the "energy leaks" (see Chapters 5 and 7)

Once an athlete can achieve the maximal strength goals, it is recommended to incorporate single-limb exercises. Single-limb exercises develop greater core stability strength and balance, and they help identify strength imbalances between sides of the body.

BRIDGING THE GAP BETWEEN STRENGTH AND POWER

After a solid base of maximal strength has been developed, an athlete is primed to produce higher levels of power. Indeed, much research has demonstrated that stronger athletes can produce more power than weaker athletes (25–28).

High levels of maximal strength will not effectively carry over to competition unless the athlete reaches peak levels of force very quickly. What matters is the athlete's RFD, a measure of how quickly the athlete can achieve peak levels of force. As stated in Zatsiorsky's text, *Science and Practice of Strength Training*: "Strong people do not necessarily possess a high rate of force development (24)."

Increasing RFD allows an athlete to engage those higher force-producing capabilities more quickly through: earlier motor unit activation, extra doublets (a motor unit that fires twice in 4 ms or less), and an enhanced firing rate of motor units (29,30).

When an athlete can quickly and simultaneously contract muscles to stiffen joint complexes, it also helps prevent injuries by restricting an excessive range of motion. This joint stabilization most likely occurs by reflex activation at the spinal level (31), but it is trainable.

Ballistic and plyometric exercises have been shown to improve explosive strength and RFD (32–35). While both types of exercise consist of fast movements with submaximal loads, a slight distinction can be made between the two. Plyometric exercises rely heavily on the stretch–shorten cycle (SSC) and are typically performed with little to no external resistance such as a single-leg hop or clap push-up (2). Ballistic exercises are not necessarily characterized by a rapid SSC (e.g., heavy medicine ball push from the chest), and they typically are performed with heavier loads than plyometric exercises (e.g., Olympic lifts). Regardless of this slight distinction, ballistic and plyometric exercises are generally considered more sport specific because of the rapid onset of muscle contraction required (36–40).

Many MMA athletes have spent considerable time performing low-load endurance exercises with little emphasis on maximal strength. Therefore, they benefit from the strength gains associated with heavier ballistic exercises. Ballistic exercises also help strengthen the connective tissues without imposing significant impact or stretch load forces on the joints.

Plyometric exercises are considered advanced training since people with low fitness levels or little experience typically benefit less from them (41,42). Many plyometric exercises, even without external resistance, induce large stretch and impact load forces. Therefore, they should be implemented only after an athlete has built a strong base of maximal strength followed by months of ballistic exercises (e.g., high pull, kettlebell swing, and medicine ball throw).

Ballistic Training Strategies

For ballistic training, two workouts per week, evenly spaced (e.g., Monday/Thursday), are recommended. Ballistic exercises can be performed at the beginning of a maximal strength workout, six or more hours away from a maximal strength workout, or on a separate day.

A circuit of the high pull, swing, and squat with a forward throw is an effective full-body ballistic training workout that improves RFD. The key point is to use a load that is heavy enough to challenge the athlete, but light enough to allow for high levels of acceleration. For many athletes, 50% to 60% of 1 RM is effective for ballistic training.

- High pull (Figure 28.7) for 3 reps and rest 30 seconds
- One-arm swing (Figure 28.8), alternate, for 10 total reps (5 reps per side) and rest 30 seconds
- Medicine ball chest throw (Figure 28.9) for 3 reps and rest 30 seconds

Repeat the three steps nine more times (10 rounds total).

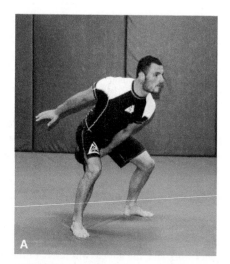

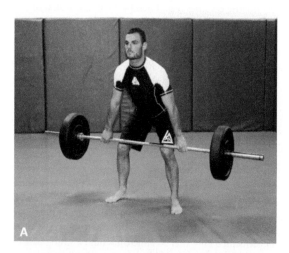

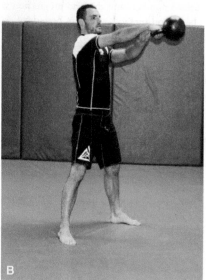

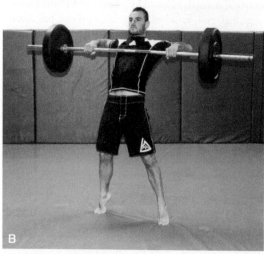

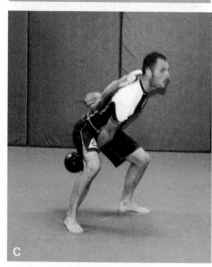

FIGURE 28-7.   (A, B) High pull.

FIGURE 28-8.   (A–C) One-arm swing.

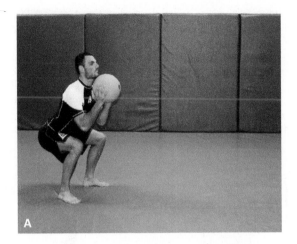

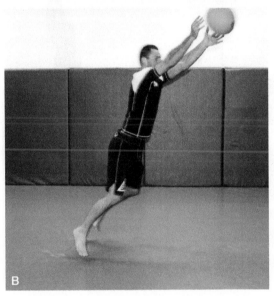

FIGURE 28-9.   (A, B) Medicine ball chest throw.

Sample Progression for Ballistic Training

The goals of ballistic training are to improve strength and RFD. Therefore, the load used for any exercise should be progressively increased, but not so much that the actual lifting velocity slows down. Indeed, there is as much art as there is science when increasing the load of ballistic exercises.

In order to boost cardiovascular endurance, an athlete should focus on decreasing the rest periods between each exercise each week. After two sessions in the first week of performing the aforementioned circuit with 30 seconds rest, each rest period should be decreased by 5 seconds over subsequent weeks in the following manner: week 2, 25 seconds of rest; week 3, 20 seconds of rest; week 4, 15 seconds of rest; week 5, 10 seconds of rest; week 6,

5 seconds of rest. Once an athlete progresses to five seconds of rest between the three exercises in a circuit, an additional ballistic exercise can be added to the circuit and the rest progression can be repeated starting with 30 seconds between exercises.

Plyometric Training Strategies

Plyometric exercises (e.g., single-leg hop) using an athlete's body weight have been shown to improve power and agility (34,35,43). A study by de Villarreal et al. (44) demonstrated that 2 days of plyometric training per week for 7 weeks was more effective than 4 days/wk for improving the vertical jump and 20-meter sprint. However, much like strength training protocols, some variety in exercise selection typically yields superior results. A meta-analysis of plyometric training suggests that combining different types of plyometric exercises produces better results for improving vertical jump height than just one form (16,44). Furthermore, this same analysis suggests that adding external load to plyometric exercises provides no additional benefit.

> **Training Tip**
>
> A key component of plyometric training is a quick reversal of muscle contractions from the stretch–shortening cycle. One popular and beneficial plyometric exercise is the depth jump. Research has demonstrated that a depth jump performed from a height of 40 cm is effective for improving power and agility in young athletes (34); however, if the contact (landing) time is too long, the benefit of this type of training will be diminished (45). Therefore, it is recommended for a coach to test the athlete to determine whether a 40-cm box is sufficient.
>
> A simple way to determine optimum height is to first test the athlete's standing vertical jump. Next, the athlete should perform a depth jump from a 40-cm box with a rebound jump. If the athlete can rebound higher off a 40-cm box, it is sufficient to train his plyometric strength qualities. If the 40-cm box results in a lower vertical jump, the height of the box should be decreased to the point where his depth jump rebound is higher than his standing vertical jump.

While it is common for trainers to increase the height of the depth jump by having athletes jump off a higher box, a thorough review of depth jump research suggests that the height of the jump is not crucial (46). Therefore, with regard to the depth jump, it is recommended to keep the height relatively low (<40 cm) so that the athlete can perform more reps per workout and reduce the risk of an impact injury.

The vertical jump and 20-meter sprint are two exercises that measure an athlete's explosive strength. A study by de Villarreal et al. (44) demonstrated that 2 days of plyometric training per week for 7 weeks was more effective than 4 days/wk for improving the vertical jump and 20-meter sprint.

A depth jump can be beneficial to an MMA athlete. However, much like strength training protocols, some variety in exercise selection typically yields superior results. A meta-analysis of plyometric training suggests that combining different types of plyometric exercises produces better results for improving vertical jump height than just one form (16,44). Furthermore, this same analysis suggests that adding external load to plyometric exercises provides no additional benefit.

For plyometric training, two workouts per week using exercises without extra external resistance are recommended.

Plyometric exercises can be performed at the beginning of a maximal strength workout, six or more hours away from a maximal strength workout, or on a separate day.

- Workout 1: 1, depth jump (see Figure 28.10) for 4 reps and rest 30 seconds; 2, clap push-up (Figure 28.11) for 4 reps and rest 30 seconds. Repeat workout 1 seven more times (8 rounds total)
- Workout 2 (3 to 4 days later): 1, split jump for 4 reps with each leg forward (8 jumps total) and rest 30 seconds; 2, medicine ball swing/slam (Figure 28.12) for 4 reps and rest 30 seconds. Repeat workout 2 seven more times (8 rounds total).

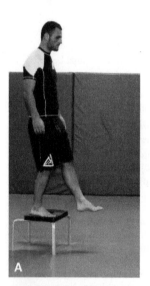
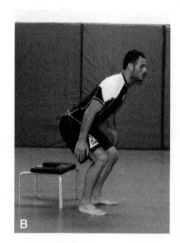
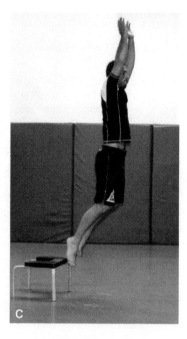

FIGURE 28-10. (A–C) Depth jump.

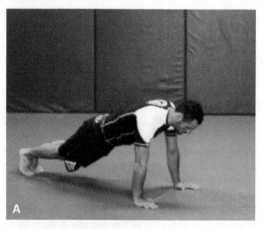
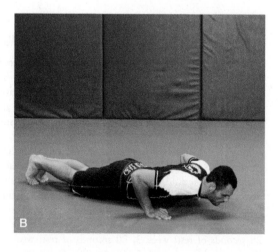

FIGURE 28-11. (A–C) Clap push-up.

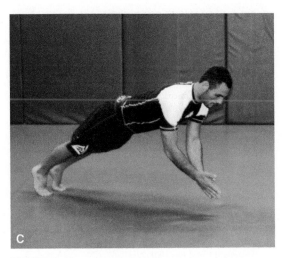

FIGURE 28-11. (*Continued*)

Sample Progression for Plyometric Training

Since adding extra load to plyometric exercises might not provide any benefit, it is recommended that plyometric training progressions for MMA athletes should focus on decreasing the rest periods over time or increasing the volume of exercise.

A sample 8-week plyometric training progression for MMA athletes follows. At the end of the 8-week progression, the athlete will perform 44 reps with each exercise.

Even though research demonstrates that 50+ reps per exercise for plyometric training produces favorable results, the research was not performed on MMA athletes who spend considerable time doing other high-impact exercises weekly, so a more conservative approach is recommended.

- Week 1: Perform 8 rounds with 30-second rest periods
- Week 2: Rest 25 seconds between each exercise, perform 8 rounds
- Week 3: Perform 9 rounds with 25-second rest periods
- Week 4: Rest 20 seconds between each exercise, perform 9 rounds
- Week 5: Perform 10 rounds with 20-second rest periods
- Week 6: Rest 15 seconds between each exercise, perform 10 rounds
- Week 7: Perform 11 rounds with 15-second rest periods
- Week 8: Rest 10 seconds between each exercise, perform 11 rounds

PUTTING IT ALL TOGETHER

Once a coach feels the athlete is ready, maximal strength, ballistic, and plyometric training can be performed in the same week. Each type of training should be performed twice per week, evenly spaced. For example, a short plyometric workout followed immediately by a maximal strength workout

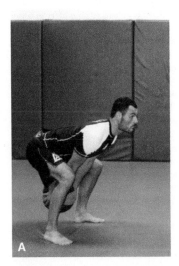
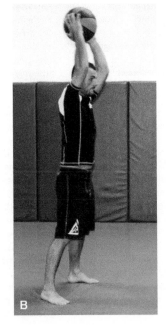
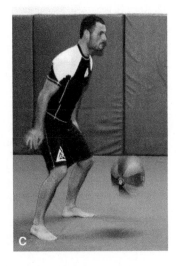

FIGURE 28-12. (A–C) Medicine ball swing/slam.

could be performed on Monday and Thursday, and ballistic training could be performed on Tuesday and Friday. The key is to spread out the training as evenly as possible and put the most demanding workouts on the days that a fighter does not have plenty of additional sparring to do.

REFERENCES

1. Zatsiorsky VM. Strength and Power in Sport. 2nd ed. Biomechanics of Strength and Strength Training. 2003 International Olympic Committee: Blackwell Science; 440–441.
2. Cormie P, McGuigan M, Newton R. Developing maximal neuromuscular power: part 1. Sports Med 2011;41(1):17–38.
3. Henneman E, Somjen G, Carpenter D. Functional significance of cell size in spinal motoneurons. J Neurophysiol 1965;28:560–580.
4. Loeb G, Ghez C. Principles of Neural Science: The Motor Unit and Muscle Action. 4th ed. New York City, NY: McGraw-Hill; 2000:674–693.
5. Nolte J. The Human Brain: An Introduction to Its Functional Anatomy. 5th ed. St. Louis, MO: Mosby; 2002:450.
6. Wakeling JM, Uehli K, Rozitis A. Muscle fibre recruitment can respond to the mechanics of the muscle contraction. J R Soc Interface 2006;3:533–544.
7. Yue G, Cole KJ. Strength increases from the motor program: comparison of training with maximal voluntary and imagined muscle contractions. J Neurophysiol 1992;67(5):1114–1123.
8. Gatev P, Ivanova T, Gantchev GN. Changes in firing pattern of high-threshold motor units due to fatigue. Electromyogr Clin Neurophysiol 1986;26(2):83–93.
9. Behm DG, Sale DG. Intended rather than actual movement velocity determines velocity-specific training response. J Appl Physiol 1993;74(1):359–368.
10. Ewing J Jr, Wolfe D, Rogers A, Amundson M, Stull G. Effects of velocity of isokinetic training on strength, power, and quadriceps muscle fibre characteristics. J Appl Physiol 1990;61:159–162.
11. Kanehisa H, Miyashita M. Specificity of velocity in strength training. Eur J Appl Physiol 1983;52:104–106.
12. Dinn N, Behm DG. A comparison of ballistic-movement and ballistic-intent training on muscle strength and activation. J Sports Physiol Perform 2007;2:386–399.
13. Storen O, Helgerud J, Stoa EM, Hoff J. Maximal strength training improves running economy in distance runners. Med Sci Sports Exerc 2008;40(6):1087–1092.
14. Guglielmo L, Greco C, Denadai B. Effects of strength training on running economy. Int J Sports Med 2009;30:27–32.
15. Millet G, Jaouen B, Borrani F, Candau R. Effects of concurrent endurance and strength training on running economy and VO$_2$ kinetics. Med Sci Sports Exerc 2002;34:1351–1359.
16. Kraemer WJ, Adams K, Cafarelli E, et al. American College of Sports Medicine position stand: progression models in resistance training for healthy adults. Med Sci Sports Exerc 2002;34(2):364–380.
17. Campos GE, Luecke TJ, Wendeln HK, et al. Muscular adaptations in response to three different resistance-training regimens: specificity of repetition maximum training zones. Eur J Appl Physiol 2002;88:50–60.
18. Lamas L, Aoki MS, Ugrinowitsch C, et al. Expression of genes related to muscle plasticity after strength and power training regimens. Scand J Med Sci Sports 2010;20(2):216–225.
19. Ryan AS, Ivey FM, Hurlbut DE, et al. Regional bone mineral density after resistive training in young and older men and women. Scand J Med Sci Sports 2004;14(1):16–23.
20. Almstedt HC, Canepa JA, Ramirez DA, Shoepe TC. Changes in bone mineral density in response to 24 weeks of resistance training in college-age men and women. J Strength Cond Res 2011;25(4):1098–1103. (Epub ahead of print).
21. Sánchez-Medina L, González-Badillo JJ. Velocity loss as an indicator of neuromuscular fatigue during resistance training. Med Sci Sports Exerc 2011;43(9):1725–1734.
22. McGill S. Ultimate Back Fitness and Performance. 4th ed. Ontario: Wabuno Publishers, Backfitpro Inc 2004;290–291.
23. Alcaraz P, Sanchez-Lorente J, Blazevich A. Physical performance and cardiovascular responses to an acute bout of heavy resistance circuit training versus traditional strength training. J Strength Cond Res 2008;22(3):667–671.
24. Zatsiorsky VM. Science and practice of strength training. Champaign, IL: Hum Kinet.1995;34.
25. Baker D, Newton R. Comparison of lower body strength, power, acceleration, speed, agility, and sprint momentum to describe and compare playing rank among professional rugby players. J Strength Cond Res 2008;22(1):153–158.
26. Cormie P, McGuigan M, Newton R. Influence of strength on magnitude and mechanisms of adaptations to power training. Med Sci Sports Exerc 2010;42(8):1566–1581.
27. McBride JM, Triplett-McBride N, Davie A, et al. A comparison of strength and power characteristics between power lifters, Olympic lifters, and sprinters. J Strength Cond Res 1999;13(1):58–66.
28. Stone M, O'Bryant H, McCoy L, et al. Power and maximum strength relationships during performance of dynamic and static weighted jumps. J Strength Cond Res 2003;17(1):140–147.
29. Duchateau J, Hainaut K. Mechanisms of muscle and motor unit adaptation to explosive power training. In: Komi PV, ed. Strength and Power in Sport. 2nd. Malden, MA: Blackwell Sciences; 2003:326.
30. Hakkinen K, Komi P, Alen M. Effect of explosive type strength training on isometric force and relaxation time, electromyographic and muscle fibre characteristics of leg extensor muscles. Acta Physiol Scand 1985;125(4):587–600.
31. Gollhofer A. Proprioceptive training: considerations for strength and power production. In: Komi PV, ed. Strength and Power in Sport. 2nd ed. Oxford, UK: Blackwell; 2003:331–342.
32. McBride JM, Triplett-McBride T, Davie A, et al. The effect of heavy- vs. light-load jump squats on the development of strength, power, and speed. J Strength Cond Res 2002;16(1):75–82.
33. Newton RU, Kraemer WJ, Hakkinen K. Effects of ballistic training on preseason preparation of elite volleyball players. Med Sci Sports Exerc 1999;31(2):323–330.
34. Thomas K, French D, Hayes PR. The effect of two plyometric training techniques on muscular power and agility in youth soccer players. J Strength Cond Res 2009;23(1):332–335.
35. Wagner DR, Kocak MS. A multivariate approach to assessing anaerobic power following a plyometric training program. J Strength Cond Res 1997;11:251–255.

36. Baker D. A series of studies on the training of high-intensity muscle power in rugby league football players. J Strength Cond Res 2001;15(2):198–209.

37. Holcomb WR, Lander JE, Rutland RM, et al. The effectiveness of a modified plyometric program on power and the vertical jump. J Strength Cond Res 1996;10(2):89–92.

38. Lyttle AD, Wilson G, Ostrowski KJ. Enhancing performance: maximal power versus combined weights and plyometrics training. J Strength Cond Res 1996;10(3):173–179.

39. Newton RU, Kraemer WJ, Hakkinen K, et al. Kinematics, kinetics, and muscle activation during explosive upper body movements. J Appl Biomech 1996;12:31–43.

40. Van Cutsem M, Duchateau J, Hainaut K. Changes in single motor unit behaviour contribute to the increase in contraction speed after dynamic training in humans. J Physiol 1998;513:295–305.

41. Allerheiligen B, Rogers R. Plyometrics program design. Strength Cond J 1995;17(4):26–31.

42. Holcomb WR, Kleiner DM, Chu DA. Plyometrics: considerations for safe and effective training. J Strength Cond Res 1998;20:36–39.

43. McBride JM, McCaulley GO, Cormie P. Influence of pre-activity and eccentric muscle activity on concentric performance during vertical jumping. J Strength Cond Res 2008;22(3):750–777.

44. de Villarreal ES, Gonzalez-Badillo JJ, Izquierdo M. Low and moderate plyometric training frequency produces greater jumping and sprinting gains compared with high frequency. J Strength Cond Res 2008;22(3):715–725.

45. Bobbert MF, Huijing PA, Van Ingen Schenau GJ. Drop jumping I. The influence of jumping technique on the biomechanics of jumping. Med Sci Sports Exerc 1987;19:332–338.

46. de Villarreal ES, Kellis E, Kraemer WJ, Izquierdo M. Determining variables of plyometric training for improving vertical jump height performance: a meta-analysis. J Strength Cond Res 2009;23(2):495–506.

29

Joseph Przytula

Off-Season Considerations for Soccer

You would be hard-pressed to find a sport that requires the degree of physical competency that soccer demands. It requires the ability to avoid tackles and leap over fallen players, as in American football; the spatial awareness to manipulate a ball through a defense, as in basketball; and the explosive change in speed to pass an opponent, as in a 400-meter sprint—all this expressed in a climate of fatigue. It is no wonder why so many professional athletes have a soccer background and often continue the sport in their off-seasons to stay game fit. No other sport requires the combination and mastery of so many fundamental movement skills—and no sport is as unforgiving when they are lacking.

A one-size-fits-all conditioning approach should be avoided. Doing a game analysis of the British Premier League soccer would produce failure in an athletic development program for a high school team. Unlike American football, position requirements are not written in stone. They fluctuate from team to team depending on that team's strengths or weaknesses. This means a program that was written for one team may not work with another. Individualization in the context of a team is an oxymoron, but a must (1).

Injury prevention strategies need to be incorporated into the soccer player's training. This too may vary from team to team and require adjustment (2,3). Ankle sprains are common to every level and gender (4). While anterior cruciate ligament (ACL) tears of the knee are common at all levels, female athletes suffer a disproportionate amount (5–8). Fortunately, the evidence supporting a well-designed neuromuscular training program in prevention is well supported by scientific literature (9–11). Men are more prone to hip and groin strains, including athletic hernia (12). Again, the research toward this injury category points to a well-designed athletic development program for prevention (13).

Although remedial exercises are helpful, often it is lack of movement skills that are precursors to injury. For instance, groin muscle strains may be a result of poor footwork—an athlete reaching for the ball. Soccer's classification as a contact sport is also an important consideration. The athlete's ability to brace upon impact to the ground is important to head, neck, and back injury (14,15). The popularity of artificial playing surfaces is also something

that needs to be considered (5). Even when considering the injury epidemiology, the lifelong health benefits of participation in the sport far outweigh the risks (16).

FUNCTIONAL SOCCER BIOMECHANICS

Soccer Flexibility

The sport does not require us to hold the static positions required for gymnastics or dance. Replace it with *mostibility*, or the ability to use just the right amount of motion, at just the right time, at just the right speed, in just the right plane, in just the right direction (17).

Soccer Strength

We do not need to overcome tremendous amounts of external resistance as a rugby player would; therefore, time spent developing maximal strength should be kept at a minimum. That means most of our strength training can and should take place outside of the weight room (1,18).

Soccer Core

The muscles of the spine, torso, abdomen, and hips must be able to accelerate and decelerate motions of the upper and lower extremities in smooth, coordinated flowing synchrony. Just the same they need to rapidly brace to protect the body from a fall or collision (19). Think *reactive core* and avoid exercises that attempt to isolate it from the rest of the body.

Soccer Balance

While static may be a good place to start, your dynamic balance is what controls your posture and center of gravity while running, kicking, or heading a ball. Think of dynamic balance as a bubble that surrounds your base of support. Your goal is to expand that bubble while maintaining your center of gravity.

Soccer Agility

Running the gambit from walking to full-speed sprinting or from backpedaling to cross-stepping, soccer is classified as a transition sport. These rapid changes in tempo and direction occur multidirectionally as a reaction to visual, auditory, and kinesthetic stimuli (20).

Soccer Sense

Although long forgotten in traditional strength and conditioning programs, enhanced movement awareness is what separates the common athlete from the exceptional one. The ability to estimate where opponents and teammates are around you, to react (or ignore) touch and timing are examples. Though difficult to measure objectively, soccer sense is often the difference between those on the bench and those on the pitch.

RUDIMENTARY STAGE—PLAY TO TRAIN

ACL prevention begins here (21). The modality of choice is games that provide the child with movement tasks to solve (22). The biomotor qualities of focus will be coordination and speed. Boredom from familiarity and frustration from difficulty means that the nervous system is inappropriately loaded. Address this with frequent changes in pace, allotted time, surfaces, closing the eyes, or reacting to signals. Coordination ready exercises include crawls, skips, hops, jumps, juggling, tag games, and obstacle courses (23).

The "Func-A-Delic" Train

Line up the athletes on the sideline of a field, about 10 feet from one another. One line is designated the "Func-Masters" and the others the "Beat Hustlers." The goal of the "Func-Master" is to use one movement skill or combination of movement skills to get to the end of the line. The job of the "Beat Hustler" is to mirror them. This continues until the "train" reaches the other side of the field. Switch roles and continue to the opposite end of the field (see Figure 29.1).

The relevancy of this drill is its promotion of agility. Also, it aims to improve the ability to react to visual stimuli (mirroring skills) as well as to make tempo and direction changes.

Shin Tag

Athletes are divided into groups of two. Each group is confined to a 5-foot square area. One person is designated offense, the other defense. The offense attempts to tap a hand to their opponent's lower leg without getting their own touched. The defense avoids their shins being touched

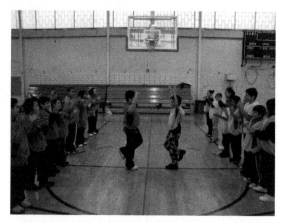

FIGURE 29-1. "Func-a-delic" train.

without leaving the 5-foot square. Repeat in 30-second intervals, then switch (see Figure 29.2).

This drill is relevant because it encourages reaction to touch and reaction time. It also should help athletes avoid being kicked.

Hopping (17)

The athlete stands on two feet and then hops onto one foot in a direction predetermined by the coach. Upon landing, the athlete quickly hops back to the original starting position onto two feet. Repeat for 3 sets of 10, changing directions each set (see Figure 29.3).

Variations include

- Sticking the landing and holding for a 5 count
- Jumping in the direction the ball is moving (the coach can dribble a soccer ball in place)
- Jumping a preset time

The relevancy of this drill involves its promotion of agility, the core (acquisition of whole-body shock absorption mechanics as they relate to the lower extremity), and balance. It also seeks to prevent ankle and ACL injury.

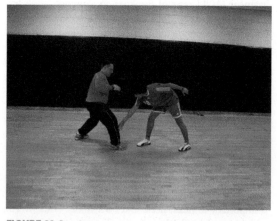

FIGURE 29-2. Shin tag.

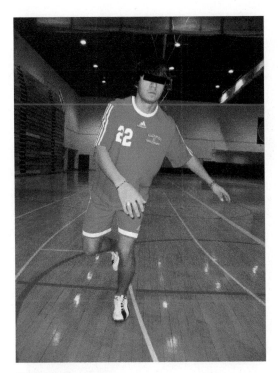

FIGURE 29-3. Hopping.

Brooklyn "Stromboli"

Place a soccer ball 5 yards from a side line or goal line. Lie perpendicular to the ball on the line. Begin by pencil rolling five times away from the ball, then back to the line. Upon reaching the line, quickly get up and sprint to the ball, touching it with the right or left foot. Sprint to the line, roll, then repeat five times (see Figure 29.4).

Variations include

- Juggling the ball five times before continuing
- Running backward

This drill intends to promote speed, the core, and movement (spatial) awareness.

Jumping Joes

Move the feet in the traditional jumping jack pattern. Swing the arms in an alternating fashion forward and back 20 times (do not let the feet move forward and back). Without stopping, swing the arms at shoulder height from right to left (Figure 29.5A).

Variations include

- Performing with legs in split stance (Figure 29.5B, C)
- Rotating the feet rapidly toward each other (pigeon toed) and then away (duck toed) (Figure 29.5D, E)
- Moving the arms forward in synchrony (sync) or right to left out of sync

This drill aims to promote the reactive core and improve agility.

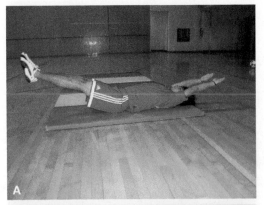
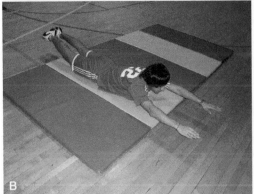

FIGURE 29-4. Brooklyn "Stromboli." (A) Start. (B) Finish.

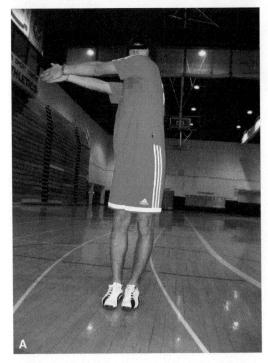

FIGURE 29-5. Jumping Joes. (A) Jumping jack rotational. (B) Split stance rotational. (C) Scissor rotational. (D) Toed in. (E) Toed out.

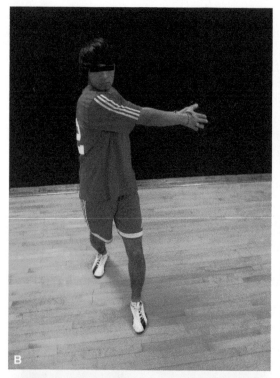

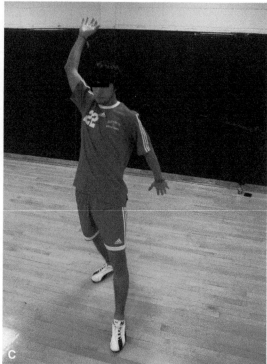

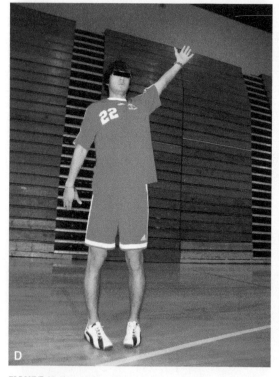

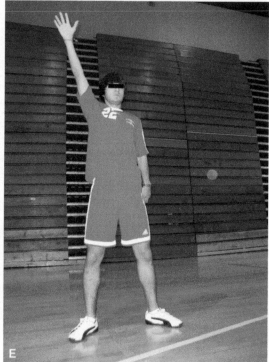

FIGURE 29-5. (*Continued*)

INTERMEDIATE STAGE: TRAIN TO COMPETE

The window of opportunity to develop speed, strength, and power begins this training period. Coordination and flexibility may suffer a temporary decline as the athlete goes through puberty, and remedial exercises may need to be prescribed. The development of the athlete's work capacity during this phase allows them to maintain a high level of coordination and skill in a climate of fatigue. The concept of the 24-hour athlete begins here. This means that although a formal conditioning program is crucial, social and academic issues must be factored into planning. Keep it simple and smart—push, pull, squat, reach, and rotate. Do not forget to keep it fun. The rudimentary games can be tweaked as to add a welcome psychological break from the rigors of training.

Four-Way Single-Leg Squat Matrix

Stand on one leg with the arms extended straight at chest height. Beginning with the hips first, squat as low as you can without the knee wiggling or an excessive torso lean forward (19). On the next repetition (rep), reach forward with the nonweight-bearing leg as far as you can with good form. On the third rep, reach the same leg laterally in the same manner. On the fourth rep, do a same side rotational reach. Begin with three sets of two each, and work up to four sets of four each (see Figure 29.6) (24,25).

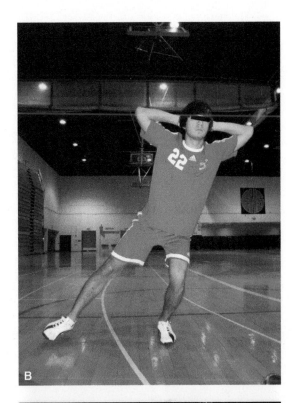

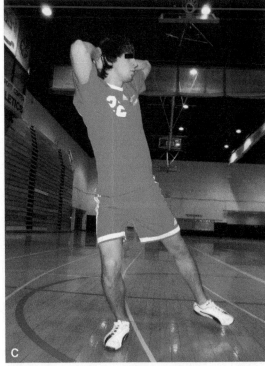

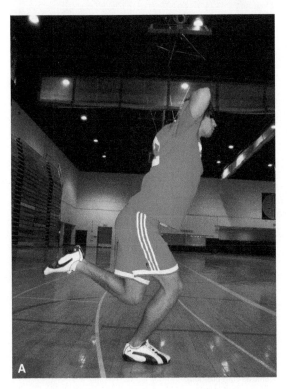

FIGURE 29-6. Single-leg squats. (A) Standard. (B) Frontal. (C) Rotational.

Variations include

- Do not let the hips translate forward—keep the butt tucked in tight (ankle dominant).
- Place the hands in a "prisoner squat" position (knee dominant), holding the bottom position for a 5-second count.
- Add a sandbag or weight vest to increase intensity (26).

This drill is relevant because it aims to produce strength and flexibility. It also seeks to prevent groin, ankle, and ACL injury.

Pivot Push–Pulls

Partners face each other in a right stride stance, with the right arm extended forward. Lock hands with your partner. Forcefully pull your partner toward you while lunging forward with the rear (left) leg. Quickly return to the starting position and repeat 10 times. Now do the same in a left stride stance with the left arm extended forward. Repeat for 3 sets (see Figure 29.7).

Variations include

- Instead of lunging onto the rear leg, do a soccer-style kick behind your partner.

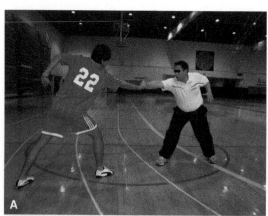

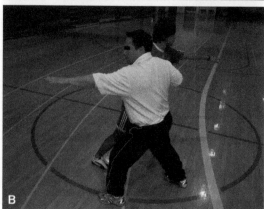

FIGURE 29-7.   (A, B) Pivot push–pulls.

- Hold a dumbbell in the freehand and throw a punch as the rear leg lunges forward.

This drill aims to promote strength and the reactive core.

Myrland Super Turtle

From a push-up position, point the right arm straight forward, then lift the straightened left leg off the ground. Now simultaneously rotate the right arm posteriorly to the floor while sneaking the left leg underneath the right so that you are now facing the sky. Without allowing the left leg or hips to touch the ground, return to the starting position. Repeat 5 times to each side for 3 sets (see Figure 29.8).

Variations include

- Begin the exercise supine rather than the "pointer" position.
- Add a weight vest to increase intensity.
- Have a partner attempt to push you off balance.

The relevancy of this drill is its promotion of the core (bracing against a fall onto the ground or another player), strength, and balance.

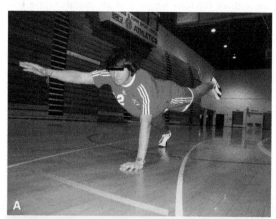

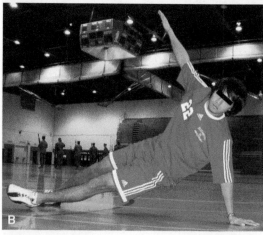

FIGURE 29-8.   Super turtle. (A) Start. (B) Rotate. (C) Middle. (D) Finish (same as start position).

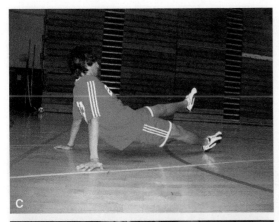

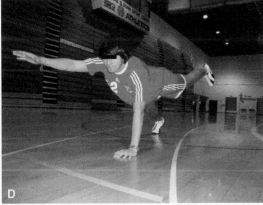

FIGURE 29-8. (Continued)

5 × 5 Cone Drill

The athlete stands at the "home" cone. The coach calls out a cone number to which the athlete must sprint, then return to the home cone. Upon reaching the home cone, the coach calls out a new random cone number to which the athlete sprints. Repeat 5 times (see Figure 29.9).

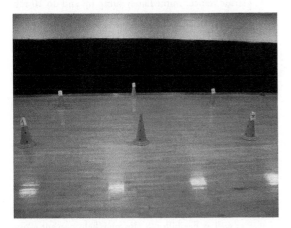

FIGURE 29-9. Drill cone setup.

Variations include

- The athlete is only permitted to power (cross) step at the cone, or speed (open) step.
- Instead of a coach calling out cone numbers, the athlete mirrors an athlete who is performing the same drill directly across from him.

This drill aims to promote agility, speed, and movement awareness (reacting to visual, auditory cues). It also may help prevent groin, ankle, and ACL injury (27).

ADVANCED OR ELITE STAGE: TRAIN TO WIN

What sets this phase of training apart from the others is the combining of physical qualities into the athlete's exercises and drills, rather than addressing them in isolation. All of the exercises described above are appropriate for the elite level. Tweaking the movements with a weight vest or closing the eyes are examples of combining these qualities. This level is the gestalt of everything that has come before it (or been neglected). The warm-up is a good place to address any movement skills that are lacking.

Jump and Go

Perform a forward jump as described above (see Hopping section). Instead of returning to the start position, the coach will give some type of verbal or hand signal indicating right or left. At that point, the athlete does a 10-yard sprint in the appropriate direction. The coach should be looking for the correct cutting technique. For instance, if the athlete is jumping onto the left leg and cutting right, an open (speed) step would be expected. If they are cutting left, a cross (power) step would be expected. Aberrant movement patterns may indicate injury or the need for remedial work (see Figure 29.10).

Variations include

- Sprint right or left diagonal (forward or backward)
- Sprint from a dead stop by sticking and holding the jump for 5 seconds before cutting
- Do the sprint from the two foot start position

This drill is relevant because it promotes multidirectional speed and agility as well as movement awareness (reacting to visual, auditory cues). It also seeks to prevent ankle and ACL injuries.

Atomic Barrel Roll

The athlete lies down on the grass supine, legs straight, and feet off the ground, with the arms extended over the head even with the ears. Hold a soccer ball in the hands. Do three continuous rolls right or left without allowing the legs

FIGURE 29-10. Jumps. (A) Start. (B) Sagittal land. (C) Right frontal land. (D) Right rotational land.

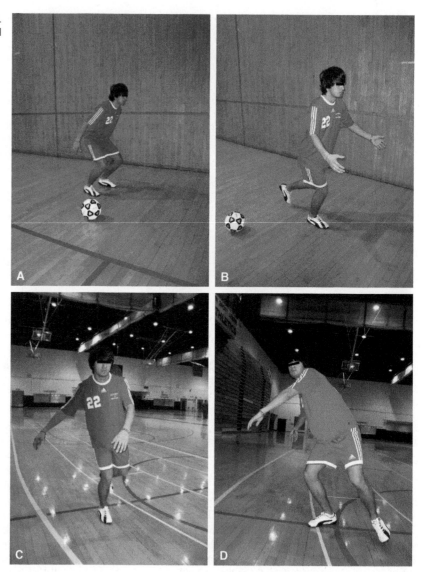

or arms to touch the ground. At completion, pull the ball to the chest (legs still off the ground) and toss it into the air. Scramble up off the ground and head it. Repeat to the opposite side. Do 3 sets (see Figure 29.11).

Variations include

- Scramble up and catch the ball (goalkeeper).
- Scramble up and dribble 5 yards.

Relevancy involves the core, speed, and balance. This drill also aims to improve the ability to rapidly recover from a fall.

3D Jump Matrix

Three types of drills that involve jumps are the following:

- Scissor jumps: From a right lunge position, jump up, cycle the left leg forward, and land in a left

stride stance. Immediately jump up and do 10 reps (Figure 29.12A, B).
- Skater jumps: From a left lunge position, drive off the right leg onto the left. Immediately jump up and do 10 reps (Figure 29.12C, D).
- Rotational jumps: From a right same side rotational lunge position, jump into the air, explosively "snapping" the hips to the left to land in a left rotational lunge position (Figure 29.12E, F).

Variations include

- Hold the hands in a "prisoner squat" position.
- Hold the bottom position for 5 seconds upon landing.
- Add a sandbag or weight vest to increase intensity.

This drill seeks to improve multidirectional speed and power as well as flexibility. It also may help prevent groin, ankle, and ACL injury.

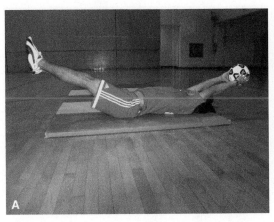
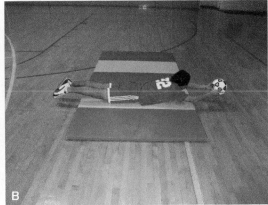

FIGURE 29-11. Atomic barrel roll. (A) Start. (B) Finish.

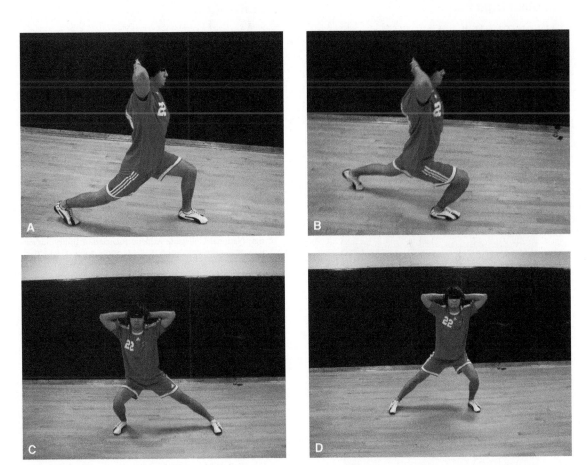

FIGURE 29-12. 3D jumps. (A) Scissor start. (B) Scissor finish. (C) Lateral lunge (skater) start on right. (D) Lateral lunge (skater) land on left. (E) Rotational lunge start on right. (F) Rotational lunge land on left.

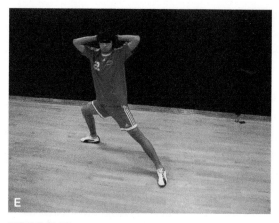

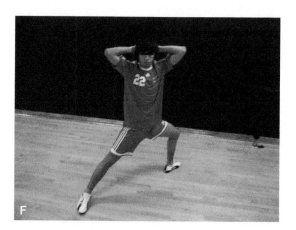

FIGURE 29-12. *(Continued)*

Dumbbell High Pull

Hold a pair of dumbbells with your elbows turned out. Triple bend from the ankles through the hips until the dumbbells are lined up with the lower thighs. Letting the arms hang like a pair of ropes, explosively drive the feet through the floor. As the lower extremity is reaching triple extension, explosively pull the dumbbells up toward the lower chest. Immediately return to the starting position, get set, and repeat. Do 4 sets of 8 reps (see Figure 29.13).

This drill is relevant because it promotes specific strength to develop a powerful jump to head the ball while being challenged by defenders.

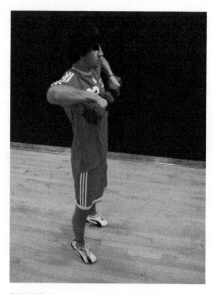

FIGURE 29-13. Dumbbell high pull.

REFERENCES

1. Gambetta V. Athletic Development. The Art & Science of Functional Sports Conditioning. Champaign, IL: Human Kinetics. 2007.
2. Adams AL, Schiff MA. Childhood soccer injuries treated in U.S. emergency departments. Acad Emerg Med 2006;13(5):571–574.
3. Yard E, Schroeder M, Fields S, Collins C, Comstock R. The Epidemiology of United States High School Soccer Injuries, 2005–2007. Am J Sports Med 2008;36(10):1930–1937.
4. Barber-Westin SD, Noyes FR, Smith ST, Campbell TM. Reducing the risk of noncontact anterior cruciate ligament injuries in the female athlete. Phys Sports Med 2009;37(3):49–61.
5. Dick R, Putukian M, Agel J, Evans TA, Marshall SW. Descriptive epidemiology of collegiate women's soccer injuries: National Collegiate Athletic Association Injury Surveillance System, 1988–1989 through 2002–2003. J Athl Train 2007;42(2):278–285.
6. Giza E, Mithofer K, Farrell L, Zarins B, Gill T, Drawer S. Injuries in women's professional soccer. Br J Sports Med 2005;39(4):212–216.
7. Le Gall F, Carling C, Reilly T. Injuries in young elite female soccer players: an 8-season prospective study. Am J Sports Med 2008;36(2):276–284.
8. Tegnander A, Olsen OE, Moholdt TT, Engebretsen L, Bahr R. Injuries in Norwegian female elite soccer: a prospective one-season cohort study. Knee Surg Sports Traumatol Arthrosc 2008.
9. Hägglund M, Waldén M, Atroshi I. Preventing knee injuries in adolescent female football players—design of a cluster randomized controlled trial. BMC Musculoskeletal Disord. 2009;23(10):75.
10. Imwalle LE, Myer GD, Ford KR, Hewett TE. Relationship between hip and knee kinematics in athletic women during cutting maneuvers: a possible link to noncontact anterior

cruciate ligament injury and prevention. J Strength Cond Res 2009;23(8):2223–2230.

11. Kiani A, Hellquist E, Ahlqvist K, Gedeborg R, Michaëlsson K, Byberg L. Prevention of soccer-related knee injuries in teenaged girls. Arch Internal Med 2010;170(1):43–49.

12. Gabbe BJ, Bailey M, Cook JL, et al. The association between hip and groin injuries in the elite junior football years and injuries sustained during elite senior competition. Br J Sports Med 2009.

13. Garvey JF, Read JW, Turner A. Sportsman hernia: what can we do? Hernia 2010.

14. McCrory P. Brain Injury & Heading in Soccer. Br Med J 2003;327:351–352.

15. Mehnert MJ, Agesen T, Malanga GA. "Heading" and neck injuries in soccer: a review of biomechanics and potential long-term effects. Pain Physician 2005;8(4):391–397.

16. Vicente-Rodriguez G, Jimenez-Ramirez J, Ara I, Serrano-Sanchez JA, Dorado C, Calbet JA. Enhanced bone mass and physical fitness in prepubescent footballers. Bone 2003;33(5):853–859.

17. Gray G. Speed/Reaction. Fast Function Video Series. Adrian, MI: Functional Design Systems; 2007.

18. Baechle T. Essentials of Strength Training & Conditioning. Champaign, IL: Human Kinetics; 1994.

19. Radcliffe J. Functional Training for Athletes at All Levels. Ulysses Press; 2007; Spratford W, Mellifont R, Burkett B. The influence of dive direction on the movement characteristics for elite football goalkeepers. Sports Biomech 2009;8(3): 235–244.

20. Lees A, Nolan L. The biomechanics of soccer: a review. J Sports Sci 1998;16(3):211–234.

21. Distefano LJ, Padua DA, Blackburn JT, Garrett WE, Guskie-wicz KM, Marshall SW. Integrated injury prevention program improves balance and vertical jump height in children. J Strength Cond Res 2010.

22. Gabbard C, LeBlanc B, Lowy S. Physical Education for Children. Englewood Cliffs, NJ: Prentice Hall; 1994.

23. Drabik J. Children & Sports Training: How Your Future Champions Should Be Healthy, Fit, and Happy. Island Pond, VT: Stadia Publishing Company; 1996.

24. Ellenbecker T. Closed Kinetic Chain Exercise. Champaign, IL: Human Kinetics; 2001.

25. King I. How to Write Strength Training Programs. Queensland: King Sports Publishing; 2000.

26. Fleck S, Kramer W. Designing Resistance Training Programs. Champaign, IL: Human Kinetics; 2004.

27. Gambetta V. Soccer Speed: The 3S system. Gambetta Sports Training Systems; 1998.

CHAPTER 30

Michael Fredericson, Cameron Harrison,
Adam Sebastin Tenforde, and Venu Akuthota

Injury Prevention in Running Sports

Athletes in running sports have unique and specific training programs emphasizing strength, power, and endurance. The rigors of running and training, however, place tremendous demands upon the muscles, joints, and bones of the lower limb that may result in injury to these structures.

Common running injuries of the lower quadrant include stress fractures, hamstring tendinopathy, patellofemoral syndrome, iliotibial band friction syndrome, medial tibial stress syndrome, Achilles tendinitis, plantar fasciitis, and lateral ankle sprain (1,2). Although the symptoms of particular injuries vary, the development of each is usually the cumulative effect of several distinct themes. The most common instigating factor is often rapid change in the duration, frequency, or intensity of a training program. Other factors include the use of inappropriate or old running shoes, insufficient stretching of key muscle groups of the lower limb, postural misalignment, and muscle imbalance. Running is predominantly a sagittal plane activity that tends to promote strong/tight hip flexors, knee extensors, and plantarflexors with relatively inhibited (weak) hip abductors and hip extensors.

The prevention of these injuries lies in the nature of their development. Avoiding rapid changes in training intensity, investing in quality running shoes, and consistently utilizing proper stretching techniques are relatively simple measures that can be taken to prevent overuse injuries. In addition, stress fractures have a lower incidence in athletes limiting their running distance to less than 20 miles per week (3). Recreational athletes should be encouraged to cross-train to strengthen different muscles.

More sophistication, however, is required to correct postural misalignment and muscle imbalances that are thought to be significant contributors to these injuries. Balance between the prime movers, synergists, and stabilizers of the hip, knee, and ankle joints is crucial to proper joint function and injury prevention. Stretching exercises are not extensively described as they have not been shown to clearly prevent injury (4,5). Many of the following functional exercises stretch muscles dynamically. For example,

gastrocsoleus or Achilles stretching may be helpful in the treatment of plantar fasciitis (6). Theoretically, stretching the gastrocsoleus may prevent excessive midfoot pronation that biomechanically occurs with tight heel cords (7). The exercises described in this chapter focus on proper timing and coordination of muscle movements. They are divided into three groups: exercises encouraging lumbopelvic stability, actions promoting fine balance and motor control, and functional movement training (8).

EXERCISES EMPHASIZING LUMBOPELVIC STABILITY

The purpose of fundamental core stabilization exercises is to improve the stability, coordination, and timing of the deep abdominal wall musculature. The use of the physioball further enhances proprioception and encourages higher levels of core stabilization. Clinicians can determine whether core stability exercises are appropriate by having athletes perform functional tasks such as timed plank tests to determine their core "ability" (9). Recent randomized trials have confirmed the role of core strengthening exercises, particularly in athletes experiencing low back pain (10). These core strengthening exercises should be performed two to three times weekly to maximize results. The athlete begins with one or two sets of 15 repetitions and progresses to three sets of 15 to 20 repetitions (Figures 30.1–30.6).

EXERCISES EMPHASIZING THE DEVELOPMENT OF BALANCE AND MOTOR CONTROL

Various devices and exercises are useful in the development of muscles responsible for postural maintenance and gait. These exercises encourage balance, coordination, precision, and skill acquisition in a process that transfers control of

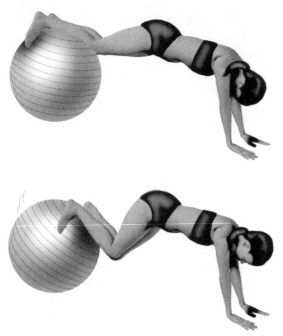

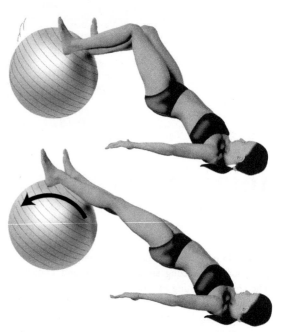

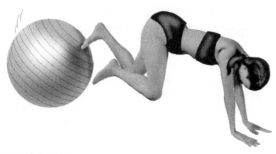

FIGURE 30-1. Squat ball thrust. The lower back and shoulder blades are kept in a neutral position while the abdominal muscles contract to move the ball forward and backward. The spine should be kept in neutral alignment throughout the movement.

FIGURE 30-3. Leg curls on a physioball. The purpose of this test is to recruit both actions of the hamstrings: hip extension and knee flexion while maintaining dynamic stability of the lumbar spine. The arms should be kept on the floor and at the sides of the body while the hips are raised off the ground until the knees, hips, and shoulders create a straight line. This position is then maintained as the ball is pushed forward with the feet.

FIGURE 30-2. Progression. The exercise is performed with only one foot on the ball.

these muscles from conscious to unconscious regulation. Balance and motor control training is particularly important for running sports that require quick changes in direction, such as football, or running on uneven surfaces, such as trail running (Figures 30.7–30.9).

EXERCISES IMPROVING FUNCTIONAL STRENGTH

Functional movements during running require acceleration, deceleration, and dynamic stabilization. All of this

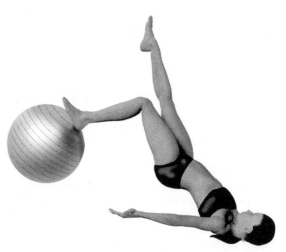

FIGURE 30-4. Progression. The knee is extended while in the bridge position. Again, care should be taken to ensure proper dynamic stability of the lumbar spine.

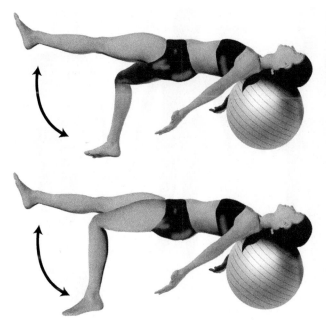

FIGURE 30-5. Alternate leg bridge with shoulders on the ball. The exercise begins in a sitting stance. The feet should then be moved forward on the ground until the head, neck, and shoulder blades are supported on the ball. Knees should be bent at a 90° angle. The foot is then raised off the ground with abdominal muscles braced. Weight should be shifted from side to side emphasizing the stability of the lumbopelvic region. The position should be held for 10 seconds and with alternation of the lower limbs.

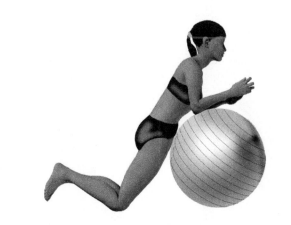

FIGURE 30-6. Abdominal rollout: The purpose of this exercise is to train the abdominals eccentrically. The exercise begins in a kneeling position with both hands on the ball. The ball is then rolled away from the body while keeping the abdominals braced and lower back in a neutral position. The ball is then pushed backward and forward a short distance with the movement only occurring at the shoulders and not at the back. Progression: the legs are gradually straightened until the weight of the body rests on the toes in an attempt to make a straight line from the back of the head to the knees.

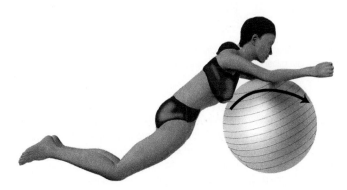

FIGURE 30-7. Single-leg balance with rocker board in three planes. Forward and backward steps mimicking the running motion are performed on a rocking board in the three planes of motion. The goal is to maintain alignment and balance while on the rocker board.

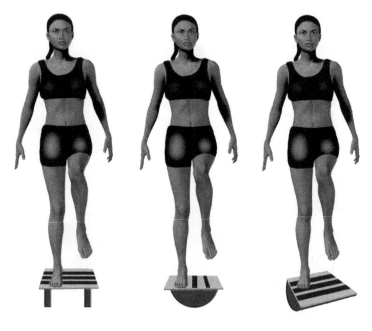

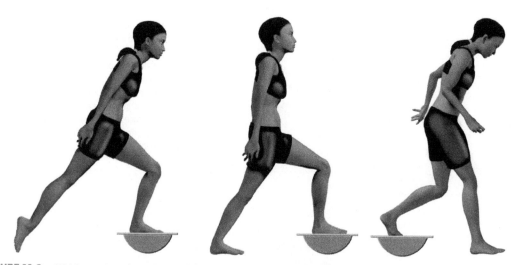

FIGURE 30-8. Weight transfers using rocker board. The athlete steps forward quickly and catches herself from falling over with a quick forward movement of the leg onto a circular balance board. The goal is to maintain spinal alignment from head to sacrum.

depends upon the neuromuscular system's ability to produce dynamic eccentric, concentric, and isometric contractions during movement patterns. A resistance cord training of shoulder and hip flexion is utilized in the following exercises that stimulate the key muscles used with running. Single-leg exercises are particularly important because they encourage recruitment of muscles that are potentially weak in runners. Hip abductor strengthening, such as with the power runner exercise (Figures 30.10 and 30.11), has been shown to prevent iliotibial band syndrome (11). The multidirectional step-up exercise (Figure 30.12) encourages muscles stimulated in the transverse plane like the vastus medialis obliquus which may be important in treating and preventing patellofemoral pain (12). In summary, utilizing these tools of proper prevention may add years of quality to an athlete's life.

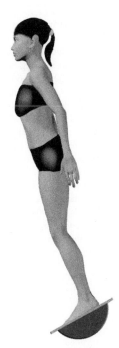

FIGURE 30-9. Forward/backward rocking: The athlete gently rocks forward and backward in an attempt to maintain postural alignment throughout the exercise.

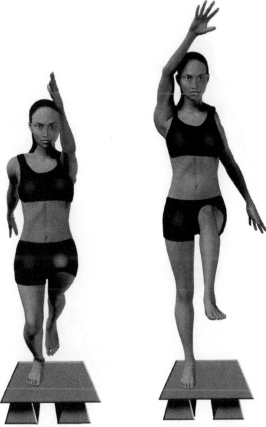

FIGURE 30-10. Power runner with resistance and step-up. The athlete performs step-ups mimicking a runner's gait with a sports cord to resist shoulder and hip flexion. The opposite arm and leg are resisted simultaneously to increase strength and coordination of this movement pattern.

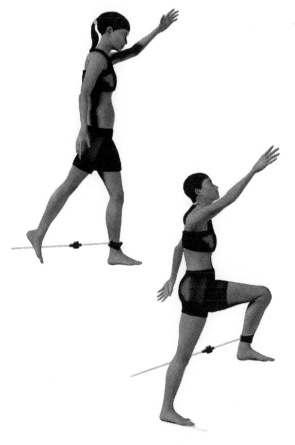

FIGURE 30-11. Power runner with resistance. This exercise is designed to develop capital plane control and to increase stability of the lower abdominal muscles during forward motion of the hip. The hips and opposite arm are flexed while attempting to maintain an erect spine in proper postural alignment.

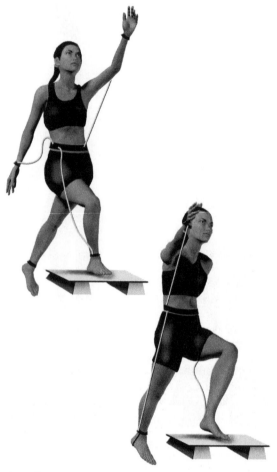

FIGURE 30-12. Multidirectional resisted alternate arm/leg step-ups. This exercise is similar to power runner with resistance as described in Figure 30.5, but is performed at a 45° angle.

REFERENCES

1. O'Conner F, Wilder R. Textbook of Running Medicine. New York, NY: McGraw-Hill Companies; 2001.
2. Lopes AD, Hespanhol Júnior LC, Yeung SS, Costa LO. What are the main running-related musculoskeletal injuries? A systematic review. Sports Med 2012;42(10):891–905.
3. Brunet ME, Cook SD, Brinker MR, Dickinson JA. A survey of running injuries in 1505 competitive and recreational runners. J Sports Med Phys Fitness 1990;30(3):307–315.
4. Pope RP, Herbert RD, Kirwan JD, Graham BJ. A randomized trial of preexercise stretching for prevention of lower-limb injury. Med Sci Sports Exerc 2000;32(2):271–277.
5. Pereles D, Roth R, Thompson D, et al. The Impact of a Pre-run Stretch on the Risk of Injury in Runners. American Academy of Orthopedic Surgeons Annual Meeting 2011. Podium No. 648.
6. Riddle DL, Pulisic M, Pidcoe P, Johnson RE. Risk factors for plantar fasciitis: a matched case-control study. J Bone Joint Surg Am 2003;85-A:872–877.
7. Brukner P, Khan K. Clinical Sports Medicine. 3rd ed. Australia: McGraw-Hill; 2006.
8. Fredericson M, Moore T. Muscular balance, core stability, and injury prevention in middle- and long-distance runners. Phys Med Rehabil Clin N Am 2005;16(3):669–689.
9. McDonald DA, Delgadillo JQ, Fredericson M, et al. Reliability and accuracy of video analysis protocol to assess core ability. Phys Med Rehabil 2011;3(3):204–211.
10. Kumar S, Sharma VP, Negi MP. Efficacy of dynamic muscular stabilization techniques (DMST) over conventional techniques in rehabilitation of chronic low back pain. J Strength Cond Res 2009;23(9):2651–2659.
11. Fredericson M, Cookingham CL, Chaudhari AM, et al. Hip abductor weakness in distance runners with iliotibial band syndrome. Clin J Sport Med 2000;10(3):169–175.
12. Cowan SM, Bennell KL, Crossley KM, et al. Physical therapy alters recruitment of the vasti in patellofemoral pain syndrome. Med Sci Sports Exerc 2002;34(12):1879–1885.

Prevention of Knee Injury in Women

THE CLINICAL DILEMMA

The majority of anterior cruciate ligament (ACL) injuries occur by noncontact mechanisms, often during landing from a jump or making a lateral pivot while running (1,2). Knee instability, due to ligament dominance (decreased dynamic neuromuscular control of the joint), quadriceps dominance (increased quadriceps recruitment and decreased hamstring strength), leg dominance (side-to-side differences in strength, flexibility, and coordination), and trunk dominance (lack of control of trunk motion) may be responsible for the increased incidence of knee injury in athletes (3–7).

DEVELOPMENT OF A NEUROMUSCULAR TRAINING PROGRAM TO DECREASE KNEE INJURY IN FEMALE ATHLETES

Applied research to decrease knee ligament injury rates in female athletes must determine the factors that make women more susceptible than men and develop treatment modalities to aid in the prevention of these injuries. The driving force behind the development of this prophylactic intervention for serious knee injury is greater than 100,000 knee injuries that are projected to occur in female athletes at the high school and collegiate levels and the 1.38 million knee injuries that occur in the general female population each year in the United States. If preventive modalities such as dynamic neuromuscular retraining could decrease the incidence of knee injury in women from five times greater than that of men to equal that of men, 40,000 knee injuries could be prevented in women in high school and college sports annually. In addition, with the ever-increasing popularity of high-risk jumping and pivoting sports such as soccer, volleyball, and basketball, even higher numbers of injuries could be avoided in the future.

NEUROMUSCULAR IMBALANCES IN WOMEN

The most common female neuromuscular imbalances are basically imbalances of four important neuromuscular parameters. With ligament dominance, there exists an imbalance between the neuromuscular and ligamentous control of the joint. With quadriceps dominance, there is an imbalance between quadriceps and knee flexor strength and coordination. With dominant leg dominance, there is an imbalance between the two lower extremities in strength and coordination. With "trunk dominance," in which the momentum of the trunk is not controlled, there is uncontrolled motion of the center of mass during deceleration and movement of the ground reaction force vector to the lateral side of the joint, which increases medially directed torques at the knee. Essentially, trainers or therapists must seek to balance these parameters.

Recent Research

"The study findings indicate that net hip rotation moment impulse, frontal plane knee range of motion during landing, asymmetries in sagittal plane knee moments at initial contact, and postural stability are collectively a strong predictor of a second ACL injury after anterior cruciate ligament reconstruction (ACLR) (with high sensitivity (0.92) and specificity (0.88)." (Paterno) (8)

Ligament Dominance: High Torques at the Knee and High Impact Forces

A common neuromuscular imbalance in women is ligament dominance, resulting in high knee valgus moments and high ground reaction forces. Typically during single-leg landing, pivoting, or deceleration, the motion at female athletes' knee joints is directed by the ground reaction forces, rather than by the athlete's musculature. Figure 31.1 shows the differences in knee valgus between female and male athletes when dropping off a box and progressing into a maximum vertical jump.

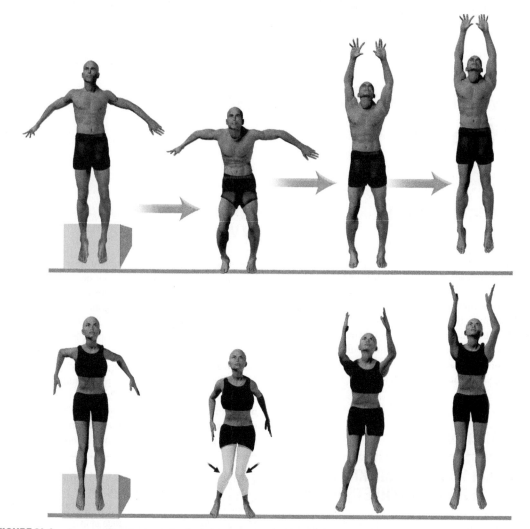

FIGURE 31-1. Representative of valgus at landing in female compared with male athlete when performing landing tasks.

Recent Research

"Participants who sustained a second ACL injury had increased 2-dimensional peak frontal plane knee motion during the landing phase of the drop vertical jump (DVJ)." (Paterno) (8)

The DVJ is performed from a 31-cm box with three trials (Figure 31.2). The participant drops off the box, landing with each foot on a separate force platform (AMTI, Watertown, MA), and then immediately performs a maximum effort vertical jump to an overhead target (8,9). High reliability has been demonstrated with this test in individuals with ACLR (10).

Correction of Ligament Dominance

In order to correct ligament dominance in female athletes, a neuromuscular training program must be designed to teach the athlete to control dynamic knee motion in the coronal (valgus and varus) plane. The first concept that the athlete and coach are taught is the knee is a single-plane hinge, not a ball-and-socket joint. Reeducation of the female neuromuscular system away from multiplanar motion of the knee to dynamic control of knee motion in the sagittal plane is achieved through a progression of single, then multiplanar exercises. Throughout the neuromuscular training program, three development phases are implemented to stress a different training focus.

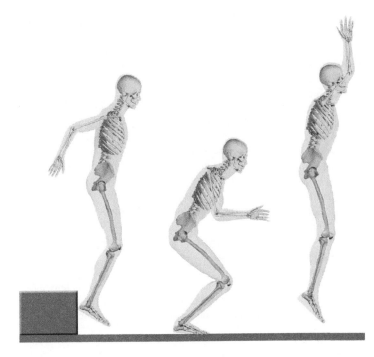

FIGURE 31-2. Drop vertical jump maneuver. (Redrawn from Paterno MV, Schmitt LC, Ford KR, et al. Biomechanical measures during landing and postural stability predict second anterior cruciate ligament injury after anterior cruciate ligament reconstruction and return to sport. Am J Sports Med 2010;38(10):1968–1978.)

The first phase targets the correction of ligament dominance by highlighting proper form and technique. The jumping and landing technique is critically evaluated by the trainer or therapist and constant feedback is given to the athlete in a manner similar to that given while learning a specific skill required for sport (Figure 31.3) (11).

Quadriceps Dominance: Low Flexor Moment and Low Hamstrings Torques

Quadriceps dominance has been documented in the literature (3,5). With quadriceps dominance, female athletes tend to activate their knee extensors preferentially over

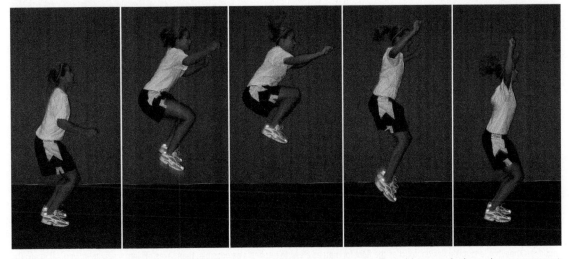

FIGURE 31-3. Tuck jumps, which are an example of an exercise to increase lower body power. The tuck jump can also be used as an assessment to grade improvement in technique. To perform the tuck jump the athlete starts in the athletic position with her feet shoulder width apart. The jump initiates with a slight crouch downward while extending her arms behind. The athlete then swings the arms forward as she simultaneously jumps straight up and pulls her knees up as high as possible. At the highest point of the jump, the athlete is in the air with her thighs parallel to the ground. When landing, the athlete should immediately begin the next tuck jump. Encourage the athlete to land softly, using a toe to mid-foot rocker landing. The athlete should not continue this jump if she cannot control the high landing force or if she demonstrates a knock-kneed landing. (Reprinted from Myer GD, Ford KR, Hewett TE. Rationale and clinical techniques for anterior cruciate ligament injury prevention among female athletes. J Athl Train 2004;39(4):352–364, with permission from the editor.)

their knee flexors to control knee stability. This over-reliance on the quadriceps muscles leads to imbalances in strength and coordination between the quadriceps and the knee flexor musculature. Quadriceps dominance must be addressed and overcome with dynamic neuromuscular training. The majority of ACL injuries (greater than 70%) occur in noncontact situations. Both inappropriate motor control about the knee joint (proper cocontraction patterns between the knee flexors and knee extensors) during landing, pivoting, and decelerating maneuvers and imbalanced contraction of the quadriceps muscles are likely contributors to the ACL injury mechanism. At low knee flexion angles (0° to 30° of knee flexion), quadriceps contractions translate the tibia forward and increase stress on the ACL. Quadriceps contractions without balanced flexor contractions significantly increase strain on the ligament. At knee flexion angles less than 45°, the quadriceps is a clear antagonist of the ACL. At knee flexion angles beyond 45°, the quadriceps translates the tibia in the opposite (posterior) direction, which reduces strain on the ligament.

Correction of Quadriceps Dominance

To decrease the tendency toward quadriceps dominance, exercises should emphasize cocontraction of the knee flexor/extensor muscles (12). At angles greater than 45°, the quadriceps is an antagonist to the ACL (13,14). Therefore, it is important to use deep knee flexion angles to put the quadriceps into an ACL agonist position. By training the athlete with deep knee flexion jumps (Figure 31.4), she learns to increase the amount of knee flexion and decrease the amount of time in the more dangerous straight-legged position. At the same time the athlete reprograms peak flexor/extensor firing patterns, increasing cofiring and quadriceps firing in deep flexion for greater protection of the ACL.

Leg Dominance: Side-to-Side Imbalances in Strength and Stability

Female athletes have been reported to generate lower hamstring torques on the nondominant than in the dominant leg (3). Side-to-side imbalances in neuromuscular strength,

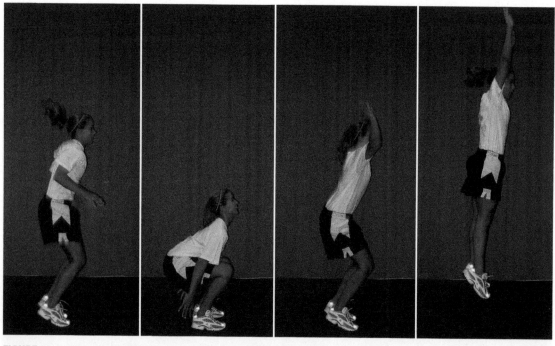

FIGURE 31-4. Squat jumps: The athlete begins in the athletic position with her feet flat on the mat pointing straight ahead. The athlete drops into deep knee, hip, and ankle flexion, touches the floor (or mat) as close to her heels as possible, then takes off into a maximum vertical jump. The athlete then jumps straight up vertically and reaches as high as possible. On landing she immediately returns to starting position and repeats the initial jump. Repeat for the allotted time or until her technique begins to deteriorate. Teach the athlete to jump straight up vertically, reaching as high overhead as possible. Encourage her to land in the same spot on the floor, and maintain upright posture when regaining the deep squat position. Do not allow the athlete to bend forward at the waist to reach the floor. The athlete should keep her eyes up, keep her feet and knees pointed straight ahead, and have her arms to the outside of her legs. (Reprinted from Myer GD, Ford KR, Hewett TE. Rationale and clinical techniques for anterior cruciate ligament injury prevention among female athletes. J Athl Train 2004;39(4):352–364, with permission from the editor.)

flexibility, and coordination represent important predictors of increased injury risk (3,15,16). Knapik et al. demonstrated that side-to-side balance in strength and flexibility is important for the prevention of injuries and when imbalances are present, the athlete is more injury prone (16). Baumhauer et al. also found that individuals with muscle strength imbalances exhibited a higher incidence of injury (17).

Correction of Leg Dominance

Correcting dynamic contralateral imbalances is addressed throughout the entire training protocol. Equal leg-to-leg strength, balance, and foot placement are stressed throughout the program. In order to correct for dominant leg dominance, the program progressively emphasizes double then single movements through the three training phases. For example, in the initial phases of training, the majority of the exercises involve both legs to safely introduce the athletes to the training movements (Figures 31.3 and 31.4). During secondary phases, a greater number of single-leg movements are introduced, though the focus is on correct technique (Figure 31.5). Final training phases utilize dynamic single-leg movements that focus on maximal performance (Figure 31.6).

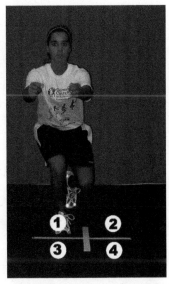

FIGURE 31-6.   Single-leg hop and hold: The starting position for this jump is a semi-crouched position on a single leg. Her arms should be fully extended behind her at the shoulder. She initiates the jump by swinging the arms forward while simultaneously extending at the hip and knee. The jump should carry the athlete up at an approximately 45° angle and attain maximum distance for a single-leg landing. Athletes are instructed to land on the jumping leg with deep knee flexion (to 90°). The landing should be held for a minimum of 3 seconds. Coach this jump with care to protect the athlete from injury. Start the athlete with a submaximal effort on the single-leg broad jump so she can experience the level of difficulty. Continue to increase the distance of the broad hop as the athlete improves her ability to stick and hold the final landing. Have the athlete keep her visual focus away from her feet, to help prevent too much forward lean at the waist. (Reprinted from Myer GD, Ford KR, Hewett TE. Rationale and clinical techniques for anterior cruciate ligament injury prevention among female athletes. J Athl Train 2004;39(4):352–364, with permission from the editor.)

Trunk Dominance

With "trunk dominance," in which the motion and momentum (inertia) of the moving trunk are not controlled sufficiently, uncontrolled motion of the center of mass during deceleration leads to movement of the ground reaction force vector to the lateral side of the joint, which increases medially directed torques at the knee. With trunk dominance, there is an imbalance between agonist and antagonist activation of the trunk musculature.

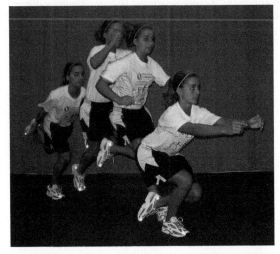

FIGURE 31-5.   X-hops: The athlete faces a quadrant pattern, stands on a single limb with the support knee slightly bent. She hops diagonally, lands in the opposite quadrant, maintains forward stance, and holds the deep knee flexion landing for 3 seconds. She then hops laterally into the side quadrant and again holds the landing. Next she hops diagonally backward and holds the jump. Finally, she hops laterally into the initial quadrant and holds the landing. She repeats this pattern for the required number of sets. Encourage the athlete to maintain balance during each landing, keeping her eyes up and visual focus away from her feet. (Reprinted from Myer GD, Ford KR, Hewett TE. Rationale and clinical techniques for anterior cruciate ligament injury prevention among female athletes. J Athl Train 2004;39(4):352–364, with permission from the editor.)

Recent Research

Hewett et al. found that the mechanism of noncontact ACL injuries in female athletes involves lateral trunk motion with the body shifted over one leg; this was associated with high knee abduction or medial knee collapse (18,19). Lateral perturbation of the trunk is also a common feature (20). Therefore, increased lateral sway of the trunk may underlie medial collapse of the knee joint in female athletes (21).

In addition, Zazulak demonstrated that trunk displacement and coronal plane knee load both predict ACL injury risk in female athletes with high sensitivity and specificity and accuracy (91%) (21,22). Trunk position and knee external abduction moment (load) may be associated mechanically; lateral positioning of the trunk can create abduction loads at the knee (Figure 31.7) (21).

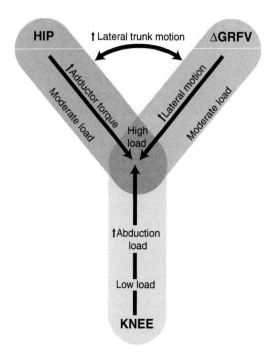

FIGURE 31-7. Conceptual model of lateral trunk motion leading to increased ground reaction force vector (ΔGRFV) and hip adductor torque and knee load. This will result in clustered load subgroups of female athletes. (Adapted from Hewett TE, Myer GD. The mechanistic connection between the trunk, knee, and anterior cruciate ligament injury. Exerc Sports Sci Rev 2011;39(4):161–166.)

Correction of Trunk Dominance

Trunk dominance neuromuscular imbalance can be addressed with dynamic core stability training (Figures 31.8 and 31.9). Therefore, the interventionist must create balance in overall trunk control during high-velocity activities. The neuromuscular training programs that have been developed to achieve this goal have shown high efficacy both in the laboratory and out on the field and court. Multiple randomized controlled trials have demonstrated the efficacy of these programs to increase control and to decrease risk. We currently have ongoing randomized controlled trials to measure the effects of trunk training on knee injury risk factors.

SUMMARY

A possible underlying mechanism for why women have more noncontact ACL injuries than their male counterparts is growth without sufficient power (21). Men experience a significant increase in neuromuscular strength and coordination as skeletal growth and maturation progresses, a so-called neuromuscular spurt not often observed in women (6). As bone length and body mass increase in men, they also demonstrate greater neuromuscular control of the knee joint than women, allowing men to better absorb loads. In lay terms, "growth results in larger machines in both sexes, but as male subjects mature, they adapt with disproportionately more muscle 'horsepower' to match the control demands of their larger machine" (21).

As a result of insufficient neuromuscular adaptation, female knees are exposed to greater ground reaction forces and high external knee abduction moments (load), particularly in landing, pivoting, and deceleration sports (6). A central hypothesis has emerged "that increased bone length and body mass, in the absence of matching adaptations in neuromuscular strength and coordinated muscle recruitment, expose the female knee to greater load and likelihood of ACL injury" (21).

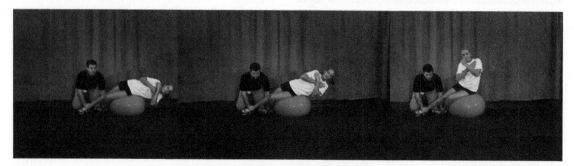

FIGURE 31-8. Swiss ball lateral crunch. The athlete starts lying on side with hip located on top of a Swiss ball. The athlete's feet and legs must be anchored during this exercise by the trainer or a stationary object. The athlete will proceed to bend laterally at the waist back and forth for the prescribed repetitions. (Reprinted from Myer GD, Chu DA, Brent JL, Hewett TE. Trunk and hip control neuromuscular training for the prevention of knee joint injury. Clin Sports Med 2008;27(3):425–448, ix, with permission from the editor.)

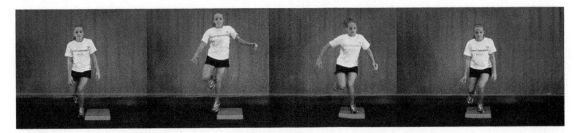

FIGURE 31-9. Single-leg lateral Airex hop-hold: The athlete starts on one side of the Airex pad and hops laterally onto the Airex. The athlete should maintain balance and hold the knee in a flexed position. The athlete then hops off the other side of the Airex onto the ground, maintains balance, and then repeats the exercise in the other direction. (Reprinted from Myer GD, Chu DA, Brent JL, Hewett TE. Trunk and hip control neuromuscular training for the prevention of knee joint injury. Clin Sports Med 2008;27(3):425–448, ix, with permission from the editor.)

REFERENCES

1. Ferretti A, Papandrea P, Conteduca F, Mariani PP. Knee ligament injuries in volleyball players. Am J Sports Med 1992;20(2):203–207.

2. Noyes FR, Mooar PA, Matthews DS, Butler DL. The symptomatic anterior cruciate-deficient knee. Part I: the long-term functional disability in athletically active individuals. J Bone Joint Surg 1983;65A(2):154–162.

3. Andrews M, Noyes FR, Hewett TE, Andriacchi TP. Lower limb alignment and foot angle are related to stance phase knee adduction in normal subjects: a critical analysis of the reliability of gait analysis data. J Orthop Res 1996;14(2):289–295.

4. Hewett TE, Paterno MV, Myer GD. Strategies for enhancing proprioception and neuromuscular control of the knee. Clin Orthop 2002;402:76–94.

5. Huston LJ, Wojtys EM. Neuromuscular performance characteristics in elite female athletes. Am J Sports Med 1996;24(4):427–436.

6. Myer GD, Chu DA, Brent JL, Hewett TE. Trunk and hip control neuromuscular training for the prevention of knee joint injury. Clin Sports Med 2008;27(3):425–448, ix.

7. Myer GD, Ford KR, Hewett TE. Rationale and clinical techniques for anterior cruciate ligament injury prevention among female athletes. J Athl Train 2004;39(4):352–364.

8. Paterno MV, Schmitt LC, Ford KR, et al. Biomechanical measures during landing and postural stability predict second anterior cruciate ligament injury after anterior cruciate ligament reconstruction and return to sport. Am J Sports Med 2010;38(10):1968–1978.

9. Ford KR, Myer GD, Hewett TE. Valgus knee motion during landing in high school female and male basketball players. Med Sci Sports Exerc 2003;35(10):1745–1750.

10. Paterno MV, Ford KR, Myer GD, Heyl R, Hewett TE. Limb asymmetries in landing and jumping 2 years following anterior cruciate ligament reconstruction. Clin J Sport Med 2007;17(4):258–262.

11. Prapavessis H, McNair PJ. Effects of instruction in jumping technique and experience jumping on ground reaction forces. J Orthop Sports Phys Ther 1999;29(6):352–356.

12. Fitzgerald G, Axe M, Snyder-Mackler L. Proposed practice guidelines for nonoperative anterior cruciate ligament rehabilitation of physically active individuals. J Orthop Sports Phys Ther 2000;30(4):194–203.

13. Andriacchi TP, Andersson GBJ, Fermier RW, Stern D, Galante JO. Study of lower-limb mechanics during stair-climbing. J Bone Joint Surg 1980;62A(5):749–757.

14. Daniel DM, Malcom LL, Losse G, Stone ML, Sachs R, Burks R. Instrumented measurement of anterior laxity of the knee. J Bone Joint Surg 1985;67A(5):720–726.

15. Hewett TE, Lindenfeld TN, Riccobene JV, Noyes FR. The effect of neuromuscular training on the incidence of knee injury in female athletes. A prospective study. Am J Sports Med 1999;27(6):699–706.

16. Knapik JJ, Bauman CL, Jones BH, Harris JM, Vaughan L. Preseason strength and flexibility imbalances associated with athletic injuries in female collegiate athletes. Am J Sports Med 1991;19(1):76–81.

17. Baumhauer J, Alosa D, Renstrom A, Trevino S, Beynnon B. A prospective study of ankle injury risk factors. Am J Sport Med 1995;23(5):564–570.

18. Hewett TE, Torg JS, Boden BP. Video analysis of trunk and knee motion during non-contact anterior cruciate ligament injury in female athletes: lateral trunk and knee abduction motion are combined components of the injury mechanism. Br J Sports Med 2009;43:417–422.

19. Krosshaug T, Nakamae A, Boden BP, et al. Mechanisms of anterior cruciate ligament injury in basketball: video analysis of 39 cases. Am J Sports Med 2007;35:359–367.

20. Boden BP, Torg JS, Knowles SB, Hewett TE. Video analysis of anterior cruciate ligament injury: abnormalities in hip and ankle kinematics. Am J Sports Med 2009;37:252–259.

21. Hewett TE, Myer GD. The mechanistic connection between the trunk, knee, and anterior cruciate ligament injury. Exerc Sport Sci Rev 2011;39(4):161–166.

22. Zazulak BT, Hewett TE, Reeves NP, Goldberg B, Cholewicki J. Deficits in neuromuscular control of the trunk predict knee injury risk: a prospective biomechanical-epidemiologic study. Am J Sports Med 2007;35:1123–1130.

Nonoperative Shoulder Rehabilitation Using the Kinetic Chain

INTRODUCTION

It has been recognized that young overhead athletes are at an increased risk for sustaining injury to the upper extremity due to overexposure and lack of adequate and/or appropriate training methods. Possible interventions such as activity modification and injury prevention techniques can be employed to help reduce these risks and increase the longevity of a young overhead athlete's competitive career (1–4). In our clinical experience, patient encounters have been steadily increasing in younger overhead athletes due to continuous exposure to athletic demands without incorporating adequate time for recovery (5). Additionally, these same athletes are improperly prepared to compete due to physiological inadequacies likely from the use of improper training or rehabilitation exercises. The exercises often utilized generally target muscle groups such as the deltoid, biceps, and pectoralis major muscles, which are large in size and designed to perform global movement. While these larger muscles are important for overall function and task execution, smaller local muscles whose primary role is stabilization should be addressed first because optimal stabilization allows for optimal mobilization and output. It is common for the muscles around the scapula (lower trapezius, serratus anterior, and rhomboids) to be an infrequent focal point of training in this young group of athletes. These muscles serve an important function in overhead athletes of all ages where they (the muscles) act as both dynamic movers and stabilizers of the scapula. The stability component is an essential link in the kinetic chain (the coordinated sequenced movements of the trunk, upper extremity, and lower extremity) and must be optimized prior to targeting the larger muscles of the shoulder.

Both training of a noninjured shoulder and rehabilitation of an injury should first concentrate on the intrinsic needs of the scapula for flexibility, strength, balance, and endurance, and on the function of the core in relation to its role in extremity function. Based on the location of these segments within the kinetic chain, the scapula and core fall under the premise of achieving proximal stability for distal mobility. Achieving optimal performance demands a thorough upper extremity training program that addresses the core, scapula, and shoulder.

The initial focus should be on any deficiencies discovered during a pretraining exam. These usually include altered patterns of motion at the hip, trunk, and shoulder as well as actual weakness or inflexibilities of muscles at those segments. Specific inflexibilities and weaknesses may be addressed locally with exercise, but motion patterns should be addressed on a global level involving the entire kinetic chain.

This chapter considers a kinetic chain–based approach to training and rehabilitation of an overhead athlete's upper extremity. Descriptions of kinetic chain function and dysfunction will be discussed accompanied by three levels of exercise training with rationale.

THE KINETIC CHAIN

Optimal athletic function results from physiological motor activations creating specific biomechanical motions and positions using intact anatomical structures to generate forces and actions. Sport-specific function occurs when the activations, motions, and resultant forces are specific and efficient for the needs of that sport. For example, upper extremity dominant athletes such as baseball pitchers and tennis players must have the specific physical components of proximal trunk and pelvis (core) stability, glenohumeral joint flexibility, scapular control, and global shoulder muscle strength in order to be proficient in their activity (6).

These components are collectively known as the links in the kinetic chain. The kinetic chain is a coordinated sequencing of mobilization and stabilization of body segments to produce an athletic activity (7). Kinetic chain–based training or rehabilitation activities can be grouped into open and closed chain (8). Characteristics of open chains generally include free movement of the terminal segment, large terminal segment velocities, and relatively many degrees of freedom in the proximal segments. Characteristics of closed chains generally include fixed or minimal movement of the terminal segment, low terminal segment velocities, minimal degrees of freedom, and coupling of movements of the segments. Typically, closed chain exercises are implemented early in the training or rehabilitation phases due to the decreased amount of force generated and stress applied to the involved joints, which is especially important to control in skeletally immature athletes. These types of exercises are best suited for reestablishing the proximal stability and control in the links of the kinetic chain such as the scapula and pelvis. Open chain exercises, which generate greater force, should be utilized later in shoulder training or rehabilitation programs due to a longer lever arm and increased demand on the body's joints.

Physiologic muscle activation results in several biomechanical effects that allow efficient local and distal function. The preprogrammed muscle activations result in anticipatory postural adjustments (APAs), which position the body to withstand the perturbations to balance created by forces of kicking, throwing, or running (9,10). The APAs create proximal stability for distal mobility by creating interactive moments that develop and control forces and loads at joints. Interactive moments are moments at joints that are created by motion and position of adjacent segments (7). They are developed in the central body segments and are key to developing proper force at distal joints with relative bony positions that minimize internal loads at the joint.

The muscle activations create interactive moments that develop and control forces and loads at joints. Interactive moments are moments at joints that are created by motion and position of adjacent segments (7). They are developed in the central body segments and are key to developing proper force at distal joints with relative bony positions that minimize internal loads at the joint. There are many examples of proximal core activation providing interactive moments that allow efficient distal segment function (6). They either provide maximal force at the distal end, similar to the cracking of a whip, or provide precision and stability to the distal end (7). Maximum shoulder internal rotation force is developed by the interactive moment due to trunk rotation. Also, maximum elbow varus torque to protect against elbow valgus strain is produced by the interactive moment resulting from this shoulder internal rotation (7). Maximal fast ball speed is correlated with the interactive moment from the shoulder that stabilizes elbow and shoulder distraction and produces elbow angular velocity (7,11,12). In addition, accuracy of ball throwing is related to the interactive moment at the wrist produced by shoulder movement (11).

As a result of the activations and interactive moments, there is a proximal to distal development of force and motion, according to the "summation of speed" principle that includes core activation (7). This is not always a purely linear development strictly from one segment to the next. In the tennis serve, elbow maximal velocity is developed before maximal shoulder velocity. However, this general pattern of force development from the ground through the core to the distal segment has been demonstrated in the tennis serve and baseball throw (11,13–15).

Force control is also maximized through the core. The trunk is essential in reacquiring the forward momentum in throwing, and approximately 85% of the muscle activation to slow the forward-moving arm is generated in the periscapular and trunk muscles, rather than the rotator cuff (16,17).

In a closed system, alteration in one area creates changes throughout the entire system. This is known as the "catch-up" phenomenon where the changes in the interactive moments alter the forces in the distal segments. The increased forces place extra stress on the distal segments, which often result in the sensation of pain or actual anatomic injury. The site of the symptoms (victim) may not be the sole site of alterations (culprit). Without elbow elevation and extension prior to maximum shoulder rotation, increased tensile loads are seen at the elbow ligaments during arm acceleration. Baseball pitching coaches have empirically known of this deleterious situation, calling this position the "dropped elbow," their term for the elbow being positioned below the level of the shoulder in the acceleration phase, and consider this the "kiss of death" for the elbow (18). Marshall and Elliott have shown that "long axis rotation," coupled with shoulder internal rotation and elbow pronation around the long axis of the arm from the glenohumeral joint to the hand that is accentuated by maximum elbow extension before maximum arm rotation, is a key biomechanical event just prior to ball release/ball impact (15). This coupled motion creates rotation around the almost straight long axis of the arm, running from the shoulder to the hand, also minimizing the valgus loads that may be generated at the elbow.

KINETIC CHAIN BREAKAGE

Dysfunction of a particular segment in the chain can result in either altered performance or injury to a more distal segment. For example, the muscles of the shoulder girdle are not capable of generating the substantial angular velocities seen at the shoulder during throwing; the force is largely generated by the more proximal segments of the lower extremities and trunk (7,19,20). The substantial forces that are transferred to, and subsequently reabsorbed by, the distal segments at the shoulder and arm during throwing leave these segments vulnerable to injury (21). In a closed system, alteration in one area creates changes throughout the entire system. This is an example of the "catch-up" phenomenon where the changes in the interactive moments alter the forces in the distal segments, which often result in the sensation of pain or actual anatomic injury.

Glenohumeral internal rotation deficit (GIRD) is a common factor associated with injury demonstrated in throwing athletes (19,22–24). Traditional definitions suggested a side-to-side asymmetry in GIRD greater than 20°.

However, studies have demonstrated that a GIRD of as little as 11° (22) or 18° (24) is associated with shoulder injury. In addition, a prospective study demonstrated that a GIRD of 18° was related to a 1.9× increased risk of injury (24). These values would also take into account the alteration in internal rotation due to osseous adaptation. A 5° asymmetry in total range of motion (TROM) has been shown to be predictive of increased injury risk (24). A recent consensus meeting concluded that GIRD will be defined as side-to-side asymmetry greater than 18°, and TROM deficit (TROMD) will be defined as side-to-side asymmetry greater than 5° (25). While GIRD and TROMD may be considered predictive for shoulder injury, they are not causative by themselves. They alter the normal glenohumeral kinematics and place increased load on adjacent joint structures (26,27). Rotation deficits are thought to be produced by acquired posterior capsular contracture and/or posterior muscle stiffness and are frequently seen in various types of shoulder injuries (25,28). GIRD creates abnormal scapular kinematics due to the "wind-up" effect of the arm on the scapula. As the arm is forward flexed, horizontally adducted, and internally rotated in throwing or working, the tight capsule and muscles pull the scapula into a protracted, internally rotated, and anteriorly tilted position that causes downward rotation of the acromion. GIRD also affects glenohumeral kinematics by shifting the humeral center of rotation posterior superiorly in cocking and anterior superiorly in follow-through. Abnormal kinematics have been statistically significant in association with labral injuries (25).

Alteration of knee flexion has been associated with increased stresses in the arm. Tennis players who did not have adequate bend in the knees, breaking the kinetic chain and decreasing the contribution by the hip and trunk, had 23% to 27% increased loads in horizontal adduction and rotation at the shoulder and valgus load at the elbow (29). A mathematical analysis of the tennis serve showed that a decrease of 20% of the kinetic energy developed by the trunk resulted in a requirement of 34% more arm velocity or 80% more shoulder mass to deliver the same energy to the ball (14).

Another example of kinetic chain alteration more proximal to the shoulder is scapular dyskinesis. The scapula is a link in the kinetic chain of integrated segment motions that starts from the ground and ends at the hand (30). Due to the important but minimal bony stabilization of the scapula from the clavicle, dynamic muscle function must govern scapular stabilization. Muscle activation is coordinated in task-specific force coupled patterns to allow stabilization of position and control of dynamic coupled motion. The predominant clinical finding observes the prominence of the medial border of the scapula at rest or during motion. This scapular dyskinesis is a nonspecific response to a painful condition in the shoulder rather than a specific response to certain glenohumeral pathology (30). Scapular dyskinesis has multiple causative factors, both proximally (muscle weakness/imbalance, nerve injury) and distally (acromioclavicular

joint injury, superior labral tears, rotator cuff injury) (31), and it is usually treated by rehabilitation (31).

TREATMENT

Athletic performance depends upon appropriate functioning of the individual components or segments of the kinetic chain. Each segment plays a critical role in helping an individual achieve optimal athletic performance. A typical progression (32) to ensure optimization of each segment follows: (1) establish proper postural alignment; (2) establish proper motion in all involved segments; (3) facilitate scapular motion via exaggeration of lower extremity/trunk movement; (4) exaggerate scapular retraction in controlling excessive protraction; (5) utilize the closed chain exercise early; and (6) work in multiple planes. A sample set of rehabilitation guidelines utilizing this progression is illustrated in Table 32.1.

Athletes who are younger and not skeletally mature (ages 8 to 18) should focus on core strength and stability, developing strength and balance in the periscapula musculature prior to developing global shoulder muscle strength and mass. Individuals in this group also need appropriate amounts of rest between training, practices, and competition in order to allow their less developed bodies time to recover before introducing the next athletic exposure. Athletes between the ages of 18 and 22 years should also focus on similar training concepts, especially early in their training; however, this group can perform larger more dynamic movements due to their anatomical maturity. Elite athletes over the age of 22 are often well-conditioned and strong in the global shoulder muscles. In our clinical experience, this group presents with deficits in the kinetic chain (weak and tight hip and/or abdominal musculature) and the scapula (strength and stability) in the presence of injury or in the instance of decreases in performance. Therefore, this older group should be able to perform more challenging dynamic kinetic chain–based exercises (in comparison to the other two age groups) once the deficits are corrected.

Rehabilitation and training should be viewed as a "flow" of exercises that build a base of stability and force generation, culminating with maximal mobility of the distal segment. The core and scapula are the central parts of this flow. Both act as the base of stability for the shoulder, with the core being the "engine" of force generation and the scapula existing as the "platform" for the rotator cuff. Since both are involved in many aspects of overhead athletic activity, they should be evaluated as part of the workup for any upper extremity injury.

The local and global stabilizers of the trunk together provide optimal core stability. The larger global muscles including the abdominal muscles, erector spinae, and hip abductors are vital to power generation and stability for upper extremity function. The incorporation of core

TABLE 32.1	Phases of Rehabilitation

Phase I: Acute Phase (Weeks 1–3)

Pearls

- Use hips to position trunk and spine
- Glenohumeral motion has lesser priority than scapular motion
- Promote scapular retraction and depression with thoracic extension
- De-emphasize the upper trapezius
- Address soft tissue inflexibilities of pectoralis minor, upper trapezius, and levator scapulae
- Closed chain exercise for glenohumeral joint is a *must* (emphasis on glenohumeral depression)
- Avoid external rotation for 3 weeks postoperatively

Goals

- Achieve 90° abduction and flexion by end of phase I
- Establish quality scapular motion using complementary trunk and hip motion

Phase II: Recovery Phase (Weeks 4–8)

Pearls

- Increase difficulty of scapular strengthening exercises
- Open the upper extremity chain
- Address all planes of motion
- Promote glenohumeral depression
- Progress from below 90° to above 90°
- Begin to load the rotator cuff in various planes and angles (with caution)
- Address glenohumeral internal rotation deficit if present
- Avoid external rotation and horizontal abduction posterior to the plane of the body
- Address soft tissue tightness and inflexibilities more aggressively

Goals

- Good scapular control and rotator cuff strength
- Full active range of motion
- Decrease pain to greater extent

Phase III: Functional Activity Phase (Weeks 8+)

Pearls

- Fine-tune scapular motion to alleviate all dyskinesis
- Increase strength and endurance of rotator cuff and scapular stabilizing muscles

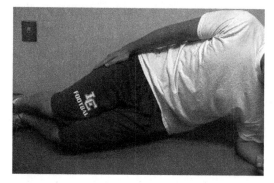

FIGURE 32-1. Horizontal side support exercise.

abdominis, and the quadratus lumborum should then be incorporated for trunk stability. Due to their direct attachment to the spine and pelvis, they are responsible for the most central portion of core stability. Exercises include the horizontal side support (Figure 32.1) and isometric trunk rotation (Figure 32.2) (25,35). This stage of rehabilitation should not be overlooked. The core, being the most proximal component of the kinetic chain (in relation to the arm), is the critical link between the development and transfer of energy (36). These exercises can be performed by athletes at all levels. This stage of rehabilitation not only serves to restore core function but also primes the first stage of extremity rehabilitation.

Flexibility of both the upper and lower extremity can be increased via standard static and/or ballistic stretching. Based on previous mobility findings in upper extremity dominant athletes, the hamstring, hip flexor,

strengthening into rehabilitation regimens has been shown to increase hip extensor muscle strength (33), resulting in pain reduction and an increase of overall strength in the pelvis and trunk postural muscles of patients with low back pain (34). In order to create a stable base, the rehabilitation protocols should focus on the primary stabilizing musculature such as the transverse abduminus and multifidi, which are responsible for segmental spinal stability and alignment. The internal/external obliques, erector spinae, rectus

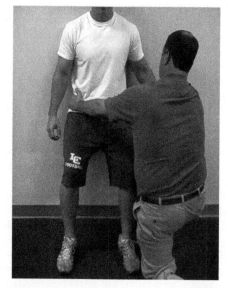

FIGURE 32-2. Isometric trunk rotation.

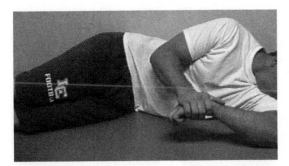

FIGURE 32-3. "Sleeper" stretch for posterior shoulder muscle tightness.

hip adductors, hip rotator, and gastrocnemius/soleus muscle groups should be targeted for the lower extremity, and the pectoralis minor and posterior shoulder muscles should be the focus in the upper extremity (28,37–40). The "sleeper" stretch (18) (Figure 32.3) can be utilized to increase posterior rotator cuff flexibility, and the "open book" (41) or corner stretch (37) (Figure 32.4) can help elongate a shortened pectoralis minor.

Periscapular muscles such as the serratus anterior and lower trapezius should be a point of focus in early training and rehabilitation. Early training should incorporate the trunk and hip in order to facilitate the kinetic chain proximal to distal sequence of muscle activation (42). Little stress is placed on the shoulder during the movements of hip and trunk extension combined with scapular retraction. All exercises are started with the feet on the ground and involve hip extension and pelvic control (Figures 32.5 and 32.6). The patterns of activation are both ipsilateral and contralateral. Diagonal motions involving trunk rotation around a stable leg simulate the normal pattern of throwing (32). As the shoulder heals and is ready for motion with load in the intermediate or recovery stage of rehabilitation, the patterns can incorporate arm motion as the final part of exercise. Specific exercises known as the low row and inferior glide have been shown to activate the serratus and lower trapezius at safe levels of muscle activation (43) (Figures 32.7 and 32.8).

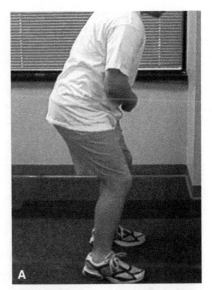

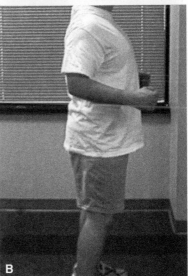

FIGURE 32-5. (A, B) Sternal lift. Begin with knees and trunk slightly flexed. Extend trunk and knees while retracting and depressing both scapulae.

A properly stabilized scapula allows for optimal rotator cuff activation. Recent studies have demonstrated that rotator cuff strength can increase as much as 24% when the scapula is stabilized and retracted (44,45). For this reason, the early phases of training should focus on scapular strengthening rather than rotator cuff strengthening. Once the scapula is properly stabilized, more advanced exercises can be incorporated to strengthen the larger global muscles around the shoulder. These exercises are depicted in Figures 32.9–32.14.

Rotator cuff rehabilitation should be emphasized when the cuff is anatomically intact or strong enough to withstand

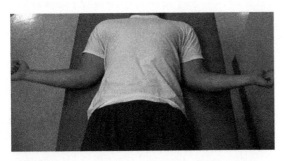

FIGURE 32-4. "Open book" stretch for pectoralis minor tightness.

FIGURE 32-6. (A, B) Step out. Begin with knees and trunk slightly flexed. Step out and rotate ipsilateral leg while retracting scapula.

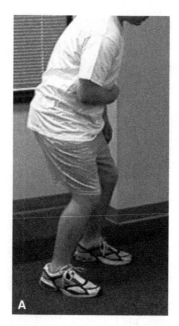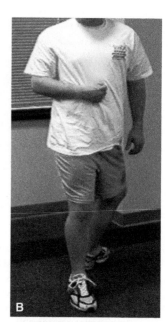

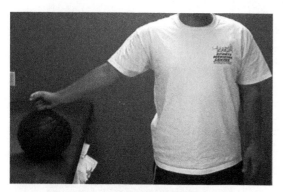

FIGURE 32-7. Inferior glide. Place arm in slightly abducted position with hand resting on firm surface or object. Depress hand in the direction of adduction while inferiorly depressing scapula and hold this position for 5 seconds.

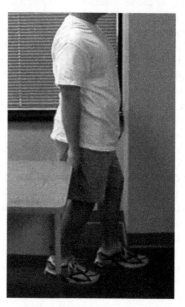

FIGURE 32-8. Low row. Place hand on the anterior edge of a firm surface with palm facing posteriorly. Simultaneously extend trunk and push hand maximally against the surface in the direction of shoulder extension while retracting and depressing the scapula—the isometric contraction is held for 5 seconds.

the applied loads and when a stable scapular base has been established for activation and for acromial clearance. The clinical evidence for scapular stability includes resolution of scapular dyskinesis, with control of scapular retraction (46). Rotator cuff activation is most efficient when it is done in an integrated manner with other potent facilitators of rotator cuff activation such as the lower trapezius and latissimus dorsi (44,45,47) (Figures 32.15 and 32.16).

Once the kinetic chain deficits have been corrected and normal kinematics have been restored, the focus should transition to muscle endurance and proprioception. Three areas should be considered: lower extremity muscle power and endurance, integrated sports-specific exercise, and upper extremity power and endurance (25,32). High-repetition exercises designed to increase lower extremity

muscle endurance should be employed first with focus on the gastrocnemius/soleus, quadriceps, hamstrings, and hip abductor muscle groups. The next component should utilize integrated sports-specific exercise to employ the improved lower extremity muscle strength and endurance for enhanced upper extremity muscle activation.

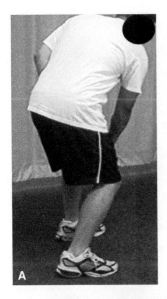
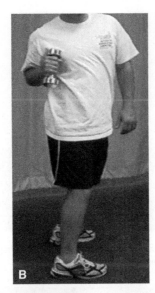

FIGURE 32-9. (A, B) Lawnmower. The lawnmower is a multijoint exercise that mobilizes joints in a diagonal pattern from the contralateral leg through the trunk to the ipsilateral arm.

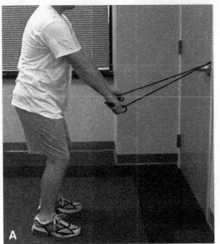
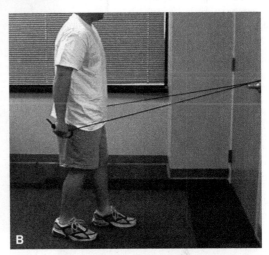

FIGURE 32-10. (A, B) Low row with resistance. This exercise incorporates hip and trunk extension with scapular retraction and depression.

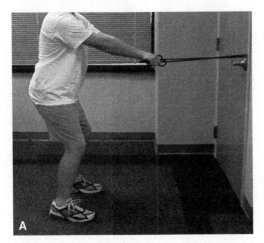
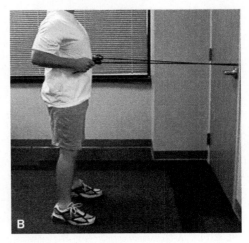

FIGURE 32-11. (A, B) Long pull with resistance. This exercise is the progression from the low row.

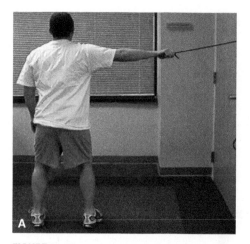
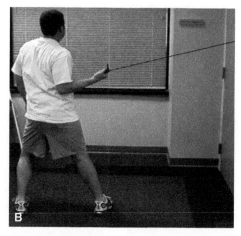

FIGURE 32-12. (A, B) Fencing. Begin with body facing laterally and arm extended away from body. Bending elbow, pull arm behind body while stepping away in order to fully retract scapula.

FIGURE 32-13. (A, B) Clean exercise. This exercise encourages scapular depression by challenging the use of hip and trunk extension.

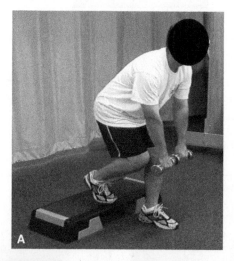
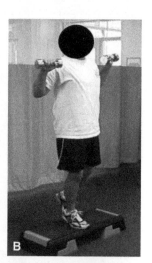

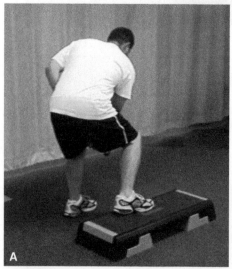
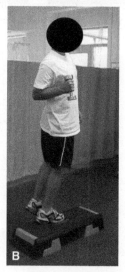
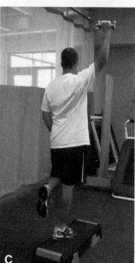

FIGURE 32-14. (A–C) Lawnmower progression. This transverse plane exercise challenges both core strength and stability while facilitating scapular retraction.

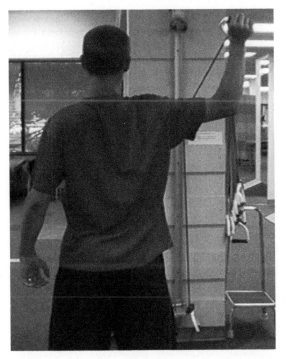

FIGURE 32-15. External rotation. Rotator cuff exercises such as resisted external rotation should be performed later in rehabilitation and should be performed with the scapula in a retracted position.

This goal is accomplished through synchronous single-leg and transverse plane exercises that improve proprioception and muscle education (25). Finally, upper extremity power and endurance are addressed by high-repetition, long-lever exercises performed both standing and prone.

Pain not generated by disrupted anatomy or kinetic chain deficit suggests that the extremity is being used excessively. Overuse leads to muscular fatigue that decreases muscular activity and force production, likely producing biomechanical abnormalities (decreased cocking, dropped elbow). Therefore, adequate rest and recovery must be allotted to avoid abnormal muscle recruitment from stress of physical activity (32).

SUMMARY

The upper extremity training program for the overhead athlete entails all components of kinetic chain function. In the presence of injury or requirements for stability, training regimens should begin with closed chain kinetic exercises, which will be progressed to open chain exercises. Skeletally immature athletes should focus on both core and scapular stability; likewise, anatomically mature athletes should correct kinetic chain deficits prior to implementing dynamic exercises. Once the scapula is stable, all groups will benefit from rotator cuff strengthening.

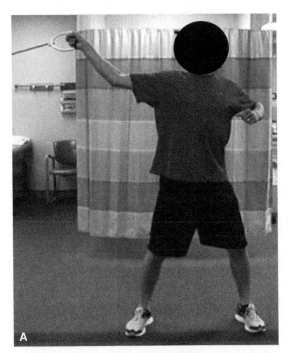
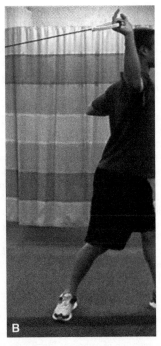

FIGURE 32-16 (A, B) Power position. This proprioceptive exercise is ideal for overhead athletes in that it utilizes both kinetic chain principles and helps establish optimal arm position for throwing.

REFERENCES

1. Fleisig GS, Andrews JR, Cutter GR, et al. Risk of serious injury for young baseball pitchers: a 10-year prospective study. Am J Sports Med 2011;39(2):253–257.
2. Lyman S, Fleisig G, Andrews JR, Osinski ED. Effect of pitch type, pitch count, and pitching mechanics on risk of elbow and shoulder pain in youth baseball pitchers. Am J Sports Med 2002;30:463–468.
3. Lyman S, Fleisig GS, Waterbor JW, et al. Longitudinal study of elbow and shoulder pain in youth baseball pitchers. Med Sci Sports Exerc 2001;33(11):1803–1810.
4. Olsen SJ, Fleisig GS, Dun S, Loftice J, Andrews JR. Risk factors for shoulder and elbow injuries in adolescent baseball pitchers. Am J Sports Med 2006;34:905.
5. Kibler WB, Sciascia A, Ellenbecker TS. Musculoskeletal aspects of recovery for tennis. In: Kovacs MS, Ellenbecker TS, Kibler WB, eds. Tennis Recovery: A Comprehensive Review of the Research. White Plains: United States Tennis Association; 2010:129–166, 978-0-692-00528-6.
6. Lintner D, Noonan TJ, Kibler WB. Injury patterns and biomechanics of the athlete's shoulder. Clin Sports Med 2008;27(4):527–552.
7. Putnam CA. Sequential motions of body segments in striking and throwing skills: description and explanations. J Biomech 1993;26:125–135.
8. Kibler WB, Livingston B. Closed-chain rehabilitation for upper and lower extremities. J Am Acad Orthop Surg 2001;9(6):412–421.
9. Cordo PJ, Nashner LM. Properties of postural adjustments associated with rapid arm movements. J Neurophysiol 1982;47(2):287–308.
10. Zattara M, Bouisset S. Posturo-kinetic organisation during the early phase of voluntary upper limb movement. 1: normal subjects. J Neurol Neurosurg Psychiatry 1988;51:956–965.
11. Hirashima M, Kadota H, Sakurai S, Kudo K, Ohtsuki T. Sequential muscle activity and its functional role in the upper extremity and trunk during overarm throwing. J Sports Sci 2002;20:301–310.
12. Stodden DF, Fleisig G, McLean SP, Lyman S, Andrews JR. Relationship of pelvis and upper torso kinematics to pitched baseball velocity. J Appl Biomech 2001;17:164–172.
13. Hirashima M, Yamane K, Nakamura Y, Ohtsuki T. Kinetic chain of overarm throwing in terms of joint rotations revealed by induced acceleration analysis. J Biomech 2008;41:2874–2883.
14. Kibler WB. Biomechanical analysis of the shoulder during tennis activities. Clin Sports Med 1995;14:79–85.
15. Marshall R, Elliott BC. Long axis rotation: the missing link in proximal to distal segment sequencing. J Sports Sci 2000;18(4):247–254.
16. Happee R. Goal-directed arm movements: I. Analysis of EMG records in shoulder and elbow muscles. J Electromyogr Kinesiol 1992;2(3):165–178.
17. Happee R, van der Helm FCT. Control of shoulder muscles during goal-directed movements, an inverse dynamic analysis. J Biomech 1995;28:1179–1191.
18. Burkhart SS, Morgan CD, Kibler WB. The disabled throwing shoulder: spectrum of pathology. Part III: the SICK scapula, scapular dyskinesis, the kinetic chain, and rehabilitation. Arthroscopy 2003;19(6):641–661.
19. Burkhart SS, Morgan CD, Kibler WB. The disabled throwing shoulder: spectrum of pathology. Part I: pathoanatomy and biomechanics. Arthroscopy 2003;19(4):404–420.
20. Burkhart SS, Morgan CD, Kibler WB. Shoulder injuries in overhead athletes, the "dead arm" revisited. Clin Sports Med 2000;19(1):125–158.
21. Fleisig GS, Barrentine SW, Escamilla RF, Andrews JR. Biomechanics of overhand throwing with implications for injuries. Sports Med 1996;21:421–437.
22. Myers JB, Laudner KG, Pasquale MR, Bradley JP, Lephart SM. Glenohumeral range of motion deficits and posterior shoulder tightness in throwers with pathologic internal impingement. Am J Sports Med 2006;34:385–391.
23. Wilk KE, Obma P, Simpson II CD, Cain EL, Dugas JR, Andrews JR. Shoulder injuries in the overhead athlete. J Orthop Sports Phys Ther 2009;39:38–54.
24. Wilk KE, Macrina LC, Fleisig GS, et al. Loss of internal rotation and the correlation to shoulder injuries in professional baseball pitchers. Am J Sports Med 2011;39(2):329–335.
25. Kibler WB, Kuhn JE, Wilk KE, et al. The disabled throwing shoulder—spectrum of pathology: 10 year update. Arthroscopy 2013;29(1):141–161.
26. Grossman MG, Tibone JE, McGarry MH, Schneider DJ, Veneziani S, Lee TQ. A cadaveric model of the throwing shoulder: a possible etiology of superior labrum anterior-to-posterior lesions. J Bone Joint Surg (Am) 2005;87(4):824–831.
27. Harryman II DT, Sidles JA, Clark JM, McQuade KJ, Gibb TD, Matsen III FA. Translation of the humeral head on the glenoid with passive glenohumeral motion. J Bone Joint Surg (Am) 1990;72(9):1334–1343.
28. Kibler WB, Sciascia AD, Thomas SJ. Glenohumeral internal rotation deficit: pathogenesis and response to acute throwing. Sports Med Arthrosc Rev 2012;20(1):34–38.
29. Elliott B, Fleisig G, Nicholls R, Escamillia R. Technique effects on upper limb loading in the tennis serve. J Sci Med Sport 2003;6(1):76–87.
30. Kibler WB, Sciascia AD. Current concepts: scapular dyskinesis. Br J Sports Med 2010;44(5):300–305. doi:10.1136/bjsm.2009.058834.
31. Kibler WB, Sciascia A, Wilkes T. Scapular dyskinesis and its relation to shoulder injury. J Am Acad Orthop Surg 2012;20(6):364–372.
32. Sciascia A, Cromwell R. Kinetic chain rehabilitation: a theoretical framework. Rehabil Res Pract 2012;2012:1–9.
33. Nadler SF, Malanga GA, Bartoli LA, Feinberg JH, Prybicien M, DePrince M. Hip muscle imbalance and low back pain in athletes: influence of core strengthening. Med Sci Sports Exerc 2002;34(1):9–16.
34. Petrofsky JS, Batt J, Brown J, et al. Improving the outcomes after back injury by a core muscle strengthening program. J Appl Res 2008;8(1):62–75.
35. Kibler WB, Press J, Sciascia AD. The role of core stability in athletic function. Sports Med 2006;36(3):189–198.
36. Sciascia AD, Thigpen CA, Namdari S, Baldwin K. Kinetic chain abnormalities in the athletic shoulder. Sports Med Arthrosc Rev 2012;20(1):16–21.
37. Borstad JD, Ludewig PM. Comparison of three stretches for the pectoralis minor muscle. J Shoulder Elbow Surg 2006;15(3):324–330.
38. McClure P, Balaicuis J, Heiland D, Broersma ME, Thorndike CK, Wood A. A randomized controlled comparison

of stretching procedures for posterior shoulder tightness. J Orthop Sports Phys Ther 2007;37(3):108–114.

39. Robb AJ, Fleisig GS, Wilk KE, Macrina L, Bolt B, Pajaczkowski J. Passive ranges of motion of the hips and their relationship with pitching biomechanics and ball velocity in professional baseball pitchers. Am J Sports Med 2010;38(12):2487–2493.

40. Wilk KE, Macrina LC, Arrigo C. Passive range of motion characteristics in the overhead baseball pitcher and their implications for rehabilitation. Clin Orthop Relat Res 2012;470:1586–1594.

41. Kibler WB, Sciascia AD. Rehabilitation of the athlete's shoulder. Clin Sports Med 2008;27(4):821–832.

42. McMullen J, Uhl TL. A kinetic chain approach for shoulder rehabilitation. J Athl Train 2000;35(3):329–337.

43. Kibler WB, Sciascia AD, Uhl TL, Tambay N, Cunningham T. Electromyographic analysis of specific exercises for scapular

control in early phases of shoulder rehabilitation. Am J Sports Med 2008;36(9):1789–1798.

44. Kibler WB, Sciascia AD, Dome DC. Evaluation of apparent and absolute supraspinatus strength in patients with shoulder injury using the scapular retraction test. Am J Sports Med 2006;34(10):1643–1647. doi:10.1177/0363546506288728.

45. Tate AR, McClure P, Kareha S, Irwin D. Effect of the scapula reposition test on shoulder impingement symptoms and elevation strength in overhead athletes. J Orthop Sports Phys Ther 2008;38(1):4–11.

46. Sciascia A, Karolich D. A comprehensive approach for nonoperative treatment of the rotator cuff. Curr Phys Med Rehabil Rep 2013;1(1):29–37.

47. Smith J, Kotajarvi BR, Padgett DJ, et al. Effect of scapular protraction and retraction on isometric shoulder elevation strength. Arch Phys Med Rehabil 2002;83:367–370. doi:10-1053/apmr.2002.29666.

Treating and Preventing Injury in the Overhead Athlete

INTRODUCTION

The overhead throwing athlete is an extremely challenging patient with unique physical characteristics as the result of sport competition. The repetitive microtraumatic stresses placed on the overhead athlete's shoulder complex challenges the physiologic limits of the surrounding tissues. Sports such as baseball, softball, tennis, volleyball, and swimming all require specific injury prevention and rehabilitation programs.

Consequently, it is imperative to emphasize the preventative care and treatment of these athletes. Injury may occur due to muscle fatigue, muscle weakness and imbalances, alterations in sports mechanics, and/or altered static stability. A comprehensive program emphasizing strength, stability, and proper mechanics designed for overhead athletes and their specific sport is necessary to avoid injury and maximize performance. This program must utilize total body conditioning to prevent fatigue leading to altered mechanics that result with increased forces on the upper extremity. Unfortunately, not all injuries may be prevented as the overhead motion is challenged by multiple external forces, which result in increased torque. These forces often exceed the ultimate tensile strength of the stabilizing structures of the shoulder (1,2).

This chapter discusses the treatment of the overhead athlete with emphasis on injury prevention and rehabilitation. The following guidelines can be individually based on the specific sport and injury that may have occurred.

PRINCIPLES OF INJURY PREVENTION PROGRAMS

Several general principles should be incorporated in the development of injury prevention and treatment programs for the overhead athlete's shoulder. Considerable overlap exists between prevention and treatment as both are based on similar principles. The primary goal of any program should maximize the balance between mobility and stability of the shoulder.

Maintain Range of Motion

The first principle involves maintaining appropriate and necessary range of motion (ROM) at the glenohumeral joint. The shoulder in overhead athletes often exhibits excessive motion. For example, professional baseball players exhibit motion ranging from 129° to 137° external rotation (ER), 54° to 61° internal rotation (IR), and 183° to 198° total ER/IR motion (3). Although the dominant shoulder has greater ER and less IR, the combined total motion should be equal bilaterally (3–5). This is termed the "total motion concept." More importantly, the act of throwing has been shown to reduce IR and total motion (Figure 33.1) (4). Studies by Ruotolo et al. (6) and Myers et al. (7) have both shown that a loss of total motion correlates with a greater risk of injury. Excessive motion has also been shown in other overhead sports such as tennis, volleyball, softball, and swimming (8–14). Measurement can be reliably quantified with a goniometer.

Thus, it is important to maintain motion over the course of a season. Reinold et al. (4) theorized that the loss of IR and total motion after throwing is the result of eccentric muscle damage as the external rotators and other posterior musculature attempt to decelerate the arm during the throwing motion. In general, total motion should be maintained equal to that of the nondominant shoulder by frequently performing gentle stretching. Caution should be emphasized against overaggressive stretching in an attempt to gain mobility, but rather consistent stretching techniques to maintain mobility.

Maintaining elbow ROM throughout a season is equally important. Repetitive overhead activities especially throwing can lead to tightening of the elbow flexors due to eccentric forces. The loss of ROM in an athlete's elbow can lead to altered mechanics and possibly result in injury due to the changes in forces applied to the upper extremity.

It is equally important to regain full ROM following injury and surgery. Time frames will vary for each injury. Athletes attempting to return to overhead activities before regaining full motion often have a difficult time returning to competition without symptoms. The clinician should

FIGURE 33.1. Screening shoulder range of motion. (A) External rotation. (B) Internal rotation.

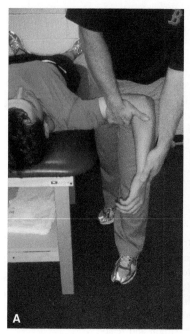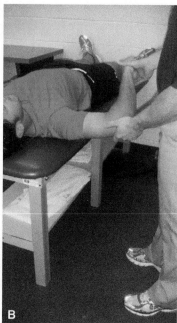

assure that full motion has been achieved before allowing the initiation of an interval sports program (ISP) designed for return to play.

Maintain Strength of the Glenohumeral and Scapulothoracic Musculature

Due to the challenges the overhead athlete's motion creates for the static and dynamic stabilizing structures of the shoulder, strengthening of the entire upper extremity, including shoulder, scapula, elbow, and wrist exercises, is essential for the overhead thrower. A proper program is designed based on the individual needs of each athlete, the unique stress of the sport motion, and the available research on strengthening each muscle (15–17). Emphasizing the external rotators, scapular retractors, and lower trapezius is important based on electromyographic studies of the biomechanics of overhead sports (15–17). Comprehensive programs should serve as a foundation for the strengthening program (see also Chapter 21) (16,17). Skilled and advanced techniques may be superimposed. A sample list of traditional strength exercises follows:

1A. Diagonal pattern D2 extension
1B. Diagonal pattern D2 flexion
2A. ER at 0° abduction
2B. IR at 0° abduction
2C. (Optional) ER at 90° abduction
2D. (Optional) IR at 90° abduction
 3. Shoulder abduction to 90°
 4. Scaption, ER
 5. Side lying ER

6A. Prone horizontal abduction (neutral)
6B. Prone horizontal abduction (full ER, 100° Abduction)
6C. Prone rowing
6D. Prone rowing into ER
 7. Press-ups
 8. Push-ups
9A. Elbow flexion
9B. Elbow extension (abduction)
10A. Wrist extension
10B. Wrist flexion
10C. Supination
10D. Pronation

Emphasize Dynamic Stabilization and Neuromuscular Control

The excessive mobility and compromised static stability observed within the glenohumeral joint often results in injuries to the capsulolabral and musculotendinous structures of the throwing shoulder. Efficient dynamic stabilization and neuromuscular control of the glenohumeral joint is necessary for overhead athletes to avoid injuries (18). This involves neuromuscular control: efferent (motor) output in response to afferent (sensory) stimulation. Dynamic stability is one of the most overlooked, yet extremely important, components of injury prevention and treatment programs for the overhead athlete.

Neuromuscular control of the shoulder involves not only the glenohumeral but also the scapulothoracic joint. The scapula provides a base of support for muscular attachment and dynamically positions the glenohumeral joint during upper extremity movement. Scapular strength and stability are essential to proper functioning of the glenohumeral joint.

A third area of concern when discussing both dynamic stabilization and neuromuscular control is the elbow joint complex. Loss of the ability to stabilize and control the elbow during the overhead motion can have deleterious effects on the entire upper extremity. Compensation for the elbow often occurs in the shoulder joint during the overhead motion. These compensations cause the shoulder joint to work harder and alter the natural biomechanics of the athlete's shoulder. These two factors can lead to an increased risk of injury in the shoulder joint over time.

Neuromuscular control techniques that should be included in rehabilitation programs for the overhead athlete include rhythmic stabilization, reactive neuromuscular control drills, closed kinetic chain (CKC), and plyometric exercises (5,15,18–21).

CKC exercises are used to stress the joint in a load bearing position, resulting in joint approximation (18). The goal is to stimulate receptors and facilitate cocontraction of the shoulder force couples (22). Plyometric exercises provide quick powerful movements by a prestretch of the muscle, thereby activating the stretch–shortening cycle (21,23,24). Plyometric exercises increase the speed of the myotactic stretch reflex, desensitize the Golgi tendon organ, and increase neuromuscular coordination (21).

Off-Season Preparation versus In-Season Maintenance

The off-season is a valuable time for the athlete to rest, regenerate, and prepare for the rigors of an upcoming season. This portion of the year allows athletes to set themselves up physically for peak-level performance during the next season. If one does not prepare appropriately in the off-season, oftentimes the athlete is at a disadvantage physically when the competitive season begins, which can result in a higher risk of injury.

An initial period of rest and progressive full-body strength and conditioning program are the main components of the player's off-season. The goal of the off-season is to build enough strength, power, and endurance to compete without the negative effects of fatigue or weakness from overtraining or undertraining. While the timing of in-season and off-season components of an athlete's yearly cycle may vary greatly between individual athletes at different skill levels and different sports, the concepts and goals for the off-season remain the same. Training is based on Matveyev's periodization concept with individualized attention to each athlete's specific goals (25).

At the conclusion of a competitive season, athletes should remain physically active, while taking time away from their specific sport. Recreational activities such as recreational swimming, golfing, cycling, and jogging are encouraged. This is also a valuable time to rehabilitate any lingering injury that may have been managed through the season.

The remainder of the off-season is used to gradually build a baseline of strength, power, endurance, and neuromuscular control, the goal of which is to maximize their physical performance prior to the start of sport-specific activities. This goal will assure adequate physical fitness to withstand the demands of the competitive season.

Equally as important to preparing for the competitive season is maintaining gains in strength and conditioning during the season. The chronic, repetitive nature of a long season often results in a gradual decline in physical performance.

While a full-body strength and conditioning program is imperative, specific attention is paid to dominant shoulder in unilateral sports such as baseball, tennis, and volleyball and the muscles of the glenohumeral and scapulothoracic joints. The nondominant arm has unique demands, and programs should be developed accordingly. In bilateral sports such as swimming, it is important to emphasize bilateral strength and stability of the shoulders. Any fatigue or weakness in these areas can lead to injury through a loss of dynamic stability.

Two other key areas of focus are the core and lower extremity. The lower extremities are extremely important in the development of force and stabilization of the body during the overhead arm motion. Core stabilization drills and lower body training are utilized to further enhance the transfer of kinetic energy and proximal stability with distal mobility of the upper extremity. Any deficits in strength, endurance, or neuromuscular control of the lower body will have a significant impact on the forces of the upper extremity and the athlete's ability to produce the specific movements needed for their sports.

Core stabilization is based on the kinetic chain concept: imbalance at any point of the kinetic chain may result in pathology. Movement patterns, such as throwing, serving in tennis, spiking a volleyball, etc., require a precise interaction of the entire kinetic chain to become efficient. An imbalance of strength, flexibility, endurance, or stability anywhere within the chain may result in fatigue, abnormal arthrokinematics, and subsequent compensation.

An in-season maintenance program should focus on strength and dynamic stability while adjusting for the workload of a competitive season.

REHABILITATION

The overhead athlete suffers unique stresses on the body, and thus there are many different injuries that can occur in overhead sports that are not as frequent in nonoverhead sports. Even with similar principles, the severity and frequency of these injuries vary from sport to sport. It is important to understand the unique biomechanics and forces that are created in the athlete's unique sport. The differences between these sports are beyond the scope of this chapter but have been referenced in numerous other research articles (26–35).

Rehabilitation Progression

In addition to eliminating pain and inflammation, the rehabilitation process for the overhead athlete must include the restoration of motion, muscular strength, and endurance, as well as restoration of proprioception, dynamic stability, and neuromuscular control (Table 33.1). As the athlete advances, sport-specific drills are added to prepare

TABLE 33.1	Treatment Guidelines for the Overhead Athlete

Phase I—Acute Phase

Goals
- Diminish pain and inflammation
- Improve posterior flexibility
- Re-establish posterior strength and dynamic stability (muscular balance)
- Control functional stresses/strains

Treatment
- Abstain from throwing until pain-free full range of motion (ROM) and full strength; specific time determined by physician

Modalities
- Iontophoresis (disposable patch highly preferred)
- Phonophoresis
- Electrical stimulation and cryotherapy as needed

Flexibility
- Improve internal rotation (IR) ROM at 90° abduction to normal total motion values
- Enhance horizontal adduction flexibility
- Gradually stretch into external rotation (ER) and flexion; do not force into painful ER

Exercises
- Rotator cuff strengthening (especially ER) with light-moderate weight
  ○ Tubing ER/IR
  ○ Side ER
- Scapular strengthening exercises
  ○ Retractors
  ○ Depressors
  ○ Protractors
- Manual strengthening exercises
  ○ Side ER
  ○ Supine ER at 45° abduction
  ○ Prone row
  ○ Side flexion in the scapular plane

- Dynamic rhythmic stabilization (RS) exercises
- Proprioception training
- Electrical stimulation to posterior cuff as needed during exercises
- Closed kinetic chain exercises
- Maintain core, lower body, and conditioning throughout
- Maintain elbow, wrist, and forearm strength

Criteria to progress to Phase II
- Minimal pain or inflammation
- Normalized IR and horizontal adduction ROM
- Baseline muscular strength without fatigue

Phase II—Intermediate Phase

Goals
- Progress strengthening exercises
- Restore muscular balance (ER/IR)
- Enhance dynamic stability
- Maintain flexibility and mobility
- Improve core stabilization and lower body strength

Flexibility
- Control stretches and flexibility exercises
  ○ Especially for IR and horizontal adduction
  ○ Gradually restore full ER

Exercises
- Progress strengthening exercises
- Full rotator cuff and scapula shoulder isotonic program; begin to advance weight
- Initiate dynamic stabilization program
  ○ Side ER with RS
  ○ ER tubing with end-range RS
  ○ Wall stabilization onto ball
  ○ Push-ups onto ball with stabilization
- May initiate two-hand plyometric throws
  ○ Chest pass
  ○ Side-to-side
  ○ Overhead soccer throws

Criteria to Progress to Phase III
- Full, pain-free ROM
- Full 5/5 strength with no fatigue

Phase III—Advanced Strengthening Phase

Goals
- Aggressive strengthening program
- Progress neuromuscular control
- Improve strength, power, and endurance
- Initiate light throwing activities

Exercises
- Stretch prior to exercise program; continue to normalize total motion
- Continue strengthening program above
- Reinitiate upper body program

(Continued)

TABLE 33.1	Treatment Guidelines for the Overhead Athlete (*Continued*)

- Dynamic stabilization drills
  - ○ ER tubing with end-range RS at 90° abduction
  - ○ Wall stabs in 90° abduction and 90° ER
  - ○ Wall dribble with RS in 90° abduction and 90° ER (90/90)
- Plyometrics
  - ○ Two-hand drills
  - ○ One-hand drills (90/90 throws, deceleration throws, throw into bounce-back)
- Stretch postexercise

Criteria to Progress to Phase IV
- Full ROM and strength
- Adequate dynamic stability
- Appropriate rehabilitation progression to this point

Phase IV—Return to Activity Phase

Goals
- Progress to throwing program
- Continue strengthening and flexibility exercises
- Return to competitive throwing

Exercises
- Stretching and flexibility drills
- Shoulder program
- Plyometric program
- Dynamic stabilization drills
- Progress to interval throwing program
- Gradually progress to competitive throwing as tolerated

Used with permission from Advanced Continuing Education Institute, LLC, www.advancedceu.com

for a gradual return to competition. Various "Interval Return to Sports Programs" are available at http://www .advancedceu.com/rehab_protocols

- Interval Throwing Program for Baseball Players: Phase I—Long Toss
- Interval Throwing Program: Phase II—Throwing Off the Mound
- Interval Football Throwing Program
- Interval Tennis Program
- Interval Softball Throwing Program

Neuromuscular control drills are performed throughout and advanced as the athlete progresses to provide a continuous challenge to the neuromuscular control system. The progression can be broken down into four different phases, each with specific goals and specific criteria to progress to the next phase. We will discuss each in detail.

Acute Phase

The acute phase of rehabilitation begins immediately following injury or surgery by abstaining from overhead activities. The duration of the acute phase is dependent on the chronicity of the injury and healing constraints of the involved tissues.

ROM exercises are performed immediately in a restricted range based on the theory that motion assists in the enhancement and organization of collagen tissue and the stimulation of joint mechanoreceptors, and it may assist in the neuromodulation of pain (36–38). The rehabilitation program should allow for progressive loads, beginning with gentle passive and active-assisted motion. Passive ROM for the elbow and wrist may be performed immediately.

Flexibility exercises for the posterior shoulder musculature are also performed early. The posterior shoulder is subjected to extreme repetitive eccentric contractions during overhead activity, which may result in soft tissue adaptations and loss of IR ROM (3,4). Thus, common stretches performed include horizontal adduction across the body, IR stretching at 90° abduction, and the sleeper stretch (Figures 33.2 and 33.3). Stretches or joint mobilizations for the posterior capsule should not be performed unless the capsule has been shown to be immobile on clinical examination. The authors caution to assess the posterior capsule before mobilization. To date, no study has shown that the posterior capsule becomes tight in overhead athletes.

The cross-body horizontal adduction stretch may be performed in a straight plane or integrated with IR at the glenohumeral joint (see Figure 33.3). Overaggressive stretching with the sleeper stretch should be avoided. Frequent, gentle stretching yields far superior results than the occasional aggressive stretch.

The rehabilitation specialist should assess the resting position and mobility of the scapula. Frequently, overhead athletes exhibit a posture of rounded shoulders and a forward head. This posture is associated with muscle weakness of the scapular retractors and deep neck flexor muscles due to prolonged elongation or sustained stretches (15,39). In addition, the scapula may appear protracted and anteriorly tilted. An anteriorly tilted scapula contributes to a loss of glenohumeral IR (40,41). This scapular position is

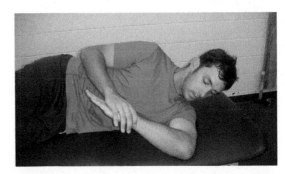

FIGURE 33.2. The sleeper stretch for glenohumeral internal rotation. The body should be positioned so that the shoulder is in the scapular plane.

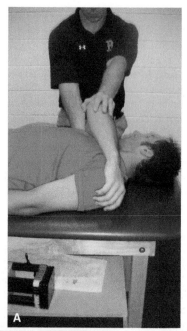

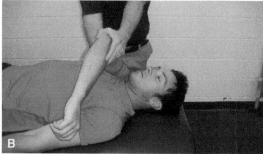

FIGURE 33.3. Cross-body horizontal adduction stretch (A). The clinician may also perform the stretch with the shoulder in internal rotation (B).

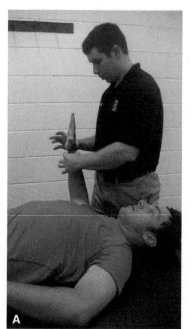

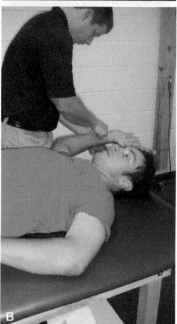

FIGURE 33.4. Rhythmic stabilization drills for internal and external rotation with the arm at 90° abduction and neutral rotation (A) and 90° external rotation (B).

associated with tightness of the pectoralis minor, upper trapezius, and levator scapulae muscles and weakness of the lower trapezius, serratus anterior, and deep neck flexor muscle groups (3,39). Tightness of these muscles can lead to axillary artery occlusion and neurovascular symptoms such as arm fatigue, pain, tenderness, and cyanosis (42–44). Muscle weakness may result in improper mechanics or shoulder symptoms. Stretching, soft tissue mobilization, deep tissue lengthening, muscle energy, and other manual techniques may be needed in these athletes.

Depending on the severity of the injury, strengthening often begins with submaximal, pain-free isometrics for all shoulder and scapular movements. Isometrics should be performed at multiple angles throughout the available ROM, with particular emphasis on contraction at the end of the available ROM.

Manual rhythmic stabilization drills are performed for internal and external rotators with the arm in the scapular plane at 30° abduction (Figure 33.4). Alternating isometric contractions facilitate cocontraction of the anterior and posterior rotator cuff musculature. Rhythmic stabilization drills may also be performed with the patient supine and arm elevated to approximately 90°–100° and 10° horizontal abduction (Figure 33.5). This position is chosen for the

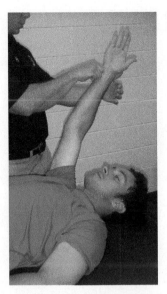

FIGURE 33.5. Rhythmic stabilization drills for flexion and extension with the arm elevated to 100° flexion in the scapular plane.

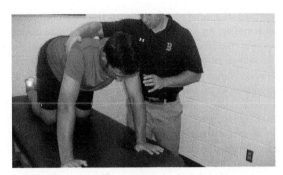

FIGURE 33.6. Rhythmic stabilization drills for the throwing shoulder while weight bearing in the quadruped position.

initiation of these drills due to the combined centralized line of action of both the rotator cuff and deltoid musculature, generating a humeral head compressive force during muscle contraction (45,46). The rehabilitation specialist employs alternating isometric contractions in the flexion, extension, horizontal abduction, and horizontal adduction planes of motion. As the patient progresses, the drills can be performed at variable degrees of elevation such as 45° and 120°.

Active ROM activities are permitted when adequate muscle strength and balance have been achieved. With the athlete's eyes closed, the rehabilitation specialist passively moves the upper extremity in the planes of flexion, ER, and IR, pauses, and then returns the extremity to the starting position. The patient is then instructed to actively reposition the upper extremity to the previous location. The rehabilitation specialist may perform these joint repositioning activities throughout the available ROM.

Also during the acute phase, basic CKC exercises are performed. Exercises are initially performed below shoulder level. The athlete may perform weight shifts on the table in the anterior/posterior and medial/lateral directions. Rhythmic stabilizations may also be performed during weight shifting. As the athlete progresses, a medium-sized ball may be placed on the table and weight shifts may be performed on the ball. Load bearing exercises can be advanced from the table to the quadruped position (Figure 33.6).

Modalities including ice, high-voltage stimulation, iontophoresis, ultrasound, and nonsteroidal anti-inflammatory medications may also be employed as needed to control pain and inflammation. Iontophoresis may be particularly helpful in reducing pain and inflammation during this phase of rehabilitation.

Intermediate Phase

The intermediate phase begins once the athlete has regained near-normal passive motion and sufficient shoulder strength balance. Lower extremity, core, and trunk strength and stability are critical to efficiently perform overhead activities by transferring and dissipating forces in a coordinated fashion. Therefore, full lower extremity strengthening and core stabilization activities are also performed during the intermediate phase. Emphasis will now be placed on regaining proprioception, kinesthesia, and dynamic stabilization throughout the athlete's full ROM, particularly at end range. For the injured athlete midseason, it is common to begin in the intermediate phase, or at least progress to this phase within the first few days following injury. The goals of the intermediate phase are to enhance functional dynamic stability, re-establish neuromuscular control, restore muscular strength and balance, and regain full ROM for overhead activities.

During this phase, the rehabilitation program progresses to aggressive isotonic strengthening activities with emphasis on restoration of muscle balance. Selective muscle activation is also used to restore muscle balance and symmetry. The shoulder external rotator muscles and scapular retractor, protractor, and depressor muscles are isolated through a fundamental exercise program for the overhead thrower (15,47–49). This exercise program is based on the collective information derived from electromyographic research of numerous investigators (15–17,50–54). These patients frequently exhibit ER weakness and benefit from side lying ER and prone rowing into ER. Both exercises elicit high levels of muscular activity in the posterior cuff muscles (17).

Drills performed in the acute phase may be progressed to include stabilization at end ranges of motion with the patient's eyes closed. Rhythmic stabilization exercises are performed during the early part of the intermediate phase. Proprioceptive neuromuscular facilitation (PNF) exercises are performed in the athlete's available ROM and progressed to include full arcs of motion. Rhythmic stabilizations may be incorporated in various degrees of elevation during the PNF patterns to promote dynamic stabilization.

Manual resistance ER is also performed during the intermediate phase. By applying manual resistance during specific exercises, the rehabilitation specialist can vary the amount of resistance throughout the ROM and incorporate concentric and eccentric contractions, as well as rhythmic stabilizations at end range (Figure 33.7). As the athlete regains strength and neuromuscular control, ER and IR with tubing may be performed at 90° abduction.

Scapular strengthening and neuromuscular control are also critical to regaining full dynamic stability of the glenohumeral joint. Isotonic exercises for the scapulothoracic joint are added along with manual resistance prone rowing. Also, neuromuscular control drills and PNF patterns may be applied to the scapula (Figures 33.8 and 33.9).

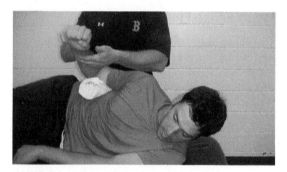

FIGURE 33.7. Manual resistance side lying external rotation with end-range rhythmic stabilizations.

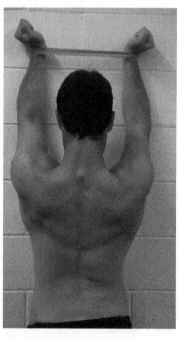

FIGURE 33.8. Arm elevation against a wall with the patient isometrically holding a light resistance band into external rotation to facilitate posterior rotator cuff and scapular stabilization during scapular elevation and posterior tilting.

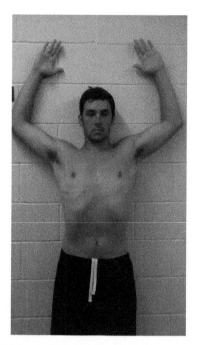

FIGURE 33.9. Arm extension wall slides to facilitate proper scapular retraction and posterior tilting.

CKC exercises are advanced during the intermediate phase. Weight shifting on a ball progresses to a push-up on a ball or unstable surface on a tabletop. Rhythmic stabilizations of the upper extremity, uninvolved shoulder, and trunk are performed with the rehabilitation specialist (Figure 33.10). Wall stabilization drills can be performed with the athlete's hand on a small ball (Figure 33.11). Additional axial compression exercises include table and quadruped using a towel around the hand, slide board, or unstable surface.

Advanced Phase

The third phase of the rehabilitation program prepares the athlete to return to athletic activity. Criteria to enter this phase include minimal pain and tenderness, full ROM, symmetrical capsular mobility, good strength (at least 4/5 on manual muscle testing), upper extremity and scapulothoracic endurance, and sufficient dynamic stabilization.

Full motion and posterior muscle flexibility should be maintained throughout this phase. Exercises such as IR and ER with exercise tubing at 90° abduction progresses to incorporate eccentric and high-speed contractions.

Aggressive strengthening of the upper body may also be initiated depending on the needs of the individual patient. Common exercises include isotonic weight machine bench press, seated row, and latissimus dorsi pull downs within a restricted ROM. During bench press and seated row, the athlete should not extend the arms beyond the plane of the

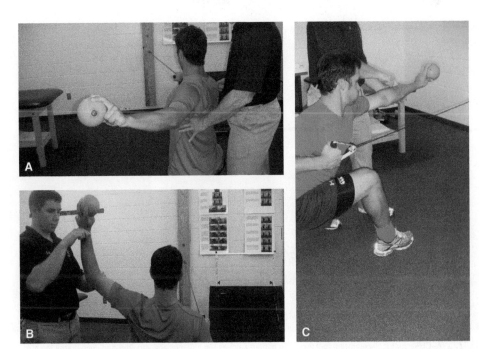

FIGURE 33.10. Transitioning weight-bearing rhythmic stabilization exercises to nonweight-bearing positions simulating the landing (A), arm cocking (B), and ball release (C) phases of the throwing motion.

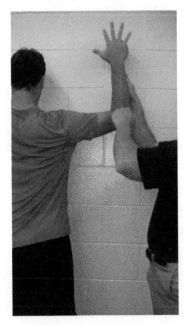

FIGURE 33.11. Rhythmic stabilization drills in the 90° abducted and 90° external rotation position on an unstable surface in the closed kinetic chain position against the wall.

body to minimize stress on the shoulder capsule. Latissimus pull downs are performed in front of the head while the athlete avoids full extension of the arms to minimize traction force on the upper extremities.

Plyometrics for the upper extremity may be initiated during this phase to train the upper extremity to dissipate forces. The chest pass, overhead throw, and alternating side-to-side throw with a medicine ball are initially performed with two hands. Two-hand drills are progressed to one-hand drills over 7–10 days. One-hand plyometrics include baseball-style throws in the 90/90 position with a 2 lb ball, deceleration flips (Figure 33.12), and stationary and semi-circle wall dribbles. Wall dribbles progress to the 90/90 position. They are beneficial for upper extremity endurance while overhead.

Dynamic stabilization and neuromuscular control drills should be reactive, functional, and in sport-specific positions. Concentric and eccentric manual resistance may be applied as the athlete performs ER with exercise tubing with the arm at 0° abduction. Rhythmic stabilizations may be included at end range to challenge the athlete to stabilize against the force of the tubing as well as the therapist and progressed to the 90/90 position (Figure 33.13). Rhythmic stabilizations may be applied at end range during the 90/90 wall dribble exercise. These drills are designed to impart a sudden perturbation to the involved shoulder near end range to develop the athlete's ability to dynamically stabilize the shoulder.

Muscle endurance exercises should be emphasized because the overhead athlete is at greater risk for shoulder and/or elbow injuries when pitching fatigued (55). Endurance drills include wall dribbling, ball flips (Figure 33.14), wall arm circles, upper body cycle, or isotonic exercises

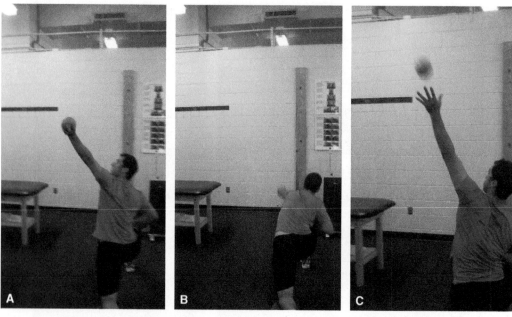

FIGURE 33.12. (A–C) Plyometric deceleration ball flips. The patient catches the ball over the shoulder and decelerates the arm, similar to the throwing motion, before flipping back and returning to the starting position.

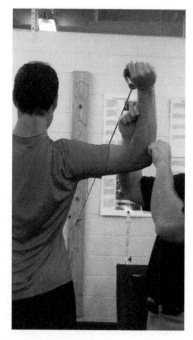

FIGURE 33.13. Rhythmic stabilization drills during exercise tubing at 90° abduction and 90° external rotation and during wall dribbles.

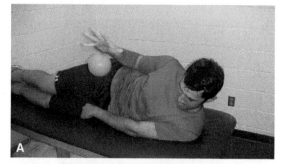

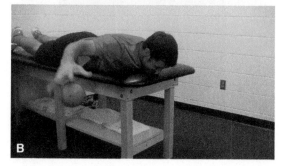

FIGURE 33.14. Ball flips for endurance of the external rotators (A) and scapular retractors (B).

using lower weights for higher repetitions. Murray et al. (56) have demonstrated the effects of fatigue on the entire body during pitching using kinematic and kinetic motion analysis. Muscle fatigue affects proprioception (57) and thus the ability to control the humeral head's position in the glenoid during the overhead throwing motion.

Once the rotator cuff muscles are fatigued, the humeral head migrates superiorly when arm elevation is initiated (58). The predisposing factor that correlated best with shoulder injuries in Little League pitchers was muscle fatigue (55), further providing evidence that endurance drills appear critical for the overhead athlete.

Return to Activity Phase

Upon completion of the rehabilitation program including minimal pain or tenderness, full ROM, balanced capsular mobility, adequate proprioception, and dynamic stabilization, the athlete may begin the return to activity phase.

The ISP is supplemented with a high-repetition, low-resistance maintenance exercise program for the rotator cuff and scapula. All strengthening, plyometric, and neuromuscular control drills should be performed three times per week (with a day off in between) on the same day as the ISP. The athlete should warm-up, stretch, and perform one set of each exercise before the ISP, followed by two sets of each exercise after the ISP. This provides an adequate warm-up but also ensures maintenance of necessary ROM and flexibility of the upper extremity.

Alternating days are used for lower extremity, cardiovascular, core stability training, ROM, and light strengthening exercises emphasizing the posterior rotator cuff and scapular muscles. The cycle is repeated throughout the week with the seventh day designated for rest, light ROM, and stretching exercises.

CONCLUSIONS

The overhead athlete can present with several different pathologies due to forces acting during overhead sport activities. The unique physical demands of each sport can cause injuries that can range in both severity and frequency. A thorough and athlete-specific off-season program should be implemented to prepare the athlete for the physical demands of the season that follows. The in-season maintenance program is just as crucial to minimize fatigue and increase the athlete's ability to recover. If an injury does occur then rehabilitation should follow a gradual and sequential progression. This progression should take into account the severity of the injury and the physical demands that are unique to that athlete's sport. Both injury prevention and rehabilitation programs should emphasize ROM, flexibility, rotator cuff and scapular strength, posture, and dynamic stabilization.

REFERENCES

1. Fleisig GS, Andrews JR, Dillman CJ, Escamilla RF. Kinetics of baseball pitching with implications about injury mechanisms. Am J Sports Med 1995;23(2):233–239.
2. Fleisig GS, Barrentine SW, Escamilla RF, Andrews JR. Biomechanics of overhand throwing with implications for injuries. Sports Med 1996;21(6):421–437.
3. Reinold MM, Gill TJ. Current concepts in the evaluation and treatment of the shoulder in overhead throwing athletes: part 1: physical characteristics and clinical examination. Sports Health. 2010;2(1):30–50.
4. Reinold MM, Wilk KE, Macrina LC, et al. Changes in shoulder and elbow passive range of motion after pitching in professional baseball players. Am J Sports Med 2008;36(3):523–527.
5. Wilk KE, Meister K, Andrews JR. Current concepts in the rehabilitation of the overhead throwing athlete. Am J Sports Med 2002;30(1):136–151.
6. Ruotolo C, Price E, Panchal A. Loss of total arc of motion in collegiate baseball players. J Shoulder Elbow Surg 2006;15(1):67–71.
7. Myers JB, Laudner KG, Pasquale MR, Bradley JP, Lephart SM. Glenohumeral range of motion deficits and posterior shoulder tightness in throwers with pathologic internal impingement. Am J Sports Med 2006;34(3):385–391.
8. Barrentine SW, Fleisig GS, Whiteside JA, Escamilla RF, Andrews JR. Biomechanics of windmill softball pitching with implications about injury mechanisms at the shoulder and elbow. J Orthop Sports Phys Ther 1998;28(6):405–415.
9. Ellenbecker TS, Roetert EP, Bailie DS, Davies GJ, Brown SW. Glenohumeral joint total rotation range of motion in elite tennis players and baseball pitchers. Med Sci Sports Exerc 2002;34(12):2052–2056.
10. Jansson A, Saartok T, Werner S, Renstrom P. Evaluation of general joint laxity, shoulder laxity and mobility in competitive swimmers during growth and in normal controls. Scand J Med Sci Sports 2005;15(3):169–176.
11. Schmidt-Wiethoff R, Rapp W, Mauch F, Schneider T, Appell HJ. Shoulder rotation characteristics in professional tennis players. Int J Sports Med 2004;25(2):154–158.
12. Thomas SJ, Swanik KA, Swanik C, Huxel KC. Glenohumeral rotation and scapular position adaptations after a single high school female sports season. J Athl Train 2009;44(3):230–237.
13. Thomas SJ, Swanik KA, Swanik CB, Kelly JD. Internal rotation and scapular position differences: a comparison of collegiate and high school baseball players. J Athl Train 2010;45(1):44–50.
14. Torres RR, Gomes JL. Measurement of glenohumeral internal rotation in asymptomatic tennis players and swimmers. Am J Sports Med 2009;37(5):1017–1023.
15. Reinold MM, Escamilla RF, Wilk KE. Current concepts in the scientific and clinical rationale behind exercises for glenohumeral and scapulothoracic musculature. J Orthop Sports Phys Ther 2009;39(2):105–117.
16. Reinold MM, Macrina LC, Wilk KE, et al. Electromyographic analysis of the supraspinatus and deltoid muscles during 3 common rehabilitation exercises. J Athl Train 2007;42(4):464–469.
17. Reinold MM, Wilk KE, Fleisig GS, et al. Electromyographic analysis of the rotator cuff and deltoid musculature during common shoulder external rotation exercises. J Orthop Sports Phys Ther 2004;34(7):385–394.
18. Davies GJ, Dickoff-Hoffman S. Neuromuscular testing and rehabilitation of the shoulder complex. J Orthop Sports Phys Ther 1993;18(2):449–458.
19. Ellenbecker TS. Rehabilitation of shoulder and elbow injuries in tennis players. Clin Sports Med 1995;14(1):87–110.
20. Reinold MM, Wilk KE, Dugas JR, Andrews JR. Internal impingement. In: Wilk KE, Reinold MM, Andrews JR, eds. The Athletes Shoulder. 2nd ed. Philadelphia, PA: Churchill Livingston Elsevier; 2009:123–142.
21. Wilk KE, Voight ML, Keirns MA, Gambetta V, Andrews JR, Dillman CJ. Stretch-shortening drills for the upper extremities: theory and clinical application. J Orthop Sports Phys Ther 1993;17(5):225–239.

22. Prokopy MP, Ingersoll CD, Nordenschild E, Katch FI, Gaesser GA, Weltman A. Closed-kinetic chain upper-body training improves throwing performance of NCAA Division I softball players. J Strength Cond Res 2008;22(6):1790–1798.

23. Heiderscheit BC, McLean KP, Davies GJ. The effects of isokinetic vs. plyometric training on the shoulder internal rotators. J Orthop Sports Phys Ther 1996;23(2):125–133.

24. Schulte-Edelmann JA, Davies GJ, Kernozek TW, Gerberding ED. The effects of plyometric training of the posterior shoulder and elbow. J Strength Cond Res 2005;19(1):129–134.

25. Matveyev LP. Perodisienang Das Sportlichen Training. Berlin: Beles and Wernitz; 1972.

26. Burkhart SS, Morgan CD, Kibler WB. The disabled throwing shoulder: spectrum of pathology Part I: pathoanatomy and biomechanics. Arthroscopy 2003;19(4):404–420.

27. Dillman CJ, Fleisig GS, Andrews JR. Biomechanics of pitching with emphasis upon shoulder kinematics. J Orthop Sports Phys Ther 1993;18(2):402–408.

28. Escamilla RF, Andrews JR. Shoulder muscle recruitment patterns and related biomechanics during upper extremity sports. Sports Med 2009;39(7):569–590.

29. Lintner D, Noonan TJ, Kibler WB. Injury patterns and biomechanics of the athlete's shoulder. Clin Sports Med 2008;27(4):527–551.

30. Meister K. Injuries to the shoulder in the throwing athlete. Part one: biomechanics/pathophysiology/classification of injury. Am J Sports Med 2000;28(2):265–275.

31. Park SS, Loebenberg ML, Rokito AS, Zuckerman JD. The shoulder in baseball pitching: biomechanics and related injuries—part 1. Bull Hosp Jt Dis 2002;61(1-2):68–79.

32. Park SS, Loebenberg ML, Rokito AS, Zuckerman JD. The shoulder in baseball pitching: biomechanics and related injuries—part 2. Bull Hosp Jt Dis 2002;61(1-2):80–88.

33. Perry J. Anatomy and biomechanics of the shoulder in throwing, swimming, gymnastics, and tennis. Clin Sports Med 1983;2(2):247–270.

34. Richardson AR. The biomechanics of swimming: the shoulder and knee. Clin Sports Med 1986;5(1):103–113.

35. Sabick MB, Kim YK, Torry MR, Keirns MA, Hawkins RJ. Biomechanics of the shoulder in youth baseball pitchers: implications for the development of proximal humeral epiphysiolysis and humeral retrotorsion. Am J Sports Med 2005;33(11):1716–1722.

36. Salter RB, Bell RS, Keeley FW. The protective effect of continuous passive motion in living articular cartilage in acute septic arthritis: an experimental investigation in the rabbit. Clin Orthop Relat Res 1981;159:223–247.

37. Salter RB, Hamilton HW, Wedge JH, et al. Clinical application of basic research on continuous passive motion for disorders and injuries of synovial joints: a preliminary report of a feasibility study. J Orthop Res 1984;1(3):325–342.

38. Salter RB, Simmonds DF, Malcolm BW, Rumble EJ, MacMichael D, Clements ND. The biological effect of continuous passive motion on the healing of full-thickness defects in articular cartilage. An experimental investigation in the rabbit. J Bone Joint Surg Am 1980;62(8):1232–1251.

39. Thigpen CA, Reinold MM, Padua DA, Schneider RS, Distefano LJ, Gill TJ. 3-D scapular position and muscle strength are related in professional baseball pitchers. J Athl Train 2008;43(2):S49.

40. Borich MR, Bright JM, Lorello DJ, Cieminski CJ, Buisman T, Ludewig PM. Scapular angular positioning at end range internal rotation in cases of glenohumeral internal rotation deficit. J Orthop Sports Phys Ther 2006;36(12):926–934.

41. Lukasiewicz AC, McClure P, Michener L, Pratt N, Sennett B. Comparison of 3-dimensional scapular position and orientation between subjects with and without shoulder impingement. J Orthop Sports Phys Ther 1999;29(10):574–583; discussion 584–586.

42. Nuber GW, McCarthy WJ, Yao JS, Schafer MF, Suker JR. Arterial abnormalities of the shoulder in athletes. Am J Sports Med 1990;18(5):514–519.

43. Rohrer MJ, Cardullo PA, Pappas AM, Phillips DA, Wheeler HB. Axillary artery compression and thrombosis in throwing athletes. J Vasc Surg 1990;11(6):761–768; discussion 768–769.

44. Sotta RP. Vascular problems in the proximal upper extremity. Clin Sports Med 1990;9(2):379–388.

45. Poppen NK, Walker PS. Forces at the glenohumeral joint in abduction. Clin Orthop Relat Res 1978(135):165–170.

46. Walker PS, Poppen NK. Biomechanics of the shoulder joint during abduction in the plane of the scapula [proceedings]. Bull Hosp Joint Dis 1977;38(2):107–111.

47. Wilk KE, Reinold MM, Andrews JR. Rehabilitation of the thrower's elbow. Clin Sports Med 2004;23(4):765–801, xii.

48. Wilk KE, Reinold MM, Dugas JR, Andrews JR. Rehabilitation following thermal-assisted capsular shrinkage of the glenohumeral joint: current concepts. J Orthop Sports Phys Ther 2002;32(6):268–292.

49. Wilk KE, Reinold MM, Dugas JR, Arrigo CA, Moser MW, Andrews JR. Current concepts in the recognition and treatment of superior labral (SLAP) lesions. J Orthop Sports Phys Ther 2005;35(5):273–291.

50. Blackburn TA, McLeod WD, White B. Electromyographic analysis of posterior rotator cuff exercises. J Athl Train 1990;25:40–45.

51. Decker MJ, Hintermeister RA, Faber KJ, Hawkins RJ. Serratus anterior muscle activity during selected rehabilitation exercises. Am J Sports Med 1999;27(6):784–791.

52. Moseley JB Jr, Jobe FW, Pink M, Perry J, Tibone J. EMG analysis of the scapular muscles during a shoulder rehabilitation program. Am J Sports Med 1992;20(2):128–134.

53. Townsend H, Jobe FW, Pink M, Perry J. Electromyographic analysis of the glenohumeral muscles during a baseball rehabilitation program. Am J Sports Med 1991;19(3):264–272.

54. Worrell TW, Corey BJ, York SL, Santiesteban J. An analysis of supraspinatus EMG activity and shoulder isometric force development. Med Sci Sports Exerc 1992;24(7):744–748.

55. Lyman S, Fleisig GS, Andrews JR, Osinski ED. Effect of pitch type, pitch count, and pitching mechanics on risk of elbow and shoulder pain in youth baseball pitchers. Am J Sports Med 2002;30(4):463–468.

56. Murray TA, Cook TD, Werner SL, Schlegel TF, Hawkins RJ. The effects of extended play on professional baseball pitchers. Am J Sports Med 2001;29(2):137–142.

57. Voight ML, Hardin JA, Blackburn TA, Tippett S, Canner GC. The effects of muscle fatigue on and the relationship of arm dominance to shoulder proprioception. J Orthop Sports Phys Ther 1996;23(6):348–352.

58. Chen SK, Wickiewicz TL, Otis JC. Glenohumeral kinematics in a muscle fatigue model. Orthop Trans 1995;18:1126.

Principles of Athletic Development

INTRODUCTION

Training is part of a continuum involving preparation, recovery, tapering, and competition. By enhancing overall strength and conditioning (S&C), athleticism, and sport-specific skill, any individual, especially the athlete, is in the best possible position to succeed. There are three overarching tenets that encapsulate the process necessary for maximizing one's physiological potential: first, progressive, **longitudinal training through the life span;** second, an **annual training program (i.e., periodization);** and third, **movement efficiency**. Naturally, when injury or recurrent pain rears its ugly head, diagnosis, therapy, rehabilitation, and return to sport (or activity) take precedence.

The principles described in this chapter are equally applicable to a sedentary individual, elite athlete, or injured person. Everyone is truly an athlete. Typical examples include:

- a grandmother with lower back pain wanting to lift her grandchildren
- a postal worker needing to carry heavy loads
- a weekend warrior who is a stock broker all week and plays golf on weekends
- a pain-free 13-year-old girl with poor single-leg stability playing soccer
- a professional athlete

By saying that everyone is an athlete what is meant is that everyone needs integrity (i.e., competency and capacity) of their musculoskeletal system. If there is a "stability shortfall" then overload will occur most likely at the "worst possible time." All of this occurs on a continuum so that the necessary capacity required for a sedentary person is clearly less than for an elite athlete. These universal principles will apply to health care, fitness, and S&C professionals.

Longitudinal training begins in childhood with the training of fundamental movement literacies consistent with their developmental stage. It then progresses to include general strength and finally power as an athlete approaches his or her peak performance capability. As one ages lower-load activities are utilized to maintain function throughout the life span (e.g., balance training).

Periodization consists of a variable training program to facilitate an athlete's ability to peak at key performance opportunities. It includes macro, micro, and daily program blocks or sessions designed to promote recovery, adaptation, and a residual training effect. High-intensity training (HIT) and low-intensity training are varied in a methodical way (polarized, undulating, etc.) to build an athlete up without breaking them down.

Movement efficiency is an essential underlying tenet of athletic development. It assures that skill acquisition, movement competencies, and physical capacities can be transferred into both the physical and psychological challenges (intrinsic motivation and cognitive resiliency) of one's activities, sport, or competition (see Chapter 35).

All three tenets incorporate the essential methods of training: general physical preparation (GPP) and special (or specialized or specific) physical preparation (SPP). GPP provides a foundation in a wide variety of physical traits and takes years to establish. SPP involves higher intensity more sport-specific training that is erected on the GPP base. In the context of longitudinal development SPP follows GPP. Within an annual periodized training cycle GPP and SPP alternate consecutively based on physiologic sport goals (power, intermittent, endurance), recovery needs (i.e., age of athlete), and the timing of peak performances (e.g., short vs. long season, once/week or more).

> "The intent of training is to increase the athlete's skills and work capacity to optimize athletic performance… Training is a process by which an athlete is prepared for the highest level of performance possible." Bompa and Haff (1)

With so many methods available to trainers and athletes the nightmare of choice can be overwhelming when deciding the best path to follow. Thus, a key question is who should drive a training program, the methods of the trainer, or the goals of the athlete?

> "Don't be a slave of methods, the methods should serve the goals." Lewit (2)

For instance, Olympic weightlifting, aerobic training, plyometrics, functional training, kettle bell training, and corrective exercise have their place, but a trainer who is biased toward one may fail to customize his/her training strategy to the physiological needs or goals of the athlete. In an **athlete-centered approach** it is crucial to customize programming based on each individual's *goals, sport, history, age, sex, preparedness, competencies,* and/or *capacities*. In addition, a trainer or coach who is determined to teach certain skills part by part, or in a rote manner, may succeed in having an athlete who develops well in practice. However, transfer to performance may be inefficient (see Chapter 35).

The goal of this chapter is to summarize the principles of athletic development within the context of rehabilitation and S&C. Knowing this should enhance communication and foster integration between clinicians, trainers, and coaches. Chapter 3 describes this athlete-centered model where a different professional becomes the team's quarterback depending where on the performance continuum the athlete is (see Figure 3.1). This chapter will not provide a detailed overview of training methodologies or program design. What it aims to do is summarize the current "expert" practices of leading trainers and place them within a context of the descriptive history of how they evolved alongside retrospective and prospective studies emerging from the sports science field. Just as on a professional or high-level collegiate sports team a group of professionals work together to enhance the success of the organization, this chapter seeks to illuminate the overlapping space between clinicians, trainers, coaches, and sports scientists that exists. Coordination, integration, and division of labor are essential components necessary to create an ideal ecological dynamic to enhance performance in an athlete or team (3,4).

> Gambetta prefers the term *athletic development* rather than S&C because it clearly denotes an integrated system for athletic development and sends a clear message that what is being developed is the complete athlete, not one component. "All components of physical performance: strength, power, speed, agility, endurance and flexibility must be developed in a systematic, sequential, and progressive manner to prepare the athlete. Athletic development coaches enhance athletic performance by developing athletes that are completely adaptable and prepared to handle the psychological, physical, technical and tactical demands required to compete." Gambetta. (5)

LONGITUDINAL TRAINING OVER A LIFE SPAN

The provenance of an athlete's training program, regardless of age, is dependent on matching the training program's emphasis with the competencies, capacities, and goals of the individual. In children or developing athletes, a foundation in fundamental movement skills (FMS) such as the basic ABCs of movement literacy—agility, balance, and coordination—is an essential starting point. Above all this should be in the context of play, not competition, so that a problem-solving attitude is inculcated. This will help shape a young person's attitude toward activity, thus providing an essential foundation for the journey toward athleticism (6).

A lack of movement in general and movement variety in particular is devastating to physical development (7). Children who are sedentary three-fourths of the time have up to nine times poorer motor coordination than their more active peers (8). Additionally, one's level of FMS may be predictive of activity level and be related to academic achievement (9–11). Lack of movement in childhood is also correlated with childhood diabetes, obesity, long-term health problems, and even shorter life span (12–14).

Sedentarism, activity, fitness, and athleticism represent a broad spectrum of the movement landscape. The seeds of sedentarism are planted in early childhood due to such societal neglect as reduction in physical education requirements and budget in public schools (7,12). Activity levels further suffer from increased "screen time" as we see children sitting, watching television or playing video games more and more (12). Activity in general is an important hedge against various diseases, low academic achievement, and even depression. It also provides a platform for preventing musculoskeletal ailments, and maximizing one's human potential in future athletic endeavors.

> **The Broader Context of the Role of Physical Activity and Well-Being**
>
> "Physical activity is not about sport and it is about more than just exercise. It is about the relationship between human beings and their environment, and about improving human well-being by strengthening that relationship. It is not about running on a treadmill, whilst staring at a mirror and listening to your iPod. It is about using the body that we have in the way it was designed, which is to walk often, run sometimes, and move in ways where we physically exert ourselves regularly whether that is at work, at home, in transport to and from places, or during leisure time in our daily lives." Das and Horton (15)

Developmental Windows or Sensitive Periods

It is important to have a plan for training the developing athlete from a very young age that will progress them appropriately as they age (16). Piaget (17) identified four distinct stages of development in children. The sensorimotor phase (birth to 2 years), the preoperational thought phase (2 to 7 years), the concrete operations phase (7 to 11 years), and the formal operations phase (beginning at 11 years). At the preoperational phase learning occurs via physical exploration rather than a cognitive approach. Cognitive perception begins to develop in the formal operations stage but it is more of a stimulus–response style. Once the formal operations phase is reached, a more systematic problem-solving approach begins to take hold.

Developmental Kinesiology

"Postural muscle activity is genetically pre-determined and occurs automatically in the course of CNS maturation.... The quality of verticalization during the first year of life strongly influences the quality of body posture for the rest of a person's life" (Kolár P, Kobesova A, & Valouchova P; see Chapter 4).

The stage from 2 to 7 years has been called the fundamental movement phase by Gallahue (18). In this stage the child explores, "a variety of stabilizing, locomotor and manipulative movements...." This is then followed by the specialized movement phase from 7 to 11 years where FMS are honed and progressed to incorporate more complex skills.

A few commonly agreed upon developmental landmarks according to McMorris and Hale (19) are as follows:

- By 6 years of age, normal children are capable of jumping, catching, skipping, throwing, and balancing
- At 6 years, a child can strike a stationary object but has difficulty with a moving object due to immature eye–hand and foot–eye coordination
- Boys perform better than girls at most skills, except balance
- Girls are more flexible than boys
- Perceptual skills such as visual acuity and depth perception reach maturity around the age of 12 years
- Physical development in 11- to 13-year-olds varies greatly
- Children reach adolescence at different ages[1]

Sensitive periods are best defined as "windows of opportunity and vulnerability in the skill acquisition process" (20). In Chinese and Korean immigrants whose first exposure to English occurred between the ages of 3 and 39 years of age, it was shown that the ages between 3 and 7 were the most sensitive (21), so much so that their English speaking fluency was indistinguishable from native English speakers. Similarly, proficiency in high levels of fine motor skill necessary for music is best achieved if trained by age 7 (22,23). For swimming the optimal or most efficient age to begin learning has been shown to be 5.5 years (24).

Simonton (25) reported that the greatest composers who started music lessons at a younger age took less time to hone their skills. In other words, the training was more efficient. The above insights should be tempered by research showing sensitive periods are not brief, sharply defined, or irreversible (20,26).

Some confusion in the literature exists, because the terms critical period and sensitive period are both used. Critical periods should narrowly be applied to developmental changes that occur in the neural circuitry underlying behavior and are more fixed (26,27). Sensitive periods refer to temporal phases where environmental input can have a potent effect on habitual behaviors (20,26,27).

The question of when to train specific motor skills is a "holy grail" in the early training of youth athletes. However, according to Anderson et al. (20) "our understanding of when children are best prepared to profit from specific experiences and how to create that preparation is poor." Nonetheless, the authors state, "motor skill learning must ultimately be considered within a developmental context if it is to be fully understood."

Long-Term Athletic Development

A knowledgeable coach will recognize when "optimal periods of learning" arise (28). This enables the coach to tailor skill acquisition goals to match the stage of development of the child. To guide this process, the long-term athletic development (LTAD) paradigm as elucidated by Balyi (29) was developed (Table 34.1; Figure 34.1; see Chapters 7 and 13). Bayli and Hamilton say, "If the fundamental and basic sport-specific skills are not established before ages 11 and 12 respectively, athletes will never reach their optimal or genetic potential" (32).

One of the limitations of Balyi's work is that longitudinal training, which considers sensitive periods, lacks evidence of effectiveness (33,34). Another weakness is that it is presented as a generic model.

Deliberate Practice and Early Specialization

In 1993, Ericsson (35) proposed that expert performance was related more to deliberate practice than to innate ability or talent. Also, the relationship between time spent in deliberate practice and performance is one that is linear. It was suggested that, based on observations from music and chess, approximately 10,000 hours of such practice was necessary in order to achieve "expert" status in a given activity.

Today, it is becoming more common for young athletes to specialize in selected sports at earlier ages. Early specialization involves year-round training in a single

---

[1]The Australian and New Zealand Rugby Union recognizes this and thus bases competition on height and weight rather than age.

TABLE 34.1 Long-Term Athletic Development Stages

1) Active Start (for developmental ages 0–6/boys and 0–4/girls)
- Movement skill development

2) FUNdamentals (for developmental ages 6–9/boys and 4–7/girls)
- ABCs of athleticism—agility, balance, coordination

3) Learn to Play (or Train) (for developmental ages 9–12/boys and 7–9/girls)
- Play a variety of sports, learn sport-specific skills

4) Train to Play (or Train) (for developmental ages 12–16/boys and 9–14/girls)
- GPP

5) Learn to Compete (for developmental ages 16–18/boys and 14–16/girls)
- Importance of fundamental skills and readiness
- Physical, mental, cognitive, and emotional development

6) Train to Compete (for developmental ages 18–22/boys and 16–21/girls)
- Transition from general physical preparation to special physical preparation

7) Train to Excel (or Win) (for developmental ages 22–29/boys and 21–28/girls)
- Special physical preparation and readiness

8) Active for Life (for developmental ages +23)
- Importance of recovery

Modified from Balyi's original eight phases of development. Adapted from Higgs C, Balyi I, Way R. Developing Physical Literacy: A Guide for Parents of Children Ages 0 to 12: A supplement to Canadian Sport for Life. Vancouver, BC: Canadian Sport Centres; 2008 and Way R, Balyi I, Grove J. Canadian Sport for Life: A Sport Parent's Guide. Ottawa, ON: Canadian Sport Centres; 2007 (30,31).

sport between the ages of 6 and 12. In certain sports where peak performance is achieved prior to biological maturation (female gymnastics, female figure skating), this approach is often deemed necessary, on the presumption of the necessity of high quantity of deliberate

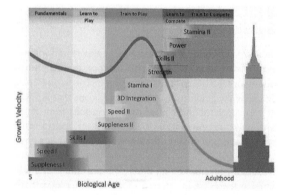

FIGURE 34-1. Junior athlete development model. Long-term athlete development. Modified from Balyi I. Phases of long-term athlete development [www.ltad.ca].

practice approaching 10,000 hours (36–39). Recently, a trend toward adopting an early specialization approach to other sports has taken hold. The question arises—will such early ripening fruits be more or less likely to have successful long-term careers?

Although the relationship between practice and performance is one of the most robust relationships in behavioral science (40), wide criticism has arisen regarding Ericsson et al.'s suggestions. Even with many studies revealing that elite performers trained more frequently than near-elite performers, the elite performer often failed to accumulate the magic number of 10,000 practice hours (41). Ultimately, there is no consensus that either early onset or early specialization is required for the development of expertise (42–44). For example, the results of Vaeyens et al. (45) reveal that there is no evidence that an early onset and a higher amount of sport-specific training are associated with greater success at a later stage.

Negative Effects of Early Specialization

A retrospective Swedish study showed that early specialization in tennis players led to burn-out and lower self-confidence with increasing age (42). The best players specialized later and practiced less than their near-elite peers between the ages of 13 and 15 but intensified their training considerably after age 15. Likewise, Lidor and Lavyan (44) found that elite athletes from different sports began specializing later than near-elite athletes. Nevertheless, the elite athletes had completed more training hours when they reached their peak performance, indicating that despite their late start, they managed to compile enough hours to perform at the top level. Barynina and Vaitsekhovskii (43) found that swimmers who specialized early spent less time on the national team and ended their sporting career earlier than athletes who specialized later.

Early specialization may lead to negative consequences for athletes, such as psychological risks (46), sense of failure (47), attrition, and negative health outcomes (48). Gould et al. (49) reported that early specialization and highly structured training reduced **intrinsic motivation** as well as led to higher dropout and burn-out among young athletes. Well-known physical consequences such as overuse have also been reported (50,51). Law et al. (52) found that Olympic-level rhythmic gymnasts who had participated in significantly more training hours in their career rated their health as lower and their participation experiences as less fun than their peers at the international level.

Further psychosocial concerns linked to early specialization include compromised social development, sport dropout, burn-out, and eating disorders (53). These concerns are even more telling when the vital need to encourage lifelong physical activity participation as well as elite performance is considered.

The social desire for early elite performance from parents, coaches, and sports organizations is being driven by ego, hunger for college scholarships, and the commercialization of youth sport (54,55). Many parents are trying to live their own unfulfilled sports fantasies through their children (51). On moral grounds alone, it can be questioned if it is logical to have children engage in serious sports training and performance when the vast majority are destined to failure (56). Early specialization often leads to dropout, which can prevent adherence to physical activity later in life (57,58).

Competition and failure are not a priori harmful experiences for children; in fact, they are essential components of the crucible of sport through which character (i.e., teamwork, sacrifice, etc.) can be built thanks to the sports experience (59). The real issue arises when adult-based concepts and values predominate leading to the eventual linking of failure to achieve with exclusion from participation (58).

The Limitations of the Long-Term Athletic Development Model

Ford states that the LTAD model is primarily a physiological view that presents an advancement of understanding of developing athletic potential together with biological growth. The model focuses on training to optimize performance longitudinally and views sensitive developmental periods known as "windows of opportunity." However, it appears that there are a number of problems with this theoretical model that are not necessarily transparent to coaches.

* the model is one-dimensional
* there is a lack of empirical evidence
* the data on which it is based rely on questionable assumptions and flawed methodologies

"Fundamentally, this is a generic model rather than an individualized plan for athletes." Ford et al. (60)

Role of Hereditary Factors

It is a long-standing argument in behavioral psychology whether nurture or nature is more significant. Ericsson et al. (35) rejected the view that innate ability is the decisive factor in whether or not a person becomes an expert. More recently Ericsson et al. (61) reiterated this contention, "individual differences in genetically determined capacities and fixed structures required for the development of elite performance appear to be quite limited, perhaps even restricted, to a small number of physical characteristics, such as height and body size." Epstein (62) in *The Sports Gene* argues in favor of genetic factors playing a significant role in expert sports performance. From long arms (relative to height) in basketball, to genetic traits of sickle-cell anemia in sprinters, to long Achilles tendons in jumpers, Epstein explains that biophysical variations exist across certain populations that may contribute to success in specific sports. He also

explains that although 10,000 is generally the average, some experts have achieved such status after 20,000+ hours of deliberate practice while others have done so with only 3,000 hours. Thus, it seems safe to conclude that while 10,000 hours may not be necessary, it may also in fact be misleading.

Marcus (63) said, "it would be a logical error to infer from the importance of practice that talent is somehow irrelevant, as if the two were in mutual opposition." Consensus is emerging that the popular, meritocratic views about deliberate practice being the decisive element in successful skill development (64,65) are simply inconsistent with the evidence (66,67). Hambrick (68) states, "deliberate practice is necessary but not sufficient to account for individual differences in performance. There is widespread skepticism, then, over Ericsson and colleagues' strong claims regarding the importance of deliberate practice for acquiring expert performance."

Late Specialization/Early Diversification

The optimal career path is not only a question of amount of training hours but also a question of when training regimes occur (69). The more recent adage "perfect practice makes perfect" (70) might need to be changed to "perfect training at the right time makes perfect." Long practice is needed. But, most likely, not early specialization in late specialization sports, which frequently leads to burn-out and overuse injuries. In fact, early specialization and a low training-to-competition ratio are correlated with an increased risk of specific injuries such as stress fractures and growth plate injuries (71).

Russian sources (72) concluded:

* Training ideally begins at age 7–8
* Initial participation is in multiple sports
* At age 10–13 participation is in various team sports
* At age 15–17 specialization begins
* Peak achieved within 5–8 years of specialization
* Early specialization athletes peak <18 years
* Late specialization athletes peak >18 years
* Only a minority of athletes who specialized early improved performance after 18 years
* Many elite performers were never junior champions or held national records

Individuals pass through three developmental phases with a progressive narrowing of sport focus during these stages (48):
1. the sampling years (6–12 years of age)
2. the specializing years (13–15 years of age)
3. the investing years (≥16 years of age

Sampling is proposed to build FMS. This provides a foundation for future movement prowess (36):

* Locomotor skills (running, jumping, etc.)
* Object control skills (throwing, catching, striking, etc.)

Participating in a variety of sports at a young age helps develop FMS and the mental advantage that comes from learning different strategies (73). Preadolescence is the optimal window to develop FMS (74–76). Ideally, this should occur in the "developmental window" prior to the period of "peak height velocity" (77) (see Chapters 7 and 13). By age 7, differences in body size due to a bifurcation in biological versus chronological age becomes apparent (78). Therefore, children who grow at a younger age should have this coordination-based training initiated earlier.

Diversifying activities in the youth has been shown to contribute to the development of FMS (79,80). These basic skills then continue to flourish from childhood to adolescence to the teenage years (81,82). FMS are thus an essential prerequisite—the building blocks—for participation in more specialized activities and sports later (80,83).

> **Movement Literacy: A Bridge between Athletic Development and Rehabilitation**
>
> "Ironically, as enhanced movement literacy becomes the goal of athletic development, training not only becomes more functional but also begins to overlap with clinical rehabilitation." Liebenson (see Chapter 1)

In the preadolescent group, training should be neither too easy nor too hard. The play aspect of early diversification should be emphasized above competition. The goal should be to have enough competition to keep children engaged and motivated, but no more (84,85).

Baker et al. (36) state that a transfer of learning occurs from one sport to another, including both cognitive and physical abilities. Current research further suggests that the effect of such a transfer is most pronounced during early stages of involvement (86), corresponding with the time frame of the sampling years.

In order to become a highly motivated, self-determined, and committed adult athlete, it is crucial to build a solid foundation of **intrinsic motivation** at early stages (87). It is hypothesized that early diversification promotes the development of intrinsic motivation (48), which in turn serves as the basis for a **self-regulated** involvement in elite sport at a later stage (38).

A crucial trait present in committed high-level performers is "grit." Paradoxically, "grit" may develop from early play and late specialization. Duckworth et al. (88) found that grit positively predicted deliberate practice and ultimately performance in spelling bee competitors. In a related study it was shown in classical musicians that "passion" was related to deliberate practice and performance (89). Further, Winner coined the phrase "rage to master," describing it as the intrinsic motivation possessed by children to obsessively master areas of interest through intense focus and voracious consumption of

new information and skills (90). Such personality factors should be considered part of the performance puzzle, but can't be said to independently predict performance (68).

> **Grit**
>
> "a personality factor reflecting persistence in accomplishing long-term goals." Hambrick et al. (68)

Howe (91) reviewed biographical details of geniuses such as Darwin, Einstein, and others and concluded, "Perseverance is at least as crucial as intelligence .... The most crucial inherent differences may be ones of temperament rather than of intellect as such." Duckworth et al. (92) described grit as encompassing both persistence and passion in the pursuit of goals in spite of adversity and challenges.

> **Early Specialization versus Early Diversification**
>
> "There is an increased likelihood of achieving a higher standard of competition when individuals participate in three competitive sports during the specializing years .... This has important implications .... for the development of young athletes who at 18 years of age may have the potential to excel in their sporting careers. The data indicate that early specialization is not necessary for performance at 18 ...." Bridge and Toms (93)

Staged Model for Motor Learning

It is hypothesized that if a young athlete follows a general progression of early diversification and sampling and later sport specialization, they will have a greater chance to succeed in high-level sports. Additionally, if they are in the vast majority who eventually leave competitive sports, they will have a greater chance to participate in long-term physical activities. A staged model for motor learning summarizes much of what we know about training progressions of an athlete or for that matter any individual wishing to enhance integrity of their musculoskeletal system (Table 34.2) (94–100).

Cognitive training is where beginners start. It is the explicit domain where the goal is to understand the nature of the movement challenge and begin to work out basic movement patterns. This is by definition very general and

TABLE 34.2	Three-Stage Model of Training Progression (after Fitts and Posner)

- Cognitive—Verbal-Motor
- Developmental—Associative
- Peak—Subcortical (autonomous)

Adapted from Fitts PM, Posner MI. Human Performance. Belmont, CA: Brooks/Cole; 1967 (94).

not highly sport-specific. This concept is encompassed in the "FUNdamentals" stage of LTAD. It will also be discussed in Chapter 35 as part of the blocked practice or part training approaches.

Key features include

- Novice
- Identification of goals
- A demonstration
- Coaches' feedback
- Allowance for errors

Developmental (or associative) is where more sport-specialized motor patterns are practiced. Read and react situations are incorporated at this stage. According to Jeffries (100) "Athletes will be seen to have completed this stage when they are able to produce effective, efficient, consistent, and fluid movement patterns in a wide range of closed and open situations, with little need to focus on the movements themselves." In an LTAD context this is the "Training to Train" stage which correlates well with both the random practice approach and whole training (see Chapter 35).

Key features include

- Intermediate
- Self-correcting
- Environmental–external cues
- Decreased errors (in contrast to the cognitive stage enhanced motor control is expected). For example:
  - a tennis player learning to hit a backhand down the line would be expected to consistently hit the ball near the target
  - a golfer should at this stage be able to put most drives in the fairway

The **peak** (or autonomous) stage is achieved when movement patterns are largely subcortical and thus both resilient and transferable (see Chapter 35). At this stage the athlete is primed for success in competition. In LTAD this stage equates to "Training to Compete" and "Competing to Win."

Key features include

- Expert
- Subconscious
- Fewest errors
- Resilient/adaptive (sustainable performance). For example,
  - proper defensive footwork in basketball even when fatigue sets in
  - golfer executing shots under pressure

Not every activity requires all the stages; certain forms of play, like climbing, are mostly instinctive and thus have little cognitive overlay. Most other activities do involve the staged model from cognitive through associative to autonomous; however, it is not age specific (94). When an elite athlete learns new skills, he or she will start at the cognitive

level in order to problem-solve. In other words, each new or novel task requires a recapitulation of the stages of motor learning.

Ecological psychologists echo Fitts and Posner's view that the stages of athletic development are not strictly tied to specific ages (19). Instead, change is spasmodic with the individual experiencing "periods of great change and periods of no change." Further to this point they say, "attempting to break a skill down to describe how different age groups perform the skill is a waste of time because each individual performs the skill differently."

Even though certain skills such as language, music, or chess are ideally learned before the age of 7, neuroscientists have found that cortical plasticity can be enhanced across the life span (101–103). In summary, research findings are equivocal for sensitive periods in sport skill development (20). Ericsson theorized that the quantity of deliberate practice is a more relevant predictor of expertise than the age of skill development (35). However, he also argues that it is hard for late starters to log the necessary 10,000 hours. Such assertions are only now being investigated (38).

New frameworks for developing FMS, movement literacies, and young athletes are emerging. Gulbin (104) presents one such model that "integrates general and specialised phases of development for participants within the active lifestyle, sport participation and sport excellence pathways". According to Gulbin it is essential that the approach be flexible and support all stakeholders.

> According to Anderson (20), "the sensitive period opens when learning a new skill begins...."

PROGRAMMING A TRAINING CYCLE—PERIODIZATION

Any person working out or playing in a sport should have a training plan. This is true for individuals exercising on their own, fitness trainers working with weekend warriors, or S&C coaches preparing athletes for competition. Programming a training cycle for an athlete has been the subject of much debate for decades.

A key principle in helping athletes achieve peak performance at the ideal time is termed **periodization** (1). Matveyev (105,106), a Russian sport scientist, published the first modern work on planning a training program for athletes. The complexity of this process is evident when one considers that some sports such as baseball, football, basketball, and hockey have longer off-seasons, while other sports like golf and tennis have very short ones. Many variables are involved, from the length of each competitive season and off-season, travel, external stressors, and secondary sports in which younger athletes may participate. Each sport also demands the training of specific metabolic attributes:

- marathon running: cardiorespiratory endurance
- soccer: occasional bursts of power interspersed with lower intensity challenge
- shot put: explosive power

These different sports engage the metabolic system (VO_2 max, lactate threshold, primarily aerobic versus anaerobic demand) in different ways (Figure 34.2). Training must be matched to the demands of the sport. Additionally, a training cycle will address components such as baseline **assessment, low-intensity training, HIT, tapering,** and **recovery.**

What Is Periodization?

Periodization is the "process of planning, sequencing and detailing various training cycles to achieve athletic improvement and peak performance at the critical times." Schexnayder (107)

Periodization is designed to incorporate phases of training structured to stimulate physiological and psychological adaptation in an ideal manner with the ultimate goal that the athlete hits their peak condition at competition.

In particular, planning included both high-volume and HIT. Ultimately, these phases were organized into blocks which were believed conducive to optimizing **transition (recovery), preparation,** and **competition** (1).

Periodization divides the season or calendar into cycles or phases (i.e., macro or meso, micro, daily) so that competency and capacity adaptations are timed to maximize the probability the athlete will achieve peak performance at key competitions. Exercise mode, intensity, and volume are varied in order to minimize the risk of overtraining and maximize the likelihood that an athletes' peak capacity is achieved at the optimal moment.

Planning a Program Is Simple. But We Often Make It Difficult

Coaches need to follow the rules and not program to their own likes or biases. "Remember the purpose of the program is to reduce injuries and improve performance. We are not trying to create power lifters, Olympic lifters, bodybuilders or strongmen. We are trying to create athletes. Strength training is simply a means to an end." Boyle (108)

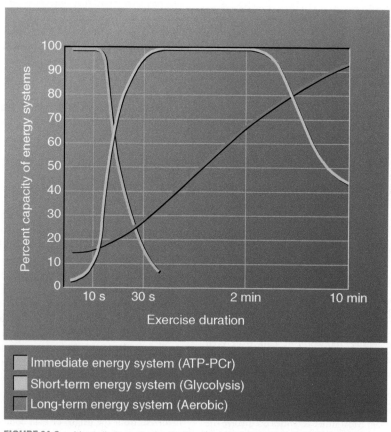

FIGURE 34-2. Metabolic demands of sport. (From McArdle WD, Katch Fl, Katch VL (2010). *Exercise Physiology. Energy, Nutrition and Human Performance* 7th ed. Baltimore, Maryland: Lippincott Williams & Wilkins. P. 226, with permission).

The transition phase occurs at the end of one competitive season and before the next and is also called the recovery phase (109). The preparatory phase is commonly subdivided into two parts—**GPP and SPP**. The competitive phase is the time when many coaches feel maximal intensity training should be cut down or eliminated (110). However, the proximity to competition of switching to submaximal work and the methods utilized to maintain a high level of competitive readiness vary based on the coach (Jamieson).

Periodization approaches have evolved over the years. Traditional approaches did not lend themselves toward preparing a modern athlete for *multipeak performances* during the year. Other issues included *insufficient training intensity* and *noncompatible workloads* being integrated together. Block periodization (BP) came about as an attempt to focus more concentrated workouts on a smaller number of motor and technical abilities (111).

> "Unlike traditional periodization, which usually tries to develop many abilities **simultaneously**, the block concept suggests **consecutive** training stimulation of carefully selected fitness components." Issurin (112)

In BP and other contemporary approaches the sequencing of specialized training blocks is orchestrated to maximize biological adaptation. Traditional and blocked approaches are compared in Table 34.3 (111,112). Four basic training mesocycles are shown in Table 34.4: restoration phase, general and special preparatory phase, sport-specific developmental phase, and competitive phase (113,114). In BP design, exercises are given in a similar order each week (microcycle) within each phase (mesocycle). They are varied slightly based on individualization and to prevent staleness. In most cycles, it is appropriate to go 3 weeks on and then 1 week off for **deloading**. Besides the BP approach, other modern periodization systems that have been popularized include nonlinear, undulating, fractal, polarized, and conjugate systems (115–117).

TABLE 34.3	Block Periodization versus Traditional Training	
	Block Periodization	**Traditional Training**
Development of motor abilities and skills	*Consecutive*	*Simultaneous*
Concentration of training loads	*High*	*Medium (low)*
Focus	*Blocks*—mesocycles	Training periods
Background	Cumulative and *residual* training effect	Cumulative training effect

TABLE 34.4	Basic Training Mesocycles		
Mesocycle Phase	**Duration**	**Core Components**	**Examples**
Restoration/transition (postseason)	4–6 weeks	Active rest	Light–moderate activities
General and special preparation (off-season training)	2–3 months (older, less and younger, more)	Nontechnical/not sport-specific	Alternating low and high neural drive
Sports-specific development (team training camp)	2 months	Technical, sport-specific	Technical work/recovery
Competitive (season)	≥5 months	Maintenance	Reduced volume but not necessarily reduced intensity

Challenges of Periodization

Periodization is a logical approach, but is it evidence-based? Recent review articles showed that a periodized program was superior to a nonperiodized program (118,119). A recent study of aerobic intervals in cyclists found that BP of training provided superior adaptations compared to a traditionally structured program despite similar training volume and intensity (120). Kiely (121) provided a counterpoint by suggesting that the main component of periodization that has been validated is variability of training as opposed to the whole system. What is clear is that a lack of variation in training (122) leads to increased incidence of overuse syndromes (123). Conversely, reductions in training monotony have been associated with increased incidence of peak performances (124).

Another limitation of more traditional periodization programs is that a rigid program structure is followed independent of outcome (i.e., the athlete's response) (125). Contemporary periodization programs have been modified after careful study of how athletes adapt to training (125). Such programs involve higher levels of individualization. Regarding when to build variety into a program Kraaijenhof (126) says, "I start training as little as possible and look for improvement, and only when the athlete does not improve anymore or the performance levels off, I will start to change things, and not necessarily train more, but look at the quality of training first."

> "It is critical that this peak form should arrive at exactly the right time when peak form matters most, presumably during championship competition." Jamieson (127)

Jamieson asks very critical questions such as "how long can one carry competitive form?" and "how many peaks can one achieve in a year?" One modern approach is that of Tschiene (128) who has influenced many modern coaches. His approach is necessitated by athletes with shorter off-seasons who maintain a state of readiness year-round. This approach has shorter cycles and includes more high-intensity work year-round to keep the athletes closer to a state of readiness.

Mujika (129) has reported that this type of consistent HIT is successful. It maintains and even enhances, via a residual training effect, training-induced adaptations while athletes gradually taper their training before a major competition. Additionally, training volume can be significantly reduced without a negative impact on athletic performance.

Various researchers have shown that a **polarized** training program with a high volume of low-intensity training (below lactate threshold) combined with a smaller percentage (>10%) of HIT (>90% VO$_2$ max) and little or no middle zone training is optimal for endurance (e.g., marathon) and intermittent (e.g., soccer) athletes (130–135). According to Sandbakk (135), a longer duration of HIT at 90% is better than shorter one at 95%. According to Guelllich (136), the best responders had the most low-intensity training and least HIT, while the worst responders had the reverse. In season, the ratio stays constant between high and low intensity, but overall training volume drops (137). According to Seiler et al. (137), the key is to avoid the middle zone at the lactate threshold which he terms "the black hole."

The Novice versus the Advanced Athlete

Periodization typically applies to elite athletes. However, the concepts are applicable to active people or athletes independent of their stage of development (Table 34.5).

Novice athletes can be defined as people who have never been through a structured training program. Generally, their competencies and capacities test at the lower end of the spectrum. Intermediate athletes can be defined as people who have trained either in poorly supervised programs or sporadically. They will test in the mid-range of your norms for the various training components. An advanced athlete can be defined as someone who has a solid training background and possesses high qualities of strength and power. Hopefully, they have good movement competencies, but this is far from guaranteed.

According to Vermeil (6), "The major difference between a novice and advanced athlete is that a novice can stay with the same training emphasis, i.e. work capacity or strength, for a substantial period of time and still make gains that will relate to performance." In contrast, an advanced athlete will require more variations.

> Periodization models have made a significant contribution to the development of training–planning practice. "However, there is a logical line of reasoning suggesting an urgent need for periodization theories to be realigned with contemporary elite practice and modern scientific conceptual models... Although the assumption of training generalizability is alluring, in the light of biological complexity this allure is revealed as illusory." Kiely (121)

GENERAL PHYSICAL PREPARATION

For developing athletes it is crucial to build a strong base without them burning out or experiencing an injury. This process can take years to achieve. Thus, a progressive approach beginning with a strong foundation in multilateral training or GPP is a key to maximizing sports performance (1,11,29,72,138,139) (Figure 34.3). The same principles can be applied to "weekend warriors" to prevent injury.

> On the whole, the development of athletes involves reaching a balance between multilateral development and specialized training. "In general, the early development of athletes should focus on multilateral development, which targets the overall physical development of the athletes.... The temptation to deviate from a multilateral development plan and begin specialized training too soon can be very great, especially when a young athlete demonstrates rapid development in a sporting activity." Bompa and Haff (1)

TABLE 34.5	Distinguishing Novice, Intermediate, and Expert Athletes	
Background	**Experience**	**Norms**
Novice	Never been trained	Lowest level
Intermediate	Trained for a few years	Room for improvement
Expert	Trained for many years	High-end training capacity

Adapted from Vermeil A, Hansen D, Irr M. Periodization: Training to develop force that applies to sports performance. Lecture Notes.

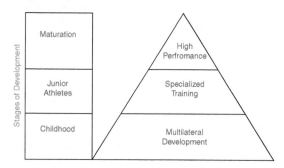

FIGURE 34-3. Sequential model for long-term athletic training. Adapted from Bompa TO, Haff GG. Periodization: Theory and Methodology of Training. 5th ed. Champaign, IL: Human Kinetics; 2009 (1).

The goal of GPP is to establish a foundation for future athletic development. For most, this should precede athletic specialization, high neural drive exercises for power, or SPP. Approximately, 80% of a young athlete's training should be dedicated to GPP (140), whereas in elite athletes the majority of training time focuses on a minimal number of targeted abilities in SPP (140). Unfortunately, according to Simmons (141), "GPP work is very common in track and field overseas, but is still very much overlooked in the United States."

The Overlap of GPP and SPP in LTAD and Periodization

The development of a young athlete progresses from GPP to SPP in much the same way that a periodized program may start with GPP and progress to SPP during the Preparation phase of the annual training cycle. However, one significant difference is that the young athlete should master GPP first, before going on to SPP, while the mature athlete performs both during the Preparation phase of the training year or cycle. One other big difference is that the developing athlete establishes a base in GPP and only then progresses to SPP *over a period of years*, while the mature athlete *alternates* GPP (low-intensity neural drive) and SPP (high-intensity during drive) in *consecutive* training microcycles during the Preparation phase of a larger training mesocycle.

Most of our youth athletes or "weekend warriors" have a low baseline level of fitness. They lack the quantity, quality, and variety of movement skills as a result of over and/or early specialization. This often results in repetitive strain injuries. Ward (142) says, "some are still stuck in that concept of 'strength' and 'conditioning', meaning we lift some weights for strength and we go for a run to condition.... both the 'strength' and 'conditioning' are not separate entities but rather work together to develop the athlete's fitness level to the highest capacity in order to succeed in their particular sport."

According to Tsatsouline, "GPP is training aimed at raising one's many fitness components applied to wide range of tasks" (140). GPP should include a broad base in different motor skills, attributes, or qualities such as *speed, power, strength, mobility, coordination, stamina,* and *suppleness* (139). Skills can be defined as "movements that are dependent on practice and experience for their execution, as opposed to being genetically defined" (143). Variety is crucial, since there is no guarantee that a training skill will transfer to performance. For example, there is limited transfer from maximum speed to agility (144,145). Most of the GPP of an individual involves exercises without any external resistance added (141). However, GPP does progress to include weights, although not exceeding 80% of maximum output (see Special Physical Preparation section below for more specific information about determining maximum strength values (146)). If broad-based movement literacy

training is added to a traditional conditioning program, improvement in athleticism (balance ability and vertical jump height) in children has been noted (147).

Gender-specific issues also should be considered (see Chapters 7 and 31). Girls and women have different fitness attributes than males. During puberty, vertical jump height in boys increases more than it does in girls (148,149). The same is true with respect to hip abduction strength, which should necessitate a training program geared toward building up this predictable "weak link" (150,151). Ford (152,153) identified that pubertal girls have a tendency toward abnormal landing mechanics, which can worsen over time. Too much jumping or plyometrics in females can increase their injury risk. Noncontact anterior cruciate ligament injuries are more common in females than in males in childhood and at the collegiate athletic level (154,155). Various risk factors in postpubertal females have been identified, and integrative neuromuscular training programs that remediate the predictable functional deficits has been shown to reduce injury risk (156–159).

"Five to eight years of correct training is required before an athlete's potential becomes apparent ... ages 14–20 are spent laying the foundation for high performance." Francis (146)

General Strength Training (Lower Demand/Intensity)

General strength training is important for young developing athletes. According to Schexnayder, "General strength exercises are exercises that develop strength, using the athlete's body weight as the sole load or resistance.... The absence of external loading keeps injury risks minimal" (160). Benefits include the following:

- No equipment requirement
- Low injury risk
- Efficient management of large groups, with minimum individualization
- Training of coordination and endurance
- Ideal training for recovery

Core training is an ideal approach for developing athletes. It establishes a base from which power can be trained. It also provides stability from the spine/torso that allows the limbs to generate power without risking injury.

Injury Prevention Is Job One

"In order to prevent injuries in the actual training process, we need to minimize risk. This does not mean eliminate risk, only minimize it. Everything you want to include in the program must be analyzed in terms of risk-to-benefit ratio." Boyle (108)

In the active individual or developing athlete—within the context of LTAD—GPP is lower intensity, whereas in the elite athlete—within the context of periodization—GPP bridges the gap to higher intensity strength work. According to Francis, in more mature athletes, the focus of core work is on development of power—explosive power—through high-intensity work. However, "when working with youngsters both circuit and core work are directed at building muscle or increasing muscle cross-section via high volume, medium intensity work (e.g., 3 to 5 sets of 5–15 repetitions at 65–75% of maximum load)" (160).

According to Verkoshansky (116), exercises with submaximal loads prepare the nervous systems for explosive activities. It may not matter if we use a bar, sandbag, or kettle bell to achieve this. Studies are now beginning to evaluate how these different methods compare. For instance, the kettle bell swing has been found to be as effective as jump squat training for improving maximal strength and explosive strength (vertical leap) (161).

A strong GPP base has been shown to improve throwing velocity (161,162). Plyometric power in the legs, specifically frontal plane leaping power, has been shown to correlate with throwing velocity in collegiate baseball players (163). Similarly, power as demonstrated in an overhead medicine ball toss (greater distance thrown) has a strong direct relationship with throwing velocity in both collegiate baseball and softball players (164). The medicine ball chest pass (4 kg) with legs extended has become part of the standard National Hockey League Combine testing (165).

Tempo Running

For the trained athlete, general strength training or tempo runs are also ideal for recovery days or weeks (Tables 34.6 and 34.7). According to Francis, "Tempo running does not have much of a CNS demand because it is performed at 75% intensity—or even lower. It is similar to performing body-building weight training methods at 65–80% loads." Tempo training is usually at distances of 100, 200, or 300 meters for a total of 2,000–3,000 total meters/workout (146).

Excessive running to build endurance or overemphasizing endurance training can be detrimental to building an athlete. As Francis states, "Endurance work must be

TABLE 34.7	Tempo Training

- 3 times/week
- 100–400 m
- Intensity 65–75% max velocity
- Smooth running
- <16 years of age: <200 m
- Variety of exercises

Adapted from Francis C. The Charlie Francis Training System. 2012. http://shop .charliefrancis.com/products/the-charlie-francis-training-system-cfts (146).

carefully limited to light-medium volumes to prevent the conversion of transitional or intermediate muscle fibre to red, endurance muscle fibre." Of course, this is not what we see at schools around the world. In contrast, cross-training in a running sport such as soccer or basketball can help develop the endurance component as well as agility that so often is lacking in overly specialized young athletes.

> **The Myth of Running in High School Sports**
>
> "Using general strength to develop endurance has the added advantage of minimizing injury risk when compared to using running workouts for the same purpose." Schexnayder (160)

SPECIAL PHYSICAL PREPARATION

As athletes mature, they are ready to specialize more in activities related to their preferred sport. About the same time a GPP base has been established, the safe development of **power** can begin. Regulating training intensity is one of the cornerstones for building power. Learning not only how to train at high intensity but also when to do so, via assessment of readiness, is critical for both safety and success.

> SPP is "the degree to which the athlete's GPP becomes directed towards the sport/positional/tactical/philosophical structure." Smith (139)

Training Intensity

Programming of athletes should be divided between lower and higher intensity training. Lower intensity basically means general strength training or interval endurance training, whereas higher intensity is roughly equivalent to neuromuscular training or power/speed training. Good training programs alternate consecutively between lower and higher intensity days versus the traditional periodization philosophy of simultaneously training lower and higher intensity exercises. In modern periodization approaches this allows

TABLE 34.6	Tempo Runs (Aerobic/Endurance Work)

- Facilitate recovery
- 60–80% of maximum
- Improve recovery
- Enhance capillarization of muscle
- Improves muscle contraction speed

Adapted from Francis C. The Charlie Francis Training System. 2012. http://shop .charliefrancis.com/products/the-charlie-francis-training-system-cfts (146).

higher intensity training, more compatible workloads, and **residual training effects** (carryover) to be achieved (111,112,128). Cardinale (166) says, "Understanding how to apply the correct modality of exercise, the correct volume and intensity and the correct timing of various interventions is in fact the 'holy grail' of S&C."

> "The objective of injury prevention strategies is to ensure that tissue adaptation stimulated from exposure to load keeps pace with, and ideally exceeds the accumulated tissue damage." McGill (167).

Dan Pfaff (168) summarizes the movement competencies that he feels are essential for physical preparation of an athlete as follows:

- Cardiovascular efficiency (i.e., intervals, steady-state running)
- Local muscle endurance (i.e., circuit training)
- Elastic strength
  - endurance lifting at 60–75% of 1 repetition maximum (RM)
  - progressing to power lifting at 70–85% of 1 RM

> "A slow methodical build up through this type of regime helps to stave off injuries and gives a foundation for future training loads." Pfaff (168)

The intensity level selected is based on a number of factors such as age, ability level, competitive schedule, readiness or recovery status, etc., the most important variable being ability level. According to Schexnayder "... the athlete (as much as the training design) determines the intensity of the workout." (169) Athletes who are younger, of lower ability, or in their competitive season will train at lower training intensity levels (see General Physical Preparation section above). In contrast, older, more elite athletes, and those in their off-season will train at higher intensity levels.

> "Since neural development is key to speed and power gains, and prevention of neural fatigue is a priority ... organize the program ... according to their neural demand." Schexnayder (169)

If high-intensity exercises are attempted with poor quality there can no benefit. In deciding between the two approaches, erosion of quality is the surest guide that high-intensity "neural" training should be limited.

> "Any CNS training with less than the highest quality can reinforce neuro-muscular patterns which are counter productive." Francis (146).

Readiness

When mental or physical fatigue is present, training should not include strong technical or high-intensity components. In such cases, particularly in the presence of unexpected fatigue or life and environmental stressors, training speed or power is useless. When an athlete is not ready to train, default to less technical and lower intensity workouts, which are ideal for recovery. In addition, supportive components such as manual therapy may be beneficial.

> "The ability to diagnose CNS fatigue and to adjust high intensity workloads accordingly is the central element in high level coaching." Francis (146).

If athletes are trained when they are not ready, injury risk is increased, and the value of training is reduced. Elite, more mature athletes train at greater horsepower and thus have a greater recovery need (Boo, Francis). They are also the most motivated.

> "Ninety percent of my time is spent holding an athlete back to prevent overtraining, and only 10% is spent motivating them to do more work." Francis (146)

Heart rate variability (HRV) testing is a recommended tool for assessing readiness or recovery. According to Kraaijenhof, "a simple HRV-test can give you some more insight into the autonomic nervous system which is at the interface between body and mind" (170). As Schexnayder says, "Assessing this state of training readiness for each athlete is an important part of training management ... it should be an ongoing process once an athlete has reached a training age where the improvement curve seems to level off and genetic potential is approached" (169).

Especially in older athletes, recovery is crucial to avoid injuries, but it is equally important in an overly eager young athlete. People can always train more, but most athletes' careers are limited by underperformance, overtraining, or injuries. Undertraining injuries seldom occur, and they are quickly solved.

Kraaijenhof says, "No matter how good you are and how hard you train, injuries keep you from performing at your very best and they always appear at the wrong time. One might say it is part of the game; well, it might be part of your game, it is certainly is not part of my game. Consistency over time pays" (126).

Sleep is one of the underrecognized keys to adequate recovery. Insufficient sleep will negatively influence recovery from training, thus interfering with training adaptation and competition performance (171). Poor sleep is a modifiable factor that may contribute to overtraining.

This is the ideal place where an integrated team of experts bridging the gap between rehabilitation and performance can prevent the tendency to overtrain, thus enhancing durability in the motivated athlete.

> "The main error that coaches all over the world make is the tendency to over train: training too often, too much and/or too hard. My important rule: train as much as necessary, not as much as possible. As much as necessary means: necessary in order to improve." Kraaijenhof (126)

High-Intensity Training

As an athlete matures, the focus is more on building power, and thus greater intensities along with lower volumes of training are necessary. According to Francis, "High volume training will never develop the specific **capacity** to generate a high work output in a short time (power)."

> "If you have a Ferrari you don't plough fields with it." Francis (146)

As Schexnayder says, "if speed and power development are not adequately addressed, an athlete is doomed to produce poor performances …" (169). Some of the fundamental qualities to focus on are **accelerative power, absolute speed, speed endurance, power, elastic or reactive strength, and absolute strength** (169).

Typically, **maximal strength** is defined in terms of 1 RM in a standardized movement, for example, the squat exercise (Table 34.8). **Power is defined as force divided by time, or the ability to produce as much force as possible in the shortest possible time.**

Maximal strength influences power. Strength establishes the athlete's capacity ceiling (Figure 34-4) (see Chapter 26).

TABLE 34.8	The 1 RM Test

- Warm-up of 10 reps at 50% of 1 RM (estimated)
- 5 reps at 70% of 1 RM
- 3 reps at 80% of 1 RM
- 1 rep at 90% of 1 RM
- 3 attempts to determine "true" 1 RM

Adapted from McBride JM, Triplett-McBride T, Davie A, Newton RU. A comparison of strength and power characteristics between power lifters, Olympic lifters, and sprinters. J Strength Cond Res 1999;13(1):58–66 (172).

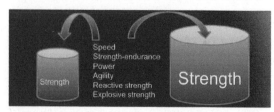

FIGURE 34-4. Strength diagram—analogy of strength to other attributes as cup volume is to contents.

A significant relationship has been observed between the 1 RM, acceleration, and movement velocity (173). The relationship of maximal strength and power is supported by studies evaluating strength and performance in jump tests as well as in 30-m sprints (174,175). Wisløff et al. (176) found that maximal strength in half squats determined both sprint performance and jumping height in high-level soccer players.

While determining the 1 RM is a "gold standard" of strength training, its practical utility may be somewhat limited. While it is a direct measure of maximal strength it is controversial weather 1 RM or multiple RM testing is safer (177). Many S&C coaches prefer 3 or 5 RM and consider it as a standard measure of maximum strength (178) (Table 34.9). An additional limitation of such testing is that due to the typical training effect that occurs when first performing a strength exercise, a 1, 5, or 10 RM will change each session as a neural adaptation or a training effect occurs during the first sessions.

Expression of power is highly dependent on a foundation of **relative strength** and a guiding principle of building strength is to train at 80–95% of the 1 RM (140). This is dependent on the athlete and the sport in which he or she participates. However, the safeguard from Tsatsouline always applies, "if there is any degradation in training, stop." Vladimir Dyachkov (legendary Russian coach who preceded Verkoshansky) recommended stopping training when the following occurs:

- Athlete starts to feel fatigue
- Speed drops
- Athlete feels loss of flexibility

Do not train to failure!

A trainer can monitor a drop in load or power with Keiser machine's power display or a Tendo unit. The Tendo unit is a tool to assess velocity of a loaded movement, or timed set drop offs (179).

Schexnayder (180) recommends, "recovery opportunity between these efforts must be long enough to ensure high quality on successive efforts." Elite athletes require shorter repetitions and routines, since they typically are generating maximum "horsepower" during their repetitions. According to Francis, "The prescription and monitoring of CNS work must be very precise … adjust this volume in accordance with the energy status of the athletes …. Complete recovery from CNS work is critical" (146).

Bear in mind that the goal is not to become the best weight lifter but to lift weights in order to build strength,

TABLE 34.9	The 3 RM Test

- General warm-up followed by static stretching
- 4–5 submaximal sets of 3–5 repetitions
- Attempt 3 repetitions at the estimated load
- Following each successful 3 RM attempt, the load is increased in 5-kg increments until the maximum lift is achieved

Adapted from Cronin JB, Hansen KT. Strength and power predictors of sports speed. J Strength Cond Res 2005;19(2):349–357 (178).

armor, and most of all power in one's sport or activities. Using the bench press as an example, safety is more important than lifting the most weight possible.

> "Iron is the means not the goal... The strength regimen must deliver great strength gains without exhausting the athlete's energy or time." (140)

The importance of building strength cannot be overestimated. According to Vermeil, "If your athlete lacks the 'burst' in their initial acceleration, strength deficits should be looked at as a possible contributor.... remember you can't get to third gear if you can't get out of first gear. Strength and starting strength are absolute prerequisites before other, more advanced training modalities" (181).

Vermeil has recommended the following standards (181). Certainly, this may not apply to all athletes, but it can give us a general guideline:
  a. Males should be able to (back) squat 150–200% their body weight
  b. Females should be able to (back) squat 140–180% of their body weight
Fleck recommends the following exercises as a staple (182):

* Bench press
* 1/2 squat
* Power cleans
* Reverse leg presses
* Hip raises

> "You can be strong without being powerful (because you can't get that strength into motion quickly), but you can't be powerful without having underlying strength of muscles and muscle groups." Verstegen and Williams (183)

Developing an athlete's ability to generate power is a crucial goal. Once **movement competency** is assured via an appropriate mobility/stability program that demonstrates good quality fundamental movement patterns, then load can be applied through the range to build **strength**. Once load can be added without compromising the quality of the movement patterns, then speed can be added to build **power** (Figure 34.5). Turner says, "Developing an athlete's ability to generate power is a key goal of periodization." He goes on, "athletes first increase force output and then the ability to apply this force under progressively time constrained movement skills specific to their sport" (184). Sports vary in terms of their explosiveness and as can be seen the sprinter is one of our most powerful athletes (Table 34.10).

According to Fleck, "Even small changes in **rate of force development** could significantly affect sprinting ability... Interesting to note, from a velocity standpoint, it's been shown that power output increases as the weight lifted decreases from 100% of 1 RM to 90% of 1 RM" (186). Performing a small number of high-intensity, high-velocity repetitions can play a role in

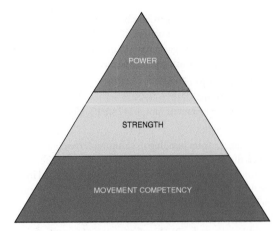

FIGURE 34-5.   Basic training progressions.

TABLE 34.10	Duration of Explosive Force Production
Sport	**Time**
Sprint	0.101
High jump	0.1500.23
Ski jump	0.25–0.30
Shot put	0.22–0.27

Adapted from Zatsiorsky VM. Biomechanics of strength and strength training. In: Komi PV, ed. Strength and Power in Sport. 2nd ed. Oxford, UK: Blackwell Science; 2003:114–133 (185).

training for power via enhancing the rate of force development (RFD) (see Chapter 28).

Jumping

Vertical jumping is an integral part of track-and-field events and sports such as volleyball, diving, and basketball. Some form of jumping is involved in most sports, even O-lifting. In fact, running is a series of alternating single-leg jumps. For this reason the vertical jump-and-reach test has become a commonly used measure of athletic ability in evaluations such as from the National Football League's Draft Combine (187).

Therefore, a staple of power training is to establish the goal of enhancing the vertical leap. Numerous studies have demonstrated that to build leaping power strength training of 80–95% a person's 1 or 3–5 RM is effective (188–192). Sotiropolous et al. (193) demonstrated that half squats performed as a dynamic warm-up at low to moderate intensity, but maximum velocity, improved vertical countermovement jump (CMJ) performance significantly.

Most jumping is preceded by a countermovement, which can be described as a quick bend of the knees during which the body's center of mass drops somewhat before being accelerated upward. Enoka (194) reported a 12% jump height advantage with the countermovement. The countermovement utilizes the stretch-shortening cycle (SSC) in which eccentric muscle stretching stores elastic energy which is then partially released during subsequent concentric muscle contraction.

Numerous researchers have found that jumping ability correlates with sprinting performance:

Squat jumps (SJ) (178,195–199)
Drop jumps (DJ) (200–202)
Countermovement jumps (178,196–198,203,204, 205,206)

This transfer from jumping to sprinting is thought to occur since the SSC is a key factor in both activities (207,208). Marques et al. (208) quantified that power expressed in vertical jumping explained approximately 36% of the sprint performance.

Young et al. (209) suggest that strength qualities during SJ, such as the RFD or force applied at 100 ms, may be more important than maximal strength in the initial acceleration phase (0–2.5 m) of sprinting.

Horizontal (i.e., long or broad) jumps have also been shown to correlate with sprinting ability. Nesser and colleagues (210) using a five-step horizontal jump reported a strong relationship with 40-m sprint performance. Maulder (211) reported that horizontal jump tests correlated better than vertical jumps with 20-m sprint performance. McGill et al. have reported that preseason long jumping predicted in season basketball performance (rebounding and blocked shots) better than vertical leap tests (212), while Meylan et al. (213) found that a horizontal single-leg CMJ had a superior ability to predict sprint (10 m) and change of direction ability than either single-leg lateral or vertical jump. Horizontal jumping is highly functional as most power in sport is generated in a horizontal direction; however, the greater decelerative forces involved in landing horizontal jumps limit its training value. Alternate exercises to train horizontal power include hip thrusts and kettle bell swings.

In testing vertical leap ability there are a few different forms of jumps that are evaluated. Four common ones are the SJ, CMJ, DJ, and Depth Jump (Table 34.11) (214). The instructions given for jumping influence performance (214) recommends for DJ and CMJ the athlete should attempt maximum jump height while minimizing ground contact time.

Landing of jumps involves potentially injurious forces (216,217). Athletes expose their lower extremity to ground reaction forces up to 5–7 times their body mass when landing or decelerating (218,219). The **double-leg DJ** is valuable for assessing valgus alignment of the knee upon landing and has been shown to demonstrate improvements following training (220). Females have been shown to have increased valgus position of the knee than males during the landing phase of both double-leg DJ (221) as well as single-leg DJ (222).

According to Vermeil, a special type of strength that is essential for acceleration from 10–30 yards is elastic strength (6). To individualize an athlete's specific training needs (see Chapter 26) compare two jumps: 1. CMJ and 2. vertical jump with approach. "If there is a greater than 4-inch difference between the two, the athlete can focus

---

TABLE 34.11 Jump Tests

Depth Jump—reactive strength

With hands on hips, step down from a 75-cm box leading with one foot. Land with legs resilient and elastic. Then jump up to maximum height with arms free to reach up.

Drop Jump—elastic energy recoil

With hands on hips throughout the test, step down from a 20- to 60-cm box. Perform a "hard" landing with the legs stiff, minimizing ground contact time, and then jump up for maximum height.

Squat Jump—concentric only

Squat down to self-selected depth, hold for 3–4 s, and then jump up to maximum height without preparatory or countermovement

Counter Movement Jump—eccentric, functional strength

Standing with hands on hips, squat quickly until knees are approximately 120 degrees, or to whatever depth they feel would allow them to jump up as high as possible with hands remaining on hips. Then immediately jump up as high as possible. Leave the ground and land with knees extended.

Adapted from Young W. A simple method for evaluating the strength qualities of the leg extensor muscles and jumping abilities. Strength Cond Coach1995;2(4):5–8; Cronin JB, Hansen KT. Strength and power predictors of sports speed. J Strength Cond Res 2005;19(2):349–357; and Verkoshansky N. Depth Jump vs. Drop Jump. 2013. http://www.cvasps.com/depth-jump-vs-drop-jump-dr-natalia-verkhoshansky/ (178,214,215)

---

more on developing strength (they are more elastic). If there is less than a 4-inch difference, the athlete can spend more time devoted to developing power (strength–speed, speed–strength methods)." The strength–speed continuum described in Chapter 26 highlights some key training nuances to appreciate in order to individualize an athlete's program (see Figure 34.6). In a relative sense as we move to the left side speed is more important, and as we move to the right strength is more important.

Plyometric training has been shown to have a positive effect on the development of vertical jump performance (223,224). Plyometrics should be performed with good quality movement patterns, limiting contacts, especially in heavier athletes (225). To train elastic strength Vermeil suggests the following:

- Jumps with short contact times (on/off box, box to ground to box, hurdle jumps, hops)
  - Increase height only if short contact times can be maintained
  - 5–10 repetitions
- Speed bounds
  - 20–30 yards
- Backboard touches
- More vertical jumping for volleyball/basketball players
- More horizontal work for speed (226)

Speed Training

Speed development is of crucial importance for most athletes (see Chapter 23). There are three phases to sprinting:

Speed–strength continuum			
ABSOLUTE SPEED	**SPEED–STRENGTH**	**STRENGTH–SPEED**	**ABSOLUTE STRENGTH**
Vertical jumps/Basketball	*Weight vest jumpss (10% body weight)*	*Jump squats (30–40% of squat mas*)*	*1 repetition maximum*

*Wilson, GJ, Newton, RU., Murphy, AJ., Humphries, BJ. The optimal training load for the development of dynamic athletic performance. *Medicine and Science in Sport and Exercise* 1993;25:1279–1286.

FIGURE 34-6.   Speed–strength continuum. On the far left is absolute speed. On the right is absolute strength. In between is the interplay of the two and how they affect power.

acceleration, maximal speed, and speed endurance. In sport we can also add in two more aspects: deceleration and change of direction ability (see Chapter 9). Determining the effectiveness of training requires a rigorous testing approach (227). Valle suggests we consider the following tests:

> Acceleration—first 10–30 m
> Maximal speed—usually one half to two-thirds range of the 100-m sprint
> Speed endurance—150-m sprint

Training approaches used in speed development include plyometrics, resistance training, weighted sleds, hill sprinting, etc. (see Chapter 23; Table 34.12) (227).

Many sports such as soccer, tennis, football, basketball, rugby, baseball, etc. require high-intensity sprints of short duration followed by brief recovery times between efforts (178,228). According to Bishop and Girard, "The ability to recover and reproduce performance in subsequent sprints is therefore important for team-sport athletes and has been termed repeated-sprint ability (229)." RSA is a surrogate measure that validly predicts both distance of high-intensity running and total sprint distance during professional soccer games (230).

Sprint training typically requires training at 95–100% of maximum speed (6). Such sprints should be ≤10 s so long as peak intensity can be maintained throughout (231,232). If a longer duration maximum intensity exercise is performed, then a decrease in performance will occur. This is referred to as an "all-out" exercise (231,232).

TABLE 34.12	**Speed Training Modalities**	
Method	**Key Points**	**Goal**
Plyometrics	Horizontal and vertical jumps	Lower body power Foot and ankle stiffness
Resistance training	Power and O-lifting Unilateral training	Hypertrophy and maximal strength Injury preventive stabilization work
Weighted sleds	Low to moderate weight Note velocity decay	Acceleration
Hill sprinting	Low-grade uphill	Acceleration

Adapted from Valle C. Introduction to Sprints and Hurdles Course Notes. Boston, MA: Spikes Only Workshop; 2013 (227).

TABLE 34.13	**Intermittent versus Repeated Sprint Exercise**		
Term	**Rest Duration**	**Recovery**	**Performance Drop**
Intermittent-sprint exercise	>1 min	Near-complete	Minimal
Repeated sprint exercise training (RSET)	<1 min	Partial	Significant

Adapted from Bishop D, Girard O. Repeated Sprint Ability (RSA). In: Cardinale M, Newton R, Nosaka K, eds. Strength and Conditioning: Biological Principles and Practical Applications. Oxford, UK: Wiley-Blackwell; 2011 (229).

When sprints are repeated, the rest duration between repetitions can either be long enough to allow near-complete recovery (>1 min) (232,233) or shorter resulting only in partial recovery (<1 min) (231) (Table 34.13).

RSA requires generating explosive power repeatedly over time. Sprint training is a high-intensity neural drive activity aimed at enhancing the RFD and the effects of fatigue (see Chapter 28). Failure to fully activate appropriate musculature will reduce force production and RSA (234). A drop off in speed with RSET has been attributed to the following (235):

- limitations in energy supply
- metabolic byproduct accumulation
- reduced excitation of the sarcolemma

Studies show that other options for enhancing RSA include the following (235):

- High-intensity interval training (80–90% VO_2 max) with rest periods shorter than the work periods
- High-intensity interval training >VO_2 max (repeated 30 s "all-out" efforts with 1.5–3 min recovery bouts)

Acceleration

For athletes in sports other than sprinting first-step quickness (5-m time) is the most functional measure to improve (178). The average duration of high-intensity running during basketball games is 1.7 s with only 27% of all high-intensity running lasting longer than 2 s (236). A similar situation has been shown to occur in soccer (237,238).

According to Holmberg (239), "straight line sprinting is not expected to translate and, therefore, enhance agility." The transfer from speed training to agility is very limited (240–242). Verstegen was one of the first S&C professionals to place relatively less emphasis on linear training of speed, and to directly train lateral and multidirectional movement (243). Accelerating, decelerating, sliding (i.e., cutting), cross-over steps, drop-steps, etc. are part of most sports (i.e., basketball, tennis, soccer, football). Functional skill training involving agility and maneuverability is a key to sport-specific speed ability (see Chapters 9 and 23).

Summary

SPP is a potent approach to enhance athleticism. It requires a foundation in GPP and an expert S&C professional to guide the variability of training stimuli to achieve maximal adaptation and positive residual effects. Most important is not to overtrain especially with highly motivated athletes, which if injuries are created will have devastating consequences on goal achievement. As Boyle (108) says, "Every good strength and conditioning coach should be paranoid about injuries."

RELATED ISSUES

Strength versus Endurance Training

Verkoshansky was the first coach to call into question the pursuit of maximum oxygen consumption (VO_2 max) as the "Holy Grail" to measure endurance (115). Instead of emphasizing VO_2 max Verkoshansky was interested in the ability of the muscles to effectively use oxygen, a concept known as *local muscular endurance* (115).

Tabata et al. (244) compared the effects of moderate-intensity endurance (MIE) exercise with HIT on VO_2 max and anaerobic capacity. The MIE group increased their VO_2 max by about 10% compared to the HIT group's 14% improvement. The HIT group also increased their anaerobic capacity by 28%, whereas the MIE group had zero improvement in this quality.

Nelson et al. (245) concluded that endurance training inhibits or interferes with strength development. He warned that simultaneous training of strength and endurance inhibits the normal adaptation to either training regimen when performed alone. At moderate levels of challenge, in terms of intensity of strength training or duration of endurance training, the inhibition is most likely minimized. But, at higher levels of challenge Nelson suggests it is beneficial to choose which goal is most important. This is the essence of the modern criticism of traditional periodization approaches where simultaneous training of different physical components was promoted. Issurin's (111) BP was the first programming approach to promote *consecutive* rather than *simultaneous* training of high-intensity power work and lower intensity work in order to maximize the residual training effect.

So what is the athlete's goal? *If it is to develop speed and power, then one may want to be wary of an overemphasis on endurance training.* According to Schexnayder (246), "chronic slow movements erode fast muscle contraction qualities". However, as Francis states, "A pitcher should have a pretty good aerobic component. They need to recover … which the aerobic **capacity** allows them to do. The power component is big, but the aerobic component is big too" (146).

Thus, finding the right balance is a key. If the goal of enhancing peak performance and preventing injury is kept in mind, then the coach can determine the right mix of high-intensity versus low-intensity work. According to Seiler (247), "Successful endurance training involves the manipulation of training intensity, duration, and frequency, with the implicit goals of maximizing performance, minimizing risk of negative training outcomes, and timing peak fitness and performances to be achieved when they matter most."

Conditioning pushes the tolerance line higher, thus widening the margin of safety. "Endurance training" is training for endurance. For example, while a speed-power athlete may not be endurance training, they may condition themselves to improve general fitness. By establishing a minimum aerobic base this will aid recovery and allow for repetitive production of power.

The Capacity Dilemma

Once movement competency is assured, then capacity can become a focus (see Figure 34.4). There is a debate between those that emphasize high-intensity, low-volume work to increase specific **work capacity** and low-intensity, high-volume work to increase cardiac output (10,248). Even among elite athletes there is limited training time available to spread between the various athletic competencies and capacities. Therefore, prioritizing the goals of training becomes a critical programming step.

According to Boyle, successful athletes' dominance in their sport has more to do with speed and power than with endurance (48). Boyle contends that in sports such as hockey or football, training should emphasize high intensity because there is a high rest to work pattern. For instance, it is 3-1 in hockey (45 s shifts/1 on 2 off) and 8-1 in football (5 s play/40 s rest). However, in sports such as mixed martial arts, boxing, cycling, or soccer, a trainer or coach may need to emphasize increasing cardiac output.

Steady-state aerobic training is a mainstay of endurance training, but given the limited time that a coach has to train an athlete this may be an inefficient use of athlete's time (5,248). Therefore, conditioning should be programmed strategically.

Capacity has within it the foundation for power. Perhaps, this is why more static athletes like baseball players can benefit so much from the overall fitness created by cross-training in sports such as soccer, tennis, or basketball which work not only their aerobic capacity but also their stopping and starting ability. As Ward says, "Capacity is the ability to either do something for a long time, such as run a marathon, or to be able to express high, powerful efforts repeatedly with minimal or incomplete rest."

Most sports involve a combination of power and **endurance**, while some are clearly at one end of the spectrum or the other (Table 34.14). *A power lifter or discus thrower would be at the power end, and a long-distance runner would be at the endurance end.* Programming for an athlete begins with evaluation of their sport to see where on the continuum it is. Ward says, "As you develop the training program keep in mind where on the continuum the sport falls and ensure you are preparing the athlete for those sports demands... Once you analyze where the sport is on the continuum you must then determine ways of going about testing the athlete to see what qualities they currently possess and what sort of qualities they are currently lacking..." This allows planning of training (49).

TABLE 34.14	Power-Endurance Spectrum in Sport	
Extreme Power	**Medium Power**	**Endurance**
Few reps/Long rest	*Frequent reps/ short rest*	*High volume/No rest*
Anaerobic	*Mix (intermittent)*	*Aerobic*
O-lifts	Mixed martial arts	Distance running
Power lifting	Boxing	Swimming
Sprint	Tennis	Rowing
Jumps	Baseball pitching	Cross-country skiing
Shot put	Football	Cycling (distance)
Javelin	Rugby, soccer	
Baseball hitting	Basketball	
Throwing	Cross-fit	
	Hockey	
	American football	
	Lacrosse	

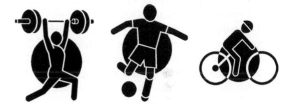

Both power athletes, such as a shot putter, and endurance athletes, such as a distance runner, need capacity, but that capacity is specific to their sport and thus can be termed their **work capacity**. Capacity is usually thought of in reference to doing a longer bout of work (i.e., endurance), and power is shorter and time dependent. But work capacity is the capacity to repeat efforts even at the power end of the spectrum.

Thus, endurance athletes require some power and power athletes require some endurance. Each sport lies within a spectrum on the continuum between power and endurance, but there is a great deal of overlap due to bioenergetic demand (i.e., lactic, alactic, etc.).

Most team sports (football, soccer, basketball, etc.) are in the middle group of the spectrum of the power-endurance spectrum and are referred to as intermittent sports. The demands of these sports are characterized by high-intensity, intermittent activity interspersed with lower intensity activity. The cardiovascular and metabolic demands of these sports can be assessed by simple physiological measurements such as of heart rate and blood lactate (50). Players in these sports experience high demands placed on both their aerobic and anaerobic metabolic pathways. Physiologically muscle glycogen is crucial for energy production (see Figure 34.2). Depletion of glycogen is theorized to play a role in fatigue toward the end of a training session or competition. However, new research suggests fatigue during intense intermittent short-term exercise is unrelated to muscle CP, lactate, pH, or glycogen (51). Different sports have different physical demands, and even within the same sport there are major individual differences related to physical capacity and tactical role. Therefore, leading S&C coaches integrate the tactical and physical demands of the players into their fitness training. According to Bangsbo et al. (250), "Training of elite players should focus on improving their ability to perform intense exercise and to recover rapidly from periods of high-intensity exercise. This is done by performing aerobic and anaerobic training on a regular basis."

Intermittent sports such as football, rugby, swimming, soccer, and cycling involve energy from aerobic and anaerobic sources. According to Laursen (252) aerobic energy supply dominates the total energy requirements after 75 s of near-maximal effort. Therefore, the majority of training for such sports is aimed at increasing aerobic metabolic capacity. Laursen reports that six to eight sessions over 2–4 weeks of HIT (at or above the maximal oxygen uptake intensity), alternated with low-intensity exercise or rest, increased intense exercise performance in well-trained athletes.

The **polarized** approach to training, whereby 75% or more of total training volume is performed at low intensities and 10–15% is performed at high intensities, has been suggested as an optimal training intensity distribution for elite athletes who perform intense exercise events (252).

Discipline Your Athlete to Avoid the "Black Hole"

For the intermittent or endurance athlete Seiler et al. (137):

- Easy days should be easy
- Hard days should be hard but not too hard
- Avoid the middle zone ("black hole")—just above lactate threshold

---

Athletes such as soccer players compete in the middle of the continuum between extreme power and endurance (253). During a soccer match, elite players run over 8 km at an average intensity close to their lactate threshold (238,254). Frequently players engage in high-intensity work such as sprints that are dependent on anaerobic or alactic energy. According to Reilly (238), such sprints:

- occur approximately every 90 s
- last 2–4 s
- make up <11% of game distance

The number of such sprints in a game is estimated to be 6–12 for a good junior team player (255). Therefore, training an athlete should pay attention to their bioenergetic demands.

A "gold standard" test for athletes who play sports which require both endurance and occasional bursts of power is the Yo-Yo Intermittent Recovery (IR) test (256). It is ideal for athletes who play soccer, tennis, basketball, etc. The test evaluates an individual's ability to repeatedly perform intervals over a prolonged period of time. It is a relatively simple and valid way to measure an athlete's capacity to perform repeated intense exercise and to examine changes in performance over time (256).

The Yo-Yo IR test has been shown to be a more sensitive measure of changes in performance than physiologic maximum oxygen uptake measurements (256). During the Yo-Yo IR test, aerobic loading was shown to approach maximal values, while the anaerobic energy system was also highly challenged (256). A modified test called the Yo-Yo Intermittent Endurance Test 2 has been shown to reliably distinguish intermittent exercise performance in players (257):

- of elite versus non-elite status
- at different stages of the season
- who play different positions

How to "develop aerobic capacity without killing the beast and turning them into an endurance athlete." Ward (249)

The Endurance Athlete

The endurance athlete presents a unique challenge. Running performance in endurance events such as the marathon is related to a number of factors such as high cardiac output, a high rate of oxygen delivery to working muscles, high VO_2 max, and the ability to move efficiently (258). Moving efficiently is termed running economy (RE). RE has become a major focus as this has been shown to be a critical factor accounting for performance differences among elite runners even when VO_2 max numbers are nearly identical (259). Additionally, it has been shown to be quite variable (258). Dumke et al. (260) showed that this is especially true in distances above 800 m. Dumke et al. also reported that VO_2 max did not relate to performance times above 800 m or events lasting longer than a few minutes. Similarly, Lucia et al. (259) found an inverse relationship between VO_2 max and cycling economy.

RE is defined as the energy demand (oxygen consumption) for a given velocity of submaximal running (260,261). It is determined by measuring the steady-state consumption of oxygen (VO_2) and the respiratory exchange ratio (260).

RE Is Influenced by Both Physiological and Biomechanical Factors

Physiological factors: metabolic adaptations within the muscle such as increased mitochondria and oxidative enzymes

Biomechanical factors: ability of the muscles to store and release elastic energy by increasing the stiffness of the muscles

Interventions claimed to improve RE are a "holy grail" among endurance athletes and their coaches. Factors showing the ability to enhance RE include HIT, plyometric training, training at altitude, hill running, and heat exposure (258).

Strength training is hypothesized to enable the muscles to better utilize elastic energy and make decelerations more efficient. It has been shown to improve RE in both untrained and trained subjects (262–264). Short-term plyometric or explosive strength training programs have also improved running performance and RE (262,265–269). An 8-week maximal strength training program improved RE without any change in VO_2 max (270).

Rønnestad et al. (120) showed that the organization of the endurance training program in cyclists is important to its success. The BP approach, with consecutive instead of simultaneous training of key components, provided superior adaptations despite similar training volume and intensity. Specific outcomes that improved include VO_2 max, maximum aerobic power, and power output.

A novel finding is that the greater the muscle stiffness, the greater the RE in well-trained runners (260). Specifically it has been shown that calf tendon stiffness is related to RE in runners (271). Both strength training and plyometric exercise have shown to influence tendon stiffness properties (272–274).

The Relationship of Stiffness to Running Economy

"The conversion of energy to motion involves recoil of some elastic energy in muscle and tendon. A 'stiffer' muscle or tendon thus is better at transferring energy economically or without the need for additional oxygen consumption." Dumke et al. (260)

Functional Training

Functional training (see also Chapter 7) is goal-oriented training that focuses on sport-specific skills. It is usually whole body and involves triplanar movements that are part of daily life, work, or sport. In contrast, traditional strength training usually isolates individual muscles rather than training integrated patterns.

The more similar the exercise is to the actual activity (contraction type, movement plane, speed, etc.) the greater the likelihood that improvements in function at home, sports, or work will occur. This is known as the transfer-of-training effect and follows the SAID principle (specific adaptation to imposed demands) (275–277). In concert with the SAID principle, the locomotor system will specifically adapt to the type of demand placed upon it. Training effects are known to be velocity (275,278) and position (i.e., joint angle) specific (279,280). Evidence also shows that training leads to length-, task-, and speed-specific changes (279–281).

Therefore, if training programs do not address the specific functional needs of the individual, the goal cannot be achieved. However, the intent is not to promote "mimicry" of sport during training. A good example of this is training deceleration ability with plyometrics. According to Dietz and Peterson (282), "The key to improved sport performance is producing more force in less time. This results when an athlete can absorb more force eccentrically, allowing him, in turn, to apply higher levels of force concentrically in less time."

The goal is to train movements not muscles (283). Strength increase can be obtained through modifications at the neural level alone due to neural adaptation (284). When morphologic changes occur they do so after neurophysiological changes have occurred (277,280). Enoka (284) famously said "neural changes precede morphological ones."

Train the Brain

"The nervous system knows nothing of muscles and thinks in terms of movements, not muscles." (Commonly attributed to Lord Sherrington; Chang et al. (285))

Functional training has its strengths and limitations. A strength is that stability and equilibrium are trained. A limitation is that absolute strength or power is often ignored. A balanced perspective is offered in Verkhoshansky ("father of plyometrics") and Siff's supertraining, "Research has shown that the transfer of strength developed in bilateral training (e.g., using squats or power cleans) offers specific improvement in performance of bilateral events such as the squat clean and snatch in weight lifting, while unilateral training (e.g., with dumbbells or split cleans) enhances performance more effectively in unilateral activity such as running, jumping or karate."

Tsatsouline and John emphasize that the current abandonment of bilateral exercises popular in "functional" circles is inconsistent with the goals of GPP, "the squat, bench press and dead lift greatly stimulate the neuromuscular and endocrine systems and makes one strong." According to Russian Karate expert Kocherghin, "Strength is needed, and the quickest and most available path to it is powerlifting" (140). Without a foundation in strength, functional training becomes an inefficient arrow in a young athlete's quiver.

According to Schexnayder (286), "I am a fan of functional training. But I have never gone completely that way, always keeping a base in more old school approaches." He goes on to state that a key for strength training is the "amount of muscle tissue activated in the course of a repetition." This is where most functional exercises fail. The main exception being Olympic lifts, which according to Schexnayder, "are where gross movements meet functional training and old school meets new school."

Corrective Exercise

Many trainers are acting like physical therapists or rehabilitation specialists as they focus more on corrective exercise and less and less on GPP and SPP. Corrective exercises are important as both a rehabilitation and injury prevention approach (283) (see Chapters 6 and 7). However, for athletic development, weight loss, general fitness, etc., GPP is needed first and foremost.

A proper balance between corrective exercise strategies, GPP, and SPP is needed. There is little doubt that we should avoid, as Cook says, attempting to "build strength on top of dysfunction" (283). However, Lewit explains "Don't try to teach perfect movement patterns. Correct the key fault that is causing the trouble" (287). The art of training is in walking the fine line between building the athlete up and breaking them down. Specifically, if we overemphasize corrective exercise we will hold the athlete back, whereas if we move too quickly into strengthening, then the athlete will break down. The goal is adaptation. Corrective exercises do not produce adaptation since they are subthreshold.

Echoing Lewit's thoughts, Kraaijenhof has always worked to look for the most flagrant errors that violate large biomechanical principles and that appear to be a source of recurrent injury factors that become chronic. "Some coaches are afraid to tamper with gifted athletes especially if they are producing at a high level. I think this is a huge injustice to the athlete, for major violations only lead to burn-out or chronic compensation patterns that eventually lead to poor function." The key is that corrective exercises don't replace the GPP or SPP programs, but rather become a movement prep or "warm-up."

A few examples to highlight Valle's approach follow:

- Do not rush forward into strength exercises with external loading.
- Body weight exercises result in fewer "trick" movement synergies to move excessive load and thus can prevent muscle imbalances and faulty movement patterns from developing.
- Body weight exercises also can improve coordination and strength endurance.

Measurement Issues

Decisions about training an athlete require ongoing assessment of competencies, capacities, and demands (see Chapters 5 and 6). This is the only way a program can be tweaked and progress monitored. Kraaijenhof enjoins us to learn as much as possible about different ways to assess our athletes "... in every workout we create many supercompensation curves, not only one!, since we always stimulate the central nervous system, cardio-pulmonary system, autonomic nervous system, neuro-muscular system, the hormonal system, at the same time. The problem is that they all supercompensate at different times! It is impossible to control all factors and at the other hand not one singular factor can give you the whole picture: only heart rate won't do it, nor will only lactate, nor only testosterone, nor only HRV. Dependent on the sport, the training, the athlete and the goal,

I try to capture the predominant physiological systems being challenged by the workout and monitor them."

Measurable athletic development is crucial to team success (see Chapter 2). Not only is team average jump height (CMJ and standing vertical leap) correlated with team success (289) but an inverse relationship exists between leg extension power and body composition (% body fat) with total number of injury days per team (289).

Tests should be selected that are meaningful for the athlete (see Chapter 7). They should aid the coach in individualized program design, assessing injury risk, or recovery status. Tests should be valid, reliable, specific; have normative data; be time efficient; and be cost-effective. Prior to testing a dynamic warm-up is recommended. Prolonged static stretching should be avoided as it has been shown to reduce force and power output in the near term (290).

There are diagnostic tests (see Table 7.2) (291,292). There are tests of biomechanical parameters such as functional movement patterns (i.e., squat, lunge, balance, etc.) or capacity (i.e., side plank endurance, 10-RM bench press, interval sprints, etc.). Performance-based "NFL Combine"-style evaluations can be made of vertical leap, 60 m speed, 3-cone drill for lateral agility, etc. (see Table 7.23). More nuanced performance tests are also available such as of RSA (see above). Also, of increasing value is the preseason measurement of an athlete's readiness for sport (preparedness) to determine if baseline movement literacy in FMS is present (77,293,294).

All tests of capacity are in reality psychophysical. Therefore, testing rates of perceived exertion (RPE) is of great value during or after training. The Borg Scale for RPE is a "gold standard," although it is a subjective evaluation of how much perceived effort a workout is requiring of an athlete (295,296). Both muscular and respiratory RPE have been shown to be related to anaerobic threshold (AT) during a test of dyspnea and leg fatigue (297). The AT is an accepted physiologic standard for assessing aerobic capacity as well as for prescribing exercise for different populations (298,299). The Borg Scale allows determination of intensity levels. The use of this scale is simple and low cost compared with the spiroergometry equipment utilized for AT determination (300–302). Therefore, identifying that a subjective, easy-to-administer questionnaire such as the Borg Scale is valid can lead to its field testing and possible utility in team sports.

One of the most important purposes of measurement is to identify fatigue. According to Newton, "… athletes get stronger, bigger, and faster when they rest and recover, not while they are actually training …." Cormack et al. (303) have demonstrated that weekly testing with a simple performance measure such as a vertical jump test can identify performance declines that are associated with cortisol issues. This can lead the athletic development team to engage in preemptive measures to aid the athlete, for instance, by adjusting critical variables such as volume, intensity,

or mode of training or by adding adjunctive measures to enhance recovery (i.e., rest, diet, supplements, manual therapy, etc.).

> "A programme of ongoing testing for the assessment of any athlete is essential to optimizing training programme design, reducing injury or illness risk, increasing career longevity, and maximizing sports performance. The adage 'you can't manage what you can't measure' applies equally to athletes as business." Newton and Cardinale (304)

CONCLUSIONS

Rehabilitation, training, and recovery go hand in hand. Hopefully, this chapter when read within the context of the entire book will help the reader chart a course on the sea between the islands of *rehabilitation, S&C, and athletic development*.

When the athlete's goals, competencies, and capacities are kept in mind, the gradual building of an athletic foundation over years of effort, injury management, and preparation designed to ensure peak performance can hopefully be achieved. The typical pitfalls to avoid are early specialization, excessive training volume, overemphasizing corrective exercises, emphasizing "functional" training to the exclusion of building strength and power, or allowing the ratio of aerobic versus work capacity training to get out of balance with the requirements of the individual athlete's sport.

Optimization of athletic performance is the goal of training. How we train the individual to enhance intrinsic motivation, establish a GPP base, and sharpen the tip of the spear with the right amount and timing of SPP are the fundamental pillars of the athletic development paradigm. This chapter has attempted to knit together a "Noah's Ark" of revolutionary trainers and sport scientists whose contributions enable us to "bridge the gap" from rehabilitation to athletic development.

REFERENCES

1. Bompa TO, Haff GG. Periodization: Theory and Methodology of Training. 5th ed. Champaign, IL: Human Kinetics; 2009.
2. Lewit K. Lecture Notes. Charles University, Prague; 1993.
3. Kerr NL, Tindale RS. Group performance and decision making. Annu Rev Psychol 2004;55:623–655.
4. McGarry T. Applied and theoretical perspectives of performance analysis in sport: scientific issues and challenges. Int J Perform Anal Sport 2009;9:128–140.
5. Gambetta V. Athletic Development: The Art & Science of Functional Sports Conditioning. Champaign, IL: Human Kinetics; 2007.
6. Vermeil A, Hansen D, Irr M. Periodization: Training to develop force that applies to sports performance. Lect Notes.

7. Bailey R, Hillman C, Arent S, Peitpas A. Physical activity: an underestimated investment in human capital? J Phys Act Health 2013;10:289–308.

8. Lopes L, Santos R, Pereira B, Lopes VP. Associations between sedentary behavior and motor coordination in children. Am J Hum Biol 2012;24:746–752.

9. Syväoja HJ, Kantomaa MT, Ahonen T, Hakonen H, Kankaanpää A, Tammelin TH. Physical activity, sedentary behavior, and academic performance in Finnish children. Med Sci Sports Exercise 2013. Online April 2013.

10. Kwak L, Kremers SP, Bergman P, Ruiz JR, Rizzo NS, Sjostrom M. Associations between physical activity, fitness, and academic achievement. J Pediatrics 2009;155(6):914–918.

11. Carlson SA, Fulton JE, Lee SM, et al. Physical education and academic achievement in elementary school: data from the Early Childhood Longitudinal Study. Am J Public Health 2008;98(4):721–727.

12. Nike, Inc. Designed to Move. http://www.designedtomove.org/en_US/?locale=en_US, 2012.

13. U.S. Department of Health and Human Services. Physical Activity Guidelines Advisory Committee Report, 2008. Washington, DC: USDHHS; 2008.

14. Lee I, Shiroma E, Lobelo P, Puska P, Blair S, Katzmarzyk P, for the Lancet Physical Activity Series Working Group. Effect of physical inactivity on major non-communicable diseases worldwide: an analysis of burden of disease and life expectancy. Lancet 2012;380(9838):219–229.

15. Das P, Horton R. Rethinking our approach to physical activity. Lancet 2012;380(9838):189–190. doi:10.1016/S0140-6736(12)61024–61021.

16. Drabik J. Children and Sports Training: How Your Future Champions Should Exercise. Island Pond, VT: Stadion; 1996.

17. Piaget J. The Psychology of the Child. New York: Basic; 1969.

18. Gallahue DL, Ozmun JC. Understanding Motor Development. Madison, WI: Brown and Benchmark; 1995.

19. McMorris T, Hale T. Coaching Science: Theory into Practice. West Sussex, England: Wiley; 2006.

20. Anderson DI, Magill RA, Thouvarecq Q. Critical periods, sensitive periods, and readiness for motor skill learning. In: Hodges NJ, Williams AM, eds. Skill Acquisition in Sport: Research, Theory and Practice. 2nd ed. London: Routledge; 2012.

21. Johnson JS, Newport EL. Critical period effects in second language learning. Cognit Psychol 1989;21:60–99.

22. Habib M, Besson M. What do music training and musical experience teach us about brain plasticity? Music Perception 2009;26:279–285.

23. Watanabe D, Savion-Lemieux T, Penhune VB. The effect of early musical training on adult motor performance: evidence for a sensitive period in motor learning. Exp Brain Res 2007;176:332–340.

24. Blanksby BA, Parker HE, Bradley S, Ong V. Children's readiness for learning front crawl swimming. Austr J Sci Med Sport 1995;27:34–37.

25. Simonton DK. Emergence and realization of genius: the lives and works of 120 classical composers. J Personality Social Psychol 1991;61:829–840.

26. Hensch TK. Critical period regulation. Annu Rev Neurosci 2004;27:549–579.

27. Knudsen EI. Sensitive periods in the development of brain and behavior. J Cognit Neurosci 2004;16:1412–1425.

28. Singer R. Motor Control and Human Performance. London: Macmillan; 1968.

29. Balyi I, Hamilton A. Long-term athlete development: trainability in childhood and adolescence. Olympic Coach 1993;16:4–9.

30. Higgs C, Balyi I, Way R. Developing Physical Literacy: A Guide for Parents of Children ages 0 to 12: A supplement to Canadian Sport for Life. Vancouver, BC: Canadian Sport Centres; 2008.

31. Way R, Balyi I, Grove J. Canadian Sport for Life: A Sport Parent's Guide. Ottawa, ON: Canadian Sport Centres; 2007.

32. Balyi I, Hamilton A. Long-term athlete development update: trainability in childhood and adolescence. Faster Higher Stronger 2003;20:6–8.

33. Bailey RP, Collins D, Ford P, MacNamara Á, Toms M, Pearce G. Participant Development in Sport: An Academic Review. Leeds: Sports Coach UK; 2010.

34. Bailey R, Collins D. The standard model of talent development and its discontents. Kinesiol Rev 2013;2:248–259.

35. Ericsson KA, Krampe RT, Tesch-Romer C. The role of deliberate practice in the acquisition of expert performance. Psychol Rev 1993;100:363–406.

36. Baker J, Côté J, Abernethy B. Sport-specific practice and the development of expert decision-making in team ball sports. J Appl Sport Psychol 2003;15:12–25.

37. Williams AM, Ford PR. Expertise and expert performance in sport. Int Rev Sport Exerc Psychol 2008;1:4–18.

38. Côté J, Lidor R, Hackfort D. ISSP position stand: to sample or to specialize? Seven postulates about youth sport activities that lead to continued participation and elite performance. J Sport Exerc Psychol 2009;9:7–17.

39. Emrich E, Güllich A. Zur Evaluation des deutschen Fördersystems im Nachwuchsleistungssport [Evaluation of the German support system for young elite athletes]. Leistungssport 2005;35:79–86.

40. Baker J, Deakin J, Côté J. On the utility of deliberate practice: predicting performance in ultra-endurance triathletes from training indices. Int J Sport Psychol 2005;36:225–240.

41. Van Rossum JHA. Giftedness and talent in sport. In: Shavinina LV, ed. International Handbook on Giftedness Dordrecht: Springer; 2009:751–791.

42. Carlson R. The socialization of elite tennis players in Sweden: an analysis of the players' background and development. Social Sport 1988;5:241–256.

43. Barynina II, Vaitsekhovskii SM. The aftermath of early sports specialization for highly qualified swimmers. Fitness Sports Rev Int 1992;27:132–133.

44. Lidor R, Lavyan Z. A retrospective picture of early sport experiences among elite and near-elite Israeli athletes: developmental and psychological perspectives. Int J Sport Psychol 2002;33:269–289.

45. Vaeyens R, Güllich A, Warr CR, Philippaerts R. Talent identification and promotion programmes of Olympic athletes. J Sports Sci 2009;27:1367–1380.

46. Boyd MP, Yin Z. Cognitive–affective sources of sport enjoyment in adolescent sport participants. Adolescence 1996;31:383–395.

47. Martens R. Psychological perspectives. In: Cahill BR, Pearl AJ, eds. Intensive Participation in Children's Sports. Champaign, IL: Human Kinetics; 1993:9–18.

48. Côté J, Baker J, Abernethy B. Practice and play in the development of sport expertise. In: Eklund RC, Tenenbaum G, eds. Handbook of Sport Psychology. 3rd ed. Hoboken, NJ: John Wiley & Sons; 2007.

49. Gould D, Udry E, Tuffey S, Loehr J. Burnout in competitive junior tennis players: Pt. 1. A quantitative psychological assessment. Sport Psychologist 1996;10:322–340.

50. Abbott A, Collins D. Eliminating the dichotomy between theory and practice in talent identification and development: considering the role of psychology. J Sports Sci 2004;22(5):395–408.

51. Hyman M. Until it Hurts: American's Obsession with Youth Sports and How It harms Our Kids. Boston: Beacon Press; 2009.

52. Law MP, Côté J, Ericsson KA. Characteristics of expert development in rhythmic gymnastics: a retrospective study. Int J Sport Exerc Psychol 2007;5:82–103.

53. Baker J. Early specialization in youth sport: a requirement for adult expertise? High Ability Stud 2003;14:85–94.

54. Baker J, Cobley S, Fraser-Thomas J. What do we know about early sport specialization? Not much! High Ability Studies 2009;20(1):77–89.

55. Coakley J. The 'logic' of specialization: using children for adult purposes. J Phys Educ Recreation Dance 2010;81(8): 1–58.

56. David P. Human Rights in Youth Sport: A Critical Review of Children's Rights in Competitive Sport. London: Routledge; 2004.

57. Collins D, Bailey R, Ford P, MacNamara A, Toms M, Pearce G. Three worlds: new directions in participant development in sport and physical activity. Sport Educ Soc iFirst article, 2011:1–19.

58. Bailey R, Collins D. The standard model of talent development and its discontents. Kinesiol Rev 2013;2: 248–259.

59. Shields DL, Bredemeier BL. True Competition: A Guide to Pursuing Excellence in Sport and Society. Champaign, IL: Human Kinetics; 2009.

60. Ford PR, De Ste Croix M, Lloyd R, et al. The long-term athlete development model: physiological evidence and application. J Sports Sci 2011;29:389–402.

61. Ericsson KA, Nandagopal K, Roring RW. Giftedness viewed from the expert-performance perspective. J Educ Gifted 2005;28:287–311.

62. Epstein D. The Sports Gene: Inside the Science of Extraordinary Athletic Performance. New York: Penguin Books; 2013.

63. Marcus G. Guitar Zero: The Science of Becoming Musical at Any Age. New York: Penguin; 2012.

64. Gladwell M. Outliers: The Story of Success. New York: Little, Brown, and Co.; 2008.

65. Coyle D. The Talent Code. New York: Bantam Dell; 2009.

66. Hambrick DZ, Meinz EJ. Limits of the predictive power of domain-specific experience. Curr Directions Psychol Sci 2011;20:275–279.

67. Campitelli G, Gobet F. Deliberate practice: necessary but not sufficient. Curr Directions Psychol Sci 2011;20: 280–285.

68. Hambrick DZ, et al. Deliberate practice: is that all it takes to become an expert? Intelligence (Sched. publication 2014).

69. Moesch K, Elbe A-M, Hauge M-LT, Wikman JM. Late specialization: the key to success in centimetres, grams, or seconds (CGS) sports. Scand J Med Sci Sports 2011;21:6: e282–e290.

70. Janelle CM, Hillman CH. Current perspectives and critical issues in expert performance in sport. In: Sharkes JL, Ericsson KA, eds. Advances in Research on Sport Expertise Champaign, IL: Human Kinetics; 2003.

71. Ekstrand J, Gillquist J, Moller M, et al. Incidence of soccer injuries and their relation to training and team success. Am J Sports Med 1983;11:63–67.

72. Colibaba ED, Bota I. Jocurile Sportive: Teoria si Medodica. Bucuresti: Editura Aldin; 1998.

73. Moran A. Sport and Exercise Psychology Textbook: A Critical Introduction. 2nd ed. East Sussex, England: Routledge; 2012.

74. Kraemer WJ, Fleck SJ, Callister R, et al. Training responses of plasma beta-endorphin, adrenocorticotropin, and cortisol. Med Sci Sports Exerc 1989;21:146–153.

75. Gallahue DL, Ozmun JC. Understanding Motor Development: Infants, Children, Adolescents, Adults. Boston: McGraw Hill; 2006.

76. Lubans DR, Morgan PJ, Cliff DP, et al. Fundamental movement skills in children and adolescents: review of associated health benefits. Sports Med 2010;40:1019–1035.

77. Myer GM, Faigenbaum AD, Ford KR, et al. When to initiate integrative neuromuscular training to reduce sports-related injuries and enhance health in youth? Am College Sp Med 2011;10:157–166.

78. Malina RM, Cumming SP, Morano PJ, et al. Maturity status of youth football players: a noninvasive estimate. Med Sci Sports Exerc 2005;37:1044–1052.

79. Abbott A, Easson B. The mental profile. In: Hale BD, Collins D, eds. Rugby Tough Champaign, IL: Human Kinetics; 2002:17–33.

80. Gallahue DL, Ozmun JC. Understanding Motor Development: Infants, Children, Adolescents and Adults. 5th ed. Dubuque, IA: McGraw-Hill; 2002.

81. Fulton J, Burgeson C, Perry G, et al. Assessment of physical activity and sedentary behavior in preschool-age children: priorities for research. Pediatric Exerc Sci 2001;13: 113–126.

82. Okely A, Booth M, Patterson J. Relationship of physical activity to fundamental movement skills among adolescents. Med Sci Sports Exerc 2001;33:1899–1904.

83. Payne V, Isaacs L. Human Motor Development: A Lifespan Approach. Mountain View, CA: Mayfield Publishing Company; 1995.

84. Faigenbaum AD, Kraemer WJ, Blimkie CJ, et al. Youth resistance training: updated position statement paper from the national strength and conditioning association. J Strength Cond Res 2009; 23:S6079.

85. Faigenbaum A, Farrell A, Radler T, et al. Plyo Play: a novel program of short bouts of moderate and high intensity exercise improves physical fitness in elementary school children. Phys Educ 2009;69:37–44.

86. Schmidt RA, Wrisberg CA. Motor Learning and Performance: A Problem Based Learning Approach. Champaign, IL: Human Kinetics; 2000.

87. Deci EL, Ryan RM. Intrinsic Motivation and Self-Determination in Human Behavior. New York: Plenum Press; 2000.

88. Duckworth AL, Kirby TA, Tsukayama E, Berstein H, Ericsson KA. Deliberate practice spells success: why grittier competitors triumph at the National Spelling Bee. Social Psychol Personality Sci 2012;2:174–181.

89. Bonneville-Roussy A, Lavigne GL, Vallerand RJ. When passion leads to excellence: the case of musicians. Psychol Music 2011;39:123–138.

90. Winner E. Gifted Children: Myths and Realities. New York: Basic Books; 1996.

91. Howe MJA. Genius Explained. New York: Cambridge University Press; 1999.

92. Duckworth AL, Peterson C, Matthews MD, Kelly DR. Grit: Perseverance and passion for long-term goals. J Personality Social Psychol 2007;92(6):1087–1101.

93. Bridge MW, Toms MR. The specialising or sampling debate: a retrospective analysis of adolescent sports participation in the UK. J Sports Sci 2013;31(1):87

94. Fitts PM, Posner MI. Human Performance. Oxford, England: Brooks and Cole; 1967.

95. Davids K, Button C, Bennett S. Dynamics of Skill Acquisition: A Constraints-Led Approach. Champaign, IL: Human Kinetics Publishers; 2008.

96. Davids, K. The constraints-based approach to motor learning: Implications for a non-linear pedagogy in sport and physical education. In: Renshaw I, Davids K. Savelsbergh GJP, eds. Motor Learning in Practice: A Constraints-Led Approach. Routledge: New York; 2010:3–16.

97. Renshaw I, Davids K, Savelsberg GJP, eds. Motor Learning in Practice: A Constraints-Led Approach. London: Routledge; 2010:3–17.

98. Brymer E, Renshaw I. An introduction to the constraints-led approach to learning in outdoor education. Austr J Outdoor Educ 2010;14(2):33–41.

99. Magill R. Motor Learning and Control: Concepts and Applications. 9th ed. New York: McGraw Hill; 2011.

100. Jeffries I. Motor learning—applications for agility, part 2. National Strength and Conditioning Association. Strength Cond J 2006;28(6):10–14.

101. Hensch TK. Critical period regulation. Annu Rev Neurosci 2004;27:549–579.

102. Kundsen EI. Sensitive periods in the development of brain and behavior. J Cognit Neurosci 2004;16:1412–1424.

103. Howard RW. Longitudinal effects of different types of practice on the development of chess expertise. Appl Cognit Psychol 2012;26:359–369.

104. Gulbin JP, Croser MJ, Morley EJ, Weissensteiner JR. An integrated framework for the optimisation of sport and athlete development: a practitioner approach. J Sports Sci 2013;31(12):1319–1331.

105. Matveyev L. Periodization of Sports Training. Moscow: Fizkultura I Sport; 1965.

106. Matveyev LP. Fundamentals of Sport Training. Moscow: Progress Publishers; 1981.

107. Schexnayder B. Managing Training Adjustments for Speed and Power. http://sacspeed.com/index.php?option=com_content&task=view&id=40&Itemid=58

108. Boyle M. Advances in Functional Training. Aptos, CA: On Target Publications; 2010.

109. Galvin B, Ledger P. A Guide to Planning Programmes. London: Sports Coach UK; 2003.

110. Jamieson J. The Ultimate Guide to HRV Training. Seattle, WA: Performance Sports Inc.; 2012:20.

111. Issurin VB. Block Periodization: Breakthrough in Sport Training. 1st ed. Ultimate Athlete Concepts; 2008.

112. Issurin VB. New horizons for the methodology and physiology of training periodization. Sports Med 2010;40(3):189–206.

113. Bondarchuk AP. Transfer of Training in Sports, Vol. II. Ultimate Athlete Concepts; 2007.

114. Bondarchuk AP. Transfer of Training in Sports. Ultimate Athlete Concepts; 2010.

115. Verkoshansky V, Siff M. Supertraining. 6th ed. Denver, CO: Supertraining International; 2009.

116. Verkoshansky V. Organization of the training process. New Stud Athl 1998;13(3)21–31.

117. Verkoshansky Y. The end of 'periodization' in the training of high-performance sport. Mod Athl Coach 1999;37(2):14–18.

118. Stone MH, O'Bryant HS, Schilling BK, et al. Periodization part 2: effects of manipulating volume and intensity. Strength Cond J 1999;21(3):54–60.

119. Graham J. Periodization: research and an example application. Strength Cond J 2002;24(6):62–70.

120. Rønnestad BR, Hansen J, Ellefsen S. Block periodization of high-intensity aerobic intervals provides superior training effects in trained cyclists. Scand J Med Sci Sports 2014;24(1):34-42..

121. Kiely J. Periodization paradigms in the 21st century: evidence-led or tradition-driven? Int J Sports Physiol Perform 2012;7:242–250.

122. Foster C. Monitoring training in athletes with reference to overtraining syndrome. Med Sci Sports Exerc 1998;30:1164–1168.

123. Smith DJ. A framework for understanding process leading to elite performance. Sports Med 2003;33:1103–1126.

124. Kellmann M, ed. Enhancing Recovery: Preventing Underperformance in Athletes. Champaign, IL: Human Kinetics; 2002.

125. Evely D. Past & Present Trends in Periodization. CACC Throws Conference 2013.

126. Kraaijenhof H. Introducing 2013 Seminar Presenter-Henk Kraaijenhof. http://www.cvasps.com/introducing-2013-seminar-presenter-henk-kraaijenhof/

127. Jamieson J. Periodization Models (Podcast) www.athleticscoaching.ca http://www.8weeksout.com/2013/08/07/the-bondarchuck-principles/

128. Tschiene P. A necessary direction in training: the integration of biological adaptation in the training program. Coach Sport Sci J 1995;1(3):2–14.

129. Mujika I. Intense training: the key to optimal performance before and during the taper. Scand J Med Sci Sports 2010;20(Suppl 2):24–31.

130. Seiler KS, Kjerland GØ. Quantifying training distribution in elite endurance athletes: is there evidence of an optimal distribution? Scan J Med Sci Sports 2006;16:49–56.

131. Zapico AG, Calderon FJ, Benito PJ. Evolution of physiological and haematological parameters with training load in elite male road cyclists: a longitudinal study. J Sports Med Phys Fitness 2007;47(2):191–196.

132. Esteve-lanao J, Foster C, Seiler S, Lucia A. Impact of training intensity distribution on performance in endurance athletes. J Strength Cond Res 2007;21(3):943–949.

133. Neal CM. Six weeks of polarized training-intensity distribution leads to greater physiological and performance adaptations than a threshold model in trained cyclists. J Appl Physiol 2013;114:461–471.

134. Munoz I, Seiler S, Bautista J, Espana J, Larume E. Does polarized training improve performance in recreational runners? Int J Sport Physiol Perform. 2014;9:265-272. [Epub ahead of print].

135. Sandbakk O, Sandbakk S, Ettema G, Welde B, Effects of intensity and duration in aerobic high intensity interval training in highly trained junior cross country skiers. J Strength Cond Res 2013;27(7):1974–1980.

136. Guelllich A, Seiler S. Lactate profile changes in relation to training characteristics in junior elite cyclists. Int J Sports Phys Perform 2010;5:316–327.

137. Seiler S, Joranson K, Olesen BV, Hetleiid KJ. Adaptations to interactive effects of exercise intensity and total work duration. Scand J Med Sci Sports 2013;23:74–83.

138. Schmolinsky G. Track and Field: The East German Textbook of Athletics. Toronto, ON, Canada: Sports Book Publisher; 2004.

139. Smith J. Physical Preparation. http://powerdevelopmentinc .com/wp-content/uploads/2011/02/Physical-Preparation.pdf

140. John D, Tsatsouline P. Easy Strength How to Get a Lot Stronger than Your Competition—and Dominate Your Sport. St Paul, MN: Dragon Door; 2011.

141. Simmons L. General Physical Preparation. http://www .westide-barbell.com/index.php/the-westside-barbell-university/articles-by-louie-simmons/the-conjugate-method/340-general-physical-preparedness

142. Ward P. PTC Interview with Patrick Ward. http://resultspe riod.blogspot.com/2013/02/ptc-interview-with-patrick-ward.html

143. Schmidt RA, Wrisberg CA. Motor Learning and Performance. 3rd ed. Champaign, IL: Human Kinetics; 2004: 183–275.

144. Little T, Williams AG. Specificity of acceleration, maximum speed and agility in professional soccer players. J Strength Cond Res 2005;19(1):76–78.

145. Young WB, McDowell MH, Scarlett BJ. Specificity of sprint and agility training methods. J Strength Cond Res 2001;15(3):315–319.

146. Francis C. The Charlie Francis Training System. 2012. http://shop.charliefrancis.com/products/the-charlie-francis-training-system-cfts

147. DiStefano LJ, Padua DA, Blackburn JT, et al. Integrated injury prevention program improves balance and vertical jump height in children. J Strength Cond Res 2010;24: 332–342.

148. Kellis E, Tsitskaris GK, Nikopoulou MD, Moiusikou KC. The evaluation of jumping ability of male and female basketball players according to their chronological age and major leagues. J Strength Cond Res 1999;13:40–46.

149. Quatman CE, Ford KR, Myer GD, Hewett TE. Maturation leads to gender differences in landing force and vertical jump performance: a longitudinal study. Am J Sports Med 2006;34:806–813.

150. Brent JL, Myer GD, Ford KR, Hewett TE. A longitudinal examination of hip abduction strength in adolescent males and females. Med Sci Sport Exerc 2008;40(5):731–740.

151. Lloyd DG, Buchanan TS. Strategies of muscular support of varus and valgus isometric loads at the human knee. J Biomech 2001;34:1257–1267.

152. Ford KR, Myer GD, Hewett TE. Valgus knee motion during landing in high school female and male basketball players. Med Sci Sports Exerc 2003;35:1745–1750.

153. Ford KR, Myer GD, Toms HE, Hewett TE. Gender differences in the kinematics of unanticipated cutting in young athletes. Med Sci Sports Exerc 2005;37(1):124–129.

154. Hewett TE, Myer GD, Ford KR, et al. Biomechanical measures of neuromuscular control and valgus loading of the knee predict anterior cruciate ligament injury risk in female athletes: a prospective study. Am J Sports Med 2005;33(4):492–501.

155. Myer GD, Ford KR, Barber Foss KD, et al. The incidence and potential pathomechanics of patellofemoral pain in female athletes. Clin Biomech 2010;25:700–707.

156. Hewett TE, Stroupe AL, Nance TA, Noyes FR. Plyometric training in female athletes. Decreased impact forces and increased hamstring torques. Am J Sports Med 1996;24:765–773.

157. Myer GD, Ford KR, Palumbo JP, Hewett TE. Neuromuscular training improves performance and lower-extremity biomechanics in female athletes. J Strength Cond Res 2005;19:51–60.

158. Myer GD, Ford KR, McLean SG, Hewett TE. The effects of plyometric versus dynamic stabilization and balance training on lower extremity biomechanics. Am J Sports Med 2006;34:490–498.

159. Myer GD, Ford KR, Brent JL, Hewett TE. Differential neuromuscular training effects on ACL injury risk factors in "high-risk" versus "low- risk" athletes. BMC Musculoskelet Disord 2007;8:1–7.

160. Schexnayder B. Using General Strength in the Training Regimen. http://sacspeed.com/index.php?option=com_con tent&task=view&id=40&Itemid=58

161. Lake JP, Lauder MA. Kettlebell swing training improves maximal and explosive strength. J Strength Cond Res 2012;26(8):2228–2233.

162. Hoff J, Almasbakk B. The effects of maximum strength training on throwing velocity and muscle strength in female team-handball players. J Strength Cond Res 1995;9:255–258.

163. Lehman G, Drinkwater EJ, Behm DG. Correlations of throwing velocity to the results of lower body field tests in male college baseball players. J Strength Cond Res 2013;27(4):902-908.

164. Green CM. The Relationship between Core Stability and Throwing Velocity in Collegiate Baseball and Softball Players. M.S. Thesis, California University of Pennsylvania; 2005.

165. Jason D, Vescovi JD, Teena M, et al. Office performance and draft status of elite ice hockey players. Int J Sports Physiol Perform 2006;1:207–221.

166. Cardinale M, Newton R, Nosaka K. Preface in Strength and Conditioning: Biological Principles and Practical Applications. Oxford, UK: Wiley-Blackwell; 2011.

167. McGill SM. 2002. Low Back Disorders: The Scientific Foundation for Prevention and Rehabilitation. Champaign, IL: Human Kinetics.

168. Pfaff D. European Sprints & Hurdles Conference. London, England; 13–14 November 2010.

169. Schexnayder B. Managing Training Adjustment for Speed and Power Athletes. http://www.sacspeed.com/pdf/Training%20Management.pdf

170. Kraaijenhof H. ithlete home page. http://myithlete.com/

171. Halson SL. Nutrition, sleep and recovery. Eur J Sport Sci 2008;8(2):119–126.

172. McBride JM, Triplett-McBride T, Davie A, Newton RU. A comparison of strength and power characteristics between power lifters, Olympic lifters, and sprinters. J Strength Cond Res 1999;13(1):58–66.

173. Buhrle M, Schmidtbleicher D. Der einfluss von maximal-krafttraining auf die bewegungsschnelligkeit (The influence of maximum strength training on movement velocity). Leistungssport 1977;7:3–10.

174. Schmidtbleicher D. Training for power events. In: Komi PV, ed. Strength and Power in Sport. Oxford, UK: Blackwell Scientific Publications; 1992:381–395.

175. Hoff J, Berdahl GO, Bråten S. Jumping height development and body weight considerations in ski jumping. In: Muller E, Schwameder H, Raschner C, et al., eds. Science and Skiing II. Hamburg: Verlag Dr Kovac; 2001:403–412.

176. Wisløff U, Castagna C, Helgerud J, et al. Strong correlation of maximal squat strength with sprint performance and vertical jump height in elite soccer players. Br J Sports Med 2004;38:285–288.

177. Newton in Cardinale M, Newton R, Nosaka K. Preface in Strength and Conditioning: Biological Principles and Practical Applications. Oxford, UK: Wiley-Blackwell; 2011.

178. Cronin JB, Hansen KT. Strength and power predictors of sports speed. J Strength Cond Res 2005;19(2):349–357.

179. Dietz C, Peterson, B. A Systematic Approach to Elite Speed and Explosive Strength Performance. Bye Dietz Sport Enterprise. Hudson, WI. 2012.

180. Schexnayder B. Development of Speed in the Horizontal Jumper. Practical Training Information for High School Coaches. Posted on http://completetrackandfield.com/speed-in-horizontal-jumper/ on September 19, 2011.

181. Vermeil A. Al Vermeil on Speed. http://www.bsmpg.com/Blog/bid/45635/Al-Vermeil-on-Speed

182. Fleck S. Strength training in explosive type sports: sprinting. In: Eliteviden, 5th International Conference on Strength Training. Syddansk Universitet, Denmark; 2006.

183. Verstegen M, Williams, P. Core Performance: The Revolutionary Workout Program to Transform Your Body and Your Life. Emmaeus, PA: Rodale; 2004.

184. Turner AN. Training for power: principles and practice. Prof Strength Cond 2009;14:20–32.

185. Zatsiorsky VM. Biomechanics of strength and strength training. In: Komi PV, ed. Strength and Power in Sport. 2nd ed. Oxford, UK: Blackwell Science; 2003:114–133.

186. Fleck SJ, Kraemer WJ. Designing Resistance Training Programmes. Champaign, IL: Human Kinetics; 2004;209–234.

187. Sierer SP, Battaglini CL, Mihalik JP, Shields EW, Tomasini NT. The National Football League combine: performance differences between drafted and nondrafted players entering the 2004 and 2005 drafts. J Strength Cond Res 2008;22(10):6–12.

188. Clark RA, Bryant AL, Reaburn P. The acute effects of a single set of contrast preloading on a loaded countermovement jump training session. J Strength Cond Res 2006;20:162–166.

189. Comyns TM, Harrison AJ, Hennesey LK, Jensen R. The optimal complex training rest interval for athletes from an-aerobic sports. J Strength Cond Res 2006;20:471–476.

190. Deutsch M, Lloyd R. Effect of order of exercise on performance during a complex training session in rugby players. J Sports Sci 2008;26(8):803–809.

191. Kilduff LP, Bevan HR, Kingsley MIC, et al. Postactivation potentiation in professional rugby players: optimal recovery. J Strength Cond Res 2007;21:1134–1138.

192. Weber KR, Brown LE, Coburn JW, Zinder SM. Acute effects of heavy-load squats on consecutive squat jump performance. J Strength Cond Res 2008;22(3):726–730.

193. Sotiropolous K, Smilios I, Christou M, et al. Effect of warm-up on vertical jump performance and muscle electrical activity using half-squats at low and moderate intensity. J Sports Sci Med 2012;9:326–331.

194. Enoka RM. Muscle strength and its development: new perspectives. Sports Med 1988;6:146–168.

195. Chelly MS, Chérif N, Amar MB. Relationships of peak leg power, 1 maximal repetition half back squat, and leg muscle volume to 5-m sprint performance of junior soccer players. J Strength Cond Res 2010;24(1):266–271.

196. Smirniotou A, Katsikas C, Paradisis G. Strength-power parameters as predictors of sprinting performance. J Sports Med Phys Fitness 2008;48(4):447–454.

197. Maulder PS, Bradshaw EJ, Keogh J. Jump kinetic determinants of sprint acceleration performance from starting blocks in male sprinters. J Sports Sci Med. 2006;5(2):359–366.

198. Mero A, Luhtanen P, Komi PV. A biomechanical study of the sprint start. Scand J Sports Sci 1983;5:20–28.

199. Harris NK, Cronin JB, Hopkins WG, Hansen KT. Squat jump training at maximal power loads vs. heavy loads: effect on sprint ability. J Strength Cond Res 2008;22(6):1742–1749.

200. Kale M, Aşci A, Bayrak C, Açikada C. Relationships among jumping performances and sprint parameters during maximum speed phase in sprinters. J Strength Cond Res 2009;23(8):2272–2279.

201. Barr MJ, Nolte VW. Which measure of drop jump performance best predicts sprinting speed? J Strength Cond Res 2011;25(7):1976–1982.

202. Bissas AI, Havenetidis K. The use of various strength-power tests as predictors of sprint running performance. J Sports Med Phys Fitness 2008;48(1):49–54.

203. Vescovi JD, McGuigan MR. Relationships between sprinting, agility, and jump ability in female athletes. J Sports Sci 2008;26(1):97–107.

204. Young W, Cormack S, Crichton M. Which jump variables should be used to assess explosive leg muscle function? Int J Sports Physiol Perform 2011;6(1):51–57.

205. Markström JL, Olsson CJ. Countermovement jump peak force relative to body weight and jump height as predictors for sprint running performances: (in)homogeneity of track and field athletes? J Strength Cond Res 2013;27(4):944–953.

206. Aerenhouts D, Debaere S, Hagman F, Van Gheluwe B, Delecluse C, Clarys P. Influence of physical development on start and countermovement jump performance in adolescent sprint athletes. J Sports Med Phys Fitness 2013;53(1):1–8.

207. Taube W, Leukel C, Gollhofer A. How neurons make us jump: the neural control of stretch-shortening cycle movements. Exerc Sport Sci Rev 2012;40(2):106–115.

208. Marques MC, Gil H, Ramos RJ, et al. Relationships between vertical jump strength metrics and 5 meters sprint time. J Hum Kinet 2011;29:115–122.

209. Young W, Pryor JF, Wilson G. Effect of instructions on characteristics of countermovement and drop jump performance. J Strength Cond Res 1995;9:232–236.

210. Nesser TW, Latin RW, Berg K, Prentice E. Physiological determinants of 40-meter sprint performance in young male athletes. J Strength Cond Res 1996;10:263–267.

211. Maulder P, Cronin J. Horizontal and vertical jump assessment: reliability, symmetry, discriminative and predictive ability. Phys Ther Sport 2005;6(2):74–82.

212. McGill SM, Andersen J, Horne A. Predicting performance and injury resilience from movement quality and fitness scores in a basketball team over 2 years. J Strength Cond Res 2012;26(7):1731–1739.

213. Meylan C, McMaster T, Cronin J, et al. Single-leg lateral, horizontal, and vertical jump assessment: reliability, inter-relationships, and ability to predict sprint and change-of-direction performance. J Strength Cond Res 2009;23(4):1140–1147.

214. Young W. A simple method for evaluating the strength qualities of the leg extensor muscles and jumping abilities. Strength Cond Coach 1995;2(4):5–8.

215. Verkoshansky N. Depth Jump vs. Drop Jump. 2013. http://www.cvasps.com/depth-jump-vs-drop-jump-dr-natalia-verkhoshansky/

216. Ferretti A, Papandrea P, Conteduca F, et al. Knee ligament injuries in volleyball players. Am J Sports Med 1992;20:203–207.

217. Shimokochi Y, Shultz SJ. Mechanisms of noncontact anterior cruciate ligament injury. J Athl Train 2008;43:396–408.

218. Dufek JS, Bates BT. The evaluation and prediction of impact forces during landings. Med Sci Sports Exerc 1990;22:370–377.

219. McNitt-Gray JL, Hester DME, Mathiyakom W, Munkasy BA. Mechanical demand on multijoint control during landing depend on orientation of the body segments relative to the reaction force. J Biomech 2001;34:1471–1482.

220. Noyes F, Barber-Westin SD, Fleckenstein C, et al. The drop-jump screening test difference in lower limb control by gender and effect of neuromuscular training in female athletes. Am J Sports Med 2005;33(2):197–207.

221. Hewett TE, Myer GD, Ford KR. Biomechanical measures of neuromuscular control and valgus loading of the knee predict anterior cruciate ligament injury risk in female athletes: a prospective study. Am J Sports Med 2005;33:492–501.

222. Russell KA, Palmier RM, Zinder SM, Ingersoll CD. Sex differences in valgus knee angle during a single-leg drop jump. J Athl Train 2006;41(2):166–171.

223. Wilson GJ, Newton RU, Murphy AJ, Humphries BJ. The optimal training load for the development of dynamic athletic performance. Med Sci Sport Exerc 1993;25:1279–1286.

224. Markovic G. Does plyometric training improve vertical jump height? A meta-analytical review. Br J Sports Med 2007;41(6):349–355; discussion 355. [Epub 2007 Mar 8].

225. Liebenson C. The ABC's of movement literacy. J Bodywork Movement Ther 2009;13:291–293.

226. Mero A, Komi PV. EMG, force, and power analysis of sprint-specific strength exercises. J Appl Biomech 1994;10:1–13.

227. Valle C. Introduction to Sprints and Hurdles Course Notes. Boston, MA: Spikes Only Workshop; 2013.

228. Spencer M, Bishop D, Dawson B, Goodman C. Physiological and metabolic responses to repeated-sprint activities: specific to field-based team sports. Sports Med 2005;35(12):1025–1044.

229. Bishop D, Girard O. Repeated Sprint Ability (RSA). In: Cardinale M, Newton R, Nosaka K, eds. Strength and Conditioning: Biological Principles and Practical Applications. Oxford, UK: Wiley-Blackwell; 2011.

230. Rampinini E, Bishop D, Marcora SM, et al. Validity of simple field tests as indicators of match-related physical performance in top-level professional soccer players. Int J Sports Med 2007;28:228–235.

231. Bishop D, Edge J, Davis C, Goodman C. Induced metabolic alkalosis affects muscle metabolism and repeated-sprint ability. Med Sci Sports Exerc 2004;36:807–813.

232. Bishop D, Claudius B. Effects of induced metabolic alkolosis on prolonged intermittent-sprint performance. Med Sci Sports Exerc 2005;37:759–767.

233. Balsom PD, Seger JY, Sjodin B, Ekblom B. Physiological responses to maximal intensity intermittent exercise: effect of recovery duration. Int J Sports Med 1992;13(7):528–533.

234. Ross A, Leveritt M. Long-term metabolic and skeletal muscle adaptations to short-sprint training. Sports Med 2001;31(15):1063–1082.

235. Spencer M, Dawson B, Goodman C, et al. Performance and metabolism in repeated sprint exercise: effect of recovery intensity. Eur J Appl Physiol 2008;103:545–552.

236. McInnes SE, Carlson JS, Jones CJ, et al. The physiological load imposed on basketball players during competition. J Sports Sci 1995;13:387–397.

237. Reilly T, Thomas V. A motion analysis of work-rate in different positional roles in professional football match-play. J Hum Mov Stud 1976;2:87–97.

238. Reilly T. Physiological profile of the player. In: Ekblom B, ed. Football (Soccer). London: Blackwell; 1994:78–95.

239. Holmberg PM. Agility training for experienced athletes: a dynamical systems approach. Strength Cond J 2009;31(5):73–78.

240. Little T, Williams AG. Specificity of acceleration, maximum speed and agility in professional soccer players. J Strength Cond Res 2005;19(1):76–78.

241. Young WB, McDowell MH, Scarlett BJ. Specificity of sprint and agility training methods. J Strength Cond Res 2001;15(3):315–319.

242. Jeffreys I. Motor learning—applications for agility, Part 1. Strength Cond J 2006;28(5):72–76.

243. Versteegan M, Marcello B. Agility and coordination. In: Foran B, ed. High Performance Sports Conditioning. Champaign, IL: Human Kinetics; 2001:139–165.

244. Tabata I, Irishawa K, Kuzaki M, Nishimura K, Ogita F, Miyachi M. Metabolic profile of high-intensity intermittent exercises. Med Sci Sports Exerc 1997;29(3):390–395.

245. Nelson AG, Arnall DA, Loy SF, et al. Consequences of combining strength and endurance training regimens. Phys Ther 1990;70:287–294.

246. Schexnayder B. Developing Speed in the High School Athlete. http://sacspeed.com/index.php?option=com_content&task=view&id=40&Itemid=58

247. Seiler S. What is best practice for training intensity and duration distribution in endurance athletes? Int J Sports Physiol Perform 2010;5:276–291.

248. Boyle M. Understanding (or Misunderstanding) Aerobic Training. http://www.strengthcoach.com

249. Ward P. The Power-Capacity Continuum. http://optimumsportsperformance.com/blog/?p=2556

250. Bangsbo J, Mohr M, Krustrup P. Physical and metabolic demands of training and match-play in the elite football player. J Sports Sci 2006;24(7):665–674.

251. Krustrup P, Mohr M, Amstrup T, et al. The yo-yo intermittent recovery test: physiological response, reliability, and validity. Med Sci Sports Exerc 2003;35(4):697–705.

252. Laursen PB. Training for intense exercise performance: high-intensity or high-volume training? Scand J Med Sci Sports 2010;20(Suppl 2):1–10.

253. Hoff J, Helgerud J. Endurance and strength training for soccer players physiological considerations. Sports Med 2004;34(3):165–180.

254. Bangsbo J. Physiological demands. In: Ekblom B, ed. Football (Soccer). London: Blackwell; 1994:43–59.

255. Helgerud J, Engen LC, Wisløff U, et al. Aerobic endurance training improves soccer performance. Med Sci Sports Exerc 2001;33:1925–1931.

256. Bangsbo J, Iaia FM, Krustrup P. The Yo-Yo intermittent recovery test: a useful tool for evaluation of physical performance in intermittent sports. Sports Med 2008;38(1):37–51.

257. Bradley PS, Mohr M, Bendiksen M, et al. Sub-maximal and maximal Yo-Yo intermittent endurance test level 2: heart rate response, reproducibility and application to elite soccer. Eur J Appl Physiol 2011;111(6):969–978.

258. Foster C, Lucia A. Running economy the forgotten factor in elite performance. Sports Med 2007;37(4–5):316–319.

259. Lucia A, Hoyos J, Perez M, et al. Inverse relationship between VO2max and economy/efficiency in world-class cyclists. Med Sci Sports Exerc 2002;34:2079–2084.

260. Dumke CL, Pfaffenroth CM, McBride JM, Grant O. Relationship between muscle strength, power and stiffness and running economy in trained male runners. Int J Sports Physiol Perform 2010;5:249–261.

261. Saunders PU, Pyne DB, Telford RD, Hawley JA. Factors affecting running economy in trained distance runners. Sports Med 2004;34(7):465–485.

262. Guglielmo LG, Greco CC, Denadai BS. Effects of strength training on running economy. Int J Sports Med 2009;30:27–32.

263. Yamamoto LM, Lopez RM, Klau JF, et al. The effects of resistance training on endurance distance running performance among highly trained runners: a systematic review. J Strength Cond Res 2008;22:2036–2044.

264. Millet GP, Jaouen B, Borrani F, Candau R. Effects of concurrent endurance and strength training on running economy and. VO(2) kinetics. Med Sci Sports Exerc 2002;34:1351–1359.

265. Paavolainen L, Hakkinen K, Hamalainen I, Nummela A, Rusko H. Explosive-strength training improves 5-km running time by improving running economy and muscle power. J Appl Physiol 1999;86:1527–1533.

266. Spurrs RW, Murphy AJ, Watsford ML. The effect of plyometric training on distance running performance. Eur J Appl Physiol 2003;89:1–7.

267. Saunders PU, Pyne DB, Telford RD, Hawley JA. Factors affecting running economy in trained distance runners. Sports Med 2004;34:465–485.

268. Saunders PU, Telford RD, Pyne DB, et al. Short-term plyometric training improves running economy in highly trained middle and long distance runners. J Strength Cond Res 2006;20:947–954.

269. Turner AM, Owings M, Schwane JA. Improvement in running economy after 6 weeks of plyometric training. J Strength Cond Res 2003;17:60–67.

270. Storen O, Helgerud J, Stoa EM, Hoff J. Maximal strength training improves running economy in distance runners. Med Sci Sports Exerc 2008;40:1087–1092.

271. Arampatzis A, De Monte G, Karamanidis K, et al. Influence of the muscle-tendon unit's mechanical and morphological properties on running economy. J Exp Biol 2006;209:3345–3357.

272. Reeves ND, Narici MV, Maganaris CN. Strength training alters the viscoelastic properties of tendons in elderly humans. Muscle Nerve 2003;28:74–81.

273. Burgess KE, Connick MJ, Graham-Smith P, Pearson SJ. Plyometric vs. isometric training influences on tendon properties and muscle output. J Strength Cond Res 2007;21:986–989.

274. Kubo K, Morimoto M, Komuro T, et al. Effects of plyometric and weight training on muscle-tendon complex and jump performance. Med Sci Sports Exerc 2007;39:1801–1810.

275. Moffroid MT, Whipple RH. Specificity of speed exercise. Phys Ther 1970;50:1693.

276. Rutherford OM. Muscular coordination and strength training, implications for injury rehabilitation. Sports Med 1988;5:196.

277. Sale D, MacDougall D. Specificity in strength training: a review for the coach and athlete. Can J Sport Sci 1981;6:87.

278. Caizzo VJ, Perine, JJ, Edgerton VR. Training-induced alterations of the in vivo force-velocity relationship of human muscle. J Appl Physiol 1981;51:750.

279. Bender JA, Kaplan HM. The multiple angle testing method for the evaluation of muscle strength. J Bone Joint Surg [Am] 1963;45A:135.

280. Meyers C. Effects of 2 isometric routines on strength, size and endurance of exercised and non-exercised arms. Res Q 1967;38:430.

281. Boucher JP, Cyr A, King MA, et al. Isometric training overflow: Determination of a non-specificity window. Med Sci Sports Exerc 1993;25:S134.

282. Dietz, C, Peterson, B. Triphasic Training a Systematic Approach to Elite Speed and Explosive Strength Performance. Hudson, WI: Bye Dietz Sports Enterprise; 2012.

283. Cook G. Movement: Functional Movement Systems. Aptos, CA: On Target Publications; 2010.

284. Enoka RM. Neuromechanical Basis of Kinesiology. Champaign, IL: Human Kinetics; 1988.

285. Chang H-T, Ruch TC, Ward Jr AA. Topographical representation of muscles in motor cortex of monkeys. J Neurophysiol 1947;10(1):39–56.

286. Schexnayder B. Interview: 5 Questions. http://speedendurance.com/2012/04/27/boo-schexnayder-interview-5-questions/

287. Lewit K. Manipulative Therapy in Rehabilitation of the Locomotor System. 3rd ed. Oxford, England: Butterworth Heinemann; 1999.

288. Valle C. Self-Organization and Athletic Development. http://elitetrack.com/blogs-details-4122/

289. Arnason A, Sigurdsoon SB, Gudmonnson A, et al. Physical fitness, injuries, and team performance in soccer. Med Sci Sports Exerc 2004;36(2):278–285.

290. Marek SM, Cramer JT, Fincher AL, Massey LL, et al. Acute effects of static and proprioceptive neuromuscular facilitation stretching on muscle strength and power output. J Athl Train 2005;40:94–103.

291. Craton N. In: Liebenson C, ed. Rehabilitation of the Spine: A Practitioner's Manual. 2nd ed. Philadelphia: Lippincott/Williams & Wilkins; 2007.

292. Liebenson C. In: Liebenson C, ed. Rehabilitation of the Spine: A Practitioner's Manual. 2nd ed. Philadelphia: Lippincott/Williams & Wilkins; 2007.

293. Hewett TE, Myer GD, Ford KR. Anterior cruciate ligament injuries in female athletes: Part 1, mechanisms and risk factors. Am J Sports Med 2006;34:299–311.

294. Faigenbaum AD, Myer GD. Resistance training among young athletes: safety, efficacy and injury prevention effects. Br J Sports Med 2010;44:56–63.

295. Borg G. Borg' s Perceived Exertion and Pain Scales. Champaign, IL: Human Kinetics; 1998.

296. Borg E, Kaijser L. A comparison between three rating scales for perceived exertion and two different work tests. Scand J Med Sci Sports 2006;16:57–69.

297. Zamuner AR, Moreno MA, Camargo TM, et al. Assessment of subjective perceived exertion at the anaerobic threshold with the Borg CR-10 scale. J Sports Sci Med 2011;10:130–136.

298. Svedahl K, Macintosh BR. Anaerobic threshold the concept and methods of measurement. Can J Appl Physiol 2003;28(2):299–323.

299. Sirol FN, Sakabe DI, Catai AM, Milan LA, Martins LEB, Silva E. Comparison of power output and heart rate levels in anaerobic threshold determinations by two indirect methods. Braz J Phys Ther 2005;9(2):1–8.

300. Crescêncio JC, Martins LE, Murta Jr LO, et al. Measurement of anaerobic threshold during dynamic exercise in healthy subjects: comparison among visual analysis and mathematical models. Comput Cardiol 2003;30:801–804.

301. Higa MN, Silva E, Neves VF, Catai AM, Gallo Jr L, Silva de Sá MF. Comparison of anaerobic threshold determined by visual and mathematical methods in healthy women. Braz J Med Biol Res 2007;40:501–508 (in Portuguese: English abstract).

302. Wasserman K, Hansen JE, Sue D, Whipp BJ, Casaburi R. Principles of Exercise Testing and Interpretation. 4th ed. Philadelphia: Williams and Wilkins; 1999.

303. Cormack SJ, Newton RU, McGuigan MR. Neuromuscular and endocrine responses of elite players during an Australian rules football season. Int J Sports Phyisol Perform 2008;3:439–453.

304. Newton R., Cardinale M, Total Athlete Management (TAM) and performance diagnosis. In: Cardinale M, Newton R, Nosaka K. Strength and Conditioning: Biological Principles and Practical Applications. Oxford, UK: Wiley-Blackwell; 2011.

Coaching Fundamentals—A Skill Acquisition Perspective

INTRODUCTION

High-performance sport has witnessed an explosion in scientific attention over the last few decades, in particular, in the fields of sport psychology, exercise physiology, and biomechanical performance analysis. However, translating research and theory into enhanced skill acquisition has lagged behind (1,2). This coaching section will address how to bridge this gap.

Prior sections of this book have described *what* the major constituents of a modern training program are. The purpose of this chapter is to describe *how* an individual should be coached to achieve these training goals.

> "If a child can't learn the way we teach, maybe we should teach the way they learn." Ignacio Estrada

INTRINSIC MOTIVATION AND SELF-REGULATION

An athlete's personality has an influence on his or her coachability. From a coach's perspective, there are different types of athletes. The best are **self-motivated**. In the long run, the less a coach has to push the better. This relates to such factors as *grit, passion*, and *intrinsic motivation*.

An athlete who possesses the personality characteristics of grit or passion is more likely to be persistent in goal achievement. Grit predicts both deliberate practice and performance in spelling bee competitors (3). Similarly, passion in classical musicians was also found to be related to deliberate practice and ultimately to performance (4). Gifted children typically possess the intrinsic motivation to obsessively pursue mastery in areas they are passionate about (5,6).

Discovery-based learning promotes active learning and **self-regulation**. Self-regulation is defined as awareness of one's errors and how to correct them (2). Such learning promotes problem-solving and has greater ecological validity to what occurs in performance as opposed to practice (7).

> "The coach worked on the principle that guidance should be used infrequently with the least physical restraint possible." Williams et al. (2)

The foundation of long-term, self-regulated involvement in elite sport is the development of a solid foundation of intrinsic motivation at early stages (8–10). Early diversification or sampling and late specialization facilitate this process (11,12).

Positive reinforcement enhances intrinsic motivation (13). The power of positive thinking (and coaching!) goes against the grain of much traditional "boot camp" styles of organizing practices and training sessions. However, positive feedback has been shown to work best. Participants who received feedback after their best trials learned more effectively (14).

> "Feedback emphasizing successful performance, while ignoring less successful attempts, benefited learning." Lewthwaite and Wulf (15)

Positive normative feedback improved outcomes and changed movement control. When an athlete or person learning a motor skill develops the conviction of being "good" at a particular task, or showing "better" improvement, this facilitates the learning process (16). Lewthwaite and Wulf (15) stated, "By creating conditions that enhance the learners' feelings of competence, instructors or coaches can speed the learning process and enhance performance." A coach, trainer, or rehabilitation clinician's actions that affect an athlete's perceptions of competence or autonomy can also influence intrinsic motivation (17,18).

> "A coach is someone who can give correction without causing resentment." Coach John Wooden

The best coaches follow a philosophy of less is more. Excessive feedback can be detrimental to long-term storage and retention of new neuromuscular habits (19). Frequent feedback has been thought of as analogous to a crutch (20) aiding when present but hampering when absent.

> "Practice has to take place in the absence of the crutch."
> Hodges and Campagnaro (19)

Self-regulation involves processes that enable individuals to control their thoughts, feelings, and actions (21). Self-regulatory processes will not immediately produce high levels of expertise, but can assist an individual in acquiring knowledge and skills more effectively (22).

> **Self-Regulation**
>
> ".... the degree to which individuals are metacognitively, motivationally, and behaviourally proactive participants in their own learning process. This means that individuals know how to attain their goal of performance improvement; they are motivated; and they take action to reach their goal." Zimmerman (23)

It is theorized that young athletes who self-regulate develop faster and are better able to get the maximum out of their potential. Jonker et al. (24,25) suggest they are more aware of their strong and weak points and have the ability to adapt (i.e., transfer) their learning strategies to their practice or game environment.

PRACTICE ORGANIZATION

Blocked versus Random Practice

Practice for a sport or performing art (i.e., music) involves scheduling a variety of tasks to enhance *learning*. Two basic forms of practice organization are blocked and random repetition schedules. **Blocked practice** involves maintaining a constant training environment while rehearsing the same fundamental skills until competency improves. **Random practice** involves simulating competition by varying the environment while practicing a variety of skills in a random order. Paradoxically, even though skills do not improve as quickly during training with random practice, there is greater long-term skill retention and transference to competition than with blocked practice (Figure 35.1). During variable or random practice, a sensory-motor program is formed for rapid execution of movement patterns necessary to carry out stereotypical goal-driven tasks (26).

> **The Paradox of Blocked versus Random Practice**
>
> "The paradox arises from the fact that blocked practice is in fact very ineffective for transfer of learning to competition as performance improvements measured during practice degrade rapidly, and are inefficient because retraining on the same skills will be necessary." Bain and McGown (27)

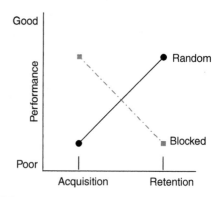

FIGURE 35-1. Paradoxical training effect predicted by contextual interference. Adapted from Battig WF. The flexibility of human memory. In: Cermak LS, Craik FIM, eds. Levels of Processing and Human Memory. Hillsdale, NJ: Lawrence Erlbaum Associates; 1979:2344.

There is a postural self-organization principle at play when we work programs of movement instead of isolated chunks of corrective exercise. As Otte and Van Zanic (28) stated that the success of the random plan originates from the Elaboration Hypothesis and the spacing of movement: the Forgetting Hypothesis. "The Elaboration Hypothesis states that when a learner performs a series of separate skills in a random order, the learner begins to recognize the distinctive nature of each skill. By understanding and feeling how each movement was distinctive, the learner is able to store the movement more effectively within long-term memory."

The superiority of random training has been demonstrated in a wide variety of sports (29)—volleyball (30,31), badminton (32,33), baseball (34,35), basketball (36), tennis (37), and soccer (38). Neurologically, it has been shown that new motor engrams are formed in this way (39).

Retention testing has shown that skill transfer is enhanced by environments that utilize contextual interference (CI; i.e., random practice) and on drill variations (40–43). Early in the learning stages, blocked training may be preferable (25,44–47). This also has psychological benefit, so the athlete (and coach!) feels something is being accomplished.

Moderately skilled learners benefit from a progressive increase in CI from a blocked to a random schedule (48). It is hypothesized that training should start with blocked if the athlete is a child, the skill level is low, or the activity involves high-skill complexity (49–51).

The neurological basis of skill acquisition depends on two different brain processes—an explicit domain (conscious) and an implicit domain (subconscious) (52). The explicit domain is concerned with the conscious goal, while the implicit domain is subconscious dealing with biomechanical and neurophysiologic properties such as limb trajectories and force generation. The implicit domain is developed by practice variability and becomes a subcortical automated movement pattern in expert performers (53–55). The explicit domain is the focus of the early stages of motor learning.

> **Purposeful Practice—What Is the Goal?**
>
> "Why do we practice? Most people would say that we practice to get better. But get better when is the question? Are we practicing to get better in practice, or are we practicing to get better in competition?" Bain and McGown (27)

> "As expert performance in sport is exemplified by the consistent execution of whole skills in game-like settings, the sooner we have the whole-skill practice algorithm in place, the faster our athletes will imprint the proper motor patterns that characterize expert performance." Bain and McGown (27)

Whole versus Part Training

Breaking a skill down into component parts should make learning a complex task easier. The **part** training approach assumes the brain can rearrange individual motor stereotypes into a final complex motor skill. However, modern neuroscience shows that the brain does not learn this way.

The brain is a processing system that converts sensory inputs to motor outputs (56). It controls voluntary movements by formatting maps that contain dense neural signatures programmed in the central nervous system (CNS) (57,58). Counterintuitively, skills requiring a high degree of interlimb coordination are best learned by practice of the **whole** skill (59–62). This has been demonstrated in a variety of disciplines—athletic, musical, or ergonomic (63–67).

> **Optimal Training Environments Require**
>
> (Bain and McGown (27)) the following:
> 1. Biomechanically correct examples when demonstrating skills
> 2. Clear functional goals for practice activities
> 3. A wide range of force production variables within the context of goal-directed functional activities
> 4. Early implementation of variable practice and whole-skill training

Jeffries has enhanced on Bain and McGown's list by adding that the coach must give appropriate feedback to the athlete during the training session (68). Jeffries emphasizes the importance of using neurolinguistically appropriate cues to aid the athlete in obtaining a general picture for the movement being trained (69,70). Wulf et al. (71) have emphasized the value of an external focus on the intended effects of the skill to enhance performance. For example:

- Training Vertical Leap
- Internal Cue: "Push from your hips"
- Preferred External Cue: "Try to touch the ceiling"

According to Schexnayder (72), for any event, "The most important drill… is the event itself. Even the best drills have relatively low rates of transfer into the events, so actually practicing the event is critical, and it's a common error to spend too much time on drills." Time and time again, research indicates that whole learning is more effective than part learning, and people should fight the temptation to break the event into small parts.

ECOLOGICAL DYNAMICS: HOW DOES ENVIRONMENT IMPACT SKILL ACQUISITION?

When we consider long-term athletic development we are interested in when certain "optimal periods of learning" arise. In contrast, ecological psychology is more concerned with how a specific skill is acquired rather than when it is.

What seems to be clear is that regardless of whether we are thinking about "whole vs. part" or "random vs. blocked," the bottom line is that motor learning or skill acquisition occurs best in a nested environment where the anticipation, ramping up, and follow-up to a skill are included in the training (73). The enemy of creating efficient, subcortical motor programs for newly acquired skills is task decomposition where a task is separated into smaller parts during practice (74). Ecological dynamics suggests that motor learning is facilitated by utilization of a nested task where perception–action coupling occurs (73).

> **Perception–Action Coupling**
>
> "…. implies that learning design should emphasize keeping information and movements together to allow athletes to couple their actions to key information sources which are available in performance and practice environments." Davids (73)

An example of a practice-training device (in common use in baseball or tennis) that is inconsistent with valid ecological dynamic is a ball machine. This may provide a tennis or baseball hitter with information about ball flight but is limited by the absence of information about the pitcher's or tennis opponent's actions (75). For the training or practice environment to be ecologically valid, it should replicate the performance environment in key areas so that perceptual **inputs** (visual, auditory, etc.) can be coupled to kinesthetic **outputs** of the individual (73).

One simple way to enhance ecological validity of a training exercise is to make it dynamic instead of static, upright instead of recumbent, or triplanar instead or uniplanar. At the end of the day, we want practice to simulate performance in sport.

> **Enhancing Ecological Validity**
>
> "Simulations are designed to facilitate the emergence of functional movement patterns in each athlete, regardless of skill level or experience." Davids (73)

In what is termed "nonlinear pedagogy," realistic performance simulations are created that present opportunities for athletes to discover their own performance solutions (75–78). In more **traditional approaches** to coaching, detailed verbal instructions and "ready-made" repetitive practice are prescribed (79), whereas in **nonlinear pedagogy**, athletes are presented with problems to solve involving unique constraints designed by their coach (79).

Discovery versus Rote Practice in Nonlinear Pedagogy

Practice is seen as "… a process of searching a perceptual-motor landscape composed of interacting personal, task and environmental constraints…. instead of attempting to change athlete behavior through highly prescriptive instructions, which might short-circuit the discovery and exploration process of learning, the coach becomes a facilitator …" who designs training and learning tasks to bring about functional changes in behavior. Davids (73)

MOVEMENT EFFICIENCY

The physical skills that are trained in general physical preparation and specialized physical preparation are necessary, but not sufficient, for performance enhancement. They must be transferable. When this integration into sport, especially during competition, occurs in a sustainable and adaptable way, we can say that the skill is programmed subcortically as an engram in the CNS. The goal of training is to create an efficient and robust neurosignature that can withstand high levels of emotional stress, cognitive challenge, or varied/high levels of external demand (80).

Successful athletes who perform at a high level depend on efficient movements where their EMG (Electromyography) output is actually subthreshold (81). In other words, they have reserve capacity or in McGill's language a "stability margin of error" (82). Examples would include:

- Golfers who choose to sacrifice 5% of their maximum distance to gain accuracy
- Baseball pitchers who can throw a fastball over 100 m.p.h. holding back until late in the game to throw their fastest pitches (i.e., Justin Verlander)
- Weight lifters use weights that are 85% of their maximum capacity so they can maintain as much speed and control as possible

Movement efficiency is epitomized by highly coordinated movement patterns specific to unique activity goals in a labile, unpredictable, or open environment—one with high levels of variability/CI (83). Individuals with high levels of movement efficiency can adapt their motor output in response to the changing needs of the task (84). Expert athletes and musicians are both quicker and more accurate partially due to their ability to identify and react to task-relevant cues—in particular visual—from their environment (85–87).

"The optimal pattern of coordination is determined by the interaction among constraints specified by the person, the environment, and the task." Newell (88)

An important irony is that while the goal is to achieve automated, efficient movement patterns, the stages by which one learns in practice are constantly recapitulated. Automatization in competition and performance is the peak our athletes (and musicians) strive to accomplish. However, in practice, cognitive and physical components are ideally both engaged in what is termed "deliberate practice" (89). This is consistent with the premise that Fitts and Posners' Stage Model for motor learning is not merely temporal, but even an elite athlete will learn a new skill via a recapitulation of all three stages as well (cognitive, developmental, and autonomous) (90).

Deliberate Practice

"Permanent gains in skilled performance capacity are only achieved when cognitive and physical training occur in tandem (Vickers) (35). This is the concept of deliberate practice, which has been presented as a key determinant of elite performance." Jeffries (80,91)

Systems theory applied to neuroscience explains the nonlinear, nonreductionist way in which our brain learns. A combination of cognitive and physical effort is required to lay down a rich and varied neural matrix with a high concentration of synaptic connections bridging pattern recognition and movement automatization centers (91–94). Thus, expertise is achieved because a relevant "weak link" is identified. Then, it is challenged so that a new software program can be "wired."

CHOKING

The ultimate saboteur of performance is **choking**, or performance anxiety. The issue of choking is one that is not only popular to speak about but is gaining the attention of sports or performance scientists. The mechanism of choking is thought to include a loss of goal-oriented focus. Precompetition routines (i.e., a free throw in basketball) have been shown to help (95).

Causer et al. (96) suggest that skilled performers in a variety of sports from basketball, golf, batting, billiards, and shooting are associated with a quiet eye (QE). Skilled athletes are more efficient with their eye movements, having longer but fewer fixations on their targets. Janelle et al. (97) have shown that a higher ratio of right hemisphere (visual-spatial) to left hemisphere (associated with verbal analytic processes) activity is associated with QE. Quieting the verbal analytic processing is part of achieving relaxed concentration. A preparatory period that precedes anticipated, imagined, or real task execution demonstrates changes in event-related potentials (ERPs) (98,99). In low-handicap golfers there was a longer prolonged QE period, greater right-central brain activation, and fewer ERPs (100).

Janelle (101) showed that heightened levels of anxiety reduce gaze efficiency. This has been shown to include more frequent and shorter QE durations (102–104). Vine (105) used QE training in elite golfers under anxiety-producing situations. QE duration predicted 43% of the variance in putting performance. Most impressively, QE training in practice was successful in transferring to performance gains.

Perceptual-cognitive training of police officers was used to train them under high-stress situations (106). The result was that the trained officers developed the ability to maintain longer duration gaze fixations on the target than the untrained group. Training included the following:

- Use normal routine
- Direct gaze to suitable target pick-up point position
- Direct eye focus quickly to target and hold as long as possible

The Science of Choking

"An increase in anxiety is associated with greater influence of stimulus-driven attentional system and a decrease in involvement of the goal-directed attentional system. However, anxiety does not normally impair performance effectiveness if compensatory strategies can be applied…." Williams et al. (2)

TALENT IDENTIFICATION

An entire industry has sprung up to support parents who strive for their children to begin "tracking" toward the rare and highly valued college athletic scholarships or professional sports careers (107,108). Early sport specialization along with a suite of personal trainers, sport-specific skill coaches, and even sport psychologists is being employed to enhance the odds that a child will be identified as "talented" or "gifted" (107,108). This is the "Holy Grail" for many families, which begs certain moral questions (109). Ironically, Gould et al. (110) reported that early specialization and highly structured training reduced **intrinsic motivation** as well as led to higher dropout and burnout among young athletes.

Hopefully, a more holistic approach will begin to evolve. Coaches are responsible not only for developing athletes but selecting those with the most potential. Traditionally, coaches selected athletes who demonstrated they were physically more mature or had high levels of physical competency or capacity while downplaying such traits as

interpersonal skills, decision-making, and understanding of the game (107–109,111–113). While physical qualities are extremely important in sport, so are psychosocial and cognitive ones. Excellence requires the development of a wide range of abilities, including interpersonal skills (114), tactical and strategic awareness (115), and grit (3). This suggests that, while performance-based approaches should of course have a part to play in the development of any youth athlete, they should not be the sole or even major focus during the formative years.

The inherent difficulty in predicting the future is highlighted by studies looking at the correlation of National Football League (NFL) combine results with draft selection order and ultimately NFL performance. Kuzmits (116) found no consistent statistical relationship between combine test results and professional football performance, with the notable exception of sprint tests for running backs. Robbins (117) reported that performance in the combine physical test battery, whether normalized or not, has little association with draft success. Of the eight performance measures investigated, straight sprint time and jumping ability seem to hold the most weight with NFL personnel responsible for draft decisions. It is suggested that it is just as important to assess and consider the mental and technical skills of the athlete as their physical characteristics (as demonstrated in the Combine testing) in order to predict future performance.

Sierer et al. (118) showed that statistical significance was found between drafted and undrafted "skilled players" (wide receivers, cornerbacks, free safeties, strong safeties, and running backs) for the 40-yard dash, vertical jump, pro-agility shuttle, and 3-cone drill. Drafted and undrafted "big skilled players" (fullbacks, linebackers, tight ends, and defensive ends) performed differently on the 40-yard dash and 3-cone drill. While undrafted "lineman" (centers, offensive guards, offensive tackles, and defensive tackles) performed significantly better than nondrafted "lineman" on the 40-yard dash, 225-lb bench press, and 3-cone drill.

Success in most sports is irreducible to a predetermined set of skills and attributes, as deficiencies in one area can be compensated for by strengths in another (119,120). Personality factors should be considered part of the performance puzzle, but can't be said to independently predict performance (6).

- They are not accurate measures of the abilities of all young people and are particularly affected by gender, ethnicity, or socioeconomic background.
- They can overlook other abilities that are also important aspects of talent.
- Until later age, they systematically discriminate against later birth date individuals.
- They ignore individuals who are potentially talented but who, due to lack of opportunity of support, are currently underachieving.

A host of factors undermine the central importance given to talent identification, as opposed to its development (121). For instance, there is the relative age effect (122,123), the unpredictability of childhood-to-adult physical measures, and childhood-to-adult performance standards (124). In addition, the arbitrary or invalid nature of most talent assessment procedures (125) exists.

Should We Question the Validity of Talent Identification in the Youth?

Researchers have suggested that many of the physical qualities that distinguish elite adult athletes do not appear until late in adolescence, therefore invalidating the talent selection methods in the youth (126–128).

This evidence suggests a radical departure is needed from standard talent identification practices. First off, we need to distinguish between valid and invalid identification measures. This should include abandoning the use of developmentally inappropriate methods of assessing young people. Instead of the current strong emphasis on identification and selection, we should replace this with an emphasis on developmentally appropriate activities and environments (129).

CONCLUSIONS

Training and coaching are complementary disciplines.

According to Kraaijenhof (130), the scientific aspect of coaching concerns applying basic rules of biology, biomechanics, and biochemistry, based on averages and statistical data. This part, which is applicable to everyone, is about being informed and intelligent. "The art of coaching is about applying all those basic rules to your unique individual athlete, about exceptions to the rule, about outliers and the other end of the spectrum. This is much more complex and cannot be learned from a book or the internet, only by hard experience and patience, it is about being smart and wise."

How a coach or trainer extrinsically creates a "nested" learning environment conducive to skill acquisition is a foundational building block of performance enhancement. Motor control is a key component in both of these processes. Training motor control is a necessary, but frequently not sufficient, step since it must be transferable to the athlete's activities and resilient to the stress and intricacies of performance. There are important neural and behavioral strategies related to how the nervous system learns, retains, and can apply new skills, which are vital to both growing and sustaining talent.

Hopefully, this book has integrated together cutting edge trainers, coaches, and sport scientists whose work crosses the divide between rehabilitation, fitness promotion, athletic development, and performance.

REFERENCES

1. Williams AM, Ford PR. Promoting a skills-based agenda in Olympic sports: the role of skill acquisition specialists. J Sports Sci 2009;27(13):1381–1392.
2. Williams AM, Ford P, Causer J, Logan O, Murray S. Translating theory into practice. In: Hodges NJ, Williams AM, eds. Skill Acquisition in Sport: Research, Theory and Practice 2nd ed. London: Routledge; 2012.
3. Duckworth AL, Kirby TA, Tsukayama E, Berstein H, Ericsson KA. Deliberate practice spells success: why grittier competitors triumph at the National Spelling Bee. Social Psychol Personality Sci 2012;2:174–181.
4. Bonneville-Roussy A, Lavigne GL, Vallerand RJ. When passion leads to excellence: the case of musicians. Psychol Music 2011;39:123–138.
5. Winner E. Gifted Children: Myths and Realities. New York: Basic Books; 1996.
6. Hambrick DZ, Oswald FL, Altmann EM, et al. Deliberate practice: Is that all it takes to become an expert? Intelligence 2013. http://dx.doi.org/10.1016/j.intell.2013.04.001
7. Masters R, Poolton JM, Maxwell JP. Stable implicit motor processes despite aerobic locomotor fatigue. Consciousness Cognit 2008;17(1):335–338.
8. Deci EL, Ryan RM. Intrinsic Motivation and Self-Determination in Human Behavior. New York: Plenum Press; 2000.
9. Côté J, Baker J, Abernethy B. Practice and play in the development of sport expertise. In: Eklund RC, Tenenbaum G, eds. Handbook of Sport Psychology 3rd ed. New Jersey: John Wiley & Sons; 2007.
10. Côté J, Lidor R, Hackfort D. ISSP position stand: to sample or to specialize? Seven postulates about youth sport activities that lead to continued participation and elite performance. J Sport Exerc Psychol 2009;9:7–17.
11. Lidor R, Lavyan Z. A retrospective picture of early sport experiences among elite and near-elite Israeli athletes: developmental and psychological perspectives. Int J Sport Psychol 2002;33:269–289.
12. Barynina II, Vaitsekhovskii SM. The aftermath of early sports specialization for highly qualified swimmers. Fitness Sports Rev Int 1992;27:132–133.
13. Badami R, Vaez Mousavi M, Wulf G, Namazizadeh M. Feedback after good versus poor trials affects intrinsic motivation. Res Q Exerc Sport 2011;82:2.
14. Chiviacowsky S, Wulf G. Feedback after good trials enhances learning. Res Q Exerc Sport 2007;78:40–47.
15. Lewthwaite R, Wulf G. Motor Learning through a motivational lens. In: Hodges N, Williams M, eds. Skill Acquisition in Sport: Research, Theory and Practice. 3rd ed., London, UK: Routledge, 2012;Chapter 10:173–191.
16. Wulf G, Dufek JS, Lozano L, Pettigrew C. Increased jump height and reduced EMG activity with an external focus. Hum Movement Sci 2010;29:440–448.

17. Ryan RM, Deci EL. Self-determination theory and the facilitation of intrinsic motivation, social development, and well-being. Am Psychologist 2000;55:68–78.

18. Ryan RM, Deci EL. Overview of self-determination theory: an organismic dialectical perspective. In: Ryan RM, Deci EL, eds. Handbook of Self-Determination Research. Rochester, NY: The University of Rochester Press; 2002.

19. Hodges N, Campagnaro P. Physical guidance research: assisting principles and supporting evidence. In: Hodges NJ, Williams AM, eds. Skill Acquisition in Sport: Research, Theory and Practice. 2nd ed. London: Routledge, 2012.

20. Salmoni AW, Schmidt RA, Walter CB. Knowledge of results and motor learning: a review and critical reappraisal. Psychol Bull 1984;95:355–386.

21. Baumeister RF, Vohs KD. Self-regulation, ego-depletion, and motivation. Social Personality Psychol Compass 2007;1(1): 115–128.

22. Zimmerman B. Investigating self-regulation and motivation: historical background, methodological developments, and future prospects. Am Educ Res J 2008;45(1):166–183.

23. Zimmerman BJ. Development and adaptation of expertise: the role of self- regulatory processes and beliefs. In: Ericsson KA, Charness N, Feltovich PJ, Hoffman RR, eds. The Cambridge Handbook of Expertise and Expert Performance. New York, NY: Cambridge University Press; 2006:705–722.

24. Jonker L, Elferink-Gemser MT, Visscher C. Differences in self-regulatory skills among talented athletes: the significance of competitive level and type of sport. J Sports Sci 2010;28:901–908.

25. Jonker L, Elferink-Gemser MT, Visscher C. The role of self-regulatory skills in sport and academic performances of elite youth athletes. Talent Dev Exerc 2011;3(2):263–275.

26. Adkins DL, Boychuk J, Remple MS, Kleim JA. Motor training induces experience-specific patterns of plasticity across motor cortex and spinal cord. J Appl Physiol 2006;101(6):1776–1782.

27. Bain S, McGown C. Motor learning principles and the superiority of whole training in volleyball. Coaching Volleyball, AVCA Tech J 2010;28(1):13–15.

28. Otte B, Zanic V. Blocked vs Random Practice with Drills for Hurdlers. http://www.coachr.org/blocked_vs_random_practice_with_drills_for_hurdlers.htm

29. Schmidt RA, Lee TD. Motor Control and Learning: A Behavioral Emphasis. Champaign, IL: Human Kinetics; 2005:555.

30. Bortoli L, Robazza C, Durigon V, Carra C. Effects of contextual interference on learning technical sports skills. Percept Mot Skills 1992;75(2):555–562.

31. Travlos AK. Specificity and variability of practice, and contextual interference in acquisition and transfer of an underhand volleyball serve. Percept Mot Skills 2010;110(1):298–312.

32. Wrisberg CA, Liu Z. The effect of contextual variety on the practice, retention, and transfer of an applied motor skill. Res Q Exerc Sport 1991;62(4):406–412.

33. Goode S, Magill R. Contextual interference effects in learning three badminton serves. Res Q Exerc Sport 1986;53: 308–314.

34. Hall KG, Domingues DA, Cavazos R. Contextual interference effects with skilled baseball players. Percept Mot Skills 1994;78(3 Pt 1):835–841.

35. Vickers JN, Livingston LF, Umeris-Bohnert S, Holden D. Decision training: the effects of complex instruction, variable practice and reduced delayed feedback on the acquisition and transfer of a motor skill. J Sports Sci 1999;17(5):357–367.

36. Landin DK, Hebert EP, Fairweather M. The effects of variable practice on the performance of a basketball skill. Res Q Exerc Sport 1993;64(2):232–237.

37. Reid M, Crespo M, Lay B, Berry J. Skill acquisition in tennis: research and current practice. J Sci Med Sport 2007;10(1):1–10.

38. Williams AM, Davids K. Visual search strategy, selective search strategy, and expertise in soccer. Res Q Exerc Sport 1998;69:111–129.

39. Wymb NF, Grafton ST. Neural substrates of practice structure that support future off-line learning. J N Physiol 2009;102(4):2462–2476.

40. Magill RA, Hall KG. A review of the contextual interference effect in motor skill acquisition. Hum Mov Sci 1990;9: 241–289.

41. Magill R. Motor Learning and Control: Concepts and Applications. 7th ed. New York: Mc Graw Hill; 2004.

42. Wulf G, Shea CH. Understanding the role of augmented feedback: the good, the bad, and the ugly. In: Williams AM, Hodges NJ, eds. Skill Acquisition in Sport: Research, Theory, and Practice. London: Rutledge; 2004:121–144.

43. Battig WF. The flexibility of human memory. In: Cermak LS, Craik FIM, eds. Levels of Processing and Human Memory. Hillsdale, NJ: Lawrence Erlbaum Associates; 1979:2344.

44. Wulf G. The effect of type of practice on motor learning in children. Appl Cognit Psychol 1991:5:123–124.

45. Jeffries I. Motor learning—applications for agility, part 1. National Strength and Conditioning Association. Strength Cond J 2006;28(5):72–76.

46. Shea, CH, DL Wright G, Wulf G, Whitacre C. Physical and observational practice afford unique learning opportunities. J Mot Behav 2000;32:27–36.

47. Wulf G, Schmidt RA. Contextual interference effects in motor learning: evaluating a KR-usefulness hypothesis. In: Nitsch JR, Seiler R, eds. Movement and Sport: Psychological Foundations and Effects. Vol. 2. Motor Control and Learning. Sankt Augustin, Germany: Academia Verlag; 1994: 304–309.

48. Porter JM, Magill RA. Systematically increasing contextual interference is beneficial for learning sport skills. J Sports Sci 2010;28(12):1277–1285.

49. Brady F. A theoretical and empirical review of the contextual interference effect and the learning of motor skills. Quest 1998;50:266–293.

50. Guadagnoli MA, Lee TD. Challenge point: a framework for conceptualizing the effects of various practice conditions in motor learning. J Mot Behav 2004;36:212–224.

51. Hebert EP, Landin D, Solomon MA. Practice schedule effects on the performance and learning of low and high skilled students: an applied study. Res Q Exerc Sport 1996;67:52–58.

52. Gentile AM. Implicit and explicit processes during acquisition of functional skills. Scand J Occup Med 1998;5:7–16.

53. Eversheim U, Bock O. Evidence for processing stages in skill acquisition: a dual-task study. Learn Mem 2001;8(4): 183–189.

54. Mazzoni P, Wexler NS. Parallel explicit and implicit control of reaching. PLoS One 2009;4(10):e7557.

55. Willingham DB. A neuropsychological theory of motor skill learning. Psychol Rev 1998;105(3):558–584.

56. Wolpert DM, Ghahramani Z, Flanagan JR. Perspectives and problems in motor learning. Trends Cogn Sci 2001;5(11):487–494.

57. Alexander GE, DeLong MR, Crutcher MD. Do cortical and basal ganglionic motor areas use "motor programs" to control movement? Behav Brain Sci 1992;15(4).

58. Houk JC. Agents of the mind. Biol Cybern 2005;92(6): 427–437.

59. Henry F, Rogers DE. Increased response latency for complicated movements and a "memory-drum" theory of neuromotor reaction. Res Q Am Assoc Health Phys Educ Recreation 1960;31:448–458.

60. Savelsbergh GJ, Van Der Kamp J. Information in learning to coordinate and control movements: is there a need for specificity of practice? Int J Sports Psychol 2000;31:467–484.

61. Savelsbergh GJ, Van Der Kamp J. Adaptation in the timing of catching under changing environmental constraints. Res Q Exerc Sport 2000;71(2):195–200.

62. Yoshida M, Cauraugh JH, Chow JW. Specificity of practice, visual information, and intersegmental dynamics in rapid-aiming limb movements. J Mot Behav 2004;36(3):281–290.

63. Palmer C, Meyer RK. Conceptual and motor learning in music performance. Psychol Sci 2000;11(1):63–68.

64. Simon DA, Bjork RA. Models of performance in learning multisegment movement tasks: consequences for acquisition, retention, and judgments of learning. J Exp Psychol Appl 2002;8(4):222–232.

65. Swinnen SP, Lee TD, Verschueren S, Serrien DJ, Bogaerds H. Interlimb coordination: learning and transfer under different feedback conditions. Hum Movement Sci 1997;16:749–785.

66. Swinnen SP, Carson RG. The control and learning of patterns of interlimb coordination: past and present issues in normal and disordered control. Acta Psychol (Amst) 2002;110(2–3):129–137.

67. Wenderoth N, Puttemans V, Vangheluwe S, Swinnen SP. Bimanual training reduces spatial interference. J Mot Behav 2003;35(3):296–308.

68. Jeffries I. Motor learning—applications for agility, part 2. National Strength and Conditioning Association. Strength Cond J 2006;28(6):10–14.

69. Schmidt RA, Wrisberg CA. Motor Learning and Performance. 3rd ed. Champaign, IL: Human Kinetics; 2004:183–275.

70. Ready R, Burton K. Neuro-Linguistic Programming for Dummies. Chichester, England: Wiley; 2004:88–96.

71. Wulf, G, McNevin N, Shea CH. The automaticity of complex motor skills learning as a function of attentional focus. Q J Exp Psychol A 2001;54:1143–1154.

72. Schexnayder B. More Training Tips. http://speedendurance.com/2012/06/25/training-tips-from-boo-schexnayder/

73. Davids K. Learning design for nonlinear dynamical movement systems. Open Sports Sci J 2012;5(Suppl 1-M2):9–16.

74. Greenwood D, Davids K, Renshaw I. How elite coaches experiential knowledge might enhance empirical understanding of sport performance. Int J Sports Sci Coaching 2012;7(2):411–422.

75. Pinder R, Davids K, Renshaw I, Araújo D. Representative learning design and functionality of research and practice in sport. J Sport Exerc Psychol 2011;33(1):146–155.

76. Davids K, Button C, Bennett S. Dynamics of Skill Acquisition: A Constraints-Led Approach. Champaign, IL: Human Kinetics Publishers; 2008.

77. Chow JY, Davids K, Hristovski R, et al. Nonlinear pedagogy: learning design for self-organizing neurobiological systems. N Ideas Psychol 2011;29:189–200.

78. Dicks M, Button C, Davids K. Examination of gaze behaviors under in situ and video simulation task constraints reveals differences in information pickup for perception and action. Atten Percept Psychophys 2010;72(3):706–720.

79. Seifert L, Davids K. The functional role of intra- and inter-individual variability in the acquisition of expertise in non-linear movement systems. Sports Med 2003;33(4): 245–260.

80. Jeffries I. Utilising a range of motor learning methods in the development of physical skills. UK Strength Cond Assoc 2011;23:33–35.

81. Wulf G, Dufek JS, Lozano L, Pettigrew C. Increased jump height and reduced EMG activity with an external focus. Hum Movement Sci 2010;29:440–448.

82. McGill SM. Low Back Disorders: The Scientific Foundation for Prevention and Rehabilitation. Champaign, IL: Human Kinetics; 2002.

83. Goodwin JE. Effect of specific and variable practice and subjective estimation on movement bias, consistency and error detection capabilities. Res Q Exerc Sport 2003;74:A31.

84. Savelsbergh GJP, van der Kamp J, Oudejans RRD, Scott MA. Perceptual learning is mastering perceptual degrees of freedom. In: Williams AM, Hodges NJ, eds. Skill Acquisition in Sport: Research Theory and Practice. London, England: Routledge; 2004:374–389.

85. Savelsbergh GJP, Williams AM, van der Kamp J, Ward P. Visual search, anticipation, and expertise in soccer goalkeepers. J Sports Sci 2002;20:279–287.

86. Williams AM, Davids K. Visual search strategy, selective search strategy, and expertise in soccer. Res Q Exerc Sport 1998;69:111–129.

87. Williams AM, Grant A. Training perceptual skill in sport. Int J Sport Psychol 1999;30:194–220.

88. Newell KM. Constraints on the development of coordination. In: Wade MG, Widing HT, eds. Motor Development in Children: Aspects of Coordination and Control. Dordrecht: Martinus Nijhoff; 1986:341–360.

89. Ericson KA. How the expert performance approach differs from traditional approaches to expertise in sport. In search of a shared theoretical framework for studying expert performance. In: Starkes JL, Ericson KA, eds. Expert Performance in Sports: Advances on Research on Sports Expertise. Champaign, IL: Human Kinetics; 2003:371–402.

90. Fitts PM Posner MI. Human Performance. Oxford, England: Brooks and Cole; 1967.

91. Vickers JN. Perception, Cognition and Decision Training—The Quiet Eye in Action. Champaign, IL: Human Kinetics; 2007:164–184.

92. Brown J, Cooper-Kuhn CM, Kempermann G, Van Praag H, Winkler J, Gage, FH. Enriched environment and physical activity stimulate hippocampal but not olfactory bulb neurogenesis. Eur J Neurosci 2003;17:2042–2046.

93. Posner MI, Raechle ME. Images of Mind. New York: Scientific American Library; 1994.

94. Singer RN. Performance and human factors: considerations about cognition and attention for self- paced and external-paced events. Ergonomics 2000;43(10):1661–1680.

95. Causer J, Holmes PS, Williams AM. Quiet eye training in a visuomotor control task. Med Sci Sports Exerc 2011;43(6):1042–1049.

96. Causer J, Janelle C, Vickers J, Williams A. Perceptual expertise: what can be trained? In: Hodges NJ, Williams AM, eds. Translating Theory into Practice in Skill Acquisition in Sport: Research, Theory and Practice. 2nd ed. London: Routledge; 2012.

97. Janelle CM, Hillman CH, Apparies RJ, et al. Expertise differences in cortical activation and gaze behavior during rifle shooting. J Sport Exerc Psychol 2000;22:167–182.

98. Fabiani M, Gratton G, Coles MGH. Event related brain potentials: methods, theory, and applications. In: Cacioppo JT, Tassinary LG, Berntson GG, eds. Handbook of Psychophysiology. Cambridge: Cambridge University Press; 2000:53–84.

99. Simonton DK. Creativity in Science: Chance, Logic, Genius, and Zeitgeist. Cambridge: Cambridge University Press; 2004.

100. Mann DTY, Coombes SA, Mousseau MB, Janelle CM. Quiet eye and the Bereitschaftspotential: visuomotor mechanisms of expert motor performance. Cognit Process 2011;12(3):223–234.

101. Janelle CM. Anxiety, arousal and visual attention: a mechanistic account of performance variability. J Sports Sci 2002;20:237–251.

102. Williams AM, Davids K, Williams JG. Anxiety, expertise and visual search strategy in karate. J Sport Exerc Psychol 1999;21:362–375.

103. Behan M, Wilson M. State anxiety and visual attention: the role of the quiet eye period in aiming to a far target. J Sports Sci 2008;26(2):207–215.

104. Causer J, Holmes PS, Williams AM. Anxiety, movement kinetics, and visual attention in elite-level performers. Emotion 2011;11(3):595–602.

105. Vine SJ, Moore LJ, Wilson M. Quiet eye training facilitates competitive putting performance in elite golfers. Frontiers Psychol 2011;2:1–9.

106. Nieuwenhuys A, Oudejans RRD. Training with anxiety: short- and long-term effects on polices officers' shooting behavior under pressure. Cognit Process 2011;12(3):277–288.

107. Baker J, Cobley S, Fraser-Thomas J. What do we know about early sport specialization? Not much! High Ability Stud 2009;20(1):77–89.

108. Coakley J. The 'logic' of specialization: using children for adult purposes. J Phys Educ Recreation Dance 2010;81(8):1–58.

109. David P. Human Rights in Youth Sport: A Critical Review of Children's Rights in Competitive Sport. London: Routledge; 2004.

110. Gould D, Udry E, Tuffey S, Loehr J. Burnout in competitive junior tennis players: Pt. 1. A quantitative psychological assessment. Sport Psychologist 1996;10:322–340.

111. Bailey RP, Dismore H, Morley D. Talent development in physical education: a national survey of practices in England. Phys Educ Sport Pedagogy 2009;14(1):59–72.

112. Bailey RP, Tan J, Morley D. Talented pupils in physical education: secondary school teachers' experiences of identifying talent within the 'Excellence in Cities' scheme. Phys Educ Sport Pedagogy 2004;9(2):133–148.

113. Morley D. Viewing Physical Education through the Lens of Talent Development. Unpublished Doctoral Dissertation, Leeds Metropolitan University; 2008.

114. Holt NL. Positive Youth Development through Sport. London: Routledge; 2008.

115. Helsen W, Hodges N, Van Winckel J, Starkes J. The roles of talent, physical precocity and practice in the development of soccer expertise. J Sports Sci 2000;18(9):727–736.

116. Kuzmits FE, Adams AJ. The NFL combine: does it predict performance in the National Football League? J Strength Cond Res 2008;22(6):1721–1727.

117. Robbins DW. The National Football League (NFL) combine: does normalized data better predict performance in the NFL draft? J Strength Cond Res 2010;24(11).

118. Sierer SP, Battaglini CL, Mihalik JP, Shields EW, Tomasini NT. The National Football League Combine: performance differences between drafted and nondrafted players entering the 2004 and 2005 drafts. J Strength Cond Res 2008;22(1):6–12.

119. Williams AM, Ericsson KA. Some considerations when applying the expert performance approach in sport. Hum Movement Sci 2005;24:283–307.

120. Williams AM, Ericsson KA. How do experts learn? J Sport Exerc Psychol 2008;30:653–662.

121. Vaeyens R, Lenoir M, Williams AM, Philippaerts R. Talent identification and development programmes in sport: current models and future directions. Sports Med 2008;38(9):703–714.

122. Helsen W, Hodges N, Van Winckel J, Starkes J. The roles of talent, physical precocity and practice in the development of soccer expertise. J Sports Sci 2000;18(9):727–736.

123. Musch J, Grondin S. Unequal competition as an impediment to personal development: a review of the relative age effect in sport. Dev Rev 2001;21:147–167.

124. Abbott A, Collins D, Martindale R, Sowerby K. Talent Identification and Development: An Academic Review: A Report for Sportscotland by the University of Edinburgh. Edinburgh: Sportscotland; 2002.

125. Burwitz L, Moore PM, Wilkinson DM. Future directions for performance-related sports science research: an interdisciplinary approach. J Sport Sci 1994;12(1):93–109.

126. French KE, McPherson SL. Adaptations in response selection processes used during sport competition with increasing age and expertise. Int J Sport Psychol 1999; 30:173–193.

127. Tenenbaum G, Sar-El T, Bar-Eli M Anticipation of ball location in low and high skill performers: a developmental perspective. Psychol Sport Exerc 2000;1:117–128.

128. Williams AM, Franks A. Talent identification in soccer. Sports Exerc Injury 1998;4:159–165.

129. Martindale RJ, Collins D, Daubney J. Talent development: a guide for practice and research within sport. Quest 2005;57(4):353–375.

130. Kraaijenhof H. Introducing 2013 Seminar Presenter-Henk Kraaijenhof. http://www.cvasps.com/introducing-2013-seminar-presenter-henk-kraaijenhof/

INDEX

Page numbers followed by t indicate table; those in *italics* indicate figure.